TEXTBOOK OF ENDOCRINOLOGY

Dr. Marie Hyacinth Chiong Tumara

ALLIED
HEALTH
PRESS

Textbook of Endocrinology

Dr. Marie Hyacinth Chiong Tumara

Allied Health Press
4164 Lakeshore Road
Burlington ON L7L 1A4
Canada
www.alliedhealthpress.com
Email: orders@arclereducation.com

ISBN: 978-1-77956-862-5

Allied Health Press publishes wide variety of books and eBooks. For more information about Allied Health Press and its products, visit our website at www.alliedhealthpress.com

ABOUT THE EDITOR

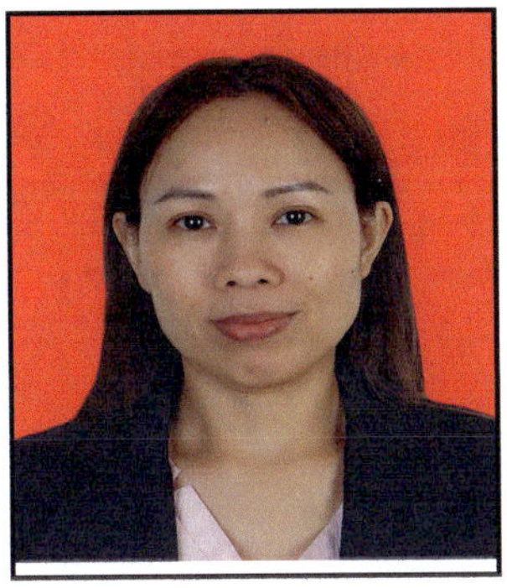

Dr. Marie Hyacinth Chiong Tumara, MD, FPCP, is an Internist with over 16 years of clinical practice and 11 years of government health service. She currently serves as Medical Director and OFW PEME Physician, with expertise in occupational and maritime medicine. A Fellow of the Philippine College of Physicians, she has authored research and medical reports and actively contributes to policy development in hospital and clinical settings. She is presently pursuing her Master's in Health and Hospital Management at Xavier University–Ateneo de Cagayan.

Brief Table of Contents

Getting Started with This Book

Chapter Openers

A list of Chapter Outline is presented providing a brief Introduction to what will be covered in the chapter.

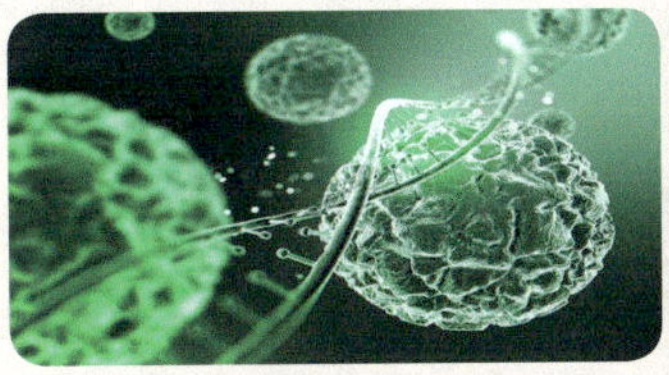

LEARNING OBJECTIVES

After studying this chapter, you will be able to:

1. Discuss the scientific method in biology;
2. Explain the cell theory;
3. Discuss the genetics and heredity;
4. Evolution and natural selection;
5. Focus on ecology and ecosystems;
6. Learn about human biology;
7. Evaluate the plant biology;
8. Explain the microbiology;
9. Focus on current trends in biology.

Introduction

Often referred to as the science of life, biology is a broad field of study aimed at comprehending the several kinds of life on Earth, from tiny creatures to sophisticated multicellular entities. Comprising several subfields, including molecular biology, ecology, and evolutionary biology, each of which advances our knowledge of living systems, this field clarifies the mechanisms controlling life events, including development, reproduction, and interaction with the surroundings, which is the central goal of biology. Moreover, biology fills in the void between the natural sciences and medicine by offering a necessary understanding of health, illness, and the interactions between organisms and their environments. Dealing with urgent global issues such as climate change, biodiversity loss, and new diseases depends on an awareness of these complex biological interactions, therefore highlighting the critical part biology plays in modern civilization. Fundamentally, biology explores and tests ideas about the living world using the scientific method. Through methodical observation and experimentation,

1.1. The Scientific Method in Biology

Learning Outcome

1. Describe the steps of the scientific method;
2. Focus on hypothesis formation;
3. Learn about experimental design.

Learning Outcomes

The beginning of each section of every chapter contains a set of Learning Outcomes that inform students of concepts they should understand. These outcomes help students understand what they should be able to do if they have mastered the material in that section.

Test Your Knowledge

Throughout each chapter, Test Your Knowledge cues you to note which topics have been covered and to self-test your understanding of the material presented.

Test Your Knowledge

1. Explain why correlation does not imply causation in scientific experiments.
2. How does the scientific method help reduce the influence of personal opinions in research?

Chapter Summary

The Summary Section appear at the end of each chapter and summarize main concepts covered throughout the chapter. These points provide key concepts in an engaging and meaningful way.

Summary

The investigation of biological principles highlights the importance of a comprehensive view of life by reflecting the intricate interactions that occur within living systems. The complexity of biology goes beyond individual species or systems, as this essay highlights; it also includes the interactions that mold ecosystems and affect biodiversity. Researchers can conduct in-depth analyses of metabolomic data using sophisticated technologies like MetaboAnalyst, which offer insights into the molecular mechanisms underlying these interactions. As demonstrated by the developments in MetaboAnalyst, for example, the integration of diverse omics data promotes a thorough understanding of metabolic pathways and helps identify important biological markers necessary for research on development and disease (Chong et al., 2018). Additionally, the phenomenon of ecological invasions is a key component of biological research and a vital field of study. The introduction of non-native species into unfamiliar habitats has significant ramifications and calls for multidisciplinary management strategies. Examining the origins and effects of these biological incursions, invasion science has become a crucial field that highlights the need to comprehend ecological dynamics and community interactions. As interest in biological invasions increases, new findings are emerging that put conventional ecological theories and practices to the test. The importance of incorporating various scientific viewpoints is shown by this developing discipline, which also highlights how invasive species shape ecosystems and advances our knowledge of ecological resilience (David et al., 2013). When taken as a whole, these discoveries from invasion science and metabolomics highlight the value of multidisciplinary biology research. Fostering cross-disciplinary collaboration and utilizing technological breakthroughs to improve our comprehension of intricate biological interactions are crucial as we look to the future of biological research. In addition to deepening our understanding of the complexities of life, this method lays the groundwork for tackling urgent environmental issues. Future studies can ensure the continued relevance of biology in a world that is constantly changing by acknowledging the interconnection of biological systems and opening the door to creative solutions that support sustainability and biodiversity conservation. We might imagine a thorough comprehension of life that serves both academia and society at large through ongoing investigation and integration of scientific knowledge.

Knowledge Assessment

The chapter includes material designed to review and reinforce each content. It includes Critical Thinking Questions to help test of your understanding of information presented in the chapter and Short answer Questions to review your understanding of the key concepts presented in the chapter.

Critical Thinking Questions

1. **Who is known as the "Father of Modern Biology"?**
   a. Aristotle
   b. Charles Darwin
   c. Gregor Mendel
   d. Louis Pasteur
2. **What is the basic unit of life?**
   a. Atom
   b. Molecule
   c. Cell
   d. Organism
3. **Which branch of biology studies the interaction of organisms with their environment?**
   a. Genetics
   b. Ecology
   c. Physiology
   d. Botany
4. **Which macromolecule is the main source of energy for living organisms?**
   a. Proteins
   b. Lipids
   c. Carbohydrates
   d. Nucleic acids
5. **DNA is primarily responsible for which function in living organisms?**
   a. Energy production
   b. Protein synthesis
   c. Storing genetic information
   d. Regulating body temperature

Short Answer Questions

1. What is biology, and why is it important to study biology?
2. What are the three main domains of life, and how are they different from one another?
3. Define homeostasis and give an example of how it works in living organisms.
4. What is the cell theory, and why is it fundamental to biology?
5. How do autotrophs and heterotrophs differ in the way they obtain energy?
6. What is the scientific method, and how is it applied in biological research?
7. Discuss how biology helps address global challenges such as climate change, disease, and food security.
8. Explain the levels of biological organization from the smallest unit to the largest. Provide examples at each level.
9. Describe the relationship between structure and function in biology, giving specific examples from cells or organs.
10. How has the discovery of genetics shaped our understanding of inheritance and variation among organisms?

Supplementary Materials

Key Terms: A list of key terms is given for quick reference

KEY TERMS FROM THIS CHAPTER

Annotation enrichment analysis
Cell theory
Ecosystems
Microbiology
Plant biology
Biological structure
Cellular structure
Genetics
Natural selection
Cell
Ecology
Human biology
Organism

Further Resources: Recommendations for additional readings, websites, and multimedia resources.

References

1. Argelaguet, R., Velten, B., Arnol, D., Dietrich, S., Zenz, T., Marioni, J. C., Buettner, F., et al. (2018). Multi-omics factor analysis—A framework for unsupervised integration of multi-omics data sets. *Molecular Systems Biology, 14.* https://doi.org/10.15252/msb.20178124.
2. Bacher, S., Blackburn, T. M., Essl, F., & Genovesi, P. (2017). *Socio-Economic Impact Classification of Alien Taxa (SEICAT).* https://core.ac.uk/download/286567949.pdf (accessed on 8th March 2025).
3. Barnett, R., Brace, S., Cucchi, T., & Dobney, K. (2013). *Divergent Evolutionary Processes Associated with Colonization of Offshore Islands.* https://core.ac.uk/download/20664364.pdf (accessed on 8th March 2025).

Detailed Table of Contents

CHAPTER 5

Endocrine Pancreas and Diabetes Mellitus 147

CHAPTER 6

Reproductive Endocrinology (Male) 185

CHAPTER 7

Reproductive Endocrinology (Female) 223

CHAPTER 8

Growth and Puberty 261

CHAPTER 9

Obesity and Metabolic Syndrome 297

CHAPTER 14

Endocrinology in Critical Illness and ICU 477

CHAPTER 15

Endocrine Tumors and Multiple Endocrine Neoplasia (MEN) 511

LIST OF FIGURES

PREFACE

The human body relies on an elaborate system of chemical messengers to regulate critical processes such as metabolism, growth, reproduction, and homeostasis. These messengers, known as hormones, are secreted by glands that form the endocrine system. The glands collectively exert widespread influences on other organ systems, maintaining the body in a state of physiological balance. Any disruption in the production, secretion, or function of these hormones may result in a range of clinical disorders, some of which can develop subtly and gradually over time, while others need immediate medical intervention. This biological control mechanism is not only important to study from the viewpoint of diagnosing endocrine disorders but also for the therapeutic management of disorders that are controlled by modulation of hormones, such as cardiovascular disease, obesity, infertility, and autoimmune syndromes.

The field of endocrinology continues to develop in parallel with advancements in molecular biology, genetics, imaging, and therapeutic technologies. New hormones have been identified, feedback mechanisms have been clarified, and insight into how derangements in hormones cause bizarre and common diseases has increased. Practitioners are expected to apply this expanding base of knowledge to make more precise diagnoses and tailor treatment to patients. Therefore, a sound understanding of endocrine physiology, pathology, and clinical practice has become essential not only for endocrinologists but also for internists, general physicians, pediatricians, gynecologists, and surgeons while they encounter endocrine-related problems in day-to-day practice.

Textbook of Endocrinology is written to provide a comprehensive and logical exposition of the endocrine system and its associated disorders. Being a comprehensive learning tool, the book restores equilibrium between basic science and clinical relevance and fills the gap between didactic knowledge and practical utility. With a strong focus on clinical applicability and simplicity, it is designed to equip readers with the capability to understand, evaluate, and manage a wide variety of endocrine disorders. The content is organized in a well-defined format, allowing learners to move from core concepts to complex disease processes logically and sequentially. Extensive coverage encompassing detailed analysis of diagnostic equipment, treatment protocols, and patient care issues, the book is an exhaustive reference for academic purposes as well as for clinical purposes.

Chapter 1 introduces the fundamental principles of endocrinology, including hormone classification, mechanisms of signaling, receptor mechanisms, and feedback control. It introduces readers to the concepts needed to describe how hormones govern cellular function and systemic physiology.

Chapter 2 addresses the hypothalamus and pituitary gland, the endocrine system's central regulators. The chapter addresses anatomical organization, regulatory hormones, feedback systems, as well as clinical conditions such as hypopituitarism, pituitary adenomas, and hyperprolactinemia.

Chapter 3 explains the role of the thyroid gland in metabolism and growth. The chapter provides a comprehensive account of thyroid hormone production, transport, and mechanism of action, along with the subjects of hypothyroidism, hyperthyroidism, goiter, thyroiditis, and thyroid nodules, supported by diagnostic and therapeutic approaches.

Chapter 4 covers the adrenal gland, detailing the adrenal cortex and medulla. It discusses steroidogenesis, mineralocorticoid and glucocorticoid function, adrenal insufficiency, Cushing's syndrome, congenital adrenal hyperplasia, and pheochromocytoma, among others.

Chapter 5 addresses the endocrine pancreas and clinical diabetes mellitus management. It addresses insulin secretion, glucose regulation, and type 1 and type 2 diabetes pathophysiology. It also highlights diabetes complications, diagnosis criteria, and management options, such as insulin therapy and newer pharmacologic therapies.

Chapter 6 covers the endocrine regulation of the male reproductive system. Discussed are the hypothalamic-pituitary-gonadal axis, testosterone physiology, and conditions such as hypogonadism, infertility, and gynecomastia, with clinical emphasis on diagnosis and treatment.

Chapter 7 presents the female reproductive endocrine system, such as the regulation of the menstrual cycle, the role of estrogen and progesterone, polycystic ovary syndrome (PCOS), amenorrhea, menopause, and hormonal therapy. It explores common reproductive disorders and their hormonal nature.

Chapter 8 covers growth and puberty. Growth patterns under normal conditions, physiology of growth hormone, pubertal growth, and the diseases growth hormone deficiency, precocious puberty, and delayed puberty are covered with specific diagnostic paradigms and treatment pathways.

Chapter 9 focuses on metabolic syndrome and obesity, describing the metabolic and hormonal derangements causing these increasingly prevalent disorders. It encompasses adipokines, insulin resistance, dyslipidemia, and endocrine consequences of obesity, and evidence-based treatment options.

Chapter 10 has the coverage of bone and mineral metabolism, including calcium and phosphate homeostasis, vitamin D physiology, and parathyroid hormone function. Conditions included are osteoporosis, rickets, osteomalacia, and hyperparathyroidism, along with diagnostic tools like DEXA scanning and laboratory tests.

Chapter 11 covers endocrine etiologies of hypertension and specifically primary aldosteronism, pheochromocytoma, and Cushing's syndrome. It provides a methodical approach to the diagnosis of secondary hypertension and discusses the implications of hormonal etiologies on the treatment of hypertension.

Chapter 12 deals with hormones of gastrointestinal function and liver physiology. The roles of gastrin, cholecystokinin, secretin, and ghrelin and other peptides are explained, and how they are involved in the diseases such as Zollinger-Ellison syndrome and hepatic insulin resistance.

Chapter 13 addresses principles of neuroendocrinology, for example, how the nervous system and hormonal mechanisms interact. Topics addressed include neuropeptides, circadian rhythms, hypothalamic disease, and syndromes for neurohormonal regulation.

Chapter 14 discusses endocrine aspects of critical illness, including the hormonal responses to stress, trauma, and infection. It outlines adrenal insufficiency in the ICU, thyroid function in critical illness, and metabolic alterations during prolonged illness.

Chapter 15 covers endocrine tumors and multiple endocrine neoplasia (MEN) syndromes. Classification of tumors, testing for diagnosis, genetics, and treatment of thyroid, parathyroid, pancreas, and adrenal functioning and non-functioning tumors are covered.

This text is accessible to a wide range of readers interested in medical practice and health sciences. Internal medicine, pediatrics, and endocrinology residents and fellows, as well as medical students, will find it useful as a basic textbook and reference. Practicing clinicians and healthcare providers, including nurse practitioners and general practitioners, will find clinician-led discussion and up-to-date guidelines useful. Secondly, the book is also a scholarly reference for academic teachers, students, and researchers seeking a structured, up-to-date review of endocrine topics to utilize in instruction or for research.

INTRODUCTION TO ENDOCRINOLOGY

1

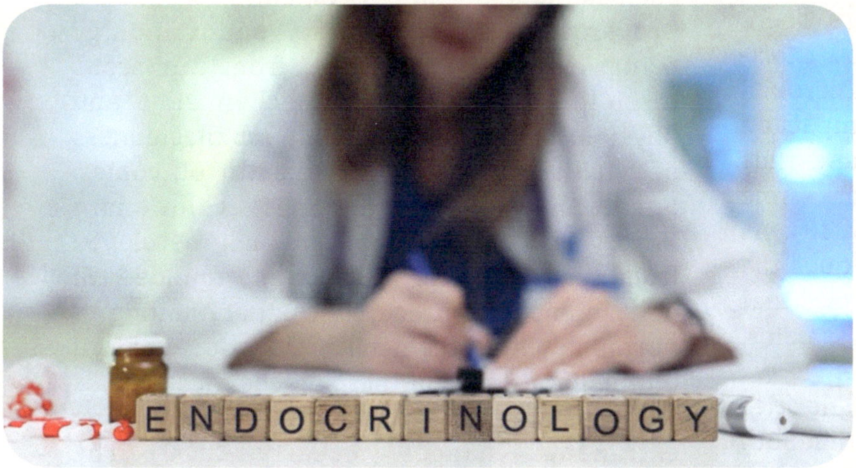

LEARNING OBJECTIVES

After studying this chapter, you will be able to:

1. Understand the history of endocrinology;
2. Discuss endocrine glands;
3. Describe hormones and their functions;
4. Define endocrine disorders;
5. Deal with diagnosis of endocrine disorders;
6. Explain treatment options in endocrinology.

Introduction

The field of endocrinology has been transformed in recent years by advances in our understanding of hormonal control and its multifaceted consequences for disease and health. Endocrinology itself is simply the physiology of hormones, the glands that make them, and the body functions they regulate. The field of endocrinology is essential to controlling big functions, including metabolism, growth, reproduction, and mood. Hormones are key signal molecules that allow for communication among different organs and systems of the body. The complexity of endocrine interactions reflects the intricate balance necessary to maintain homeostasis, illustrating the importance of studying endocrinology not only for the diagnosis and management of endocrine disease but also to study how endocrine imbalance can result in all sorts of systemic disease. This chapter shall present a detailed analysis of the fundamentals of endocrinology and its application in modern medical science. Recent literature focuses on the primary importance of the gut microbiota in endocrine and metabolic control, stressing the intricate interconnection between microorganisms and host physiology. In this context, the gut-brain axis appears as the key signaling pathway through which the gut microbiota exerts an influence on endocrine function and behavior. The quiet signaling mechanisms involved—stretching from immune reactions, neurotransmitter release, and hormonal release—open new frontiers for the pathogenesis of a wide variety of disorders, including obesity and affective disorders. There is a vast amount of evidence showing how short-chain fatty acids (SCFAs), products of microbial fermentation, could have a significant impact on neuro-immunoendocrine regulation and thus on our understanding of the microbiota's role in disease and health (Silva et al., 2020). As the recognition of this axis grows, so does the need to explore microbial-based therapies that may reshape treatment paradigms across fields, from psychiatry to metabolic disease. As we become more comfortable with the complexities of endocrinology, it becomes apparent that both environmental and biological factors interact to shape hormone function and microbiota profile throughout life. Factors such as early childhood infections, diet, and even stress levels become central in the determination of the microbiota and its subsequent interaction with the endocrine system (John et al., 2019). Additionally, the process of aging also brings variables that can diminish microbial diversity, thus impacting hormonal well-being and metabolic processes. As gut microbiota imbalances have been implicated in various neurodevelopmental and neurodegenerative disorders, understanding microbiota–gut–brain interactions is important in elucidating the pathophysiology of these conditions. With ongoing research and translational studies, the endocrinology field is poised to uncover the mechanisms behind the interactions and identify therapeutic strategies towards regaining balance in both the microbiota and hormonal systems.

Definition of Endocrinology

The word endocrinology also encompasses the study of hormones and all the ways that hormones influence body function and health. This branch of medicine looks at the endocrine glands, the pituitary, thyroid, adrenal, and pancreas, whose function is to create and secrete hormones. Hormones are chemical messengers that allow cells and organs to talk to each other so they can regulate functions such as metabolism, growth, and reproductive processes. As a discipline, endocrinology brings together knowledge from numerous disciplines like biology, biochemistry, and physiology to highlight the interconnectedness of hormonal balance with health outcomes. Furthermore, endocrinology's evolutionary history demonstrates how it gradually developed from crude medical speculations founded on body humors to its current understanding of hormonal interaction with attention focused on the importance of these biochemical signals in the homeostasis of life and responding to extraneous changes (McCarty, 2020). The relevance of endocrinology extends past academic interest; it is essential for the diagnosis and treatment of several diseases. Diseases such as diabetes mellitus, hyperthyroidism, and adrenal insufficiency reflect the negative impact of hormonal imbalance on health. Endocrinology has progressed to have very sophisticated methods to assess endocrine function, including hormone level tests and imaging studies to image endocrine organs. In order to understand these disorders, integration of the biological sciences with clinical practice, a feature of endocrinology, needs to be done. In addition, advances in research have opened up possibilities of studying new facets of the interaction of the endocrine system with other physiological systems. For example, the interaction between the endocrine system and microbiota-gut-brain axis illustrates how endocrine impact can extend beyond traditional limits and hold implications for mental health, with additional implications for the management of a number of disorders (John et al., 2019). The field of endocrinology has, in recent years, broadened to include the study of endocrine disruptors that are likely to negatively affect hormonal balance. These disruptors, which are common in many environmental substrates and consumer items, have become a focus for research to ascertain their impact on human health. Environmental interaction and endocrine functioning are especially important today, as increased awareness regarding pollution and man-made chemicals requires reassessment of existing lifestyles. This new direction places emphasis on multidisciplinary research approaches tackling not just clinical endpoints but wider sociocultural and environmental determinants of endocrine wellbeing. Therefore, endocrinology is now a changing science that aims to address not just the clinical manifestations of hormonal disease but also those root causes resulting in endocrine illnesses in modern society (McCarty, 2020) (Figure 1.1).

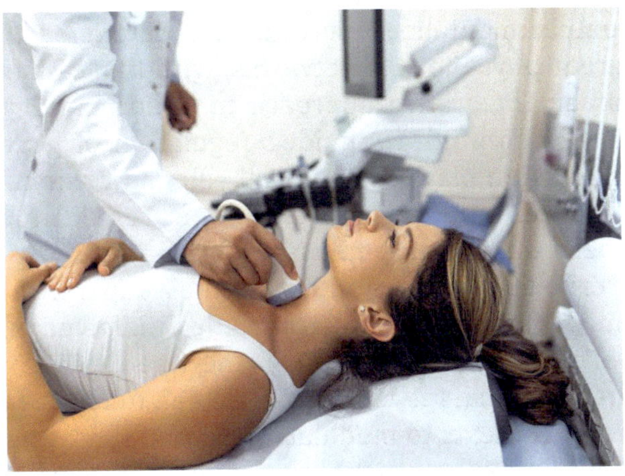

Figure 1.1. An endocrinologist investigates the glands of the endocrine system.

Source: https://texasfms.com/wp-content/uploads/2024/04/doctor-making-ultrasound-thyroid-gland-woman-patient-clinic-diagnosis-treatment-autoimmune-thyroiditis-concept-1.jpg.

Importance of Endocrinology in Medicine

Endocrinology is at the forefront of modern medicine, particularly when it pertains to the management of metabolic diseases such as polycystic ovary syndrome (PCOS). Endocrinology is more than mere diagnosis and treatment; it is about comprehending the body's hormone balance and how hormones affect overall health. The 2023 International Evidence-based Guideline for the Assessment and Management of PCOS illustrates this by highlighting the importance of multidisciplinary care, including a variety of health professionals, and addressing the diverse symptoms and complications of the condition. Such recommendations, based on evidence and consensus among specialists, enable clinicians to provide individualized therapies in accordance with the distinct needs of each patient.

Therefore, endocrinology not only trains therapeutic practice but also enhances the patient experience through individualized care and enhanced health outcomes for conditions supported by hormonal imbalance (Teede et al., 2023). Furthermore, the significance of endocrinology is also present in other facets of human health that impact human growth, reproduction, and metabolism. The field assists with the development of diagnostic criteria and treatment guidelines that are needed for the management of a wide range of endocrine diseases, including diabetes, thyroid disorders, and adrenal insufficiency.

The impact of hormonal well-being on overall health cannot be exaggerated; disruptions in endocrine function can have the capacity to produce serious health complications whose reach will extend beyond isolated symptoms. For instance, diabetes requires not just pharmacological management but also lifestyle modification, education, and long-term follow-up. This integrative approach illustrates how endocrinology is a keystone within prevention medicine by addressing not just the endocrine system but also its intricate interaction with cardiovascular and metabolic disease (Zhang et al., 2023). In a time of rapid chronic illness prevalence, the importance of endocrinology is further enhanced by advances in research and technology. The growing recognition of the role of the microbiome in metabolic well-being and endocrine function underscores the need for ongoing endocrinology research. New treatment options, such as fecal microbiota transplantation (FMT), reveal new promise for the treatment of disease resulting from microbiome dysbiosis, linking endocrine health with other systemic illnesses. These new therapies show that endocrinology is not a rigid science but a dynamic one, always shifting in accordance with new science and societal needs. The application of advanced research to the clinic not only increases our understanding of hormonal control but also encourages effects that favor the greater objectives of public health and wellness programs (Teede et al., 2023; Zhang et al., 2023).

Overview of Hormonal Functions

The hormonal functions of the body are complicated and operate in concert as components of the physiological processes that sustain homeostasis. The hormones are chemical messengers produced and secreted by endocrine glands, influencing numerous biological functions. They include growth and development, metabolism, immunity, and mood. For instance, insulin, which is released by the pancreas, plays a vital function in glucose metabolism, enabling cells to utilize sugar as an energy source. Conversely, the adrenal glands secrete the stress hormone cortisol, which controls the body's response to stress as well as plays a role in controlling blood glucose levels, thereby emphasizing the interdependence of the actions of hormones in numerous bodily functions. All of these interactions serve to show that the delicate balance of the hormones is essential not only to individual health but also to the correct functioning of the body, showing the relevance of endocrinology to the understanding of disease and health. The functions of the hormones are more than just regulating the body's functions—they are also transmitters between systems in the body. This communication is mediated by the microbiota-gut-brain axis, as the gut microbiota interacts with the central nervous system, influencing psychological outcomes and overall health. Evidence over the last fifteen years has shown the microbial community's role as a central regulator of both brain and gut function, illustrating the complexity of hormonal signaling pathways. This communication between the gut microbiota and the brain is mediated by hormones and metabolites, i.e., short-chain fatty acids, which may regulate the secretion of neurotransmitters and ultimately influence mood and behavior. This interaction illustrates that the function of hormones is not compartmentalized but, instead, entangled in larger physiological networks, with this calling for an integrative approach in endocrinology. In addition, miRNA-guided regulation of gene expression plays a significant role in hormonal function and overall hormone regulation. These small non-coding RNA molecules play a crucial role in modulating messenger RNA (mRNA) stability and translation involved in hormone synthesis, vital in the fine-tuning of the hormonal response. miRNAs can function in many contexts to modulate hormone synthesis, degradation, and signal transduction pathways integral to homeostasis. For instance, in some physiological conditions, miRNAs have been shown to suppress or induce the translation of certain target genes and thereby the secretion of hormones like insulin or cortisol. In addition, the secretory property of miRNAs that enables them to be secreted into extracellular fluids implies that they can also act as messengers in cell-to-cell communication. Consequently, understanding the complex roles of miRNAs in hormonal regulation is a promising area of research in endocrinology, particularly as it concerns therapeutic approaches to disorders with hormonal imbalances (Jacob et al., 2018; John et al., 2019).

1.1. History of Endocrinology

Learning Outcome

1. Discuss early discoveries in hormonal research;
2. Explain key figures in endocrinology;
3. Focus on the evolution of endocrine theories.

The history of endocrinology as a scientific field can be traced to advanced knowledge in the physiology of hormones. The field started out as an investigation of organ function, with systemic activities of particular glands being known. Over time, this knowledge grew, leading to specialized centers for conducting endocrinological research. For instance, the 100th anniversary of the Federal State Budgetary Institution "National Medical Research Center for Endocrinology" State Research Center will be celebrated on February 18, 2025, marking an epoch-making date in Russian endocrine research history. This center made a significant contribution, transforming from an "organotherapeutics laboratory" to one of the key sources of basic and applied research concerning endocrine diseases, thus highlighting the institutional component of assistance for scientific advancement in this field (Shestakova, 2025). With advancements in endocrinology, the discipline of endocrinology went through a paradigm shift, particularly in the domain of understanding metabolic disorders, such as obesity. Over the past half-century, researchers have come to view obesity as more of an endocrine/metabolic disorder than as merely a lifestyle consequence. Two prominent hypotheses have resulted from this development: the "Energy Storage" hypothesis and the "Energy Balance" hypothesis. Both stem from the complex mechanisms implicated in the causation of obesity, including genetic, hormonal, and environmental factors. Notably, the discovery of leptin in 1994 bridged the two paradigms, opening significant hormonal regulatory functions in the regulation of weight. Even so, the challenge of leptin resistance persists, demonstrating the endurance of complexity in endocrinology research and illustrating the discipline's intricate interconnectedness with more comprehensive metabolic disease pathology (Lustig et al., 2022). The dynamism of endocrinology is also manifested in its responsive adaptation to newer medical problems and public health crises. As the field has aged, so has its fascination with hormone disorders and has seen expanded diagnostic and therapeutic modalities. The establishment of specialized research institutions, such as the one stated in Russia, was responsible for speeding up innovation in treatment protocols for diseases like diabetes, thyroid disorders, and growth disorders. In addition, interspecialization between endocrinologists and professionals in other medical fields has expanded knowledge in hormone action. As science progresses to define further the nuances of endocrine interaction in the body, the impact of these early breakthroughs will assuredly inform future enhancements in medical science and patient care and reinforce the vital significance of endocrinology to modern medicine.

1.1.1. Early Discoveries in Hormonal Research

The foundation of endocrine research was further laid by early discoveries that described the adrenal glands' function. The importance of the adrenal gland, for instance, was not thought highly of until 1564 and its functions were not understood for centuries. The functions of the adrenals were originally known from deduction from pathologic conditions such as Addison's disease, where there was an accentuation of adrenal insufficiency. Moreover, physiologists were confused about the separation of the adrenal cortex and medulla. The purification of epinephrine in 1901 marked a shift, as it was the very first hormone to be found, which subsequently led to the identification of many adrenal cortical steroids between 1930 and 1949. These findings paved the way for the eventual clinical application of hormonal treatments, namely the historic release of cortisone during the 1950s for conditions such as arthritis and Addison's disease, marking a revolutionary period of endocrinology (Walter et al., 2022). The development of hormonal research also hinged significantly on the knowledge of congenital adrenal hyperplasia (CAH) and its related disorders. Although known in the 19th century, the underlying biochemical defects of CAH, especially the 21-hydroxylation defect, were not known until 1957. This breakthrough was followed shortly by the hormonal characterization of different CAH types, including defects in other essential enzymes, in the 1960s. These works contributed to a better understanding of steroidogenesis and its disorders; a paradigm shift in the topic. The identification of cytochrome P450 enzymes in the early 1960s also signaled an elaborate biological mechanism through which steroid hormone biosynthesis could be performed. These early findings not only enhanced understanding but also prompted advancements in genetic and, biochemical studies, ultimately leading to the identification of mutations that cause most endocrine diseases (Walter et al., 2022). As the scope of hormonal investigation expanded, the interconnectedness of body systems became more apparent. One of the interesting areas of focus was on the gut-brain axis, revealing the widespread role the microbiota plays in hormonal regulation and overall homeostasis. Recent research has indicated that the trillions of microbes found in the body have a pivotal role to play within gut-brain function, enabling communication through various mechanisms like immune system communication and metabolism. This intricate interaction has been in the limelight for its influence on a wide array of disorders, from psychiatric disorders like anxiety to neurodegenerative disorders like Alzheimer's. While scientists continue to discern more about the microbiota-gut-brain axis, it brings out the way early endocrine results provided the stage that still determines contemporary understanding of endocrine interactions and their importance with respect to health and disease (Figure 1.2).

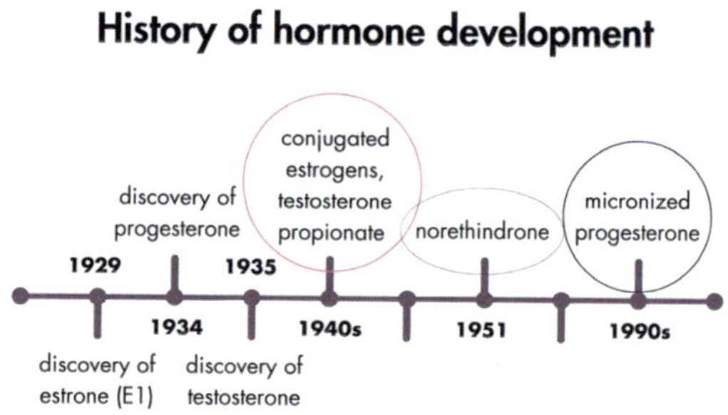

Figure 1.2. History of hormone development.

Source: https://www.larabriden.com/wp-content/uploads/history-of-hormone-development-1024x576.jpg.

1.1.2. Key Figures in Endocrinology

The endocrinology as a science has evolved long way, courtesy in large measure to the pioneering contributions of such visionary figures whose contributions have shaped our understanding of hormone function and disease. Claude Bernard is one of these visionaries, often referred to as the father of the endocrinological science in the 19th century. His research on the role of the pancreas in digestion and glucose metabolism led to the identification of pancreatic secretions, or what we now refer to as hormones. Bernard's invocation of the term *milieu intérieur* emphasized the importance of hormonal regulation in homeostasis. His work laid the groundwork for modern endocrinological research, and later generations took cues from him to delve into the complexities of the endocrine system and its relationship with general health and disease. In the 20th century, further advancements in endocrinology were made by researchers such as Rosalind Franklin and Charles Best. Franklin's work on the molecular arrangements of hormones, in the case of insulin, provided evidence that was pivotal to developing many endocrine disorder therapies. Meanwhile, Charles Best, along with Frederick Banting, discovered the therapeutic application of insulin, revolutionizing the management of diabetes mellitus.

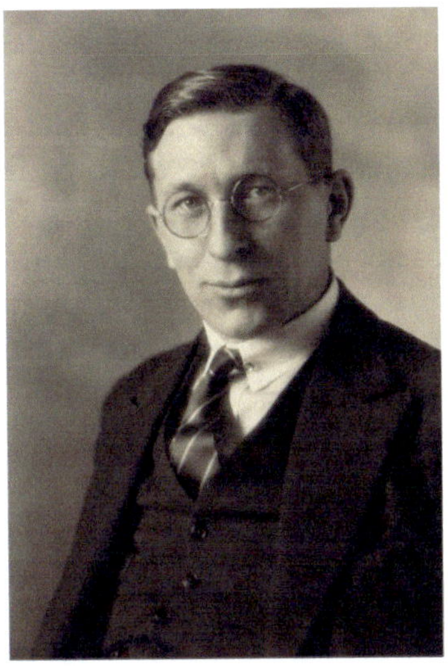

Figure 1.3. Frederick Banting, who discovered insulin's therapeutic potential.

Source: https://upload.wikimedia.org/wikipedia/commons/5/57/F._G._Banting_1923.jpg.

Through concerted collaboration, the discoveries highlighted not only the importance of the pancreas in regulating glucose metabolism but also the intricate mechanisms of hormones in modulating body functions. Their contributions have continued to shape contemporary endocrine investigation and clinical management, emphasizing collaboration and imagination in establishing medical science. Endocrine interdisciplinary research is further exemplified by current investigations of extracellular vesicles (EVs). EVs are increasingly noted for their potential as biomarkers of disease and therapy. According to recent studies, advancements in EV metrology and their biological roles are reshaping our understanding of hormonal communication and the pathological processes related to endocrine disorders (Joshua et al., 2024). As researchers continue to make progress in developing more efficient methods to purify and characterize EVs, multidisciplinary data are required to address current challenges (Mary et al., 2023). This collaborative approach not only has the ability to forward the field of endocrinology but also can lead to new treatments that enhance patient outcomes in endocrine disease (Figure 1.3).

1.1.3. Evolution of Endocrine Theories

The evolution of endocrine theories constitutes a fundamental change in our understanding of the control of hormones and how they impact human physiology. Initially conceptualized by way of crude models constructed around the idea of chemical communication between glands and target tissues, these theories have evolved to incorporate complex interactions among hormones, receptors, and cellular responses. Endocrinology research has progressed from descriptive models toward more comprehensive approaches that are concerned with feedback mechanisms and the impact of environmental factors on endocrine function. The shift was made easier due to advances in biochemistry and molecular biology that provided the possibility of investigating the endocrine system as a dynamic, interactive network rather than a set of isolated processes. Such developments have long-term implications for how we treat disease and health, in the sense that they necessitate a systems vision of endocrine pathways that regulate many physiological phenomena. Further, the application of machine learning techniques in endocrinology studies has been a revolution in drug discovery and therapeutic interventions. Machine learning techniques, which search large datasets for predictive models, have transformed the way scientists find possible drug candidates designed to tackle specified hormonal pathways. The computational approach allows unmatched precision in the understanding of endocrine disorders and the creation of customized treatments based on differences among individual patients. As noted in recent criticism, the application of these technologies has significantly reduced the cost and time needed in preclinical phases of drug development, testifying to the intersection of computer science and endocrinological inquiry. Through the combination of these advanced methodological models with traditional endocrine assumptions, today's scientists can explain the nuances of hormone activities and interactions in ways previously unimaginable, opening up new windows for productive clinical applications. Further, the evolution of endocrine theory is not merely an expression of scientific advance, but also one of shifting sociocultural perceptions of disease and health. As our understanding of the biological determinants of behavior and physiology has evolved, so have our definitions of masculinity, femininity, and their relationships to hormonal activity. The analysis of sexual dimorphic behavior and endocrine influence has begun to reveal the complexity of human identity, challenging dualistic presumptions and calling for more universalistic narratives. These reconsiderations can be heard in debates about gender identity and its biological underpinnings, suggesting that hormonal influence may extend beyond traditional roles to encompass a wider range of gender experience. Therefore, embracing such shifting hormonal theories accommodates a wider picture of human behavior and health, attuned to both scientific developments and ongoing cultural debates.

Test Your Knowledge

1. Which hormone was the first to be isolated and identified in pure form, and by whom?
2. Before hormones were understood, what were some early theories on how body functions were regulated?
3. Who first demonstrated the concept of internal secretion, marking the beginning of modern endocrinology?

1.2. Endocrine Glands

Learning Outcome

1. Describe major endocrine glands and their functions;
2. Explain the structure and location of endocrine glands;
3. Discuss the hormones produced by each gland.

The human body relies upon a complex network of endocrine glands to help regulate numerous physiological functions. They include the pituitary, thyroid, adrenal, and pancreatic glands that constitute vital components of the endocrine system. Through releasing hormones directly into the bloodstream, these glands control a variety of functions such as metabolism, growth, and mood. The importance of such glands is illustrated when one observes disorders like multiple endocrine neoplasia type 1 (MEN1), characterized by the formation of tumors in the pancreas, parathyroid, and pituitary glands. Such an inherited syndrome helps to highlight the intricate interplay between hormone regulation and genetic susceptibility, illustrating how dysfunction of endocrine glands can lead to impactful clinical presentation. It is relevant to learn about these glands and their interrelations in the diagnosis and management of most endocrine diseases that involve human health. The evolution of endocrinology as a science dates back to ancient times and has, over the centuries, evolved. Originally linked with primitive organotherapy and religious practices, the understanding of how internal secretions influence body functions created a foundation for modern endocrinology.

Revolutionary contributions of the Renaissance, in addition to the establishment of the concept of ductless glands, compelled the scientific world towards identifying the role of hormones. Systematic investigation of the endocrine glands gained momentum in the latter half of the nineteenth century through experimental research conducted by well-known scientists such as Claude Bernard and Thomas Addison. This tradition of discovery laid the groundwork for the purification and synthesis of hormones, which ultimately led to therapeutic manipulations that transformed medicine and improved public health outcomes (Eknoyan, 2004). In conclusion, the history of endocrine glands not only reveals the complexity of endocrine control but also indicates the importance of ongoing research and clinical discovery. Diseases like MEN1 illustrate the possible outcomes of molecular and genetic disturbances in such vital glands. With advancing knowledge of endocrinology, healthcare providers must be constantly aware of the manifestations of endocrine imbalance and its effects on general health. Future advances in genetics and molecular biology promise new directions for treatment and management of endocrine disorders, so there is a need for continual education and research in this important area. By fostering a broader understanding of endocrine glands and their functions, we can strive for improved healthcare outcomes and become better equipped to combat the effects of endocrine-related diseases (Gorgel et al., 2020).

1.2.1. Major Endocrine Glands and Their Functions

The endocrine system comprises several large glands that play significant functions in regulating numerous physiological processes of the body. The pituitary gland, or the master gland, controls the functions of other glands in the endocrine system and plays a vital role in regulating growth, metabolism, and reproductive functions. It secretes hormones such as growth hormone (GH) and adrenocorticotropic hormone (ACTH), which act on other glands such as the adrenal glands. The communication between these glands brings out the intricate feedback loops that maintain homeostasis. Furthermore, understanding the major endocrine gland functions is paramount in the diagnosis and treatment of endocrine disorders that can disrupt bodily functions and lead to severe health issues. The adrenal glands, which sit above each kidney, are vital in controlling stress response, metabolic processes, and immune responses. They are two distinct regions: the cortex and the medulla, each performing different functions via the secretion of different hormones. The adrenal cortex secretes glucocorticoids like cortisol that aid in metabolism and stress, and the adrenal medulla secretes catecholamines like adrenaline that prepare the body for fight-or-flight. Recent studies have provided evidence of the debilitating effects of endocrine-disrupting chemicals (EDCs) on adrenal gland function, suggesting that these chemicals can disrupt hormonal balance and affect metabolic regulation (Li et al., 2025). This is an indication that more studies are necessary to safeguard the functional integrity of adrenal glands when exposed to environmental toxins. The thyroid gland, which is located in the neck region, regulates metabolism, growth, and development through the secretion of thyroid hormones like thyroxine (T4) and triiodothyronine (T3). Thyroid hormones play a critical role in regulating metabolic rate and energy levels in the body. Additionally, the thymus gland, while sometimes overlooked, plays a crucial role in immunity, particularly during childhood, through the secretion of thymosin, which is involved in T-cell maturation. There have also been some recent reports that indicate plant-based diets can significantly influence endocrine well-being, and elements present in fruits, vegetables, and grains may make the functioning of the various endocrine glands, like the thyroid and adrenal glands, more efficient (Khalid et al., 2022). This therefore indicates an internal connection between nutrition and endocrine health, tuning diet intake in synchronization with endocrine regulation (Figure 1.4).

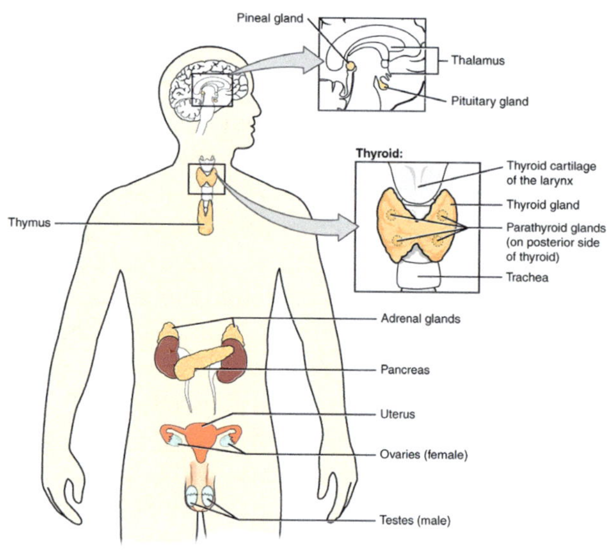

Figure 1.4. The major endocrine glands.

Source: https://upload.wikimedia.org/wikipedia/commons/thumb/1/15/1801_The_Endocrine_System.jpg/800px-1801_The_Endocrine_System.jpg.

1.2.2. Structure and Location of Endocrine Glands

The organization and strategic location of endocrine glands are essential to their function in the regulation of numerous physiological activities. Specialized organs are distributed all over the body, strategically placed so as to ensure proper secretion of hormones into the circulatory system. For instance, the hypothalamus, which is found in the brain, is a critical center for the release of hormones that regulate the anterior pituitary gland, which also controls the release of hormones from other glands, including the thyroid and adrenal cortex. Such a hierarchical organization highlights the unique organization of each gland, with the hypothalamus consisting of neurosecretory cells, and the pituitary that has anterior and posterior sections, both of which produce varying hormonal outputs required in maintaining homeostasis of body processes. Of the numerous endocrine glands, the adrenal glands demonstrate most eloquently the harmony between gland structure and hormonal activity, with their two regions—the cortex and medulla—serving distinct functions under the coordinating control of the hypothalamic-pituitary-adrenal (HPA) axis. The adrenal cortex produces essential steroid hormones, such as cortisol and aldosterone, each serving a vital function in metabolism and electrolyte homeostasis, respectively. In contrast, the adrenal medulla releases catecholamines like adrenaline and noradrenaline, which all play key functions in the body's acute stress response. The unique interrelationship between location and structure of these glands allows for rapid response to physiological demands, which is especially crucial under stress conditions, as made clear by various reactions observed in males versus females concerning their endocrine production under stress conditions (Levine, 2002). Also, endocrine glands' inter-gland communication and systemic influence are influenced by their spatial organization. For example, the thyroid gland, located in the neck, is closely related to the parathyroid glands that rest within its tissue. There is coordinated secretion of the thyroid hormones and parathyroid hormone (PTH) facilitated by this closeness, which ensures homeostasis of calcium in the body. These hormones' production must be well-regulated because any form of imbalance will lead to very serious metabolic diseases. In addition, disorders such as the Carney complex demonstrate how the interruption of endocrine function and genomic integrity can have system-wide effects, influencing a number of endocrine tissues, such as adrenal glands and the pituitary gland in a way that causes hormonal imbalance (Stratakis et al., 1996). Understanding the intricacies of these organs and their functions is of paramount importance in comprehending how endocrine glands coordinate body physiology on a whole-body scale (Figure 1.5).

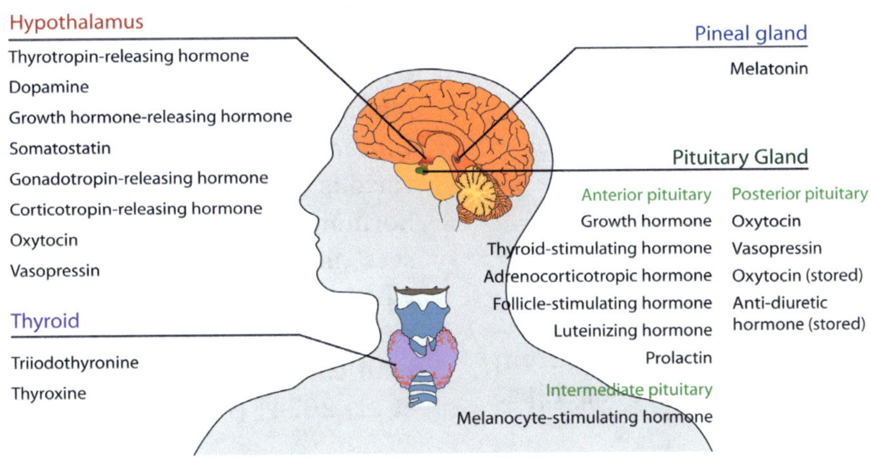

Figure 1.5. Endocrine glands in the human head and neck and their hormones.

Source: https://upload.wikimedia.org/wikipedia/commons/thumb/9/96/Endocrine_central_nervous_en.svg/1024px-Endocrine_central_nervous_en.svg.png.

1.2.3. Hormones Produced by Each Gland

The human organism's endocrine system is an endocrine organ that secretes and synthesizes hormones, playing a crucial role in the regulation of various physiological functions. For instance, the pituitary or master gland secretes GH, prolactin, and ACTH. The secretion of these hormones influences growth, metabolism, and stress response, respectively. The hypothalamus, which controls the pituitary gland, secretes corticotropin-releasing hormone (CRH) and gonadotropin-releasing hormone (GnRH), illustrating the intricate interplay between these organs for the control of body homeostasis (Drakopoulos, 2025). Furthermore, the posterior pituitary stores and releases oxytocin and vasopressin, which are critical components of delivery and fluid balance, illustrating the diverse roles of hormones secreted during this crucial portion of the endocrine system. Outside of the pituitary gland, the thyroid gland produces thyroxine (T4) and triiodothyronine (T3) hormones required for the regulation of metabolism and energy utilization. The hormones influence nearly all of the body cells, regulating metabolic rate and growth and development. Thyroid hormone production is irrevocably connected to the intake of iodine; a deficiency in iodine will lead to hypothyroidism and other thyroid disorders. Apart from thyroxine secreted by the thyroid gland, the parathyroid glands secrete parathyroid hormone (PTH), which is required to regulate blood calcium, providing insight into how hormones from different glands interact synergistically to achieve proper physiological function (Fernanda et al., 2024). Collectively, the glands demonstrate the complexity and specificity of the endocrine system, whereby each hormone has a distinctive and essential role in the maintenance of homeostasis. The adrenal glands, which sit atop the kidneys, are an example of the flexibility of hormone secretion in the endocrine system.

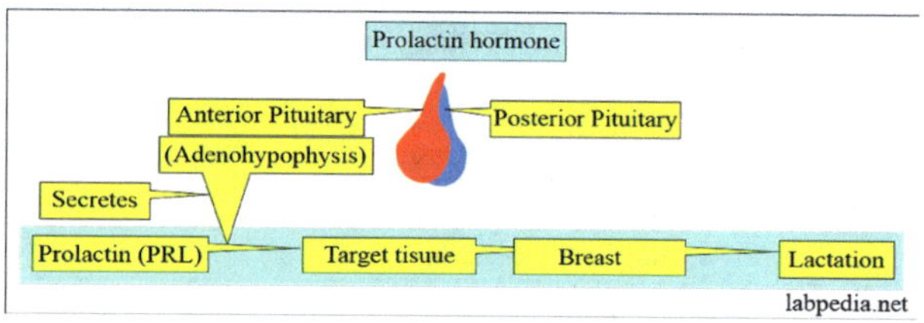

Figure 1.6. Prolactin hormone.

Source: https://labpedia.net/wp-content/uploads/2020/01/Prolactine-secretion-1.jpg.

They secrete glucocorticoids, mostly cortisol, which play a vital role in the regulation of response to stress, metabolism, and immune system function. Also, adrenal medulla produces catecholamines such as adrenaline and noradrenaline that participate in the fight-or-flight response of the body, demonstrating the chief connection between hormonal control and stress.

These processes not only indicate the role of adrenal hormones in the regular physiological process of everyday life but also show the potential implications of adrenal insufficiency, leading to diseases like Addison's disease. Understanding the hormones released by various glands enhances our understanding of hormonal balance and its impact on health, as seen through examples like Sheehan's Syndrome, which illustrates the importance of hormonal control and need for monitoring in patients with extreme hormonal imbalances (Fernanda et al., 2024) (Figure 1.6).

Test Your Knowledge

1. Which gland is often referred to as the "master gland" of the endocrine system, and why?
2. Where is the thyroid gland located, and what are its main hormones?
3. Which endocrine gland is both an endocrine and exocrine organ, and what is its key endocrine hormone?

1.3. Hormones and Their Functions

Learning Outcome

1. Explain types of hormones;
2. Understand the mechanisms of hormone action;
3. Discuss the hormonal regulation of body processes.

Hormones are vital chemical messengers of the endocrine system, guiding a vast variety of physiological functions indispensable for homeostasis. The hormones are secreted by endocrine glands into the blood and then transported to target organs, tissues, or cells where they bind to specific receptors, initiating a variety of responses. The functions of hormones are growth, metabolism, reproduction, and mood, to regulate both short-term and long-term changes in the body. For instance, upon stress, the body releases hormones like cortisol, which gear the body for fighting or flight. This intricate network of hormones underscores the importance of hormonal homeostasis, as even minor changes in the hormonal milieu can lead to numerous diseases and alterations in normal physiological processes, further emphasizing the need to understand these chemical interactions within the broader endocrinological context. Hormone research is not merely about understanding the physiological roles of hormones; it's also about observing how these chemicals influence behavior and psychological phenomena. Behavioral endocrinology takes into account two-way interactions between behavior and hormones, demonstrating that hormonal changes can significantly impact emotional and social functioning. For instance, during growth periods such as puberty and pregnancy, hormones are not merely accountable for physical changes but also for the development of behaviors and states of mind. Furthermore, research has shown that hormone levels are able to affect aggression, mate selection, and social behavior, enlightening us on how biological and psychological processes relate to each other. This is vital knowledge because it provides an understanding of how hormonal differences can impact lifestyle, mental health, and social structures in various environments, thereby enhancing our understanding of human psychology and behavior (N/A, 2019). Besides, the role of energy availability (EA) is also critical in the explanation of endocrine behaviors, particularly among sports persons and physical health. Poor EA, resulting from abnormal dietary patterns or excessive training, can have severe consequences on the hormonal milieu, resulting in conditions such as the female athlete triad and relative energy deficiency in sport (RED-S). Experiments have demonstrated correlations between low energy availability and adverse effects on reproductive endocrine function, bone metabolism, and overall physiological homeostasis. Recognition of the implications of LEA gives insight into the interaction between lifestyle, endocrine health, and reproduction and supports the creation of interventions to counteract these effects. This heightened examination of hormonal mechanisms in comparison to energy availability highlights the importance of a balanced approach towards exercise and diet that is necessary for the maintenance of not only physical sporting capability but also general well-being across various groups of individuals (José et al., 2020).

1.3.1. Types of Hormones: Peptide, Steroid, and Amine

In endocrinology, hormones are classified into three broad categories: peptide, steroid, and amine hormones. Peptide hormones, which consist of short chains of amino acids, are produced from longer precursor proteins and play important roles in many biological processes. Peptide hormones are soluble in water and interact with cell membrane receptors in general, initiating a cascade of intracellular actions without passing through the target cells.

This bonding has the ability to trigger instant physiological responses, i.e., the release of insulin by pancreatic beta cells in response to elevated blood glucose levels. Peptide hormones' function is further illustrated by their participation in such critical physiological processes as growth, metabolism, and immune response, showcasing the fine balance these molecules maintain in the endocrine system. Steroid hormones, on the other hand, are cholesterol-derived and possess a rather distinct mechanism of action compared to their peptide counterparts. Since steroid hormones are lipid-soluble, they easily cross cell membranes and possess the ability to bind intracellular receptors, thus influencing gene expression. This remains for longer since it targets protein production that is crucial in most body functions. Steroid hormones such as cortisol, testosterone, and estrogen regulate processes such as stress response, reproduction, and inflammation. Their intricate roles in homeostasis make it all the more important to identify steroid hormone signal pathways and their possible role in health and disease regulation throughout life, particularly concerning hormonal imbalance and related pathology. Amine hormones, while less frequently used as posters, form another essential component of endocrine control. These molecules, synthesized from single amino acids such as tryptophan and tyrosine, include well-known examples like epinephrine and thyroxine.

Amine hormones can be both water-soluble and lipid-soluble and create a broad range of effects. Thyroid hormones, for instance, are lipid-soluble and exert long-term effects on growth and metabolic function, while catecholamines like epinephrine quickly control the body's reaction to stress. The complexity of endocrine function and hormone production is also seen in their evolutionary background, as the thyroid hormones, with deep origins in primitive biological functions (Mazzaferro et al., 2015), have evolved. The complexity of amine hormones is indicative of their role in creating appropriate physiological responses, in addition to peptide and steroid hormones, in ensuring overall homeostasis (Figure 1.7).

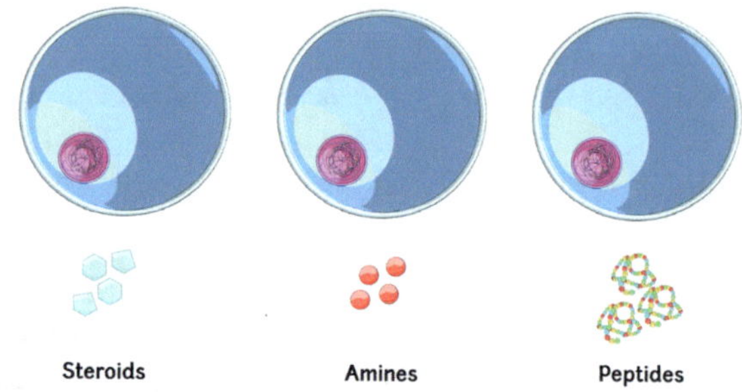

Figure 1.7. Types of hormones.

Source: https://www.jove.com/files/media/science-education/science-education-thumbs/10988.jpg.

1.3.2. Mechanisms of Hormone Action

Mechanisms of hormone action are at the core of endocrinology, as these define how hormones exert their physiological effects on target tissues. Hormones can be broadly classified into steroid hormones and peptide hormones, both of which undergo distinct mechanisms of action. Steroid hormones, being lipid-soluble, can diffuse across cell membranes and bind to intracellular receptors to generate hormone-receptor complexes that bind directly to DNA to modify gene expression. By contrast, peptide hormones, which are hydrophilic, generally interact with cell surface receptors and initiate a cascade of intracellular signaling through second messengers like cyclic AMP. This basic dichotomy in signaling mechanisms reflects the myriad ways that hormones can shape cellular function, in the long run influencing a range of physiological processes, including metabolism, growth, and developmental patterns. The complexities of hormone action are more underscored by the progress in molecular biology and genomic technologies that have explained the complexities of hormone signaling pathways. Research into GH actions serves as a good example of these mechanisms, as studies have established that GH primarily acts through the GH receptor, which initiates the activation of specific transcription factors, such as STAT5B. This interaction subsequently initiates the expression of insulin-like growth factor 1 (IGF-1), a critical mediator of GHs growth factor-like effects. An understanding of these hormonal axes not only enhances our knowledge of endocrine function but also defines therapeutic targets for GH and IGF-1 balance-related disorders. These findings are thus paramount in the treatment of conditions such as growth deficiencies or metabolic syndromes associated with altered hormone function (Basu et al., 2018).

As studies in endocrinology continue, comparative endocrinology is increasingly being emphasized as a means of comprehending the evolutionary intricacies of mechanisms of hormone actions between species. By analyzing the evolution of the hormonal signaling pathways, scientists are able to view the functional specificity and regulation of the pathways over evolutionary time. One such example is the glucocorticoid and mineralocorticoid receptors that shared a common ancestor during vertebrate evolution. This is a great example of how minimal genetic mutations have led to enormous changes in hormone specificity and function. Not only does it enhance our understanding of the physiology of normal, but it also offers important implications for human endocrinopathies. With the aid of genomics in permitting deeper exploration of the genomes of ancient man and hominins, the potential for uncovering the evolutionary origin of hormone action mechanisms opens up exciting directions for resolving present endocrine disease (Rotwein, 2015) (Figure 1.8).

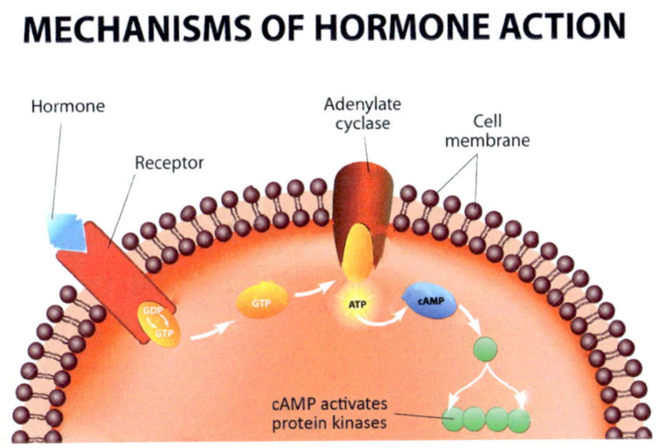

Figure 1.8. Mechanism of hormone action.

Source: https://www.onlinebiologynotes.com/wp-content/uploads/2017/03/mechanism-of-hormone-action.jpg.

1.3.3. Hormonal Regulation of Body Processes

The endocrinological regulation of body functions is not a static but a dynamic science that demonstrates how hormones regulate a multitude of physiological processes. Hormones like insulin, glucagon, and cortisol regulate metabolic pathways to deliver energy in an effective way and store it properly. Insulin, for instance, induces the uptake of glucose within cells, while glucagon induces the mobilization of glucose from storage pools within the liver and thus regulates blood sugar levels. The precise balance of these hormones is most crucial for homeostasis; any deviation might lead to metabolic diseases such as diabetes. The interaction of hormones with other tissues suggests a complex system of communication whereby signals are conveyed by receptors and biochemical cascades, underlining their role in maintaining the internal environment of the body and responding to external stimuli. The influence of environmental stimuli on hormonal regulation cannot be overstressed. External stimuli such as stress, light, and food availability affect hormone secretions that, in turn, affect physiological and behavioral responses. For example, the glucocorticoid reaction to stress illustrates how fluctuations in hormones play a vital role in survival. Elevated levels of stress hormones, such as cortisol, prepare the body to respond to threats by enhancing energy mobilization and inhibiting non-essential processes at the moment. Further, these endocrine reactions are not fixed; they are variable in response to internal conditions such as genetics, sex, and life stage. As emphasized in eco-evolutionary endocrinology, knowing how these variations beget individual and population-level differences is the key to realizing the plasticity of organisms to their environments (Stevenson et al., 2020). At the cellular level, their actions are mediated by a balance between short-term signal transduction and longer-term genomic responses that manifest the dynamic character of endocrine control. Their action is mediated by particular receptors on target cells, that trigger signaling cascades that can influence gene expression and protein synthesis. This interaction occurs in growth, reproductive function, and calcium homeostasis. For instance, parathyroid hormone and vitamin D are equally important in calcium homeostasis, managing the movement of calcium in the body (Ramy et al., 2022). Any disruptions in these hormonal processes can lead to severe health issues, including osteoporosis and cardiovascular disease, underscoring the need for highly regulated hormonal control. Understanding of the subtle balance and regulation of these hormones provides valuable information about endocrine health and disease therapy, emphasizing the role as essential components of integrative physiological homeostasis.

Test Your Knowledge

1. What is the key structural difference between peptide, steroid, and amine hormones?
2. How do peptide hormones typically exert their effects on target cells?
3. What role does negative feedback play in hormonal regulation? Give one physiological example.

1.4. Endocrine Disorders

Learning Outcome

1. Understand common endocrine disorders and their symptoms;
2. Describe causes and risk factors for endocrine disorders;
3. Discuss the impact of endocrine disorders on health.

Endocrine disorders are a group of heterogeneous diseases that target various endocrine glands and result in catastrophic health issues among the affected individuals. They disturb the normal production, control, and secretion of the hormones and manifest in a multitude of varied clinical syndromes. Endocrine disorders such as diabetes mellitus, thyroid disorders, and adrenal insufficiency have varied etiologies and management protocols. Advances in genetic research, for instance, as described in the EndoGene database, have clarified the role of genetic variants in the pathogenesis of these diseases, demonstrating the multifactorial nature of their etiology. The database holds genetic information of patients with different endocrine disorders and has yielded useful information on their molecular etiology, hence enhancing diagnostic and therapeutic approaches in endocrinology (Buzdin et al., 2025). Emergency medical conditions most often arise from endocrine disorders, which significantly affect patient morbidity and mortality. A review on the period from 2018 to 2023, conducted in Ryazan, showed that endocrinology emergency conditions accounted for approximately 0.5% of all emergencies medical calls. Among them, recently diagnosed diabetes mellitus and hypoglycemia cases were particularly prevalent, and this undeniably demands urgent intervention (Yankina et al., 2025). Type 2 diabetic women most frequently needed emergency consultations due to complications of hypo- and hyperglycemia. The research described an ominous trend toward hospitalization due to these acute-onset endocrine crises, with a 0.1% rate of mortality among the patients in the pre-hospital phase. These data illustrate the demanding nature of the management of endocrine diseases and the potential for enhanced outcomes with the utilization of effective emergency response systems. Also, genetics and environmental interactions are at the center of the development and management of endocrine diseases. The EndoGene database is a goldmine of information regarding these impacts, and conclusions are based on genomic and technical data obtained from almost 6,000 patients with varying endocrine conditions. By integrating genetic information with clinical records, researchers can better describe the etiology of such conditions as well as their clinical presentation (Buzdin et al., 2025). This integrative strategy is important because it enables the development of targeted treatments and personalized medicine strategies. Ultimately, sustained research into endocrine illnesses with the help of advanced genetic analysis and emergency treatment guidelines will have to be employed to further improve patient outcomes and make treatment processes more efficient for endocrinologists.

1.4.1. Common Endocrine Disorders and Their Symptoms

Endocrine disorders are among the most important tasks of modern medicine, as they affect diverse physiological functions due to hormonal imbalance. The most frequent diseases are diabetes mellitus, thyroid gland pathology, and disorders of the adrenal glands. Diabetes mellitus, characterized by hyperglycemia, can have symptoms such as excessive thirst, polyuria, and blurred vision. On the other hand, thyroid disorders can manifest as hypothyroidism with symptoms of fatigue, weight gain, and intolerance to heat, or hyperthyroidism with weight loss, intolerance to heat, and tachycardia. The impact of such conditions goes beyond signs and symptoms that are physical in nature and can lead to complications of long-term illness, hence necessitating early detection and intervention for optimal patient outcomes (Buzdin et al., 2025). Ovarian disorders, such as polycystic ovary syndrome (PCOS), portray another prominent category of endocrine disorders, which predominantly affect women in their childbearing years. PCOS constitutes irregular menstrual periods, hypertrichosis, and acne that arise as a consequence of hormonal imbalance, i.e., elevated levels of androgens. These symptoms, if left untreated, can lead to other problems such as infertility and the risk of metabolic syndrome. Moreover, menstrual abnormalities, including oligomenorrhea and abnormal uterine bleeding, might be combined with endocrine disorders, complicating the patient's course. Genealogical study has indicated that the hereditary burden of reproductive and endocrine pathology tends to complicate the prognosis for the patients, attesting to the interaction between the genetic and environmental loads in the pathogenesis of the mentioned diseases (Bagatska, 2024). In addition, diseases of the adrenal glands, specifically Cushing's syndrome and Addison's disease, represent the diversity of endocrine abnormalities. Cushing's syndrome, typically resulting from hypersecretion of cortisol, has side effects such as weight gain, high blood pressure, and susceptibility to bruising. Addison's disease, characterized by hyposecretion of the hormones of the adrenal glands, can lead to fatigue, muscle weakness, and low blood pressure.

The multifactorial etiology of these disorders complicates them in the sense that both lifestyle variables, environmental factors, and genetic susceptibilities cross paths to have an impact on hormone levels and general health. Given the seriousness of these endocrine disorders, a clear comprehension of symptoms and etiology of these disorders is required in order to aid proper diagnosis, control, and prevention strategies within the field of endocrinology (Buzdin et al., 2025) (Figure 1.9).

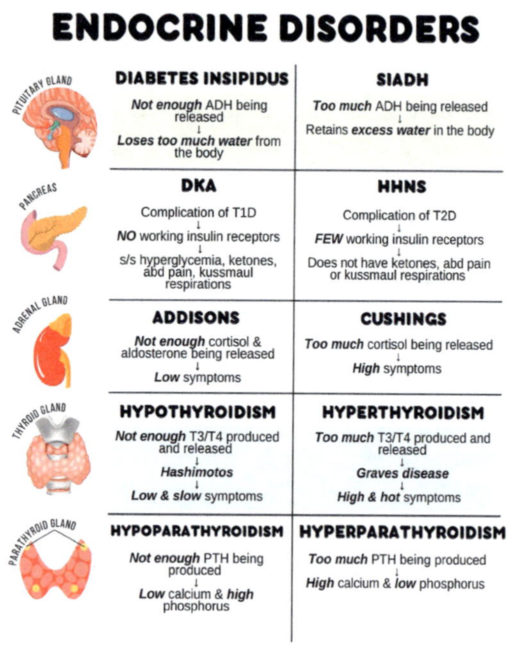

Figure 1.9. Illustration of endocrine disorders.

Source: https://encrypted-tbn0.gstatic.com/images?q=tbn:ANd9GcRLyOH1dYjolii-OYzI38UCrEux2vBi7gtM2g&s.

1.4.2. Causes and Risk Factors for Endocrine Disorders

Endocrine disorders are caused by a multi-factorial interaction between genetic, environmental, and lifestyle factors. One of the main risk factors is genetic predisposition, for example, when specific mutations lead to type 1 diabetes and specific thyroid disease. Monogenic endocrine disorders are generally caused by rare variants of genes, whereas polygenic conditions, the case of type 2 diabetes, result from the cumulative effect of many genetic variants in combination with environmental factors such as diet and physical activity level. The newer advances of molecular genetics in the form of genome-wide association studies have made these genetic predispositions clearer. These investigations underscore the importance of early risk identification to enable the presence of focused prevention strategies and to enable individuals to make well-informed lifestyle choices to minimize their risk of developing endocrine disorders (Kim et al., 2023). Environmental influences are equally crucial in the etiology of endocrine disorders. Exposure to endocrine-disrupting compounds, which are commonly found in pesticides, plastics, and industrial waste, could potentially have a significant impact on hormonal function and metabolism. These drugs have the ability to mimic or interfere with the body's own endogenous hormones, potentially leading to endocrine diseases such as obesity and diabetes. Lifestyle factors must also be taken into account; physical inactivity, poor diet heavy in processed foods, and being overweight are strongly correlated with an increased risk of developing endocrine diseases. This correlation is significant in the public health requirement to incorporate healthier lifestyle alternatives so that such risk factors are diminished. Understanding of the multifactorial etiology of endocrine disorders will not only aid in the development of effective treatment plans but also aid in devising preventive interventions targeting modifiable risk factors (Kim et al., 2023). Moreover, demographic determinants such as age, sex, and socio-economic status contribute to the risk for endocrine disease. For instance, women tend to develop certain diseases, like autoimmune thyroid diseases, possibly due to hormonal shifts and variations in the immune system. Similarly, socio-economic status influences healthcare access as well as prevention and management resources for these disorders. Recent research demonstrates that some subpopulations may face variations in the incidence of endocrine disorders following events like the COVID-19 pandemic, and so there is a requirement for in-depth studies that take into account such demographic factors. This information is critical to ensure healthcare interventions are tailored to cater to the unique needs of various populations and achieve optimal results in endocrine disorder control and care (Krueger et al., 2024) (Figure 1.10).

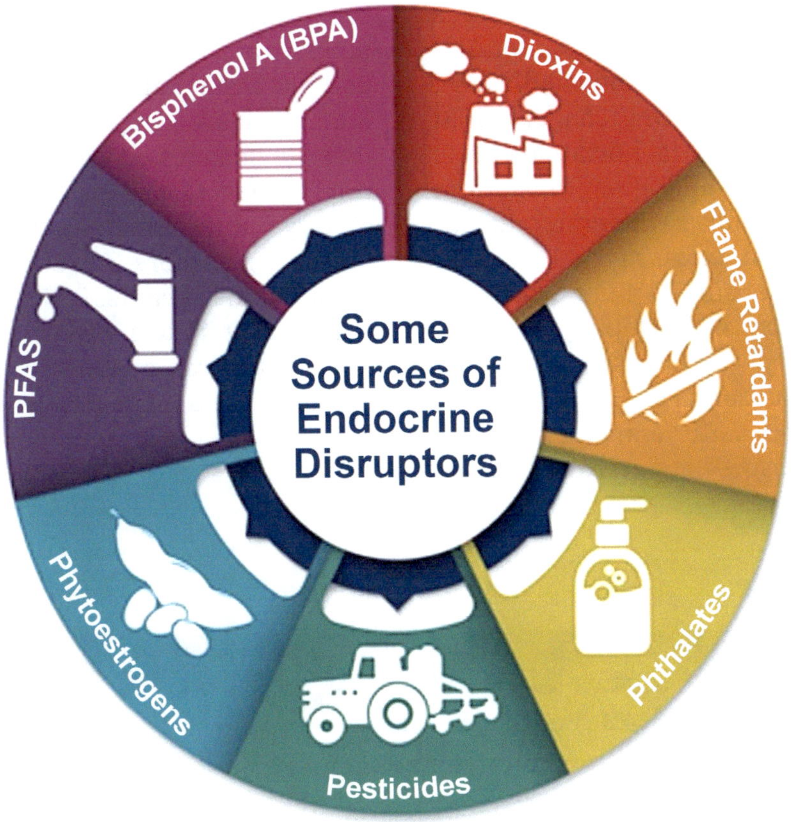
Some Sources of Endocrine Disruptors
Bisphenol A (BPA)
Dioxins
Flame Retardants
Phthalates
Pesticides
Phytoestrogens
PFAS

Figure 1.10. Endocrine disruptor sources.

Source: https://www.niehs.nih.gov/sites/default/files/health/assets/images/endocrine_disruptor_sources.jpg.

1.4.3. Impact of Endocrine Disorders on Health

The impact of endocrine disease on health is more than the quality of individual symptoms, with a significant impact on the general quality of life and long-term consequences. Diseases such as diabetes mellitus and thyroid disease profoundly impact other body systems, with complications having an impact on both body and mind. Diabetes, for instance, not only alters glucose metabolism but also enhances the risk for cardiovascular complications, neuropathy, and renal disease. Equally, hypothyroidism or hyperthyroidism may change metabolic function, influencing weight, energy, and even mood stability. This very intricate interaction deserves management by a multidisciplinary approach, with utmost priority given to healthcare providers observing the myriad ways endocrine disorders can compromise health and well-being (Pandey, 2024). The interaction between endocrine disorders and oral health is a crucial aspect that is often neglected. These patients usually endure periodontal disease, dry mouth, and compromised wound healing, which make routine dental procedures challenging and increase the likelihood of oral infection. Patients taking thyroid medication are also prone to experiencing challenges in oral health as alterations in hormone levels normally affect saliva and gum formation. Emphasizing the need for an integrated health approach, newer developments in endocrine and dental sciences have come to illuminate how the disorders interact. In developing protocols for interdisciplinary collaboration between endocrinologists and dental practitioners, the results can be significantly enhanced, noting the necessity to ensure an interdisciplinary approach to treating endocrine disorders (Pandey, 2024). Furthermore, the general impact of global warming on endocrine health cannot be downplayed, as observed by its correlation with increased endocrine disorders. As climate change continues to alter environmental conditions, humans can become vulnerable to metabolic and endocrine-based diseases. For instance, extreme temperatures can increase heat-associated illnesses and negatively impact insulin efficiency because insulin and other important endocrine medicines are temperature-sensitive. Besides, lifestyle changes caused by climatic conditions can cause increased physical inactivity and poor dietary habits, which further increase the risk for these disorders. The South Asian Federation of Endocrine Societies has stressed the need for a united effort to tackle these issues, pointing towards environmentally friendly interventions that promote both environmental and endocrine well-being.

Test Your Knowledge

1. What are the symptoms and typical physical signs of hyperthyroidism?
2. Which endocrine disorder is caused by prolonged exposure to high cortisol levels, and what are some characteristic features?
3. How can endocrine disorders like polycystic ovary syndrome (PCOS) affect reproductive and metabolic health?

1.5. Diagnosis of Endocrine Disorders

Learning Outcome

1. Describe diagnostic tests for hormonal levels;
2. Understand imaging techniques in endocrinology;
3. Explain the role of patient history in diagnosis.

Diagnosis of endocrine disorders requires a keen understanding of the subtle endocrine system interactions. Clinically, historically, diagnosis has relied significantly on clinical evaluation and biochemical investigations to ascertain hormonal levels. Diabetes mellitus, for example, could be diagnosed on the basis of fasting plasma glucose or hemoglobin A1c concentrations. The subtle nature of hormone regulation requires a multidisciplinary expert approach to effectively interpret these results. Modern practice favors a multidisciplinary approach, combining information from various specialties such as endocrinology, urology, and general practice in primary care. Multidisciplinary interaction aims to provide a more comprehensive view of patient health, particularly in diseases such as male hypogonadism, where fluctuations in diagnosis and management are significantly different, impacting outcomes (Jayasena et al., 2021). Hence, by utilizing a diverse team, there is better precision and less error in the diagnosis of endocrine disorders. During the diagnostic process, physicians must be acutely sensitive to the subtleties indicative of different endocrine disorders. Symptoms often overlap with each other, introducing complexities into the diagnostic picture. For instance, both adrenal insufficiency and hypothyroidism may present with fatigue and weight changes, and therefore, it is important that clinicians perform vigorous differential diagnoses. Advances in medical technology, like improved imaging modalities and molecular diagnostics, permit finer analysis of endocrine function. These developments make it possible for medical professionals to detect abnormalities at the cellular or genetic level, leading to more precise and earlier diagnoses. Nevertheless, as proved by ongoing research, there is still much to be learnt regarding the genetic origin for the majority of endocrine diseases, as revealed in procedures for prenatal diagnosis (Robert et al., 2020). This new knowledge is required to anticipate and address such diseases successfully. The impact of early and accurate diagnosis of endocrine disorders cannot be overstated, as an early intervention can dramatically change patient outcomes. For diseases like diabetes or thyroid conditions, delayed diagnosis or misdiagnosis can lead to severe complications like neuropathy or cardiovascular illnesses. To combat this, health care systems are starting to apply standardized diagnosis protocols, not just making the identification process more effective but also presenting practitioners of every discipline with the same fundamental information. Endocrinology educational programs play a vital role in generating awareness and knowledge among healthcare providers. Furthermore, as new diagnostic facilities and treatment modalities emerge, continuing education will be instrumental in keeping clinicians up-to-date. These initiatives not only speak of personalized care optimization but also pave the way for innovation in the whole specialty of endocrinology, resulting in more efficient management of complicated endocrine disorders (Jayasena et al., 2021).

1.5.1. Diagnostic Tests for Hormonal Levels

Hormonal imbalance diagnosis forms a core part of endocrinology, employing a set of diagnostic tests suitable for specific hormones and pathologies. Quantitative serum assays that measure the concentration of significant hormones such as thyroid-stimulating hormone (TSH), cortisol, and sex hormones are standard tests. These not only provide information regarding the function of the endocrine system but also guide therapeutic maneuvers. For instance, thyroid function tests that measure levels of thyroid hormones and TSH can be employed to distinguish between hypothyroidism and hyperthyroidism. This is important since the tests are highly essential in the early diagnosis and management of disease conditions, influencing patient health and quality of life seriously. Proper interpretation of these hormonal assays is thus essential to effective clinical management strategy development. Recent studies have highlighted the role of vitamin D status in thyroid function and revealed the complex relationship between vitamin D deficiency and thyroid disease. One such observation has been that higher vitamin D levels are inversely associated with hypothyroidism, as indicated by a strongly reduced odds ratio with increased vitamin D. These correlations validate the potential that optimal vitamin D levels could act as a prevention method for certain thyroid disorders. The reverse is not as extreme but also merits mentioning in clinical assessments (Ihsan et al., 2025). Application of vitamin D as a biomarker in the understanding of thyroid health illustrates the interactive nature of endocrinological diagnostic practice in which several factors are considered in determining the interpretation of hormonal status. In addition to the traditional hormone tests, new biomarkers are also being researched to enhance diagnoses like central precocious puberty (CPP). For instance, research has established that fasting insulin (FINS) and insulin-like growth factor-1 (IGF-1) have the potential of being effective biomarkers in the diagnosis of CPP, with a less invasive approach compared to conventional measures such as the GnRH provocation test. Elevated levels of the biomarkers correlate with increased risk for CPP, making them effective for early screening and intervention (Zhang et al., 2025). This trend towards the utilization of metabolic and growth factors in hormonal diagnosis is merely a broader tendency in endocrinology, highlighting the need for innovative methodology that will increase accuracy and patient outcomes in endocrine-related diseases (Figure 1.11).

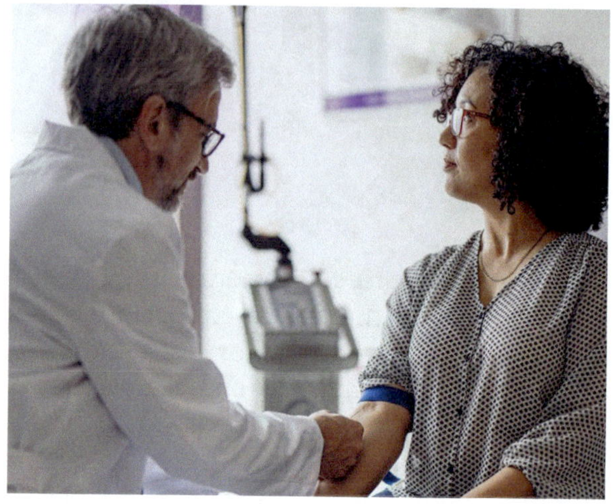

Figure 1.11. Tests for hormonal levels.

Source: https://livehealthy.muhealth.org/sites/livehealthy/files/styles/1200x900/public/2024-08/Hormon%20testing_1600x740_0.jpg?itok=VtP7rMDr.

1.5.2. Imaging Techniques in Endocrinology

Imaging modalities are a significant application in the field of endocrinology practice, aiding clinicians in diagnosing and managing various hormonal disorders. From the simple X-rays to the more advanced modalities like MRI and PET scans, imaging modalities enable visualization of the endocrine organs, including the thyroid, adrenal glands, and pituitary gland. For instance, thyroid imaging is required to evaluate nodules, hyperfunctioning tissue, or cancer, with the use of radioactive isotopes being the most common method used to assess functionality as well as structural issues. Not only does the use of imaging enhance diagnostic accuracy, but it also directs treatment, with patients being treated with care specifically tailored to their own medical condition. The constant development of imaging technologies, such as high-resolution ultrasound and functional imaging, is revolutionizing the management of endocrine disorders by healthcare providers, particularly in the fine-tuned diagnosis of complex cases. Disorders of sex development (DSDs) are significantly better managed through the integration of imaging modalities, facilitating all-rounded evaluations and evidence-based clinical decisions. As outlined in the new guidelines, imaging modalities are of pivotal importance in diagnosing anatomical anomalies and associated risk factors, enabling doctors to formulate individualized care plans. For example, MRI is particularly valuable in delineating inner structures and helping in the evaluation of indeterminate genitalia, where accurate interpretation is critical in determining appropriate management plans. Furthermore, imaging facilitates ongoing follow-up of patients, not just addressing physical problems, but psychosocial problems too, as they navigate the subtleties of their conditions. The evolution of imaging in the treatment of DSDs necessitates an interdisciplinary approach, combining hormonal evaluation with imaging findings to optimize patient outcomes and quality of life (Peter et al., 2016). In the setting of thyroid cancers, imaging techniques are essential for medullary thyroid carcinoma staging and treatment, a topic of interest in recent American Thyroid Association guidelines. Imaging techniques such as ultrasound, CT scans, and functional PET scanning assess tumor dissemination, nodal involvement, and potential metastasis, information that determines therapy. Enhanced imaging capability allows for more precise preoperative planning, as information about the degree of disease can critically affect surgery and prognosis. Since these guidelines are updated periodically, according to the recent research and technology developments, it becomes increasingly essential for the cooperation between endocrinologists, radiologists, and surgeons to provide holistic management (Samuel et al., 2015). This interdepartmental collaboration emphasizes the necessity of integrating imaging modalities into daily endocrine practice, most urgently in the event of disorders requiring strict diagnostic workups (Figure 1.12).

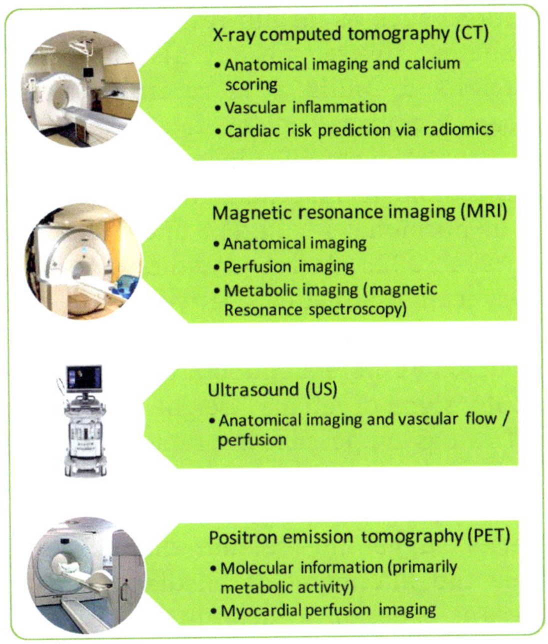

Figure 1.12. Medical imaging techniques commonly performed and their common uses.

Source: https://www.researchgate.net/publication/353827351/figure/fig2/AS:11431281250146743@1717770739697/Medical-imaging-techniques-commonly-performed-and-their-common-uses-All-photos-licenced.png.

1.5.3. Role of Patient History in Diagnosis

In endocrinology, the role of patient history cannot be overestimated in differential diagnosis and effective management of endocrine disorders. Accurate information about a patient's past medical history regarding earlier diseases, endocrine disorders, family history, drug use, and others is extremely important to clinicians. The information is pivotal in understanding risk factors and the likely etiology responsible for hormonal disturbances. For instance, one's history of metabolic syndrome, diabetes, or obesity may be a sign of susceptibility to the development of conditions such as nonalcoholic fatty liver disease (NAFLD), which is becoming more common in patients with endocrine conditions such as insulin resistance and type 2 diabetes. Hence, patient history enables physicians to build a more individualized approach to diagnosis and treatment, particularly in the context of chronic illnesses with complex pathophysiological mechanisms, such as in the case of hormonal regulation and metabolism (Mary et al., 2023). Moreover, a thorough patient history can distinguish between otherwise similar presenting symptoms that could be attributed to different endocrine disorders. For example, signs of fatigue, weight changes, and mood swings are possible in a range of disorders from hypothyroidism to adrenal insufficiency. By careful patient history, physicians can learn patterns suggesting certain diagnoses and reduce the likelihood of misdiagnosis. This process is especially crucial in endocrinology, where timely treatment can significantly alter disease course and patient outcome. In addition, lifestyle choices, diet, and psychosocial contexts, components of patient histories, can significantly influence the progression of endocrine disorders. Introducing these elements into the equation for diagnosis is essential to realizing how they may trigger or exacerbate underlying conditions or initiate new ones (Chalasani et al., 2017). Lastly, the inclusion of a patient's endocrine history can enhance overall quality of care. Patient history not only enhances the accuracy of diagnosis but can also affect the selection of appropriate screening and monitoring methods based on each patient's risk profile. With all historical information relevant to the case documented, endocrinologists can implement preventive action where necessary. For instance, patients with thyroid disease or atypical lipid profiles in their families may need to be monitored more intensively in order to enable early diagnosis of thyroid abnormality or dyslipidemia. In addition, knowledge of the patient's previous experiences of healthcare can disclose obstacles to treatment adherence or to patient engagement, so that clinicians are able to communicate information appropriately and treat their patients appropriately. Thus, a comprehensive patient history is a foundation for good decision-making in endocrinology, not only for diagnosis but also for continuation of therapeutic plans (Mary et al., 2023).

Test Your Knowledge

1. How does a patient's medical history and symptom timeline aid in diagnosing endocrine disorders?
2. What imaging technique is frequently used to evaluate the structure of the pituitary gland?

1.6. Treatment Options in Endocrinology

Learning Outcome

1. Describe hormone replacement therapy;
2. Discuss medications for managing endocrine disorders;
3. Understand surgical interventions in endocrinology.

Endocrinology treatment has evolved significantly to manage a large variety of disorders, particularly those that have a hormonal imbalance component. A significant method of treatment is pharmacological, and this can involve hormone replacement or the use of novel drugs that target specific mechanisms. Diabetic care, for example, employs insulin therapy in conjunction with novel oral agents such as GLP-1 receptor agonists and SGLT2 inhibitors. These oral drugs not only control blood glucose but also potentially have cardiovascular effects, implying an expanding role for drug therapy in the control of multifactorial endocrinologic diseases. And the research continues to unveil new and innovative treatments, expanding the clinician's arsenal. It also needs to be reviewed regularly to optimize the benefit to patients, whereby the treatment regimens should be tailored to address the particular requirements of patients, taking an integrated approach (Pellesi et al., 2024). Another area of focus in endocrinology includes the management of hypoparathyroidism (HypoPT). Traditionally, the treatment of HypoPT has been achieved by maintaining serum calcium stability with oral calcium and active vitamin D supplementation. However, this classical management is not without disadvantages, being unable to mimic the natural parathyroid hormone (PTH) action with consequent suboptimal control and potential long-term problems. More recent advances, such as the introduction of recombinant human PTH(1–84), demonstrate a trend toward directly treating the causative deficiency. This novel therapy offers an alternative to standard management, potentially leading to improved biochemical control and a reduction in associated complications. These advancements evidence the necessity of ongoing investigation in the development of efficient therapies that better address the complexity of endocrine illnesses like HypoPT (Misiorowski et al., 2023). New therapeutic modalities for migraine—a common but disabling neurological disorder—have also begun to reshape the therapeutic horizon of endocrinology. Traditional pharmacological approaches yield limited efficacy, and the quest for novel treatments that target distinct pathological pathways of the disorder is warranted. Current research identifies future prospects such as drugs against the trigeminovascular system and cannabinoid-based medicines as promising in the relief of migraine. Furthermore, incorporation of hormonal and metabolic therapies into treatment protocols has been highlighted, which mirrors a confluence between neurology and endocrinology. These developments indicate a promising approach to treating migraine, with the need for further investigation and clinical trials to establish efficacy and safety. Eventually, once these new treatments gain momentum, they can potentially improve the well-being of millions of people who suffer from migraines (Pellesi et al., 2024).

1.6.1. Hormone Replacement Therapy

Hormone Replacement Therapy (HRT) is a critical intervention within the field of endocrinology and has been used primarily to reverse the effects of hormonal deficiencies in patients, particularly menopause in females and andropause in males. Over time, the estrogen and testosterone levels drop, and the patient may develop a variety of disabling symptoms such as hot flashes, mood swings, and decreased libido. HRT not only alleviates such symptoms but also prevents long-term complications of hormonal deficiency, including osteoporosis and cardiovascular disease. HRT can significantly enhance quality of life and overall well-being by restoring hormonal balance. It is therefore crucial to have a good understanding of the mechanism and impact of HRT for healthcare practitioners managing patients experiencing hormonal changes. While HRT has been found to be advantageous, it has risks and controversies as well. Contemporary literature has triggered concerns regarding the long-term consequences of hormone replacement, linking it with increased risks of certain conditions, including breast cancer and thromboembolic events. Starting HRT must involve balancing individual risk factors and the overall condition of the patient. Current practice guidelines support individualized approaches to HRT, emphasizing ongoing follow-up and re-evaluation of therapy according to new evidence. Moreover, patients are encouraged to participate in the shared decision-making process to enable balancing possible benefits against likely risks. The collaborative process is crucial to optimizing therapeutic benefit and reconciling therapy with patient preferences. The employment of HRT to manage adrenal incidentalomas is also representative of the complexity of endocrine therapies. Adrenal incidentalomas, usually nonfunctioning tumors incidentally discovered on imaging, can rarely possess autonomous cortisol secretion and therefore share symptoms with Cushing's syndrome. In such cases, determining the appropriateness of HRT is extremely challenging. Recent guidelines suggest that assessing cortisol levels is essential to determine whether surgical resection or hormonal therapy is indicated. Clinicians must be able to differentiate between benign and possibly malignant adrenal pathology, so that planning for management is according to the given patient conditions. The complicated interrelation of adrenal and systemic levels of hormones also conveys the importance of an interdisciplinary approach to endocrinology that considers information on HRT and adrenal status for optimal patient management (Fa Mßnacht et al., 2016; Webber et al., 2016) (Figure 1.13).

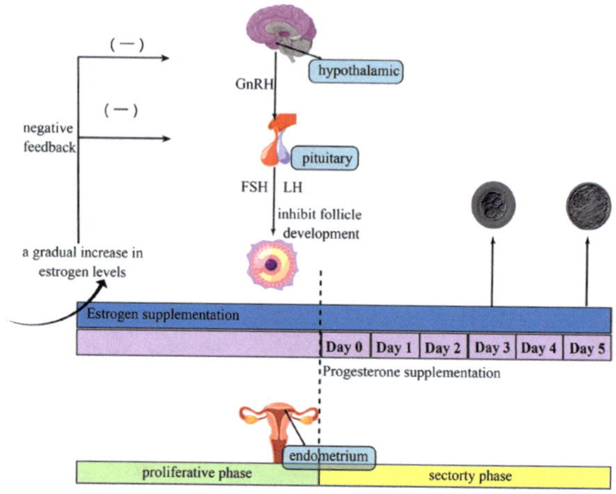

Figure 1.13. Hormone replacement therapy protocol in frozen embryo transfer (FET).

Source: https://www.researchgate.net/publication/380822832/figure/fig1/AS:11431281299801070@1735113607456/Hormone-replacement-therapy-protocol-in-FET.jpg.

1.6.2. Medications for Managing Endocrine Disorders

Effective management of endocrine diseases often involves the use of drugs since the body regulation of hormones in the human body is intricate. Drugs used in endocrinology can be broadly categorized based on their indications, such as corticosteroids for adrenal insufficiency, thyroid hormone replacement for hypothyroidism, and insulin therapy for diabetes mellitus. The selection of an appropriate drug is not merely dependent on the specific endocrine condition, but also on patient factors, including age, the presence of other disease conditions, and preferences for the route of administration. Additionally, improvement in drug delivery systems, including long-acting insulin and combination products, is designed to enhance patient compliance and minimize side effects. It is essential that health professionals have a thorough understanding of these pharmacological options because that has a direct impact on treatment efficacy and patient quality of life regarding endocrinology. In addition to the conventional drugs, more focus has been placed on changes in lifestyle and adjunct treatments that could be combined with pharmacologic therapy in endocrine disorders. For instance, diet and physical exercise lifestyle changes are essential factors in managing type 2 diabetes and endocrine disorders resulting from obesity. Proper nutrition with whole foods and reduced consumption of processed carbohydrates has been established to improve glycemic control and overall health outcomes among patients suffering from hormonal imbalance. Besides, patient education on the significance of self-monitoring blood glucose and taking medication can empower the patient to take a proactive role in his/her treatment plan. In developing effective management strategies, integrating these non-pharmacological practices is given priority in achieving long-term remission and reducing complications associated with endocrine disorders. The resulting interdependence between endocrine disorders and associated comorbidities further deepens this pharmacological context. For example, diabetic patients have associated conditions such as hypertension and dyslipidemia that necessitate the use of combination drugs. The challenge is how to maximize these combinations without inducing drug interactions while not compromising on the therapeutic benefit. Current evidence indicates that certain endocrine illnesses, like hypothyroidism or GH deficiency, may occur together with genetic syndromes and influence the choice of medication and increase postoperative complications risk (Gökberk et al., 2024). Besides, healthcare providers should be careful regarding the psychological aspects of the management of endocrine illnesses. Vulnerable populations such as people with type 1 diabetes usually have greater numbers of eating disorders, which complicate their treatment even further (Felicino et al., 2024). A proper understanding of pharmacological and psychosocial features is thus necessary for providing effective care in endocrinology.

1.6.3. Surgical Interventions in Endocrinology

Surgical interventions in endocrinology are of vital significance in treating numerous endocrine disorders, particularly those concerning hormone-secreting glands such as the thyroid, adrenal, and pituitary glands. Surgical interventions are mostly employed once a malignancy, excess secretion of hormones, or anatomical abnormalities in need of correction are identified. Thyroidectomy, for instance, is among the most prevalent surgical interventions used to treat thyroid cancers or hyperthyroidism where conservative management is ineffective. These treatments not only help alleviate symptoms and restore hormone levels to normal but also significantly enhance patients' quality of life. Surgical approaches must be tailored individually, with consideration for the patients' overall health, disease severity, and specific gland affected, demonstrating the complicated decision-making process inherent in endocrine surgery. Advances in surgical techniques and technology, such as minimally invasive surgery, have revolutionized the practice of endocrine surgery. These methods have kept recovery times to a minimum, decreased postoperative complications, and improved cosmetic outcomes. Endoscopic surgery, for example, allows surgeons to access and remove endocrine tumors through small cuts, causing less trauma to the surrounding tissues. Moreover, intraoperative instrumentation such as ultrasound and nerve monitoring improves the precision of operations, particularly in delicate areas such as the neck in thyroid surgery. Yet despite all of these innovations, the complexity and heterogeneity of endocrine disorders require a multidisciplinary team with not only surgeons but also endocrinologists and allied healthcare workers to optimize patient outcomes. Surgery is the key to treating diseases such as Cushing's syndrome and pheochromocytoma, which are often related to disorders of the adrenal gland. In Cushing's syndrome, the primary aim is excision of the adenoma causing excess cortisol production since it can lead to serious systemic complications. Pheochromocytoma must also be surgically excised to remove the catecholamine-secreting tumor that can lead to lethal hypertension. Surgical intervention not only becomes essential to treat these conditions but also the concomitant metabolic disturbances that follow because of excessive overproduction of the hormone over a prolonged period. With advancements in the science of endocrinology, it has become imperative to establish preoperative evaluation and postoperative care protocols as essential for ensuring the effectiveness of surgical interventions and enhancing patient safety (Cho et al., 2023; Nugent et al., 2024) (Figure 1.14).

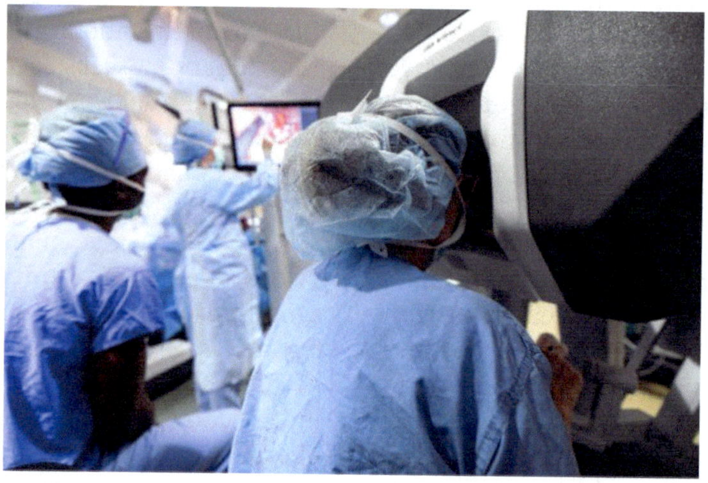

Figure 1.14. Surgical interventions in endocrinology play a pivotal role in managing various endocrine disorders.

Source: https://www.mayoclinic.org/-/media/kcms/gbs/patient-consumer/images/2025/04/10/15/50/surgeons_at_robotic_console_8-col.jpg.

Test Your Knowledge

1. What is the goal of hormone replacement therapy (HRT), and which two endocrine disorders commonly require it?
2. When might surgical removal of an endocrine gland be necessary, and name one example?

SUMMARY

In synthesizing the field of endocrinology, it is necessary to affirm the significance of educational outreach programs for enhancing public awareness and understanding of endocrine-related health issues. The implementation of targeted initiatives, i.e., the school outreach program among lower socioeconomic students, demonstrates considerable potential for health promotion in terms of conditions such as obesity, diabetes, and polycystic ovary syndrome. This course emphasized the importance of engagement strategies to reach populations of varying backgrounds, providing students with the scaffold to grasp complex medical topics. The increase in student interest in medical careers, although not statistically significant, is an encouraging trend and shows that well-designed educational initiatives can inspire future generations of healthcare professionals. The positive reaction to activities proves that interactive learning can enhance comprehension and possibly bridge health gaps in the long term (Baig et al., 2024). Additionally, the insights derived from pediatric endocrinology analysis reiterate the need to implement stringent guidelines in medical practice so that medical imaging, particularly MRI scans, is responsibly utilized. The figures provided demonstrated that a significant proportion of such scans were found to be unnecessary, 67% having normal findings. This is an important finding concerning the effectiveness and appropriateness of available diagnostic tests in pediatric endocrinology. By adopting more robust guidelines, the medical profession can help reduce the economic strain on health systems, as well as alleviate physical and emotional distress for individuals and families. The emphasis now has to be on optimizing diagnostic planning to minimize imaging done solely when clinically indicated in order to optimize patient care and utilization of resources (Marin et al., 2024). Finally, as endocrinology advances with development, future research must be set on maximizing outreach programs and optimizing clinical procedures to maximize patient outcomes. Such research can involve longitudinal research to quantify the long-term effect of education intervention on student objectives in the medical field. In addition, research on factors associated with the prevalence of incidental findings in pediatric MRI will be crucial in creating targeted initiatives for minimizing unwanted medical interventions. Through facilitating collaboration between schools of medicine and healthcare providers, we can advance the understanding of endocrinology further, finally leading to increased health literacy and better patient care efficiency. The marriage of education and clinical practice will remain a key to navigating the challenges of the endocrine system and associated diseases (Baig et al., 2024; Marin et al., 2024).

In the enormous domain of endocrinology, understanding intricate systems of hormonal control is essential to understanding many of the body's physiological processes. The function of hormones as biochemical messengers, controlling all manner of body functions, including metabolism, growth, and reproduction, cannot be overemphasized. Of particular interest in the discipline is the interaction of hormones and states of disease, most specifically in regard to the role of hormonal imbalance in diseases such as diabetes, obesity, and cardiovascular disease. The relationship between disruptions in endocrinology and overall systemic health highlights the importance of ongoing investigation aimed at elucidating these complex associations, demonstrating that optimal management of hormonal health can have a profound impact on overall well-being. As practitioners start to assess individual therapies for hormonal dysregulation, the development of integrated knowledge of hormonal pathways remains imperative to advancing medical treatment and improving patient outcomes. The study of stem cell application in endocrinology also highlights important developments in regenerative medicine. Developments recently achieved emphasize the use of various types of stem cells to correct endocrine deficiencies and restore hormonal balance. For instance, research has proved that some progenitor cells can regenerate insulin-producing beta cells in type 1 diabetes, a promising avenue in the treatment of this chronic condition. In addition, the complementary application of various stem cell types offers a novel strategy for depathologizing chronic endocrine disease and constructing individualized therapy regimens. Various aspects still need to be settled, including the best method of delivering stem cells and standardizing treatment protocols, but the therapeutic potential for applying preclinical research to clinical medicine remains a source of enthusiasm for the endocrinology community, enabling new paradigms of treatment (Kyryk, 2024). Quantitative summaries have also been an essential resource for summarizing important results in endocrinology research, offering deeper insights into complex data. Key Point Analysis (KPA) and other techniques are applied to pull major information from ample amounts of literature into rapid summaries that guide follow-up research. These summary tools leverage supervised learning as well as emerging technologies like aspects of sentiment analysis to pull and quantify key results. Since endocrinologists want to keep pace with inter-professional research that informs practice, effective summarization strategies help distill the content of research into actionable knowledge. Therefore, as methods continue to evolve, the application of such analytical tools in endocrinology could reveal the underappreciated interface between hormonal well-being and specific pathologies, resulting in a holistic approach to patient care (Tang et al., 2024).

KEY TERMS FROM THIS CHAPTER

- Endocrinology
- Endocrine disruptors
- Endocrine imbalance
- Endocrine regulation
- Adrenal insufficiency
- Blood glucose levels
- Chemical messengers
- Disorders of sex development (DSDs)
- Extracellular fluids
- GnRH provocation test
- Homeostasis
- Hormonal imbalances
- Hormone synthesis
- Hypothyroidism
- Endocrine disease
- Endocrine function
- Endocrine production
- Addison's disease
- Biochemical signals
- Calcium homeostasis
- Clinical assessments,
- Drug discovery
- Extracellular vesicles (EVs)
- Gum formation
- Hormonal disease
- Hormonal regulation
- Hyperthyroidism
- Metabolic disease

CRITICAL THINKING QUESTIONS

1. **The discovery of insulin as a hormone was made by which scientists?**
   a. Banting and Best
   b. Starling and Bayliss
   c. Watson and Crick
   d. Pavlov and Cannon
2. **Which gland is referred to as the "master gland" of the endocrine system?**
   a. Thyroid
   b. Pituitary
   c. Adrenal
   d. Pineal
3. **Which hormone is responsible for regulating metabolism?**
   a. Oxytocin
   b. Thyroxine (T4)
   c. Prolactin
   d. Aldosterone
4. **Which diagnostic test is commonly used to assess thyroid function?**
   a. Fasting blood glucose
   b. MRI scan
   c. TSH (Thyroid Stimulating Hormone) test
   d. ECG
5. **Which class of drugs is used to treat adrenal insufficiency?**
   a. Beta-blockers
   b. Antithyroid drugs
   c. Insulin
   d. Corticosteroids

Short Answer Questions

1. Name any three major endocrine glands and one hormone produced by each.
2. Differentiate between peptide, steroid, and amine hormones in terms of structure and receptor location.
3. Which diagnostic test is commonly used to evaluate thyroid function, and what does a high TSH level typically indicate?
4. How does imaging such as MRI assist in diagnosing pituitary gland disorders?
5. What is hormone replacement therapy (HRT), and for which two conditions is it most commonly used?
6. Why is it important to consider patient history and symptoms in diagnosing endocrine disorders? Provide one example.

Answers to Critical Thinking Questions

1. (a); 2. (b); 3. (b); 4. (c); 5. (d)

REFERENCES

1. Areta, J. L., Taylor, H. L., & Koehler, K. (2020). Low energy availability: History, definition and evidence of its endocrine, metabolic and physiological effects in prospective studies in females and males. *European Journal of Applied Physiology, 121*, 1–21. https://doi.org/10.1007/s00421-020-04516-0 (accessed on 22nd July 2025).
2. Azhar, S., Dong, D., Shen, W., Hu, Z., & Kraemer, F. (2020). The role of miRNAs in regulating adrenal/gonadal steroidogenesis. *Journal of Molecular Endocrinology*. https://www.semanticscholar.org/paper/fc8e35f9892d8e2e589781fe29f2600789fa6b3c (accessed on 22nd July 2025).
3. Bagatska, N. (2024). Determination of predictive factors in families of girls with menstrual disorders comorbid with endocrine system pathology. *Ukrainian Journal of Pediatric Endocrinology*. https://www.semanticscholar.org/paper/530488e0f02e11b5be200bc486b1509f5076582b (accessed on 22nd July 2025).
4. Baig, S. A., Malhotra, K., Kowsik, M., Banerjee, J., Rahman, F., Ashokkumar, A., Gillett, C., et al. (2024). Findings from a public engagement programmed for school children aged 13–15 years about endocrinology. *Endocrine Connections, 13*. https://www.semanticscholar.org/paper/d724fe2ce719a5d17805999eb3dbccabf21b336a (accessed on 22nd July 2025).
5. Bashshur, R. L., Doarn, C. R., Frenk, J., Kvedar, J. C., & Woolliscroft, J. O. (2020). Telemedicine and the COVID-19 pandemic: Lessons for the future. *Telemedicine Journal and e-Health, 26*, 571–573. https://doi.org/10.1089/tmj.2020.29040.rb (accessed on 22nd July 2025).
6. Basu, R., Qian, Y., & Kopchick, J. (2018). Mechanisms in endocrinology: Lessons from growth hormone receptor gene-disrupted mice: Are there benefits of endocrine defects? *European Journal of Endocrinology, 178*(5), R155–R181. https://www.semanticscholar.org/paper/c7e785b00694039725c50dc0b265138f6b585b61 (accessed on 22nd July 2025).
7. Bédécarrats, G., Hanlon, C., & Tsutsui, K. (2022). Gonadotropin inhibitory hormone and its receptor: Potential key to the integration and coordination of metabolic status and reproduction. *Frontiers in Endocrinology, 12*. https://www.semanticscholar.org/paper/03ce167c7d44830456831fe7eb084684ae4d4f28 (accessed on 22nd July 2025).
8. Bhattacharya, S., Sahay, R., Afsana, F., Sheikh, A., Widanage, N. M., Maskey, R., Naseri, M., et al. (2024). Global warming and endocrinology: The Hyderabad Declaration of the South Asian Federation of Endocrine Societies. *Indian Journal of Endocrinology and Metabolism, 28*, 129–136. https://www.semanticscholar.org/paper/6573769355a99ebeacca51f576e992f0d9acdf73 (accessed on 22nd July 2025).
9. Bribiescas, R. G. (2020). Evolutionary and life history insights into masculinity and warfare. *Current Anthropology, 62*, S38–S53. https://doi.org/10.1086/711688 (accessed on 22nd July 2025).
10. Buzdin, A., Zolotovskaia, M. A., Roumiantsev, S. A., Emelyanova, A. G., Golounina, O. O., Pugacheva, P., Luppov, D. V., et al. (2025). EndoGene database: Reported genetic variants for 5,926 Russian patients diagnosed with endocrine disorders. *Frontiers in Endocrinology, 16*. https://www.semanticscholar.org/paper/687475039e97b742729bc141dd942fef048143bd (accessed on 22nd July 2025).

11. Carracedo-Reboredo, P., Liñares-Blanco, J., Rodríguez-Fernández, N., Cedrón, F., Nóvoa, F. J., Carballal, A., Maojo, V., et al. (2021). A review on machine learning approaches and trends in drug discovery. *Computational and Structural Biotechnology Journal, 19*, 4538–4558. https://doi.org/10.1016/j.csbj.2021.08.011 (accessed on 22nd July 2025).

12. Çavuşoğlu, G., Boynuyoğun, E., Erek, N., Çalış, M., Canoruç Emet, D., Gönç, N., Özön, A., et al. (2024). Impact of endocrine disorders associated with cleft lip and palate. *The Turkish Journal of Pediatrics, 66*(6), 703–712. https://www.semanticscholar.org/paper/f0d8aeb0a14ae616db12e023d0aff1d340d52e9c (accessed on 22nd July 2025).

13. Chalasani, N., Younossi, Z. M., Lavine, J. E., Charlton, M., Cusi, K., Rinella, M. E., Harrison, S. A., et al. (2017). The diagnosis and management of nonalcoholic fatty liver disease: Practice guidance from the American Association for the Study of Liver Diseases. *Hepatology, 67*, 328–357. https://doi.org/10.1002/hep.29367 (accessed on 22nd July 2025).

14. Cho, Y., Choi, J. W., Kwon, H., Kim, K., Lee, B. C., Chu, H., Lee, D. H., et al. (2023). Transarterial chemoembolization for hepatocellular carcinoma: 2023 expert consensus-based practical recommendations of the Korean Liver Cancer Association. *Clinical and Molecular Hepatology, 29*, 521–541. https://www.semanticscholar.org/paper/ae207281a620305a959258c5a69889b45ba6bc78 (accessed on 22nd July 2025).

15. Creasy, R. K., & Resnik, R. (2020). *Maternal-Fetal Medicine*. American Academy of Pediatrics eBooks. https://doi.org/10.1542/9781610023993-2-ch27 (accessed on 22nd July 2025).

16. Cryan, J. F., O'Riordan, K. J., Cowan, C. S. M., Sandhu, K. V., Bastiaanssen, T. F. S., Boehme, M., Codagnone, M. G., et al. (2019). The microbiota-gut-brain axis. *Physiological Reviews, 99*, 1877–2013. https://doi.org/10.1152/physrev.00018.2018 (accessed on 22nd July 2025).

17. Csaba, G. (2016). The immunoendocrine thymus as a pacemaker of lifespan. https://core.ac.uk/download/42947412.pdf (accessed on 22nd July 2025).

18. Drakopoulos, P. (2025). Balancing hormonal symphony: The dynamics of reproduction and pregnancy. *BMC Endocrine Disorders, 25*. https://www.semanticscholar.org/paper/e2d2f9db21e4e1c6353c8c6a09694a60a58af23b (accessed on 22nd July 2025).

19. Eknoyan, G. (2004). Emergence of the concept of endocrine function and endocrinology. *Advances in Chronic Kidney Disease, 11*(4), 371–376. https://www.semanticscholar.org/paper/8cd9d72432c86d73ba9700b7cf84a4f990ce1411 (accessed on 22nd July 2025).

20. Faßnacht, M., Arlt, W., Bancos, I., Dralle, H., Newell-Price, J., Sahdev, A., Tabarin, A., et al. (2016). Management of adrenal incidentalomas: European Society of Endocrinology Clinical Practice Guideline in collaboration with the European Network for the Study of Adrenal Tumors. *European Journal of Endocrinology, 175*, G1–G34. https://doi.org/10.1530/eje-16-0467 (accessed on 22nd July 2025).

21. Gorgel, A., Gorgel, S. N., Demirpençe, M., & Bahçeci, M. (2020). A rare combination: Multiple endocrine neoplasia type 1 and follicular thyroid carcinoma. *The Turkish Journal of Endocrinology and Metabolism*. https://www.semanticscholar.org/paper/ec8acd0ffccbf81254d62c23900b529e6221c86e (accessed on 22nd July 2025).

22. Hanna, R. M., Ahdoot, R. S., Kalantar-Zadeh, K., Ghobry, L. M., & Kurtz, I. (2022). Calcium transport in the kidney and disease processes. *Frontiers in Endocrinology, 12*. https://www.semanticscholar.org/paper/3493aca3fe60dd60c9010d7a3308060361b3c109 (accessed on 22nd July 2025).

23. Hong, N., Park, H., & Rhee, Y. (2020). Machine learning applications in endocrinology and metabolism research: An overview. *Endocrinology and Metabolism, 35*, 71–84. https://doi.org/10.3803/enm.2020.35.1.71 (accessed on 22nd July 2025).

24. Jayasena, C., Anderson, R. A., Llahana, S., Barth, J. H., MacKenzie, F., Wilkes, S., Smith, N., et al. (2021). Society for Endocrinology guidelines for testosterone replacement therapy in male hypogonadism. *Clinical Endocrinology, 96*, 200–219. https://doi.org/10.1111/cen.14633 (accessed on 22nd July 2025).

25. Khalid, W., Maqbool, Z., Arshad, M., Kousar, S., Akram, R., Siddeeg, A., Ali, A., et al. (2022). Plant-derived functional components: Prevent from various disorders by regulating the endocrine glands. *International Journal of Food Properties, 25*, 976–995. https://www.semanticscholar.org/paper/769c88835b2a76b307e292586322e6305f8e1622 (accessed on 22nd July 2025).

26. Kim, J. H., & Choi, J. H. (2023). Applications of genomic research in pediatric endocrine diseases. *Clinical and Experimental Pediatrics, 66*, 520–530. https://www.semanticscholar.org/paper/94796a644990f10045dbf3a22510186da1033689 (accessed on 22nd July 2025).

27. Krueger, N., Alfar, H., Shaka, A., Seares, M. J., Lanka, L., & Shaka, H. (2024). 9374 Gender disparities in endocrinology and metabolism-related readmissions following COVID-19 hospitalization. *Journal of the Endocrine Society, 8*. https://www.semanticscholar.org/paper/76af092659dc48ef34020d220623e115ee8ae5b4 (accessed on 22nd July 2025).

28. Kyryk, V. (2024). Stem cell therapy for cardiac regeneration: Key points. *Cell and Organ Transplantology*. https://www.semanticscholar.org/paper/6a1b536f3691ad0d162e4187a4a2e2ffd1507b5f (accessed on 22nd July 2025).

29. Lee, P. A., Nordenström, A., Houk, C. P., Ahmed, S. F., Auchus, R. J., Baratz, A. B., Dalke, K. B., et al. (2016). Global disorders of sex development update since 2006: Perceptions, approach and care. *Hormone Research in Pediatrics, 85*, 158–180. https://doi.org/10.1159/000442975 (accessed on 22nd July 2025).

30. Levine, J. (2002). Editorial: Stressing the importance of sex. *Endocrinology, 143*(12), 4502–4504. https://www.semanticscholar.org/paper/31e5d92acd0a24bdd5896a7665de6697c7e876f7 (accessed on 22nd July 2025).

31. Li, Z., & Robaire, B. (2025). Effects of endocrine-disrupting chemicals on adrenal function. *Endocrinology, 166*. https://www.semanticscholar.org/paper/b6d42a0487f515be3698aa7b6eb21c7542778c44 (accessed on 22nd July 2025).

32. Lustig, R., & Fennoy, I. (2022). The history of obesity research. *Hormone Research in Pediatrics, 95*, 638–648. https://www.semanticscholar.org/paper/08416b356f88178333c12a0b8338431929c82b65 (accessed on 22nd July 2025).

33. Marin, M., Murru, F., Baldo, F., Tamaro, G., Faleschini, E., Barbi, E., & Tornese, G. (2024). Minimizing unnecessary brain magnetic resonance imaging in pediatric endocrinology: A retrospective cohort analysis. *Frontiers in Endocrinology, 15*. https://www.semanticscholar.org/paper/2bd9c8a3c916adab2458283e70dd9734d59dc6c9 (accessed on 22nd July 2025).

34. Mazzaferro, S., & Pasquali, M. (2015). Vitamin D: A dynamic molecule. How relevant might the dynamism for a vitamin be. https://core.ac.uk/download/74320782.pdf (accessed on 22nd July 2025).

35. McCarty, R. (2020). *Evolution of the Stress Concept.* Oxford University Press eBooks. https://doi.org/10.1093/med-psych/9780190697266.003.0003 (accessed on 22nd July 2025).

36. Miller, W. L., & White, P. C. (2022). History of adrenal research: From ancient anatomy to contemporary molecular biology. *Endocrine Reviews, 44*, 70–116. https://doi.org/10.1210/endrev/bnac019 (accessed on 22nd July 2025).

37. Misiorowski, W., Dedecjus, M., Konstantynowicz, J., Zygmunt, A., Kos-Kudła, B., Lewiński, A., Ruchała, M., et al. (2023). Management of hypoparathyroidism: A position statement of the expert group of the Polish Society of Endocrinology. *Endocrinologic Polska, 74*(5), 447–467. https://www.semanticscholar.org/paper/aeee157562f0abd02e9c7de75c7b93d4ef25ce18 (accessed on 22nd July 2025).

38. Nam, G. (2025). Clinical and preclinical obesity: Cardiovascular implications of a new diagnostic paradigm. *Cardiovascular Prevention and Pharmacotherapy*. https://www.semanticscholar.org/paper/cc20ee8616f8b28449b757213d557301ae82c897 (accessed on 22nd July 2025).

39. Nugent, Z., Paice, E., Jensen, A., & Peffers, M. J. (2024). Equine odontoclastic tooth resorption and hypercementosis. *UK-Vet Equine*. https://www.semanticscholar.org/paper/ce2e8257bf95e08cfb2fce02cf5f41722dc3c5ae (accessed on 22nd July 2025).

40. O'Brien, J. A., Hayder, H., Zayed, Y., & Peng, C. (2018). Overview of microRNA biogenesis, mechanisms of actions, and circulation. *Frontiers in Endocrinology, 9*. https://doi.org/10.3389/fendo.2018.00402 (accessed on 22nd July 2025).

41. Pandey, A. (2024). The interplay between dentistry and endocrinology: Implications, innovations, and future directions. *Endocrinology and Disorders*. https://www.semanticscholar.org/paper/6d62065108684b6cf48e95d24366d6bb044d133f (accessed on 22nd July 2025).

42. Pellesi, L., Do, T. P., & Hougaard, A. (2024). Pharmacological management of migraine: Current strategies and future directions. *Expert Opinion on Pharmacotherapy, 25*, 673–683. https://www.semanticscholar.org/paper/b2f855b018f7aa7b415a48b1b26cfa12fcbc178f (accessed on 22nd July 2025).

43. Pulatova, D. (2024). Impact of gut microbiota on the gut-brain axis in neurological disorders and the role of endocrine and metabolic markers. *The American Journal of Medical Sciences and Pharmaceutical Research*. https://www.semanticscholar.org/paper/b9cc616d6f2a1fac46e0d06096f38210ac107a5e (accessed on 22nd July 2025).

44. Rinella, M. E., Lazarus, J. V., Ratziu, V., Francque, S., Sanyal, A. J., Kanwal, F., Romero, D., et al. (2023). A multisociety Delphi consensus statement on new fatty liver disease nomenclature. *Journal of Hepatology, 79*, 1542–1556. https://doi.org/10.1016/j.jhep.2023.06.003 (accessed on 22nd July 2025).

45. Rinella, M. E., Neuschwander-Tetri, B. A., Siddiqui, M. S., Abdelmalek, M. F., Caldwell, S. H., Barb, D., Kleiner, D. E., et al. (2023). AASLD practice guidance on the clinical assessment and management of nonalcoholic fatty liver disease. *Hepatology, 77*, 1797–1835. https://doi.org/10.1097/hep.0000000000000323 (accessed on 22nd July 2025).

46. Rodrigues, F. S., Silva, C. C., Da Silva, W., Caldas, T. M., & Rocha, L. K. (2024). 6705 Sheehan syndrome: A case report. *Journal of the Endocrine Society, 8*. https://www.semanticscholar.org/paper/64d605d4c65aa1e4e7eb356982d8504f5c8d3169 (accessed on 22nd July 2025).

47. Rotwein, P. (2015). Editorial: Is it time for an evolutionarily based human endocrinology? *Molecular Endocrinology, 29*(4), 487–489. https://www.semanticscholar.org/paper/d08b56257e40e3b8f08ebf6c3818e420283435ba (accessed on 22nd July 2025).

48. Sahi, I. S., Hasan, I. J., & Zamil, A. L. (2025). Association between vitamin D levels and thyroid status; diagnostic insights into hyperthyroidism and hypothyroidism–A cross-sectional diagnostic study. *Journal of Parathyroid Disease*. https://www.semanticscholar.org/paper/ab711dd3e70e1c11b8a4fe38e0d5d9cd7364c3a5 (accessed on 22nd July 2025).

49. Shestakova, M. (2025). A century history of Russia's first Endocrinological Research Centre (to the 100th anniversary of the Endocrinology Research Centre). *Annals of the Russian Academy of Medical Sciences*. https://www.semanticscholar.org/paper/c47f2cc7309f09fcf91ea2ed4aeb70407699d798 (accessed on 22nd July 2025).

50. Silva, Y. P., Bernardi, A., & Frozza, R. L. (2020). The role of short-chain fatty acids from gut microbiota in gut-brain communication. *Frontiers in Endocrinology, 11*. https://doi.org/10.3389/fendo.2020.00025 (accessed on 22nd July 2025).

51. Stevenson, T. J., Hanson, H., & Martin, L. B. (2020). Theory, hormones and life history stages: An introduction to the symposium epigenetic variation in endocrine systems. *Integrative and Comparative Biology, 60*(6), 1454–1457. https://www.semanticscholar.org/paper/dc662310f067f933bdc46bdc7e4f8f17694abd90 (accessed on 22nd July 2025).

52. Stratakis, C., Jenkins, R., Pras, E., Mitsiadis, C. S., Raff, S., Stalboerger, P., Tsigos, C., et al. (1996). Cytogenetic and microsatellite alterations in tumors from patients with the syndrome of myxomas, spotty skin pigmentation, and endocrine overactivity (Carney complex). *The Journal of Clinical Endocrinology and Metabolism, 81*(10), 3607–3614. https://www.semanticscholar.org/paper/5f5a53587c1ff6ff3141558d2900db4ceaaed4b5 (accessed on 22nd July 2025).

53. Tang, A., Zhang, X., Dinh, M., & Cambria, E. (2024). Prompted aspect key point analysis for quantitative review summarization. *ArXiv, abs/2407.14049*. https://www.semanticscholar.org/paper/ed73a37eb5200c4864e622947c4299886cdfe7a1 (accessed on 22nd July 2025).

54. Teede, H., Tay, C. T., Laven, J. J. E., Dokras, A., Moran, L., Piltonen, T., Costello, M., et al. (2023). Recommendations from the 2023 international evidence-based guideline for the assessment and management of polycystic ovary syndrome. *The Journal of Clinical Endocrinology & Metabolism, 108*, 2447–2469. https://doi.org/10.1210/clinem/dgad463 (accessed on 22nd July 2025).

55. Viera Felicino, N., & Lam, D. (2024). 6482 Knowledge and comfort in addressing eating disorders in people living with Type 1 Diabetes in an academic endocrinology center. *Journal of the Endocrine Society, 8*. https://www.semanticscholar.org/paper/edac0448a3a7ed4ca1e7a0fd3e3d75fcd6a36ad9 (accessed on 22nd July 2025).

56. Webber, L., Davies, M., Anderson, R. A., Bartlett, J. R., Braat, D., Cartwright, B., Cífková, R., et al. (2016). ESHRE guideline: Management of women with premature ovarian insufficiency. *Human Reproduction, 31*, 926–937. https://doi.org/10.1093/humrep/dew027 (accessed on 22nd July 2025).

57. Wells, S. A., Sylvia, L., Dralle, H., Elisei, R., Evans, D. B., Gagel, R. F., Lee, N. Y., et al. (2015). Revised American Thyroid Association guidelines for the management of medullary thyroid carcinoma. *Thyroid, 25*, 567–610. https://doi.org/10.1089/thy.2014.0335 (accessed on 22nd July 2025).

58. Welsh, J. A., Goberdhan, D. C. I., O'Driscoll, L., Buzás, E. I., Blenkiron, C., Bussolati, B., Cai, H., et al. (2024). Minimal information for studies of extracellular vesicles (MISEV2023): From basic to advanced approaches. *Journal of Extracellular Vesicles, 13*. https://doi.org/10.1002/jev2.12404 (accessed on 22nd July 2025).

59. Wintermyer, G., & Gillis-Funderburk, S. (2024). 6370 New-onset autoimmune diabetes following COVID-19 infection and its implications for identical twin siblings. *Journal of the Endocrine Society, 8*. https://www.semanticscholar.org/paper/d5ba8f6d1cec643131b271bdd959c6d19b8a6dab (accessed on 22nd July 2025).

60. Wong, L., & McMahon, L. (2023). Crosstalk between bone and muscle in chronic kidney disease. *Frontiers in Endocrinology, 14*. https://www.semanticscholar.org/paper/903e6dfbafce01f59f686b0ae92cf018895a2d48 (accessed on 22nd July 2025).

61. Yankina, S. V., Minaeva, N. V., Obereshin, V., & Bolobonkina, T. (2025). Emergencies in endocrinology in the pre-hospital period: From the experience of emergency medical teams in Ryazan in 2018–2023. *Disaster Medicine*. https://www.semanticscholar.org/paper/b9ef345815b32356a2ddb1adaa67077bd10eb9dc (accessed on 22nd July 2025).

62. Zhang, F., Wang, W., Nie, Y., Li, J., & He, X. X. (2023). From microbial technology to microbiota medicine as a clinical discipline: Sustainable development goal. *Microbial Biotechnology, 16*, 1705–1708. https://doi.org/10.1111/1751-7915.14317 (accessed on 22nd July 2025).

63. Zhang, H. R., Xiao, Y., Jiang, S. Q., Sun, J., Shi, W. H., Li, J. B., & Wang, W. (2025). Diagnostic value of fasting insulin and insulin-like growth factor-1 levels in girls with central precocious puberty. *Journal of Pediatric Endocrinology and Metabolism, 38*, 240–247. https://www.semanticscholar.org/paper/4b5f954388fbe624510eb6d6c8f6889e56904679 (accessed on 22nd July 2025).

HYPOTHALAMUS AND PITUITARY GLAND

2

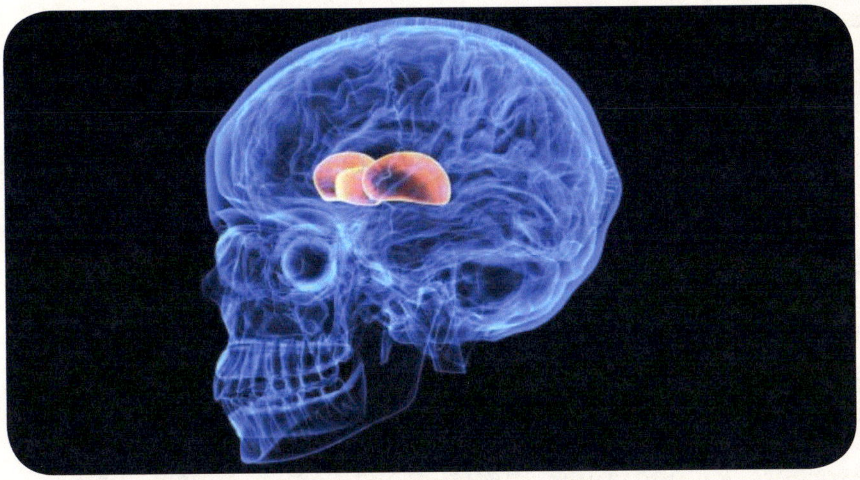

LEARNING OBJECTIVES

After studying this chapter, you will be able to:

1. Understand the anatomy and functions of hypothalamus;
2. Describe the anatomy and functions of pituitary gland;
3. Discuss the interaction between the hypothalamus and pituitary gland;
4. Explain disorders related to the hypothalamus and pituitary gland.

Introduction

The hypothalamus and pituitary gland play a role in maintaining homeostasis within the human body through an intricate network of signaling that integrates various endocrine as well as physiological functions. Located at the base of the brain, the hypothalamus serves as a master controller, integrating autonomic, endocrine, and behavioral responses to various stimuli. It releases inhibiting and releasing hormones, which control the activity of the anterior pituitary gland, releasing hormones that influence growth, metabolism, and reproduction. This interlocking system reveals the importance of the hypothalamus not only as a command center but also as an important player in the regulation of bodily function, dynamically responding to internal as well as external changes to keep the organism in balance. To realize how the hypothalamus and pituitary gland are essential, one must understand how they are involved in numerous physiological processes, such as stress response, temperature, and appetite. How these two function together is the best example of a meticulously fine-tuned feedback mechanism wherein the hypothalamus monitors hormone levels and physiological state and adjusts neuroendocrine output accordingly. For instance, when the body is stressed, the hypothalamus initiates the release of corticotropin-releasing hormone (CRH), which in turn stimulates the pituitary gland to secrete adrenocorticotropic hormone (ACTH), also affecting the activity of the adrenal glands. This process illustrates how the hypothalamus and the pituitary gland are essential mediators of the body's response to environmental stresses to sustain life and adaptability amidst changing environments. Moreover, the latest studies highlight the intricate interrelationship between the pituitary gland, hypothalamus, and other systems of the body, particularly in relation to neurodegenerative diseases and mental illness. Understanding the role played by these structures is crucial, as they not only influence bodily health but also impact mental well-being. The hypothalamic-pituitary-adrenal axis, for example, has been shown to be pivotal in anxiety and mood disorders, linking stress response with long-term health outcomes. With recent research investigating the complexity of the microbiota-gut-brain axis, the relationship between such endocrine hubs and other mental disorders becomes increasingly relevant, illustrating the intricate web of interconnection between our physical and psychological status (John et al., 2019). The potential implications of this research may lead to new therapies addressing the hypothalamus and pituitary, ranging from the treatment of metabolic syndrome to stress reactions (Peter et al., 2017).

Definition of the Hypothalamus

The hypothalamus, a compact yet critical region in the brain, plays a crucial role in promoting homeostasis throughout the body. It serves as a command center, processing inputs from numerous systems and carrying out responses that control the fundamental physiological processes, including temperature, hunger, thirst, and circadian rhythms. This cluster of nuclei, situated beneath the thalamus, is part of the diencephalon and has a vital association with the pituitary gland, forming a key link in endocrine signaling. Regulating the body's internal environment and reacting to changes, the hypothalamus keeps the body in homeostasis, which is essential for good health. Its function encompasses direct neural control and endocrine control, making it an integrative center for sensory input as well as a central player in hormonal homeostatic response that affects many bodily functions. Furthermore, the hypothalamus possesses a unique structural organization to enhance its diverse functions. Composed of multiple nuclei, each with designated functions, it regulates autonomic functions by affecting the sympathetic and parasympathetic nervous systems. The hypothalamic-pituitary axis is a prime example of such interaction since it itself controls the release of pituitary gland hormones and thus affects growth, metabolism, and reproduction. For instance, the release of CRH by the hypothalamus stimulates the pituitary to secrete ACTH, which goes on to stimulate the adrenal glands to release cortisol, one of the key stress hormones. This interaction not only showcases the regulatory capability of the hypothalamus but also emphasizes its role in responding to internal and external stressors, thus creating an onerous balance necessary for survival. In endocrine disorders, the role of the hypothalamus gains even more importance. Dysfunction in the regulation of the hypothalamus can lead to several clinical conditions like obesity, diabetes, and reproductive disorders. For instance, gonadotropin-releasing hormone (GnRH) secretion anomalies can disturb the hypothalamic-pituitary-gonadal axis and lead to menstrual and fertility abnormalities. The role of the hypothalamus in metabolic functions, including glucose regulation, demonstrates its general contribution to global health. It is essential to understand the intricacies of hypothalamic function and its interaction with the pituitary gland, enabling the development of therapeutic strategies for treating these endocrine disorders and, more importantly, advancing our overall knowledge of human biology, particularly in the domains of neuroendocrinology and metabolic health (Figure 2.1).

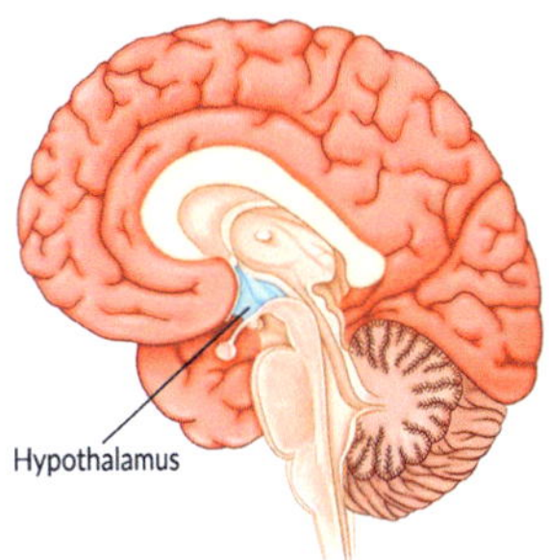

Figure 2.1. Illustration of hypothalamus.

Source: https://cdn.flintrehab.com/uploads/2020/03/hypothalamus-damage-1.png.

Definition of the Pituitary Gland

The pituitary gland, or master gland, plays a vital role in the endocrine system as it controls a variety of physiological processes. Located at the base of the brain, the pea-sized organ functions as a go-between between the hypothalamus and other endocrine glands in the remainder of the body. It accomplishes this by producing and secreting an array of hormones that influence growth, metabolism, and reproductive functions. The anterior pituitary releases hormones such as the growth hormone (GH), which is vital in normal growth and development, and ACTH, which stimulates the adrenal glands. The posterior pituitary, by contrast, is simply a storage and release site for hypothalamic hormones such as vasopressin and oxytocin. Overall, the coordination by the pituitary gland of hormonal messages underscores its central role in homeostasis and in facilitating communication between the endocrine system. Besides, there should be communication between the pituitary and hypothalamus to regulate body functions according to intrinsically and extrinsically originated stimuli. The hypothalamus releases hormones that regulate the activity of the pituitary gland, thus producing a feedback mechanism that is vital for homeostasis. This communication not only illustrates the complexity of endocrine signaling but also the impact that disturbances within this axis have on overall health. For instance, exposure to endocrine-disrupting chemicals can impair the hypothalamus-pituitary-adrenal (HPA) axis, resulting in adverse health outcomes such as metabolic syndrome or reproductive disease.

The regulation of this interaction highlights the significance of the pituitary gland, further solidifying its position as a central regulator in endocrine control. Later years have witnessed scientific exploration extend the function of the pituitary gland beyond the secretion of hormones. Recent studies indicate the impact of environmental stimuli on the pituitary gland, that is, the hypothalamic-pituitary-gonadal axis. For example, endocrinologists have gotten interested in knowing the impact of endocrine-disrupting chemicals on this vulnerable axis, which could lead to infertility or developmental issues (John et al., 2019). Moreover, the communication between gut microbiota and the endocrine system has given a new dimension to this research because microbial metabolites could control hormone production, thereby affecting the function of the pituitary (John et al., 2019). As science explores the interconnections of these structures, the understanding of the pituitary gland's definition and function becomes increasingly valuable, enabling the formulation of site-specific therapies for endocrine disorders and improving overall health outcomes (Figure 2.2).

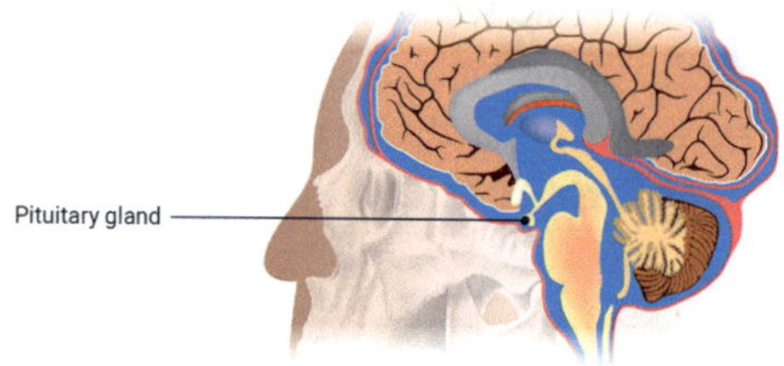

Figure 2.2. Pituitary gland.

Source: https://media.healthdirect.org.au/images/inline/original/pituitary-gland-5d0767.jpg.

Importance of the Hypothalamus and Pituitary Gland in the Endocrine System

Hypothalamus and the pituitary gland, both being prominent components of the endocrine system, play crucial roles in the regulation of various physiological processes and homeostasis. The hypothalamus, situated below the brain, acts as the primary connection between the endocrine and nervous systems. It releases hormones that stimulate or inhibit the release of pituitary hormones, thereby regulating functions such as body temperature, thirst, hunger, and sleep-wake patterns. The pituitary or master gland responds to the hypothalamic stimuli by secreting a cascade of hormones that affect growth, metabolism, reproduction, and responses to stress. The intricate coordination facilitates a coordinated response to internal and external stimuli, emphasizing the role of the hypothalamus and pituitary glands to sustain overall health and function of the endocrine system. In addition, the influence of the hypothalamus and pituitary gland carries over into the area of reproductive well-being, in which they play a role in controlling fertility. Abnormalities in the hypothalamic and pituitary activities may result in hormonal imbalances affecting reproductive function, which is increasingly being found in research on infertility. For instance, hypopituitarism or specific tumors that affect pituitary actions can disrupt the secretion of reproductive hormones normally, and this, in turn, can cause infertility in both men and women. The character of these conditions illustrates how endocrine disruptors of this axis can affect reproductive health because infertility affects millions of individuals globally and is often associated with endocrine disorders. Addressing these issues does not only encompass medical interventions but also public health interventions for improving fertility awareness and supporting affected individuals with infertility issues (N/A, 2021). Beyond the process of reproduction, the pituitary gland and hypothalamus are also involved in stress regulation and metabolism, highlighting their widespread influence on bodily functions. Hypothalamus releases CRH, which in turn stimulates the pituitary gland to release ACTH, which then stimulates the adrenal glands to release cortisol, a key stress hormone. This process is crucial for responding to stressors, ensuring that energy metabolism is regulated appropriately to meet increased demands. Further, these glands regulate metabolic hormones such as thyrotropin and GH, which have a core function in energy balance as well as in the growth of the body. Dysregulation in these hormones may result in several metabolic diseases, and thus, the role of the hypothalamic-pituitary axis cannot be overemphasized when it comes to metabolic health and homeostasis (John et al., 2019).

2.1. Anatomy of the Hypothalamus

Learning Outcome

1. Define the location of the hypothalamus within the brain;
2. Understand the structure and components of the hypothalamus;
3. Explain how the hypothalamus serves as a critical bridge connecting various brain regions.

The hypothalamus, tiny in size, is a key controller of many of the physiological processes required to deliver homeostasis to the body. Comprised of many groups of nuclei, the hypothalamus coordinates the nervous and endocrine systems with one another, indicative of its integrative function. In feedback and feedforward regulation, it is intimately associated with the pituitary gland, controlling hormonal regulation of growth, metabolism, and stress responses. In addition, the hypothalamus is most important in the maintenance of circadian rhythms, which govern many of the body's processes throughout the day. Such complex interactions among hypothalamic nuclei render this structure essential in coordinating the body's response to external stimuli, leading one to consider it the central coordinator of neuroendocrine functions. Anatomically, the hypothalamus is comprised of a number of discrete nuclei, each possessing unique regulatory functions. These nuclei, e.g., the suprachiasmatic nucleus, play a part in circadian regulation, while others, like the arcuate and ventromedial nuclei, play central functions in appetite control and energy homeostasis. Interestingly, it has been shown in recent research that the Ca^{2+}/calmodulin-dependent protein kinases (CaMKs) present in these nuclei play significant functions in endocrine activity, most significantly, neuropeptide control over vasopressin. These findings illustrate that the microanatomy of the hypothalamus is directly associated with its multiplicity of signaling roles, thus contributing to the secretion of pituitary hormones and, by extension, influencing other metabolic activities (Cimini et al., 2022). Functional diversity in such a minute brain region is typical of the critical role the hypothalamus has in physiological homeostasis. The hypothalamus is also a major contributor to the body's behavioral and affective responses as a site for internal and external environment signal integration. It is connected to many areas of the brain that allow it to modulate aggression, social behavior, and reward reaction. This is significant because it allows the hypothalamus to interact with the autonomic nervous system, which governs stress reactions and emotional states. Besides, the identification of newer methods, such as genetic modification and optogenetic excitation, has enabled scientists to study the unique functions and interactions of specific hypothalamic neurons. A greater understanding emphasizes clinical conditions of hypothalamic dysfunction and points out the areas pivotal role in not only somatic but also emotional regulation, which has a substantial impact on well-being (Morris, 2021).

2.1.1. Location Within the Brain

Hypothalamus and pituitary gland are found very close to each other in the brain, the space they share being as important to endocrine regulation as it is populated with neural pathways. The hypothalamus is located below the thalamus and forms the floor of the third ventricle, and is a major regulatory influence on several physiological activities through its tracts to the pituitary gland. This gland is located within the sella turcica, a cavity at the base of the skull, alongside important structures such as the optic chiasm and cavernous sinuses. This strategic position enhances the functionalities of the hypothalamic-pituitary axis to convey signals rapidly and efficiently throughout the body, thus highlighting the role of these regions in maintaining homeostasis and coordinating hormone secretion according to physiological requirements. Secondly, the anatomical sophistication of the sellar and parasellar regions underscores the necessity for precise localization in medical imaging and diagnosis. The sellar area is not just limited to the pituitary gland proper but extends to vital structures like the ventral adenohypophysis and dorsal neurohypophysis. Sellar and parasellar areas are subject to a variety of pathologies, such as neoplasms and vascular abnormalities, which may manifest as growths or lesions of both pituitary and contiguous structures. The pituitary gland and the hypothalamus are linked together by the infundibular stalk, which is a thin tissue bridge that carries hormonal messages crucial for growth control, metabolism, and reproduction. Hence, understanding the relative position of these organs is important in order to diagnose and treat any disorder that could be caused by a defect in either gland or the link between them (Simão, 2018). The third ventricle's position, surrounded by the hypothalamus and thalamus, again highlights the interconnectivity of these key brain areas. The ventricle is of particular importance as a location where more than one pathology can occur in the form of extrinsic masses influencing surrounding brain areas.

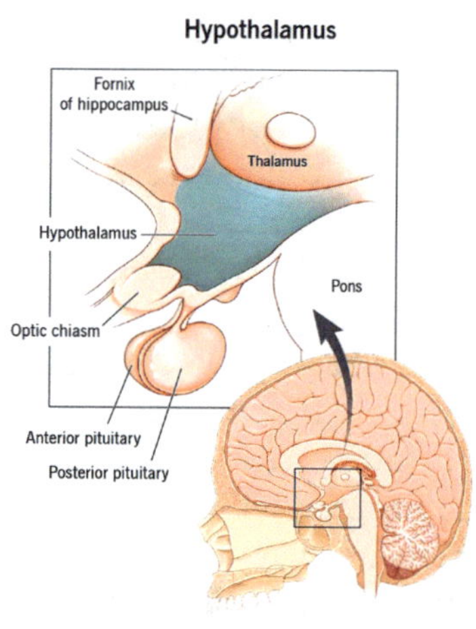

Figure 2.3. Location of the hypothalamus.

Source: https://my.clevelandclinic.org/-/scassets/images/org/health/articles/22566-hypothalamus.

Third ventricle abnormalities can be indicators of occult disease compromising the hypothalamus or pituitary and may require keen diagnostic insight to assess the significance of various mass formations. The architectural structure around the ventricle can be altered by a variety of conditions such as tumors or congenital malformations, profoundly influencing hormonal balance and neurophysiological function. By defining the third ventricle and surrounding structure anatomical boundaries, professionals can create targeted differential diagnoses, allowing for a comprehensive method of providing care to patients with endocrine dysfunctions (Glastonbury et al., 2011) (Figure 2.3).

2.1.2. Structure and Components

The pituitary gland and hypothalamus are very interconnected components of the endocrine system and function as a master controller of hormonal activity. The hypothalamus, which lies at the base of the brain, is a vital relay station, linking many signals from the nervous system to control homeostasis. It comprises several nuclei, each of which is responsible for processing different hormonal signals, thereby allowing for the release of regulatory hormones. These hormones either stimulate or inhibit the release of the pituitary gland's own hormones. The diverse shape of the hypothalamus enables it to control complex physiological processes, including stress, temperature regulation, and metabolic regulation, ultimately maintaining the body's internal homeostasis and responding to external environmental changes. The pituitary gland, also referred to as the master gland, is situated directly beneath the hypothalamus and is composed of two distinct lobes: the anterior and posterior pituitary. The anterior pituitary is composed of glandular tissue that secretes and produces a range of hormones, including GH, prolactin, and ACTH. Such an arrangement of the lobes enables it to react effectively to the hypothalamic releasing hormones, highlighting the fundamental interdependence of the two glands. The posterior pituitary stores and secretes the hypothalamus's secreted hormones, namely oxytocin and vasopressin. This anatomical differentiation highlights the functional sophistication and command by the hypothalamus of the anterior and posterior pituitaries in its endocrine regulation functions. Awareness of the anatomy and composition of the hypothalamus and pituitary gland is applied to their role in physiological function and dysfunctions. For instance, alterations in glycosylation-related processes are likely to influence hormone function of both the pituitary gland and hypothalamus, as illustrated by their influence on the production of thyroid hormone (Poche et al., 2018). In addition, extrinsic factors, like exposure to endocrine disruptors, can interfere with neuroendocrine regulatory processes, demonstrating the ways in which outside forces interfere with hormonal balance, especially at delicate developmental stages (Bellingham et al., 2016). Thus, the organizational complexity of the pituitary and hypothalamus is as essential in normal physiological control as for understanding how multiple pathologies can affect hormonal regulatory processes, underscoring the role of these structures in both disease and health.

2.1.3. Connections to Other Brain Regions

The hypothalamus is an important bridge between various regions of the brain, integrating complex body activities through its extensive neural networks. It involves close interaction with the pituitary gland to enable the body's hormonal and metabolic responses. Other than this collaboration, the hypothalamus comes into contact with the limbic system, whose fundamental role is to control emotions. For instance, their connections with the amygdala have a deep influence on stress response and emotional behavior, often impacting on hypothalamic–pituitary–adrenal (HPA) axis function. This axis dysregulation, which is widespread in most psychiatric diseases, such as depression, underscores the importance of hypothalamic connections. Evidence has revealed that gene expression alterations in response to stress, such as FKBP5, are linked to these interactions in important brain regions, illustrating how the hypothalamus integrates both emotional and physiological information to maintain homeostasis (Mikołaj et al., 2025). Furthermore, the hypothalamus' connectivity is not limited to the limbic system but also to the brainstem, which plays an essential role in autonomic and motor processes. By this system, the hypothalamus can control functions such as hunger, sleep, and body temperature. Of special mention are interactions with the brainstem by which the hypothalamus can influence cardiovascular and respiratory control in the face of internal and external stimuli. By these pathways, there is a sensitive response to stressors and environmental stimuli with a systemic mechanism of maintaining body balance. Additionally, evidence suggests that estrogen receptors are present in the pituitary and hypothalamus, and their modulation can influence connectivity with the brainstem, thereby impacting overall physiological responses (Ghazanfari et al., 2024). Thus, interconnectivity among these brain regions is the best demonstration of the central role of the hypothalamus in synthesizing different physiological signals. Thus, the intricate interplay of the hypothalamus, pituitary gland, and other components of the brain is crucial to understanding the regulation of states of physiology and psychology. The above implies a multi-functioning process where the hypothalamus does not merely transmit information but also integrates sensory information to yield correct hormonal outputs. The evidence that long-term treatments like lithium are able to affect gene expression across these areas also suggests that hormonal signal pathways are regulated by broader neural interactions. As studies dig deeper into the expression of the likes of FKBP5 and how the ERs work in the brain, it is gradually becoming clear that interrupting these mechanisms results in various disorders, confirming the need for further research into the interrelatedness of the hypothalamus-pituitary axis (Ghazanfari et al., 2024; Mikołaj et al., 2025) (Figure 2.4).

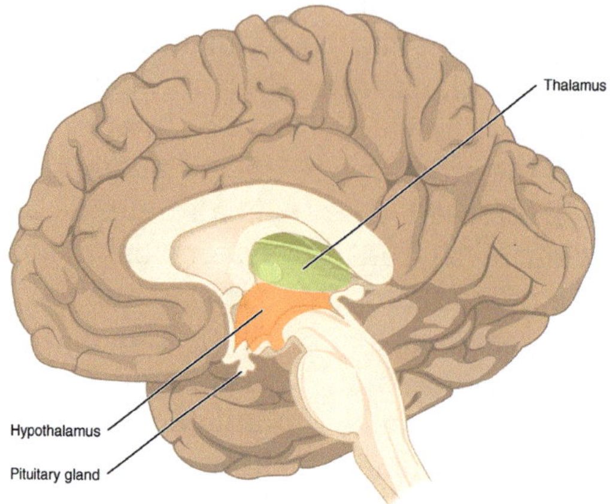

Figure 2.4. Hypothalamus serves as a critical bridge connecting various brain regions.

Source: https://cdn.lecturio.com/assets/hypothalamus-within-the-brain.jpg.

Test Your Knowledge

1. Where is the hypothalamus located within the brain?
2. What are the main structural components or nuclei of the hypothalamus involved in endocrine regulation?
3. Which major brain region does the hypothalamus connect to directly via the pituitary stalk (infundibulum)?

2.2. Functions of the Hypothalamus

Learning Outcome

1. Explain how the hypothalamus regulates body temperature;
2. Discuss how the hypothalamus controls hunger and thirst;
3. Regulate sleep-wake cycles.

The hypothalamus is a necessary regulatory location in the brain that controls many of the physiological processes associated with homeostasis. One of its primary functions is the regulation of endocrine function through its interaction with the pituitary gland. Through the release and secretion of various releasing and inhibiting hormones, the hypothalamus regulates the secretion of the anterior pituitary hormone. This active interaction is essential to the regulation of most body functions, including growth, metabolism, and stress response. The hypothalamus is similarly key to maintaining body temperature, blood pressure, and fluid balance, a demonstration of its integrative role in responding to internal and external stimuli. The timely coordination of these hormonal messages is reflective of the significance of the hypothalamus in maintaining homeostasis and overall organism function. Furthermore, the hypothalamus plays a critical role in sustaining autonomic nervous system functions. The region gets sensory input corresponding to emotional and physiological states and translates the inputs into the appropriate autonomic response. It, for instance, regulates heart rate, breathing rate, and digestion by modifying sympathetic and parasympathetic circuits. Moreover, the function of the hypothalamus in heat regulation is an illustration of its critical role in maintaining the body in equilibrium. Research indicates that the hypothalamus, in conjunction with the anterior pituitary, acts to stimulate the hypothalamic-pituitary-thyroid axis, which has key functions in the metabolic rates of organisms and energy use. Patterns of development of such hormonal interactions in avian species find the timelines to indicate the central role of the hypothalamus in thermoregulation processes and emphasize the sophistication of its functions in different organisms as indicated in available literature (Baarendse et al., 2008).

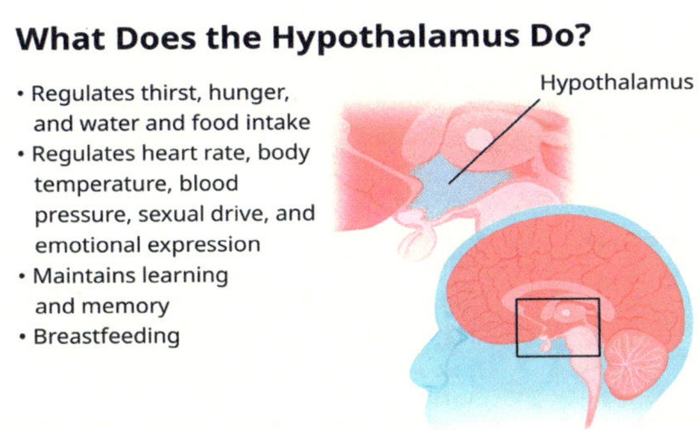

Figure 2.5. What does the hypothalamus do?

Source: https://www.verywellhealth.com/thmb/njIn5G2d7yQg0YTQQxDrNQ02_wI=/1500x0/filters:no_upscale():max_bytes(150000):strip_icc()/VWH-What-to-Know-About-the-Hypothalamus-final-1-33954b4531ca4d2bbfe5224d450756bc.png.

In addition, the hypothalamus cannot be replaced in regulating appetite, thirst, and temperature, which are all vital for survival. Some of the hypothalamic nuclei, such as the arcuate nucleus, have a role in integrating the body's energy status signals, consequently influencing hunger or satiation. Its regulatory function helps maintain balance in energy intake and expenditure, which impacts metabolic well-being. Similarly, osmoregulatory responses in the hypothalamus controlled by nuclei like the supraoptic and paraventricular nuclei demonstrate their role in fluid balance via control of thirst and release of the posterior pituitary's antidiuretic hormone (ADH). The complexity of these processes is further increased by genetics that can lead to conditions like hypopituitarism, implying normal functioning of the hypothalamus is a function of complicated developmental processes (Aarskog et al., 2009). This convergence of neurologic and hormonal processes exemplifies the multifunctional role of the hypothalamus in regulating vital biological processes, emphasizing its importance in the hypothalamus-pituitary axis (Figure 2.5).

2.2.1. Regulation of Body Temperature

Hypothalamic control of body temperature is a critical process involving complex interactions between the hypothalamus and the pituitary gland. The thermostat of the body is the central nervous system component that acts to sense changes in internal and external temperatures. By receiving signals from thermoreceptors throughout the body, the hypothalamus coordinates and regulates homeostasis. When the set point is departed from, the hypothalamus triggers such processes as sweating or shivering, leading to loss of heat or production of heat, respectively. The pituitary gland also plays a crucial role in regulating endocrine responses that influence thermogenesis and metabolism, thereby integrating temperature regulation into broader metabolic pathways. The relationship between body temperature control and the hypothalamic–pituitary–thyroid axis is especially significant. Thyroid hormones, secreted by the pituitary gland, significantly affect metabolic rate, which then has an impact on body temperature as well as heat production. In particular, triiodothyronine (T3) is reputed to accelerate metabolic processes, increasing thermogenesis and thereby affecting body temperature levels. Research indicates that impairment of this axis can lead to abnormal thermoregulation and metabolic dysfunction, and the importance of both the pituitary and hypothalamus in the thermal homeostasis of the body. In hypothyroidism, the deficiency of thyroid hormone production means decreased function in temperature adjustment, and therefore the balance of these systems in thermoregulation. Moreover, circadian rhythms controlling body temperature are strongly associated with hypothalamic function. The suprachiasmatic nucleus (SCN) within the hypothalamus is the master clock for circadian rhythms and influences many physiological functions, such as the regulation of body temperature. Experiments have shown that modifications in the SCN lead to altered rhythms of temperature and metabolism, and therefore, a functioning circadian system plays an essential role in effective thermoregulation. Circadian desynchronizations can result in metabolic syndromes, including obesity and other endocrine illnesses. Investigations into interactions between body temperature, the SCN, and the hypothalamus provide additional understanding into metabolic and thermoregulatory well-being, particularly in terms of conditions like hypothyroidism, whereby the rhythms can become significantly deranged (Emrich et al., 2024) (Figure 2.6).

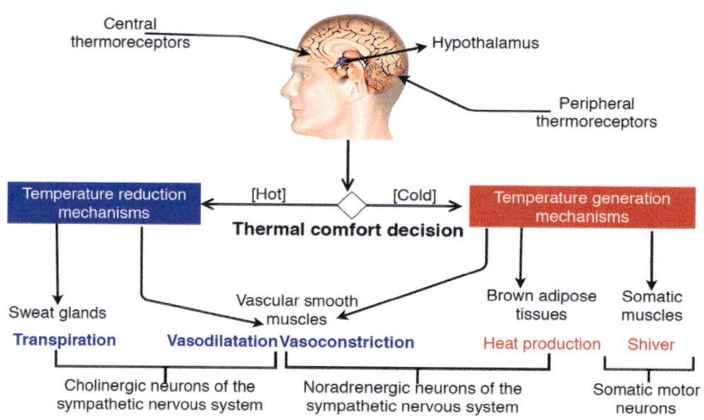

Figure 2.6. A simplified view of human thermoregulation—the hypothalamus checks the body's core temperature and initiates necessary thermogenic or heat-dissipating processes to maintain thermal balance.

Source: https://www.researchgate.net/profile/Kizito-Nkurikiyeyezu/publication/333743297/figure/fig1/AS:769135491444736@1560387599390/A-simplified-human-thermoregulation-the-hypothalamus-checks-the-bodys-core-temperature.png.

2.2.2. Control of Hunger and Thirst

Regulation of hunger and thirst has its roots deeply within the hypothalamus and pituitary gland, two of the key structures in homeostatic regulation within the human body. The hypothalamus, located below the thalamus, is centrally responsible for the integration of a multitude of signals corresponding to energy balance and hydration level. Within its neuronal architecture, certain nuclei—such as the arcuate and paraventricular nuclei—are centers for hunger and thirst, respectively. These regions process hormonal inputs and neural signals that communicate the body's energy reserves and fluid status. Therefore, the hypothalamus responds not only to changes in the availability of nutrients but also modulates behavior and physiological response to keep the organism in both energy balance and fluid homeostasis, essential for survival. Among the key players in hunger control is the hormone leptin, released by the adipocytes on the condition of excess fat storage. Leptin sends signals to receptors in the hypothalamus, influencing not just appetite but also the body's energy expenditure as a whole. The primary role of leptin is to generate the feeling of satiety; when the level of leptin is adequate, it leads to reduced food intake, thereby preventing obesity. Conversely, a lack of leptin or dysfunction in its signaling process could result in uncontrollable hunger and consequent weight gain.

This relationship highlights the intricate neuroendocrine interaction between the hypothalamus, pituitary gland, and peripheral hormones that regulate energy, as evidenced by research demonstrating how hormones like QRFP43 influence the secretory activity of the HPT axis, ultimately controlling the body's metabolic activities (Przybył et al., 2025). Control of thirst also involves intricate hormonal interaction, especially with the anti-diuretic hormone (ADH). Synthesized in the hypothalamus and secreted by the posterior pituitary, ADH is necessary for water retention and osmotic balance maintenance. By dehydration or increased plasma osmolality, osmoreceptors in the hypothalamus stimulate thirst sensation and stimulate the release of ADH.

This stimulates reabsorption of water by the kidneys, effectively maintaining the fluid of the body. In addition, the stimulation of the low blood volume-sensitive hormone angiotensin II also stimulates thirst and endocrine pathways to prioritize water. The intricate regulation system demonstrates the way in which the hypothalamus and pituitary gland interact to coalesce several signals in maintaining energy balance as well as fluid homeostasis, a fundamental aspect of overall physiological health (Najla et al., 2017) (Figure 2.7).

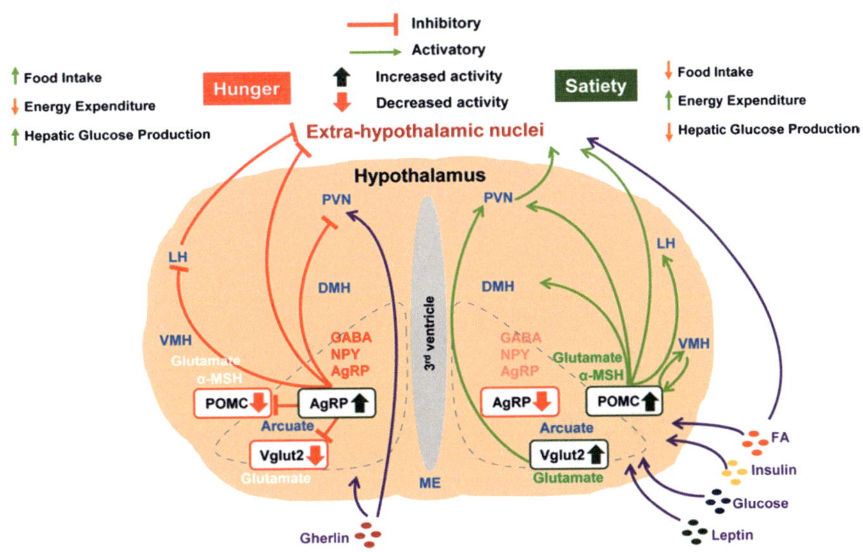

Figure 2.7. Hypothalamic control of hunger and satiety.

Source: https://www.researchgate.net/publication/326088008/figure/fig1/AS:960999653904393@1606131580259/Hypothalamic-control-of-hunger-and-satiety-A-schematic-representation-of-the-nuclei-of.png.

2.2.3. Influence on Sleep-Wake Cycles

The regulation of sleep-wake cycles has a close relationship with the hypothalamus, particularly its suprachiasmatic nucleus (SCN), or the body's master circadian clock. At the bottom of the brain, the SCN receives direct input from photoreceptors in the retina, thereby being able to orchestrate physiological reactions to light-dark ambiance. Orchestration is necessary in order to provide normal sleep habits and overall health. Disruption of the activity of SCNs, either due to exposure to artificial light or shift work, can lead to desynchronized circadian rhythms. Therefore, the people will experience sleep disorders or chronic fatigue, highlighting the vital function of the hypothalamus in the control of sleep-wake cycles. These interruptions can have further effects on metabolic well-being, hormones, and even mental processes, emphasizing the role of the hypothalamus in controlling various body systems and its pivotal role in the maintenance of homeostasis. The hypothalamus also controls sleep-wake cycles via its link to the pituitary gland, through hormonal regulation. The pineal gland's secretion of hormones such as melatonin is controlled by inputs from the SCN, with direct effects on falling asleep and sleep continuity. Other hormones that regulate arousal and wakefulness, such as cortisol, are also controlled by the hypothalamus, which includes a circadian rhythm that typically peaks in the early morning. Elevated levels of cortisol will increase wakefulness, while reduced levels at night will promote sleep. The delicate balance that these hormones maintain illustrates the critical function of the hypothalamus in controlling our sleep-wake cycle and its broader implications for overall health. Disruption of this balance, via stress, lifestyle adjustments, or neurological disease, can produce desperate disruption to sleeping patterns, illustrating the co-dependency of the hypothalamus, pituitary gland, and the control of sleep. In studying the pathophysiology of neurodegenerative diseases such as Alzheimer's disease, the activity of the hypothalamus in the regulation of sleep-wake cycles comes increasingly to the fore. Research has indicated that abnormality in the hypothalamus may hasten the progression of Alzheimer's disease, affecting not just cognitive function but also sleep and overall metabolic function. Alzheimer's patients often endure significant sleep disturbances, with an abnormal circadian rhythm that mirrors the underlying hypothalamic pathology. These changes can also further exacerbate the symptoms of the disease, as inappropriate sleep further accelerates cognitive decline and metabolic derangement. Therefore, defining the dual function of the hypothalamus as both regulating sleep and disease pathology opens new therapeutic areas of intervention and drug targeting. Anti-hypothalamic intervention holds the promise not only to improve sleep but to reverse associated cognitive and metabolic impairment in affected individuals (Iadecola et al., 2015).

Test Your Knowledge

1. How does the hypothalamus help regulate body temperature in response to changes in the environment?
2. Which part of the hypothalamus is primarily responsible for triggering the sensation of hunger?
3. What role does the hypothalamus play in regulating the sleep-wake cycle?

2.3. Anatomy of the Pituitary Gland

Learning Outcome

1. Discuss the location of the pituitary gland in relation to the hypothalamus;
2. Understand the structure and lobes of the pituitary gland;
3. Describe the blood supply and innervation.

The pituitary gland, which is frequently referred to as the master gland of the endocrine system, is a small but significant organ that sits at the base of the brain, beneath the hypothalamus. Structurally, the gland has two primary lobes: the anterior (front) lobe and the posterior (rear) lobe, each of which is responsible for particular functions in the secretion and production of hormones. The anterior pituitary is in charge of the synthesis and release of several crucial hormones, such as GH, prolactin, and ACTH. In contrast, the posterior lobe releases and secretes hormones produced by the hypothalamus, i.e., oxytocin and vasopressin. The intricate structure and position of the pituitary gland underscore its critical role in the hormonal regulation of numerous physiological functions, highlighting a complex association between structure and function that is essential for maintaining homeostasis within the body (Knight et al., 2021). The anatomic association between the hypothalamus and pituitary gland is critical for optimal endocrine coordination. The hypothalamus, located immediately above the pituitary gland, is a regulating center that controls the release of hormones produced by the pituitary using various mechanisms for signaling. The hypothalamus houses specialized neurons that secrete releasing and inhibiting hormones, which, in the bloodstream, transport themselves to the anterior pituitary to influence its activity. This neuroendocrine connection illustrates the dynamic nature of hormonal regulation, whereby the hypothalamus integrates neural signals and bodily feedback to regulate pituitary function. Therefore, dysregulation of this connection might lead to gigantic hormonal deficiencies, affecting growth, metabolism, and reproductive functions, highlighting the importance of understanding the anatomy of the pituitary gland within the broader context of the hypothalamic-pituitary axis (Knight et al., 2021). Research is ongoing to uncover more nuances of the pituitary glands function, particularly in relation to health diseases such as obesity. More current research has demonstrated a very robust association between the pituitary gland's functional connectivity and body mass index (BMI), and marks particular regions of the brain that converse with pituitary hormones that are involved with metabolic function and weight regulation.

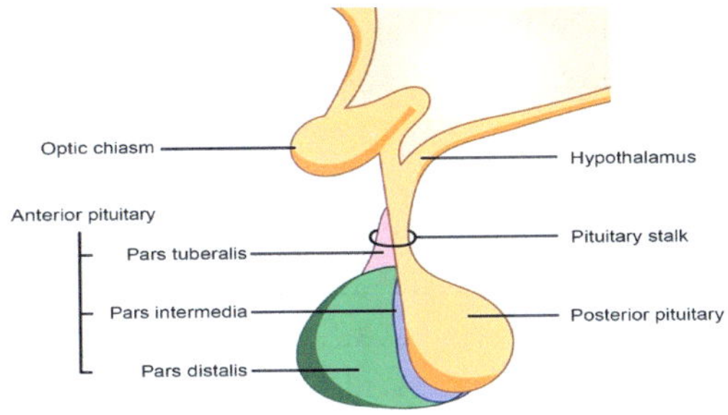

Figure 2.8. Pituitary gland anatomy.

Source: https://prod-images-static.radiopaedia.org/images/52193989/e53dddef9ba02e2fb86bad2d0e22ff_big_gallery.jpeg.

For instance, connections between the pituitary and areas such as the hippocampus, lingual gyrus, and orbitofrontal cortex have been discovered to describe how the function of the pituitary gland extends beyond hormone secretion to involve roles in shaping complex biological behaviors and processes involving hunger and satiety. This increasing awareness accentuates the pituitary gland's significant role in mediating not just endocrine function but also overall implications on metabolic well-being that necessitate more studies of its anatomical and functional relationships with the hypothalamus (Figure 2.8).

2.3.1. Location in Relation to the Hypothalamus

The location of the hypothalamus is central to its role in regulating various physiological activities and its connection with the pituitary gland. Below the thalamus and above the brainstem, the hypothalamus is a critical link in the neuroendocrine system. Its physical proximity to significant structures such as the optic chiasm, pituitary stalk, and brainstem further underscores its major function in the central nervous system. This spatial organization allows the hypothalamus to adequately communicate with the pituitary gland, providing adequate release of hormones essential to numerous body functions. The location of the hypothalamus relative to these structures also plays an important part in how sensory information and hormonal signals are treated, ultimately influencing homeostasis and behavioral response. Having knowledge of the location of the hypothalamus is of particular importance in clinical practice, especially during surgical planning. The interaction of tumors, such as craniopharyngiomas, with the hypothalamus can significantly influence the result of surgery and patient recovery. To illustrate, careful preoperative assessment of a tumor's spatial relationship to the hypothalamus and nearby structures, as well as its size and configuration, is essential. This includes consideration of how the tumor is related to the pituitary stalk and optic chiasm, which can impact endocrine function and vision. The data acquired from imaging and anatomy are useful in surgical planning, allowing for the delicate tissues surrounding the hypothalamus to be spared and the tumor to be successfully removed (Dizdarevic et al., 2024). This precision enhances postoperative outcomes and minimizes the risk of hypothalamic dysfunction. Also, the hypothalamus is a command center for the hypothalamic-pituitary-adrenal (HPA) axis, and its location in the brain betrays its role in stress processes. By receiving input from messages related to internal and external stressors, the hypothalamus can initiate a hormonal cascade of activity. It secretes CRH and arginine vasopressin (AVP), which stimulate the anterior pituitary gland to secrete ACTH, with the last step being secretion of cortisol by the adrenal cortex (Milleniari, 2023). The close physical proximity of the hypothalamus to the pituitary gland is necessary for the speedy and efficient transfer of these hormone signals for the body to achieve homeostasis under stress. The physiological implications of such a position highlight the delicate relationships between these significant structures, supporting the hypothalamus' role in coordinating endocrine functions according to various physiological demands (Figure 2.9).

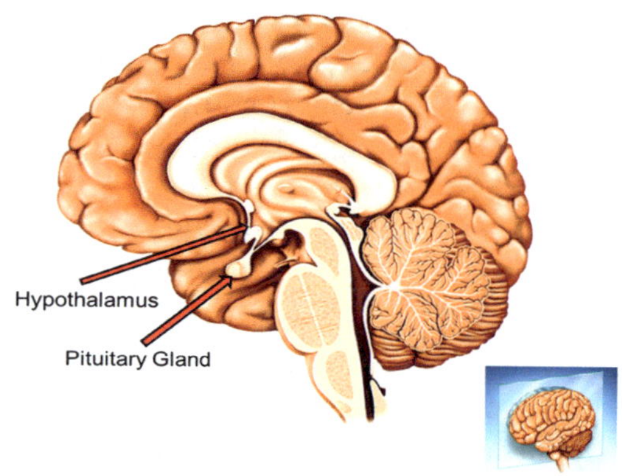

Figure 2.9. The location of the hypothalamus is instrumental to its role in regulating various physiological functions and interacting with the pituitary gland.

Source: https://i0.wp.com/www.timeofcare.com/wp-content/uploads/2016/10/hypothalamus-and-pituitary.png?resize=808%2C659.

2.3.2. Structure and Lobes of the Pituitary Gland

The pituitary gland, which is a small but essential endocrine gland, is made up of two distinct lobes: the anterior and posterior lobes. The roles of each of these lobes are distinct when it comes to the secretion and regulation of distinct physiological processes. The anterior pituitary, or adenohypophysis, secretes and releases six of the most significant hormones, including GH, prolactin, and ACTH. On the contrary, the posterior pituitary or neurohypophysis is not a gland that secretes hormones but a storage and release site for hormones synthesized in the hypothalamus, i.e., oxytocin and vasopressin. This close functional relationship with the hypothalamus reflects the integrated character of hormonal regulation and demonstrates the responsiveness of the anterior lobes to hypothalamic stimuli, thereby regulating homeostasis within the body (Agam et al., 2018). The anatomical position of the pituitary gland in the sella turcica, a bony depression on the base of the skull, is complemented by its anatomical relationship to neighboring structures. The protective capsule is encircled by fulcrum neurovascular structures, like the internal carotid arteries and cranial nerves, which highlight the anatomical significance of the gland. Interestingly, the pituitary gland is connected to the hypothalamus through the pituitary stalk, a pathway for important communication. The anterior and posterior lobes are distinguished in terms of embryological origin; while the anterior lobe is derived from the Rathke's pouch ectoderm, the posterior lobe is an outgrowth of the neural ectoderm. It is critical to the surgical techniques and treatment options for pituitary disease to have an appreciation of this unique anatomy and of the structures around it (Peter et al., 2017). Pituitary gland integrity and functioning are critical to numerous endocrine processes and overall health. In transsphenoidal surgery, the most common procedure for treating pituitary adenomas, the anatomical knowledge of the gland can have significant implications for surgical success. Complications may arise due to the gland's close proximity to surrounding vascular and nervous tissues, vindicating the necessity of meticulous surgical techniques to minimize risks. As an example, surgical maneuvering around the sella turcica anatomy may prevent accidental damage to the essential surrounding structures, leading to complications such as diabetes insipidus or hypopituitarism. Thus, the physiological and anatomical nuances of the pituitary gland not only determine its crucial role in the endocrine system but also reflect the intricacies of surgical intervention involving the critical organ (Agam et al., 2018) (Figure 2.10).

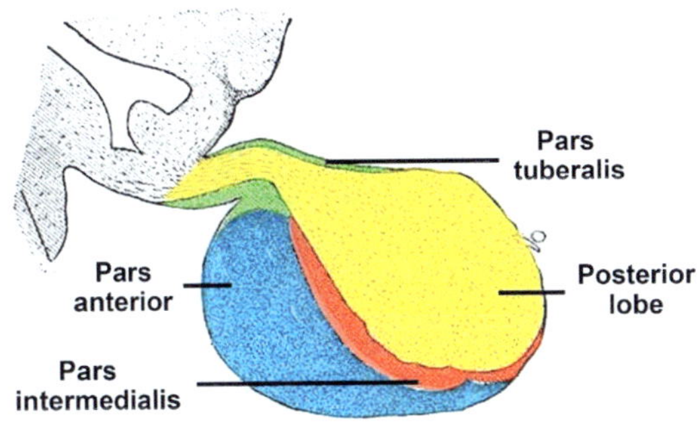

Figure 2.10. The structure of the pituitary gland.

Source: https://teachmeanatomy.info/wp-content/uploads/Structure-of-the-Pituitary-Gland.jpg.

2.3.3. Blood Supply and Innervation

Perfusion and innervation of the pituitary gland and hypothalamus are vital to their function in the regulation of various physiological activities. The anterior pituitary receives its blood supply through the hypophyseal portal system, a unique vascular structure that allows effective delivery of hormones secreted by the hypothalamus to the pituitary gland. This system ensures that neurohormones such as CRH and gonadotropin-releasing hormone have little dilution in their action on pituitary cells. Additionally, the posterior pituitary, where neuropeptides such as vasopressin and oxytocin are released and stored, is directly innervated by hypothalamic magnocellular neurons. The rich innervation of nerve fibers and blood vessels again underlines the essential role of the hypothalamus in ensuring homeostasis by complex endocrine communication. In addition to their blood supply, the hypothalamus and pituitary are supplied with an abundance of neural inputs that govern their function based on various stimuli. The hypothalamus receives rich supplies of afferent fibers from the brainstem, limbic system, and other sensory tracts, contributing to its role as an integrating central center for endocrine and autonomic regulation. For example, sensory and affective stimuli may influence the release of hypothalamic hormones, which in turn may modulate pituitary hormone secretion. Such a dynamic interrelation not only facilitates the adaptation of the body's internal milieu to environmental changes but also reflects the important role of the nervous system in regulating endocrine function. All these mechanisms underscore the significance of neural connections in orchestrating the intricate interplay between the hypothalamus and the pituitary gland. New technology has revealed that conventional *in vitro* culture models can have profound limitations when modeling accurately the bidirectional neuroendocrine interactions between the hypothalamus and pituitary gland. Two-dimensional and three-dimensional models that currently exist are often unable to mimic the complex multicellular organization necessary for optimal function. Due to such deficiencies, researchers have developed new platforms, such as the 'hypothalamic–pituitary (HP) axis-on-a-chip,' which incorporates many cellular components of both glands. This microchip not only enhances the understanding of neuroendocrine toxicity but also provides a more realistic simulation of blood supply and representation of the hypothalamic-pituitary axis, allowing better drug candidate toxicities to be assessed. Through the application of these advanced techniques, the analysis of blood supply and innervation can yield significant information about the intricate dynamics of endocrine signaling in the pituitary gland and hypothalamus (Park et al., 2024; Singh et al., 2023) (Figure 2.11).

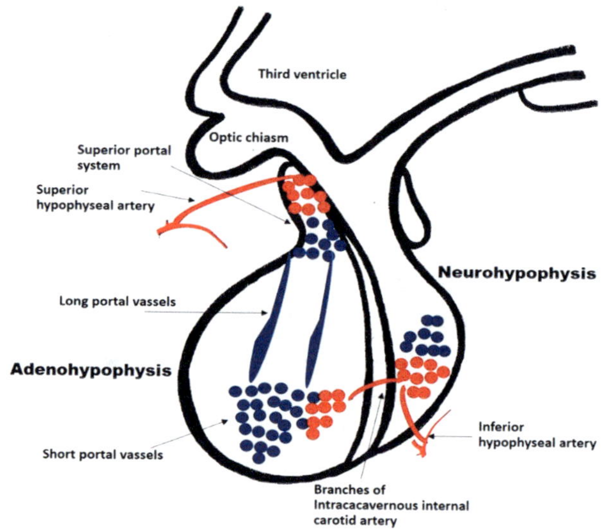

Figure 2.11. Pituitary blood supply and portal system.

Source: https://www.researchgate.net/publication/362551693/figure/fig1/AS:11431281387283358@1745106011125/Pituitary-blood-supply-and-portal-system-The-adenohypophysis-and-neuro-hypophysis.tif.

Test Your Knowledge

1. Name the two main lobes of the pituitary gland and briefly describe their functions.
2. What type of tissue composes the anterior pituitary compared to the posterior pituitary?
3. Describe the primary blood supply system of the pituitary gland and its significance.

2.4. Functions of the Pituitary Gland

Learning Outcome

1. Understand the process of hormone production and secretion;
2. Explain the role in growth and development;
3. Regulate reproductive functions.

The pituitary gland, or "master gland," is a crucial controller of many endocrine activities of the body. Situated below the brain, it responds to the signals from the hypothalamus by secreting and releasing hormones that control many of the body's functions. One of the many functions that it carries out is the secretion of ACTH, which stimulates the adrenal glands to secrete cortisol. This interaction is required to regulate the stress responses, exemplifying the pituitary's key role in the HPA axis. The secretion of other hormones, such as GH and prolactin, also exemplifies the pituitary's function in growth, metabolism, and reproductive functions. The ability of the gland to integrate systemic hints from the body further confirms its role in homeostasis regulation and coordination of complex biological reactions among various systems (Yan et al., 2023). One other exceptional characteristic of the pituitary gland is its ability to communicate with the immune system, which demonstrates the sophistication of its regulatory functions. Research indicates that in systemic inflammatory states, there is an intense response by pituitary hormone-secreting cells (HPCs), which means the gland modulates its hormonal output according to physiological demands. For instance, during inflammation, corticotropes are activated to produce ACTH, influencing immune mechanisms. This reveals that the pituitary is not only a passive recipient in endocrine signaling but also an active participant in the modulation of immune homeostasis in both canonical and non-canonical pathways. The pituitary's release of bioactive molecules such as Nptx2 by corticotropes shows how the pituitary gland is a critical intermediary between neuroendocrine control and the immune system, making its activity two-dimensional and irreplaceable for overall health (Yan et al., 2023). Further elucidating the role of the pituitary gland, more recent work has underlined the significance of recently identified hormones like Spexin2 (SPX2), underlining the gland's ongoing role in metabolic regulation. Although a great deal of work has hitherto focused upon traditional pituitary hormones, SPX2 has been shown to influence feeding behavior and energy balance, with notable effects being observed in models like chickens. SPX2 expression in the pituitary and hypothalamus suggests its role in appetite regulation, where it acts on some receptors to modulate feeding behavior. This finding highlights the broadening understanding of the functions of the pituitary beyond traditional endocrine roles, where it integrates signals for energy homeostasis and nutritional status. Thus, the study of hormones like SPX2 is a critical move towards understanding the general function of the pituitary glands in endocrine and metabolic processes.

2.4.1. Hormone Production and Secretion

The intricate relationship between the pituitary gland and the hypothalamus lies at the very heart of endocrine function of hormone secretion and production as an imperative regulatory cycle of the endocrine system. Located at the base of the brain, the hypothalamus secretes and synthesizes various releasing hormones that directly impact the secretion of the pituitary gland's own hormones. For instance, thyrotropin-releasing hormone (TRH) stimulates the pituitary gland to release thyroid-stimulating hormone (TSH), which in turn prompts thyroid hormone release from the thyroid gland. The intricate feedback system is not only vital for growth and metabolism but also in thermoregulation, highlighting the hypothalamus' role in maintaining the body in homeostasis through hormone regulation (Baarendse et al., 2008). Understanding this relationship explains how various physiological processes are controlled within the body. The hormonal axes regulated by the pituitary gland and hypothalamus extend beyond metabolic control to stress reactions and reproductive functions. The HPA axis is also of special interest since it is responsible for the body's stress response by releasing CRH, which stimulates the release of ACTH from the pituitary. ACTH induces the release of cortisol from the adrenal glands, a hormone involved in controlling stress and influencing many metabolic processes. Similarly, in men's reproductive physiology, the hypothalamus releases gonadotropin-releasing hormone (GnRH), which regulates the release of luteinizing hormone (LH) and follicle-stimulating hormone (FSH) from the pituitary to allow the generation of sperm and overall reproductive health (Clavijo et al., 2018). These associated mechanisms illustrate the diverse roles of hormone synthesis and secretion to adapt to internal and external changes. Knowledge of hormone production and secretion, particularly through the hypothalamic-pituitary axis, not only forms an essential part of rudimentary physiology but also an essential part of endocrine clinical practice in hormonal diseases. Dysregulation within these hormonal processes may cause abnormalities such as hyperthyroidism, adrenal insufficiency, or hypogonadism, thereby showing the necessity to maintain hormonal homeostasis. For healthcare professionals, a strong grasp of the mechanisms governing these endocrine systems underlies effective treatment programs via hormonal therapy and intervention. Through the incorporation of knowledge of the regulatory roles of the pituitary gland and the hypothalamus, practitioners are better equipped to deal with the complexity of hormonal disorders, presenting a more comprehensive approach to male reproductive medicine and beyond (Clavijo et al., 2018). The dynamics of secretion and hormone production highlight the central role these brain structures play in promoting health and stability throughout the body's various systems (Figure 2.12).

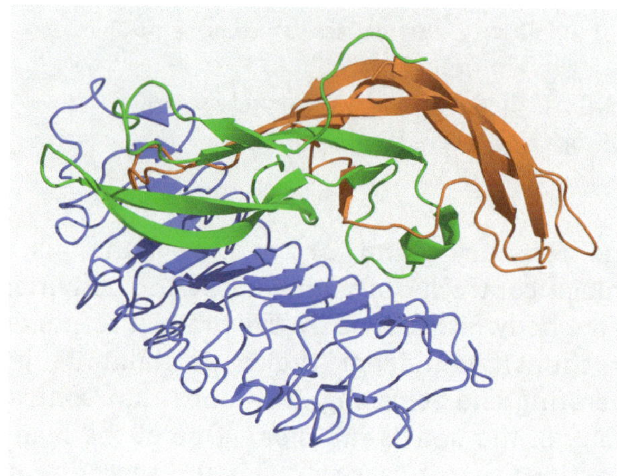

Figure 2.12. 3D structure of FSH (A chain in green, B chain in orange) complexed with the FSH receptor (blue).

Source: https://upload.wikimedia.org/wikipedia/commons/thumb/d/d9/FSHA%2BB%2Breceptor_1XWD.png/800px-FSHA%2BB%2Breceptor_1XWD.png.

2.4.2. Role in Growth and Development

The pituitary gland and hypothalamus are central to biological mechanisms that control growth and development in mammals by virtue of a complex neuroendocrine interaction. GH-releasing hormone and somatostatin secretion from the hypothalamus regulate the secretion of the anterior pituitary GH. GH is generally regarded as the master regulator of somatic growth since it not only controls growth but also metabolic homeostasis by controlling carbohydrate and lipid metabolism via intricate signaling pathways. IGF-1-mediated feedback mechanisms, as the major mediator of GH action, illustrate the plasticity of the growth axis based on physiological demand, with evidence provided by genetically modified mouse models highlighting the significance of this endocrine signaling towards maintenance of growth and homeostasis (Al-Samerria et al., 2021). In addition, the relationship between the pituitary gland and the hypothalamus is also important in regulating seasonal variations in growth and physiological activity. This is particularly evident for organisms that inhabit temperate climates, where fluctuating periodic changes in day length affect appetite, body fat content, and growth rates, all of which are regulated by neuroendocrine signals. The pars tuberalis of the pituitary gland responds to melatonin levels, which provide tanycytes in the hypothalamus with nutritional cues vital for nutrient sensing and endocrine regulation. In addition to facilitating the entry of important hormones into the hypothalamus, these tanycytes also exhibit seasonal gene expression change for thyroid hormone metabolism, which is vital for the correct growth and development response in a fluctuating environment (Jo et al., 2017).

Additionally, the adaptiveness of the hypothalamic-pituitary axis underscores its central role in developmental processes. Experiments illustrate the manner in which thyroid hormone level manipulations within the hypothalamus produce profound effects on seasonally occurring behaviors in various species, such as sheep and Siberian hamsters. The ability of the hypothalamus to make use of growth pathway utilization in adults illustrates how growth and development transcend being mere anatomical additions; they consist of physiological compensations to environmental stimuli. These findings suggest that growth and development processes are interactive and adaptive, with the pituitary and hypothalamus as the masters of the stroke in the intricate system and offering insights regarding potential therapeutic direction in metabolic disorders and growth-related illness (Jo et al., 2017).

2.4.3. Regulation of Reproductive Functions

The regulation of reproductive functions is, in fact, governed by the intricate feedback mechanisms of the hypothalamic-pituitary-gonadal (HPG) axis. Central to this regulation is the hypothalamus, which orchestrates the pulsatile release of gonadotropin-releasing hormone (GnRH). Such pulsatility is crucial, as it ensures the appropriate timing and quantity of gonadotropins—i.e., follicle-stimulating hormone (FSH) and luteinizing hormone (LH)—released by the pituitary gland. These hormones then stimulate the gonads, influencing mechanisms like sex steroidogenesis and development of gametes. The dynamic nature of the HPG axis highlights the coordination of diverse internal and external factors like nutritional status, age, and environmental influences, which play significant roles in modulating reproductive function and health within the organism, as indicated by the fine balance but very crucial interaction between hormonal messages (Kaminska et al., 2024). The essential function of the pituitary gland in reproductive regulation is underlined by its receptiveness to both hypothalamic and peripheral signals. Adipocytokines derived from adipose tissues play an important role in pituitary functions, as a reflection of the gland's sensitivity to both reproductive and energy homeostasis signals. Adipose tissue-secreted hormones, leptin and adiponectin, are not only expressed in the pituitary gland but can also alter patterns of gonadotropin secretion. This highlights the importance of metabolic status in reproductive health since an insufficient energy supply may encourage the deterioration of reproductive functions, illustrating the imperative dependence of energy balance and endocrine control of reproductive physiology. Moreover, the synthesis and morphological adaptation of the pituitary to various reproductive signals further confirm its role as a crucial endocrine nodal point in the HPG axis (Kaminska et al., 2024). Recent developments in understanding the neurophysiological mechanisms controlling GnRH release have brought into the picture the complexity of reproductive processes. Recent evidence suggests that neural circuits, particularly the kisspeptin-neurokinin-dynorphin axis, play significant roles in controlling GnRH release, thereby dictating reproductive outcomes. Photoperiod and photoperiod-induced melatonin release also contribute to modulating GnRH and ensuing LH production required for male and female reproductive function. Behavioral responses related to hormonal reproduction are yet another illustration of how integrated regulatory mechanisms become at the level of the hypothalamus and pituitary. They not only enhance our understanding of hormonal control during reproduction but also present potential directions for the maximization of reproductive efficiency in farm animals and emphasize the applied significance of such information (Zhao et al., 2023) (Figure 2.13).

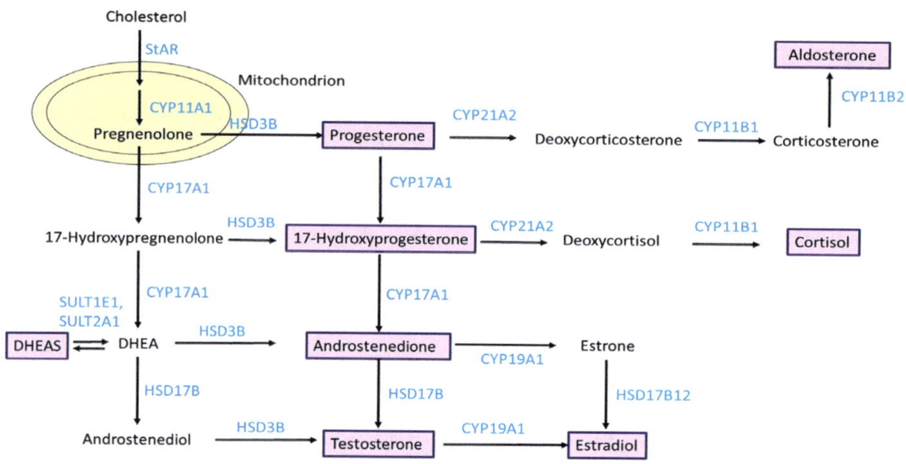

Figure 2.13. Sex steroid hormone metabolism pathway.

Source: https://www.researchgate.net/publication/364272351/figure/fig1/AS:11431281088748674@1665281662144/Sex-steroid-hormone-metabolism-pathway-Metabolites-hormones-are-displayed-in-black-text.png.

Test Your Knowledge

1. Which hormones are produced by the anterior pituitary gland, and what are their primary target organs?
2. What hormone is secreted by the posterior pituitary to regulate water balance in the body, and how does it work?
3. Describe the role of the pituitary gland in regulating female reproductive functions such as the menstrual cycle.

2.5. Interaction Between the Hypothalamus and Pituitary Gland

Learning Outcome

1. Discuss hormonal signaling pathways;
2. Explain how feedback mechanisms play a pivotal role in maintaining homeostasis within the endocrine system;
3. Define the role of the pituitary gland in maintaining homeostasis.

The pituitary gland and hypothalamus, also referred to as the master controllers of the endocrine system, share information in a complex manner to maintain homeostasis within the body. This communication is depicted by the hypothalamic-pituitary-thyroid (HPT) axis, where the hypothalamus secretes thyrotropin-releasing hormone (TRH), thereby stimulating the pituitary gland to secrete thyroid-stimulating hormone (TSH). The role of TRH extends simply to stimulating TSH secretion; it influences the overall metabolic rate and thermoregulatory activities in organisms. Notably, in the case of bird species, the functionality of the HPT axis develops differently in precocial and altricial birds, which emphasizes the complexity of the interaction between the two glands in growth and environmental adaptation. These differences demonstrate the adaptations developed to optimize hormonal control in various situations and profoundly influence thermoregulation at different stages of life (Baarendse et al., 2008). Also, the communication between the hypothalamus and pituitary gland is not only via the HPT axis. The hypothalamus also regulates the hypothalamic-pituitary-adrenal (HPA) axis, involved in stress response and metabolic regulation. When an individual is faced with a stressor, the hypothalamus secretes CRH, which prompts the pituitary gland to secrete ACTH. ACTH then stimulates the adrenal cortex to secrete glucocorticoids, primarily cortisol, which helps to modulate the body's stress response and metabolic activities. This process highlights the necessity for precise feedback mechanisms that not only enable the body's adaptation to stress but also its total endocrine equilibrium. Significantly, even though TRH and CRH mechanisms are well understood, there remain a number of areas to explore, most significantly, how these mechanisms interact with cellular metabolic processes (Baarendse et al., 2008). In addition to their role as regulators of other endocrine glands, the pituitary and hypothalamus also utilize complex glycosylation pathways, which have an impact on hormone production and function. For instance, thyrotropin-stimulating hormone (TSH) and thyroglobulin (Tg) are both prone to glycosylation, and this affects their stability and functionality. The complex interaction implies that alterations in glycosylation can lead to abnormal hormonal activities and consequently contribute to various metabolic diseases. The evidence indicates that alterations in the glycosylation of thyroid proteins might be linked with long-term diseases such as thyroid cancers and autoimmune diseases. Therefore, the glycosylation complexity can provide more insight into the interaction of the pituitary gland and hypothalamus and further detail the biochemical foundation of endocrine control of hormones.

2.5.1. Hormonal Signaling Pathways

The hypothalamus and pituitary gland play a central part in the regulation of hormonal signal pathways that influence most of the physiological processes within the body. The hypothalamus serves as the integration center, integrating the signals from the endocrine system as well as the nervous system to maintain homeostasis. It releases the releasing and inhibiting hormones that regulate the secretion of hormones of the anterior pituitary gland. This dynamic interaction maintains bodily functions such as growth, metabolism, and stress responses in a precise balance. For instance, when the body's stress level elevates, the hypothalamus releases CRH, which stimulates the pituitary gland to release ACTH, which ultimately results in the synthesis of cortisol by the adrenal glands. These circuits demonstrate the crucial function played by hypothalamic signaling in the regulation of metabolic balance and response to environmental stress, reaffirming its importance as part of the extended network of hormonal signaling (Al-Kufaishi et al., 2024). Hormonal signaling pathways from the pituitary gland are also indicative of its essential function in the endocrine system. The anterior pituitary releases different critical hormones, including thyroid-stimulating hormone (TSH), luteinizing hormone (LH), and follicle-stimulating hormone (FSH). They act on multiple target organs, including the thyroid, ovaries, and testes, to regulate a wide range of physiological functions, from reproductive health to metabolism. Notably, release of the gonadotropins LH and FSH is under tight regulation by the hypothalamic hormone gonadotropin-releasing hormone (GnRH). This interaction is a tightly regulated feedback loop in which hypothalamic signaling has a direct impact on pituitary function, thereby impacting downstream cascades of hormones that regulate reproductive processes. The interdependence of the organs emphasizes the complexity of hormonal communication as well as the central role that the pituitary and hypothalamus play in endocrine regulation (Xu et al., 2023). An appreciation of these pathways of hormonal signaling also sheds light on their involvement in health and disease. Dysregulation of the hypothalamus-pituitary axis results in a number of endocrine disorders, including stress response, growth, and reproductive disorders. For example, elevated cortisol due to chronic stress alters the metabolic function and hormonal balance and results in disease states like Cushing's syndrome. Pathophysiology of such diseases relies heavily on continued exploration of the signaling pathways of hormones. As technology improves, molecular research has identified the differentially expressed genes in the pituitary and hypothalamus responsible for numerous physiological effects, illustrating how hormone signaling pathways can be targeted for treatment. Thus, knowing about these pathways is not just important for gaining insight into normal physiological regulation but also to address clinical issues arising from endocrine disturbances (Al-Kufaishi et al., 2024; Xu et al., 2023).

2.5.2. Feedback Mechanisms

In the intricate pituitary gland-hypothalamus interaction, feedback mechanisms play a vital role in the regulation of homeostasis of the endocrine system. The hypothalamus, the master control unit, produces releasing and inhibiting hormones specific to the action on the pituitary gland. These hormones stimulate or inhibit the secretion of anterior pituitary hormones, which in turn influence numerous bodily physiological functions. Most significantly, the pituitary gland's reaction to these hypothalamic stimuli is controlled by feedback from hormones of target organs. When peripheral hormone secretion is best, it informs the hypothalamus and pituitary to reduce hormone synthesis. This demonstration illustrates how the hypothalamus and pituitary work together to regulate essential functions, ensuring endocrine homeostasis and allowing body systems to function smoothly. The hypothalamic and pituitary interactions are also made more complicated by the action of adipocytokines, which serve as significant peripheral signals. These hormones, which are released from fat, influence pituitary gland activity, thereby forming a further layer of regulatory feedback. Research indicates that various adipokines, such as adiponectin and resistin, are expressed in the pituitary gland and can influence the secretion of its hormones. For example, increased levels of certain adipokines may enhance the pituitary's sensitivity to hypothalamic signals and hence augment hormonal releases involved in metabolism as well as reproduction. This interaction also validates the delicate balance between endocrine regulation and energy homeostasis. Having caused appropriate physiological responses, such hormones provide negative feedback to the pituitary and hypothalamus in order to limit further secretion, hence overall system balance, showing the complexity of involved feedback processes for hormonal health in the body (Kaminska et al., 2024). Advances in research technology have brought into focus the importance of studying feedback processes within the hypothalamic–pituitary axis through novel models, such as the hypothalamic–pituitary (HP) axis-on-a-chip. Conventional 2D culture models never model the complex neuroendocrine communication between these essential tissues. The HP axis-on-a-chip incorporates cell types from the hypothalamus and pituitary domain, enabling more realistic simulations of their interactions under changing conditions. This model enables the examination of feedback mechanisms in real time, hence offering information on neuroendocrine crosstalk, which could be influenced by factors external to the system, e.g., toxins. For instance, the understanding of how SERPINB2 is a strong neuroendocrine toxic marker demonstrates the way in which feedback loops are disrupted by undesirable environmental conditions, bringing to the fore the advantages and liabilities of the hypothalamic and pituitary response (Park et al., 2024) (Figure 2.14).

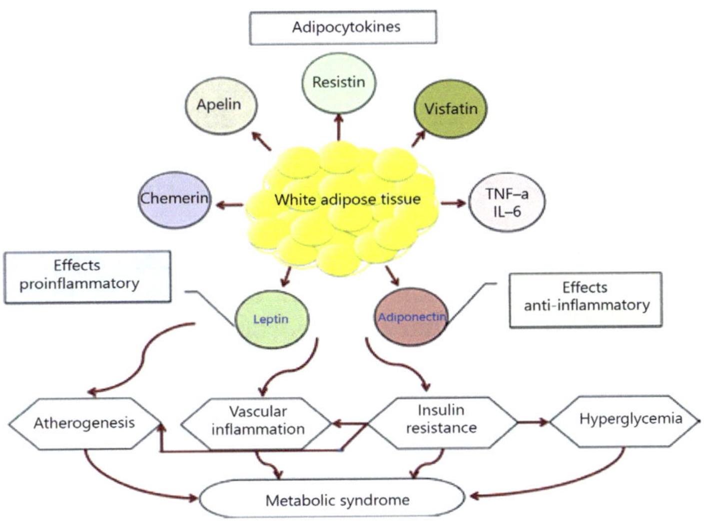

Figure 2.14. Functions of adipocytokines. Several adipocytokines produced by white adipose tissue are shown, along with their roles in inflammatory processes, insulin resistance, and atherogenesis, as well as their correlation with metabolic syndrome.

Source: https://www.researchgate.net/profile/Maria-Gunturiz/publication/348060231/figure/fig1/AS:974835228352512@1609430238487/Some-functions-of-adipocytokines-Several-of-the-different-adipocytokines-produced-by.png.

2.5.3. Role in Maintaining Homeostasis

The hypothalamus is a crucial component in maintaining homeostasis in the human body by regulating various physiological activities. This small but efficient structure is a bridge between the endocrine and nervous systems. It integrates complex feedback systems that are responsible for regulating body temperature, hunger, thirst, sleep, and circadian rhythms in a manner that maintains internal conditions stable regardless of changes in the environment. For example, thermoregulation is predominantly controlled by the hypothalamus, which responds to a change in body temperature and triggers mechanisms like sweating or shivering to restore the body to its normal temperature range. Via its complex system of neuroendocrine feedback, the hypothalamus constantly scans the body's status and adjusts as needed to keep the body at homeostasis, demonstrating its crucial contribution to physiological balance. The pituitary gland assists the hypothalamus in maintaining homeostasis by regulating the release of hormones. The pituitary has been referred to as the master gland because it releases a variety of hormones that influence other endocrine glands and bodily functions. The anterior pituitary, for example, secretes hormones such as ACTH, which stimulates the adrenal glands to secrete glucocorticoids that play a crucial role in stress response and metabolic regulation. This interaction between the pituitary and the hypothalamus is a quintessential example of the feedback loop that is required for homeostasis. Glucocorticoids, through their effect on the glucocorticoid receptor, play crucial roles in the regulation of metabolism, homeostasis, and making adaptive responses to environmental challenges (Piechota et al., 2025). The concerted secretion of hormones is indicative of the interconnectedness of the hypothalamic-pituitary axis in regulating critical physiological parameters essential for survival. Moreover, pituitary and hypothalamic regulation of the reproductive hormones is important for homeostatic control, particularly in women. The prolactin and estrogen interaction is a good example of such interaction; the estrogen regulates the amount of prolactin in the pituitary, which, in turn, is vital during reproduction and lactation. Interestingly, administration of estrogen centrally during lactation has been reported to reduce prolactin levels in lactating women, indicating a refined feedback mechanism that supports homeostasis of hormones (Yu et al., 2024). This mechanism illustrates how the hypothalamus, through modulation of estrogen receptors, can influence the secretion of prolactin and, consequently, reproductive health. These regulatory mechanisms are not only vital to the provision of adequate reproductive function but also to the upkeep of overall physiological balance, indicating the significance of the hypothalamic-pituitary axis in homeostatic control.

Test Your Knowledge

1. How does the hypothalamus communicate with the anterior pituitary gland to regulate hormone secretion?
2. What is the function of the hypothalamic-pituitary portal system in endocrine signaling?
3. How do the hypothalamus and pituitary gland work together to maintain homeostasis?

2.6. Disorders Related to the Hypothalamus and Pituitary Gland

Learning Outcome

1. Define hypopituitarism;
2. Describe diabetes insipidus disorder;
3. Explain Cushing's disease.

Hypothalamus and pituitary gland disease encompasses a range of conditions with profound impacts on hormonal equilibrium and body function as a whole. The hypothalamus plays a pivotal part in the regulation of endocrine function via control of the pituitary gland, which subsequently secretes hormones that influence a number of body physiological processes, including growth, metabolism, and reproduction. Dysfunction of this complex system may lead to a variety of disorders such as hypopituitarism, which is a deficiency of one or more of the pituitary hormones and is characterized by symptoms such as fatigue, weight alteration, and reproductive dysfunction. Such disorders are significant as they can greatly hamper an individual's quality of life and require substantial medical care for management. Besides hormone deficiency, the pituitary gland and hypothalamus are also implicated in conditions leading to excess of hormones. For instance, benign tumors arising in the pituitary gland, known as pituitary adenomas, can lead to oversecretion of hormones, such as Cushing's disease or acromegaly following excess cortisol and GH, respectively. Such conditions carry significant health consequences, like metabolic and psychosocial complications. Additionally, since these conditions are likely to progress over time, patients may not experience symptoms immediately, resulting in delays in diagnosis and treatment. Continuous monitoring and earlier intervention can improve patient outcomes through the treatment of hormonal imbalance prior to progression to more complicated health issues. Pharmacological treatment is a fundamental intervention in the management of disorders of the hypothalamus and pituitary gland, particularly in treating hormonal abnormalities resulting from external agents, e.g., drugs. Research has depicted an immediate need for information regarding the effect of various drugs on thyroid function, which is closely tied to the hypothalamic-pituitary-thyroid axis. Antiepileptics and glucocorticoids, among other drugs, have been shown to induce thyroid dysfunction, which creates a challenge to clinicians in how to effectively treat patients with such medication (Bacinschi et al., 2024). Additionally, advancements in radiation therapy techniques, particularly in the use of protons as opposed to photons, highlight the importance of minimizing the exposure of radiation to strategic sites such as the pituitary and hypothalamus in cancer treatments (Regentova et al., 2024). This highlights the importance of interdisciplinary treatment methods in endocrinology, pharmacology, and oncology to enhance patient care in disorders related to these areas of the brain.

2.6.1. Hypopituitarism

The intricate interplay of the hypothalamus and pituitary gland is critical in maintaining hormonal homeostasis within the body. Hypopituitarism, characterized by decreased secretion of pituitary hormones, typically results from endocrine axis dysfunction. Hypopituitarism is caused by varied etiologies such as pituitary adenoma, head trauma, infection, and genetic disorders. When approximately 75% of the gland is involved, there is a spectrum of clinical presentations ranging from mild to severe. Furthermore, the prevalence of this disorder is very low, with studies demonstrating approximately 45.5 per 100,000 individuals. Because of its multiple causes, the diagnosis of hypopituitarism can be delayed for several years, emphasizing the need for greater awareness of its clinical presentations and implications. One of the implications of hypopituitarism is that it has a link to mental health disorders. Research has argued that individuals with the condition are at increased risk of depression and anxiety, particularly in women and adults over 18 years of age, in which women's risk of depression was ten times that of men (Mikołaj et al., 2025). The GH deficiency with hypopituitarism has also been linked with cognitive impairment and other forms of atypical depression, further illustrating the ways in which pituitary failure can affect not only physical, but mental, health as well. Historical accounts, such as the 1949 Sheehan and Summer report, have documented that nearly one-third of hypopituitary patients demonstrated reduced drive and social withdrawal, bearing witness to the extremely devastating effect of endocrine dysregulation on mental health (Mikołaj et al., 2025).

The treatment context for hypopituitarism is complex because it needs a multi-dimensional approach specifically tailored to each patient's hormone deficiencies. Hormone replacement therapy is the cornerstone of management that restores hormonal balance and alleviates physical and psychological symptoms. Of particular interest, treatment with GH is effective in improving cognitive function and in decreasing the severity of depression in patients with this condition, particularly those with traumatic brain injury (Mikołaj et al., 2025). Though some patients do have an acute response to treatment, withdrawal from these treatments worsens psychiatric symptoms as well as cognitive impairment, which underscores the necessity for long-term treatment. Ultimately, addressing the psychosocial challenges that afflict individuals with hypopituitarism is necessary, encouraging a holistic treatment in favor of physical as well as psychological well-being (Mikołaj et al., 2025) (Figure 2.15).

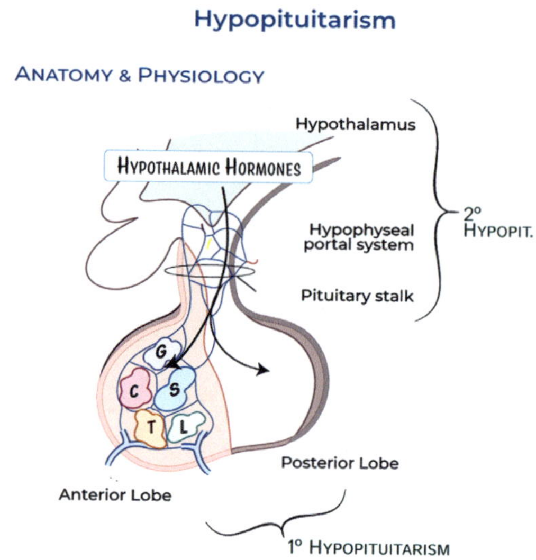

Figure 2.15. Hypopituitarism illustration.

Source: https://d1j63owfs0b5j3.cloudfront.net/term/images/hypopituitarism-5842.png.

2.6.2. Diabetes Insipidus

Diabetes insipidus (DI) is an endocrine disease characterized by polydipsia and the formation of large quantities of watery urine, fundamental issues caused by a deficiency of the antidiuretic hormone (ADH), or vasopressin. The hormone, synthesized in the hypothalamus and secreted from the posterior pituitary gland, is the one accountable for ensuring balanced amounts of water within the body. The lack of ADH causes a failure of the kidneys to concentrate urine, and there is a hyperosmolar state. It is essential to understand the neuroendocrine mechanism that controls ADH production and release so one can understand how disturbances in these mechanisms lead to the clinical presentation of DI. Ultimately, this relationship between the hypothalamus and the pituitary gland is an impetus for why endocrine control of homeostasis is so important. The pathophysiology of DI is classified into central and nephrogenic forms. Central diabetes insipidus is typically the consequence of damage to the pituitary gland or hypothalamus by various causes such as trauma, tumors, or genetic abnormalities associated with the secretion of ADH. Nephrogenic diabetes insipidus, however, is due to resistance of the kidneys to ADH, primarily due to genetic conditions or the consumption of certain drugs that are antihormonal in action. Both refer to the key roles of the hypothalamus and pituitary gland in body water balance.

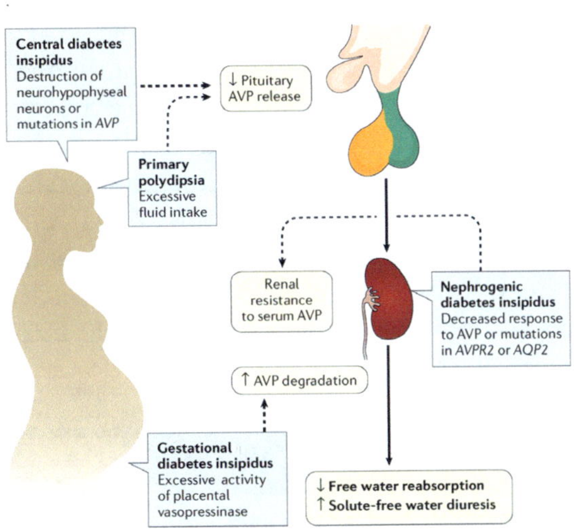

Figure 2.16. Diabetes insipidus (DI) is a form of polyuria–polydipsia syndrome caused by various acquired or hereditary lesions or disorders.

Source: https://www.researchgate.net/profile/Morris-Goldman/publication/335054047/figure/fig1/AS:941116233154 57@1601389904314/Pathophysiology-of-DI-Diabetes-insipidus-DI-is-a-form-of-polyuria-polydipsia.png.

Moreover, as elaborated in more recent literature, understanding genes and proteins that contribute to water balance can provide insight into mechanisms behind these disorders in order to enable more mechanistic diagnosis and management (Mark et al., 2015). In the clinical scenario, the treatment and assessment of diabetes insipidus are highly dependent on the underlying cause and symptoms of the patient. Although the usual treatments involve desmopressin infusion for central DI, the treatment of nephrogenic forms is usually a combination of dietary management and the use of thiazide diuretics. Monitoring the intake of fluid and the output of urine still plays a crucial role in managing these patients, so as to avoid putting them at risk of dehydration or electrolyte imbalance. One should also investigate any potential complications that may arise from an untreated DI, including hypernatremia or renal injury. Advances in research are essential to comprehend the complexities of ADH and regulation that can further enhance therapeutic interventions and patient care (Briet et al., 2015) (Figure 2.16).

2.6.3. Cushing's Disease

Cushing's disease is a typical pathological condition expressed by hypercortisolism, usually due to an ACTH-secreting pituitary adenoma. This form of hypercortisolism displays the intricate interaction between the pituitary gland and hypothalamus in regulating endocrine function. The hypothalamus releases CRH, which results in the release of ACTH from the pituitary gland. ACTH then causes the release of cortisol from the adrenal glands. When this feedback mechanism is interrupted by tumors of the pituitary gland, cortisol levels get excessively high to cause an abundance of complications, including metabolic syndrome, cardiovascular disease, and immune suppression. This maladaptation response not only illustrates the importance of pituitary output but also signifies the great significance of hypothalamic input, leading to the pathophysiology of Cushing's disease. Understanding of the importance of Cushing's disease is pivotal beyond its direct effect on physiology, to encompass important psychological and emotional effects. The patient will present with changes in mood, depression, and anxiety secondary to hypercortisolemia, reflecting the long-documented effect of the hormone on the central nervous system. The hypercortisolism also impacts corticosteroid-sensitive neurotransmitter systems that exacerbate mental illnesses. Perhaps most notably, the intricate feedback loop between the hypothalamus, the pituitary gland, and the adrenal cortex is further complicated in the context of stress-related conditions such as the long-term conundrum of the COVID-19 pandemic. For instance, glucocorticoids like cortisol can alter the homeostatic balance of the hypothalamic-pituitary-adrenal (HPA) axis, and in the most severe conditions, lead to adrenal insufficiency due to inherent disorders aggravated by conditions like infection and inflammation (Jensterle et al., 2022). Treatment for Cushing's disease is typically achieved through the remission of the underlying pituitary tumor and regulation of normal cortisol levels. Surgical intervention, through transsphenoidal resection, is generally the treatment of choice in cases of localized pituitary adenomas. Where surgery is contraindicated or where adjuvant treatment is needed, therapy can be applied to manage cortisol secretion. Agents such as ketoconazole, metyrapone, and pasireotide interfere with adrenal hormone synthesis or block ACTH action. These therapeutic actions exemplify the significance of hypothalamic-pituitary interaction, as it is necessary to regulate the pituitary function to enhance the signs of Cushing's disease and restore the overall hormonal balance of the patients. In addition, the interaction between the hormonal axis and peripheral factors such as adipokines renders the condition even more complex to treat, and the need to follow a multifaceted approach will become unavoidable (Kaminska et al., 2024).

Test Your Knowledge

1. What is hypopituitarism, and what are some common symptoms caused by this disorder?
2. Describe the cause and primary symptoms of diabetes insipidus related to the hypothalamus or pituitary gland.
3. What hormone is overproduced in Cushing's disease, and which gland is typically responsible for this overproduction?

SUMMARY

The intricate interaction between the pituitary gland and the hypothalamus is essential to the body's homeostasis and regulation of key physiological processes. As the hub for endocrine signaling, this duo integrates a myriad of functions, from metabolism to stress response and reproductive function. Their interconnectedness affords us a profound understanding of how hormonal imbalance may underlie a range of disorders. Medical imaging, particularly MRI, has enhanced our ability to image these glands significantly, allowing us to better delineate their anatomy and variability across populations, as research aimed at defining normative measurements within diverse populations exemplifies (Krishna et al., 2024). Such studies highlight the importance of placing hormonal function within anatomical and physiological contexts. In addition, recent studies place greater focus on estrogen receptors within the hypothalamic-pituitary region, particularly in psychiatric conditions. More recent research employing positron emission tomography (PET) has examined the quantification of these receptors, collecting valuable knowledge regarding how changing hormones can influence mood and cognition. For instance, results of studies involving [18F]FES PET scans illustrate quantifiable receptor availability change, particularly after selective estrogen receptor degrader use (Ghazanfari et al., 2024). Such an observation not only advances our comprehension of the impact of hormones on mental health but also calls attention to the potential of targeted therapies that might be realized from such insight. So, it is imperative to integrate research at both the anatomical and biochemical levels to develop precise and integrated treatment modalities. An integrative understanding of the hypothalamic-pituitary axis provides a solid foundation for addressing a wide range of health issues. The exploration of anatomical differences and receptor dynamics provides valuable information that can guide clinical practices and therapeutic interventions. As science progresses, it becomes clearer that factors such as gender, age, and receptor availability ensnare each other to influence overall health. This intricate process highlights not only the need for more research into the pituitary gland and hypothalamus but also for collaborative models integrating endocrinology and neurobiology. Ultimately, a greater understanding of such systems can lead to improved patient outcomes for patients suffering from hormone-disorder conditions and mental illness.

The pituitary and the hypothalamus form core parts of the endocrine system, serving as significant controllers of several physiological processes. The hypothalamus serves as a liaison between the endocrine system and nervous system, integrating neural messages to create and release some hormones. They have a direct action on the pituitary gland, which is referred to as the master gland due to its ability to govern other endocrine glands in the body. The intricate feedback pathways and mechanisms created by these two organs reflect their fundamental role in homeostasis, with their regulation extending to processes such as metabolism, growth, and stress. Understanding the mechanisms by which the pituitary and hypothalamus operate sheds light on the greater complexities of endocrine regulation and physiological adaptation. One such area of study has identified the role of long non-coding RNAs (lncRNAs) in the regulation of gene expression, particularly in relation to the HPA axis. The evidence suggests that lncRNAs can control the activity of genes, providing insight into the complexity of phenotypes in various species. For instance, studies that have involved the use of RNA-Seq data have provided evidence for differential expression patterns among lncRNAs in primary organs such as the hypothalamus and pituitary gland. This is particularly relevant in the context of feed efficiency in livestock, where some lncRNAs have been associated with the regulation of hormone production and metabolism. Research into such interactions not only promotes greater understanding of endocrine interactions but also leads to the doorway of enhanced animal management and selection processes, revealing the promise of genomic information in improving productivity. In conclusion, the coordinated function of the pituitary gland and hypothalamus plays a key role in body balance, as well as impacting various physiological and metabolic processes. The emerging role of lncRNAs along this axis is an emerging research area, marking potential mechanisms of regulation that show the intricacies of hormonal control. As further studies continue to uncover new lncRNAs associated with traits of individuals, for example, feed efficiency, the impact on human health and livestock management is far-reaching. Through the discovery and understanding of the regulatory networks that are present, scientists can better describe how genetic expression is connected to phenotypic outcomes, eventually advancing endocrinology and its practices within agriculture and medicine.

KEY TERMS FROM THIS CHAPTER

- Anterior pituitary
- Behavioral responses
- Differential diagnoses
- Endocrine function
- Environmental stresses
- Glucose regulation
- Growth hormone (GH)
- Hormonal messages
- Hormone production
- Autonomic nervous system functions
- Blood pressure
- Endocrine dysfunctions
- Endocrine signaling
- Fertility abnormalities
- Gonadotropin-releasing hormone (GnRH)
- Hormonal activity
- Hormonal therapy
- Hypothalamic-pituitary axis

CRITICAL THINKING QUESTIONS

1. **Which hormone is secreted by the hypothalamus to stimulate the anterior pituitary?**
    a. Oxytocin
    b. Thyrotropin-releasing hormone (TRH)
    c. Antidiuretic hormone (ADH)
    d. Growth hormone (GH)
2. **Which part of the pituitary gland stores and releases hormones produced by the hypothalamus?**
    a. Anterior pituitary
    b. Intermediate lobe
    c. Posterior pituitary
    d. Pars distalis
3. **The hormone responsible for stimulating milk production in mammary glands is:**
    a. Prolactin
    b. Luteinizing hormone (LH)
    c. Follicle-stimulating hormone (FSH)
    d. Corticotropin
4. **Which of the following hormones is released directly by the posterior pituitary gland?**
    a. Thyroid-stimulating hormone (TSH)
    b. Oxytocin
    c. Adrenocorticotropic hormone (ACTH)
    d. Growth hormone (GH)
5. **The hypothalamus controls the pituitary gland mainly through:**
    a. Neural signals only
    b. Direct hormone secretion into the general circulation
    c. Electrical impulses in the spinal cord
    d. Blood vessels called the hypothalamo-hypophyseal portal system

Short Answer Questions

1. Where is the hypothalamus located, and how is it anatomically connected to the pituitary gland?
2. Name three major nuclei of the hypothalamus involved in endocrine regulation and their functions.
3. What are the main differences between the anterior and posterior lobes of the pituitary gland in terms of hormone production?
4. How does the hypothalamic-pituitary portal system facilitate hormone signaling?
5. Which hormones are secreted by the posterior pituitary, and what are their primary physiological roles?
6. Explain the negative feedback loop involving the hypothalamus, pituitary gland, and adrenal cortex.
7. What are the clinical consequences of damage to the hypothalamus or pituitary gland? Provide two examples.
8. How do the hypothalamus and pituitary gland coordinate the body's response to stress?

Answers to Critical Thinking Questions

1. (b); 2. (c); 3. (a); 4. (b); 5. (d)

REFERENCES

1. Aarskog, T., Acampora, D., Agarwal, N., Aijaz, N., Alba, R., Ambrosetti, D., Ambrosetti, G., et al. (2009). Genetic regulation of pituitary gland development in human and mouse. https://core.ac.uk/download/1688593.pdf (accessed on 22nd July 2025).
2. Agam, M., & Zada, G. (2018). Complications associated with transsphenoidal pituitary surgery. *Neurosurgery, 65*, 69–73. https://doi.org/10.1093/neuros/nyy160 (accessed on 22nd July 2025).
3. Alexandre, P. A., Reverter, A., Berezin, R. B., Porto-Neto, L. R., Ribeiro, G., Santana, M. H. A., Ferraz, J. B. S., et al. (2020). Exploring the regulatory potential of long non-coding RNA in feed efficiency of indicine cattle. *Genes, 11*, 997–997. https://doi.org/10.3390/genes11090997 (accessed on 22nd July 2025).
4. Alexandre, P. A., Reverter, A., Porto-Neto, L. R., Berezin, R. B., Ribeiro, G., Santana, M. H. A., Ferraz, J. B. S., et al. (2020). Exploring the regulatory potential of long non-coding RNA in feed efficiency of indicine cattle. https://doi.org/10.20944/preprints202007.0711.v1 (accessed on 22nd July 2025).
5. Al-Kufaishi, A., & Al-Musawi, N. J. T. (2024). Hypothalamus-pituitary-adrenal axis in patients with post-traumatic stress disorders and related to oxidative stress. *Hormone Molecular Biology and Clinical Investigation, 45*, 157–164. https://www.semanticscholar.org/paper/d2d0b94e75d5d4f804bda985098599c69881194d (accessed on 22nd July 2025).
6. Al-Samerria, S., & Radovick, S. (2021). The role of insulin-like growth factor-1 (IGF-1) in the control of neuroendocrine regulation of growth. *Cells, 10*, 2664–2664. https://doi.org/10.3390/cells10102664 (accessed on 22nd July 2025).
7. Baarendse, P. J. J., Brand, H., van den Bruggeman, V., et al. (2008). Involvement of the hypothalamic-pituitary-thyroid axis and its interaction with the hypothalamic-pituitary-adrenal axis in the ontogeny of avian thermoregulation: A review. https://core.ac.uk/download/pdf/29259797.pdf (accessed on 22nd July 2025).
8. Bacinschi, S., Chicu-Hadirca, C., & Vudu, L. (2024). Drug-induced thyroid gland dysfunctions. *Public Health, Economy and Management in Medicine*. https://www.semanticscholar.org/paper/dab9bf51cce7a738e6c3aa40ecfb9a20d4cfc00b (accessed on 22nd July 2025).
9. Bellingham, M., Cotinot, C., Evans, N. P., Fowler, P. A., et al. (2016). Timing of maternal exposure and fetal sex determine the effects of low-level chemical mixture exposure on the fetal neuroendocrine system in sheep. https://core.ac.uk/download/74230048.pdf (accessed on 22nd July 2025).
10. Briet, C., Salenave, S., Bonneville, J. F., Laws, E. R., & Chanson, P. (2015). Pituitary apoplexy. *Endocrine Reviews, 36*, 622–645. https://doi.org/10.1210/er.2015-1042 (accessed on 22nd July 2025).
11. Butt, A., & Azhar, M. J. (2024). Unveiling the psychiatric dimensions of hypopituitarism: Investigating associations, challenges, and treatment strategies. *JPMA. The Journal of the Pakistan Medical Association, 74*(10), 1898–1899. https://www.semanticscholar.org/paper/e190c3e8fdd4e165bdead6f58ff79565c7303d85 (accessed on 22nd July 2025).
12. Cardon, S. Z., & Iberall, A. S. (2025). A study on dynamic systems response of the performance characteristics of some major biophysical systems. https://core.ac.uk/download/pdf/80680406.pdf (accessed on 22nd July 2025).

13. Cimini, V., Van Noorden, S., Terlizzi, C., & Altobelli, G. G. (2022). Calcium/calmodulin-dependent kinases in the hypothalamus, pituitary, and pineal gland: An overview. *International Journal of Endocrinology, 2022*. https://www.semanticscholar.org/paper/ed0bff28d3ad2d0550772403c4430ed61a96cd4b (accessed on 22nd July 2025).

14. Clavijo, R., & Hsiao, W. (2018). Update on male reproductive endocrinology. https://core.ac.uk/download/323070097.pdf (accessed on 22nd July 2025).

15. Cryan, J. F., O'Riordan, K. J., Cowan, C. S. M., Sandhu, K. V., Bastiaanssen, T. F. S., Boehme, M., Codagnone, M. G., et al. (2019). The microbiota-gut-brain axis. *Physiological Reviews, 99*, 1877–2013. https://doi.org/10.1152/physrev.00018.2018 (accessed on 22nd July 2025).

16. Dizdarevic, K., Alsuwat, M. A., Alrubie, S. S., & Alrubaei, F. S. (2024). Pear-shaped craniopharyngioma: Selection of the transcranial approach with respect to topographical classifications. *Cureus, 16*. https://www.semanticscholar.org/paper/92415aeffe1411883d13dbddabce898d4a5c7c1e (accessed on 22nd July 2025).

17. Emrich, F., Gomes, B. H., Selvatici-Tolentino, L., Lopes, R. A., Secio-Silva, A., Carvalho-Moreira, J. P., Bittencourt-Silva, P. G., et al. (2024). Hypothyroidism alters the rhythmicity of the central clock, body temperature and metabolism: Evidence of Bmal1 transcriptional regulation by T3. *The Journal of Physiology, 602*. https://www.semanticscholar.org/paper/4248116e68d07502bebcf587cf36e0bb9e1be934 (accessed on 22nd July 2025).

18. Ghazanfari, N., Doorduin, J., van der Weijden, C. W. J., Willemsen, A., Glaudemans, A., van Waarde, A., Dierckx, R. A., et al. (2024). Pharmacokinetic analysis of [18F]FES PET in the human brain and pituitary gland. *Molecular Imaging and Biology, 26*, 351–359. https://www.semanticscholar.org/paper/105793d3f644b3f6810f2c8d2808b7d59b921cc3 (accessed on 22nd July 2025).

19. Glastonbury, C., Osborn, A., & Salzman, K. (2011). Masses and malformations of the third ventricle: Normal anatomic relationships and differential diagnoses. *Radiographic: A Review Publication of the Radiological Society of North America, Inc., 31*(7), 1889–1905. https://www.semanticscholar.org/paper/1345a1a3d011b4c783a8c3a755f80563031cfb31 (accessed on 22nd July 2025).

20. Goadsby, P. J., Holland, P. R., Martins-Oliveira, M., Hoffmann, J., Schankin, C. J., & Akerman, S. (2017). Pathophysiology of migraine: A disorder of sensory processing. *Physiological Reviews, 97*, 553–622. https://doi.org/10.1152/physrev.00034.2015 (accessed on 22nd July 2025).

21. Iadecola, C., & Ishii, M. (2015). Metabolic and non-cognitive manifestations of Alzheimer's disease: The hypothalamus as both culprit and target of pathology. https://core.ac.uk/download/pdf/82094082.pdf (accessed on 22nd July 2025).

22. Janicka, L., Dajnowska, A., & Arciszewski, M. (2025). Role of proopiomelanocortin (POMC) derivatives in body weight regulation: A review of current knowledge and significance in the pathogenesis of obesity in mammals. *Medycyna Weterynaryjna*. https://www.semanticscholar.org/paper/e05ea4d08172099fabcfc71aacbc8a86d1fbaa0b (accessed on 22nd July 2025).

23. Jensterle, M., Herman, R., Janež, A., Mahmeed, W., Al-Rasadi, K., Al-Alawi, K., Banach, M., et al. (2022). The relationship between COVID-19 and hypothalamic–pituitary–adrenal axis: A large spectrum from glucocorticoid insufficiency to excess—The CAPISCO International Expert Panel. *International Journal of Molecular Sciences, 23*. https://www.semanticscholar.org/paper/65a128435ed1d0852f5888f73ad6baa53f165c2e (accessed on 22nd July 2025).

24. Kaminska, B., Kurowicka, B., Kieżun, M., Dobrzyn, K., Kisielewska, K., Gudelska, M., Kopij, G., et al. (2024). The role of adipokines in the control of pituitary functions. *Animals: An Open Access Journal from MDPI, 14*. https://www.semanticscholar.org/paper/a1feda9a72de0265ccc9f38597ea68315e0209f3 (accessed on 22nd July 2025).

25. Knepper, M. A., Kwon, T. H., & Nielsen, S. (2015). Molecular physiology of water balance. *New England Journal of Medicine, 372*, 1349–1358. https://doi.org/10.1056/nejmra1404726 (accessed on 22nd July 2025).

26. Knight, J., Andrade Sienz, M., & Bayram-Weston, Z. (2021). Endocrine system 2: Hypothalamus and pituitary gland. https://core.ac.uk/download/478091231.pdf (accessed on 22nd July 2025).

27. Krishna, G. K., Bopaiah, H., Sakalecha, A. K., & Joy, L. (2024). Morphometric analysis of pituitary gland using magnetic resonance imaging in Indian subjects. *Asian Journal of Medical Sciences*. https://www.semanticscholar.org/paper/7c08e8a053e59e17170cd9a47dfdeaf50ded0a46 (accessed on 22nd July 2025).

28. Kubiak, M., Majewska, W., Kachel, M., Dola, A., Koga, W., Nowakowska, J., Langwiński, W., et al. (2025). Lithium treatment increases FKBP5 protein but not mRNA expression in the pituitary gland of depressive-like rats. *Brain Sciences, 15*. https://www.semanticscholar.org/paper/975404a2cb442656d945fb42951727a502135582 (accessed on 22nd July 2025).

29. Lauretta, R., Sansone, A., Sansone, M., Romanelli, F., & Appetecchia, M. (2019). Endocrine disrupting chemicals: Effects on endocrine glands. *Frontiers in Endocrinology, 10*. https://doi.org/10.3389/fendo.2019.00178 (accessed on 22nd July 2025).

30. Lewis, J. E., & Ebling, F. J. P. (2017). Tanycytes as regulators of seasonal cycles in neuroendocrine function. *Frontiers in Neurology, 8*. https://doi.org/10.3389/fneur.2017.00079 (accessed on 22nd July 2025).

31. Meng, F., Wu, Y., Yu, Y., Bu, G., Du, X., Liang, Q., Cao, X., et al. (2023). Spexin2 is a novel food regulator in *Gallus gallus*. *International Journal of Molecular Sciences, 24*. https://www.semanticscholar.org/paper/b48301840337415de000766f21cbb392c48efb34 (accessed on 22nd July 2025).

32. Milleniari, Rr. F. D. I. (2023). Neuroendocrine: The hypothalamus-pituitary-adrenal axis and the relation to stroke. *Ganesha Medicine*. https://www.semanticscholar.org/paper/bc92f9b0f3d2b5758bce6e689f0a62fee1f871df (accessed on 22nd July 2025).

33. Morris, J. (2021). Functional anatomy of the hypothalamus and pituitary. *Oxford Textbook of Endocrinology and Diabetes 3e*. https://www.semanticscholar.org/paper/b4a836473e06922ca9e3facc756987d8343ff338 (accessed on 22nd July 2025).

34. Najla, A., Majed, A., & Abdulhameed, A. (2017). A novel mutation leading to leptin receptor deficiency and subsequent childhood morbid obesity. *4*, 1, 2. https://www.semanticscholar.org/paper/d1d7171d48323b3dd46eef81f6725e6eeb76a256 (accessed on 22nd July 2025).

35. Park, S. R., Kook, M. G., Kim, S. R., Lee, J., Yu, Y. S., Park, C. H., Lim, S., et al. (2024). A microscale 3D organ on a chip for recapitulating reciprocal neuroendocrine crosstalk between the hypothalamus and the pituitary gland. *Bio Fabrication, 16*. https://www.semanticscholar.org/paper/d919b8280719d6dc046295ade944bee693dc7b63 (accessed on 22nd July 2025).

36. Piechota, M., Zięba, M., Borczyk, M., Gołda, S., Hajto, J., Skupio, U., Slezak, M., et al. (2025).

A cross-tissue transcriptomic approach decodes glucocorticoid receptor-dependent links to human metabolic phenotypes. *BMC Genomics, 26.* https://www.semanticscholar.org/paper/56e9301f49880a58c222f076afbb9b22299fd7f7 (accessed on 22nd July 2025).

37. Pocheć, E., Kozłowska, K., & Ząbczyńska, M. (2018). Glycosylation in the thyroid gland: Vital aspects of glycoprotein function in thyrocyte physiology and thyroid disorders. https://core.ac.uk/download/161347823.pdf (accessed on 22nd July 2025).
38. Przybył, B., Szlis, M., Misztal, A., & Wójcik-Gładysz, A. (2025). QRFP43 modulates the activity of the hypothalamic-pituitary-thyroid axis in female sheep. *Scientific Reports, 15.* https://www.semanticscholar.org/paper/d56bc12f6e9e0052d462961b5bc01cc169865c87 (accessed on 22nd July 2025).
39. Regentova, O., Shcherbenko, O., Kumirova, E., Antonenko, F., & Solodkiy, V. (2024). Proton therapy in pediatric neuro-oncology: Potential advantages and the relationship between cost and results. *Siberian Journal of Oncology.* https://www.semanticscholar.org/paper/2a40fb2211a71e5612d2e8119859ca07b01443ac (accessed on 22nd July 2025).
40. Rosenfield, R. L., & Ehrmann, D. A. (2016). The pathogenesis of polycystic ovary syndrome (PCOS): The hypothesis of PCOS as functional ovarian hyperandrogenism revisited. *Endocrine Reviews, 37,* 467–520. https://doi.org/10.1210/er.2015-1104 (accessed on 22nd July 2025).
41. Rucker, E. P. (2017). Pituitary gland functional connectivity and BMI. https://core.ac.uk/download/148695960.pdf (accessed on 22nd July 2025).
42. Simão, G. (2018). Sellar and parasellar abnormalities. *Radiologic Brasileira, 51,* IX–IX. https://www.semanticscholar.org/paper/7b5eda8b0e031c8b31ef7b4e497686b8b430f493 (accessed on 22nd July 2025).
43. Singh, G., & Gautam, V. (2023). Pituitary gland size estimation and lesion detection using segmentation-based color thresholding technique. *2023 International Conference on Sustainable Computing and Smart Systems (ICSCSS).* https://www.semanticscholar.org/paper/8472ecb3077c1e22bd1bafe59c1448406233fd20 (accessed on 22nd July 2025).
44. Xu, W., Mu, R., Gegen, T., Ran, T., Wu, Q., Wen, D., Wang, F., et al. (2023). Transcriptome analysis of hypothalamus and pituitary tissues reveals genetic mechanisms associated with high egg production rates in Changshun green-shell laying hens. *BMC Genomics, 24.* https://www.semanticscholar.org/paper/cd65935707c8370fc01f68d7d7bfffb86f3662a2 (accessed on 22nd July 2025).
45. Yan, T., Wang, R., Yao, J., & Luo, M. (2023). Single-cell transcriptomic analysis reveals rich pituitary–immune interactions under systemic inflammation. *PLOS Biology, 21.* https://www.semanticscholar.org/paper/3b5632e43c16cd4b4b951f75fa4b57ed404b1014 (accessed on 22nd July 2025).
46. Yu, M., Wang, C., & Xu, Y. (2024). 7411 Hypothalamic estrogenic signal regulates prolactin homeostasis and reproduction in female. *Journal of the Endocrine Society, 8.* https://www.semanticscholar.org/paper/5892e84ce8b4c45ff7f3b550d470e413b145479e (accessed on 22nd July 2025).
47. Zhao, W., Adjei, M., Zhang, Z., Yuan, Z., Cisang, Z., & Song, T. Z. (2023). The role of GnRH in Tibetan male sheep and goat reproduction. *Reproduction in Domestic Animals = Zuchthygiene.* https://www.semanticscholar.org/paper/e6cb8021e86df71643780b7079495771936c6fdc (accessed on 22nd July 2025).

THE THYROID GLAND

3

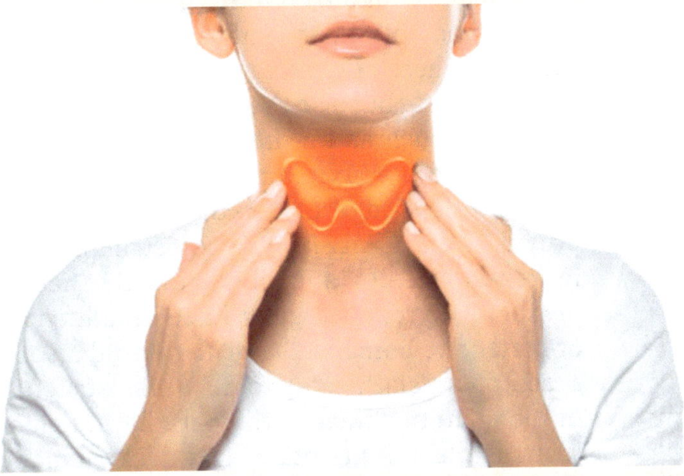

Introduction

The butterfly-inverted thyroid gland located at the base of the neck is held accountable for homeostasis as well as the body's regulation of metabolism. The function of the thyroid goes further beyond the regulation of metabolic rate; it regulates numerous functions of the body by the secretion of thyroid hormones, primarily thyroxine (T4) and triiodothyronine (T3). These hormones are essential for processes such as growth, development, and the balance of metabolic interactions between various organ systems. With a time when more individuals are suffering from metabolic disorders, being aware of the thyroid's intricate signal processing becomes all the more imperative. Evidence has validated that communication between organs, the pillar of metabolic health, relies to a great extent on thyroid gland-secreted hormones and supporting the need to explore its different roles in managing energy homeostasis and responding to outside stimulation (Castillo et al., 2019). The thyroids' function is related to quite a number of other

LEARNING OBJECTIVES

After studying this chapter, you will be able to:

1. Understand the anatomy of the thyroid gland;
2. Discuss the functions of the thyroid gland;
3. Describe thyroid hormones and their regulation;
4. Define common thyroid disorders;
5. Explain how to diagnose thyroid disorders;
6. Focus on treatment options for thyroid disorders.

organs and, hence, is an important intermediary in the endocrine system. Through synthesizing and secreting hormones that control most of the body's metabolic functions, the thyroid guides action encompassing not only metabolic regulation but also action with the central nervous system and other peripheral organs. Regulating interaction between systems allows the body to adapt to fluctuating energy needs and to attain homeostasis. Over the last few years, technological advancements have brought to light how the thyroid gland and hormones interact with some of the other most important metabolic organs like the liver, muscles, and adipose tissue (Castillo et al., 2019). Such connections highlight the necessity of an interdisciplinary investigation of the thyroid, particularly as we struggle to devise therapeutic interventions in conditions such as obesity and type 2 diabetes, where this communication may be disrupted. In addition, the understanding of thyroid physiology concerns not only the individual hormones themselves but also the more general implications of thyroid dysfunctions and their systemic ramifications. Diseases such as hypothyroidism and hyperthyroidism are classic examples of how imbalances in thyroid hormones may lead to severe metabolic disturbances, affecting a large number of functions in the body. Hypothyroidism, for instance, causes decreased expenditure of energy and weight gain, while hyperthyroidism may lead to increased metabolism and weight loss. The fact that thyroid diseases are on the rise makes it essential to study both the pathogenetic mechanisms and potential intervention techniques at length. With progressing knowledge in the area, emphasis is laid on the interaction of thyroid hormones and newly found metabolic signals that enter global energy homeostasis, thus setting the stage for future breakthroughs in the regulation of thyroid function in a more metabolic-focused medical landscape.

Definition of the Thyroid Gland

The thyroid gland, located at the back of the neck, is an essential component of the endocrine system and a pivotal role in regulating metabolism, growth, and development. The butterfly-shaped gland is composed of two lobes connected by a thin isthmus and enveloped by a fibrous capsule that underscores its function in physiological processes. One of its major functions is the production and secretion of thyroid hormones, thyroxine (T4) and triiodothyronine (T3), which play a vital role in the metabolic functions of the body. These hormones influence not only the metabolic rate but also the efficacy of other body functions, such as the heart rate, temperature control, and the functioning of other endocrine glands. Knowledge of the thyroid's definition provides insight into its widespread implications in general health and highlights the need to preserve thyroid integrity in the maintenance of metabolic homeostasis. The thyroid also has a complex relationship with other structures in the anatomy, such as the parathyroid glands responsible for maintaining calcium balance. The fact that the parathyroid glands are in close proximity to each other makes their preservation a significant factor during thyroid surgeries since any damage can contribute to massive complications like hypoparathyroidism. New imaging modalities aim to improve the identification and preservation of the parathyroid glands during thyroidectomy, suggesting the significance of this relation in surgery. Advanced methods such as near-infrared autofluorescence (NIRAF) with indocyanine green are poised to maximize surgical success by ensuring the functionality of the parathyroid glands is intact. This parathyroid-thyroid gland interaction is indicative of the intricacy and dependency of the endocrine system, warranting a multiderivative approach in surgery and clinical practice to reduce thyroid disease- and intervention-related morbidity (Karcioglu et al., 2023). The definition of the thyroid glands extends beyond its anatomical structure to encompass its physiological functions and regulatory mechanisms. The pituitary and hypothalamus control the release of thyroid hormones by a feedback mechanism that maintains levels within a narrow range. Dysregulation of this control mechanism results in thyroid pathology, hyperthyroidism, and hypothyroidism, which have a profound impact on metabolic processes and overall health. Recent studies emphasize the necessity of examining environmental and genetic factors affecting thyroid function, as shown by reports of glyoxalase 1 expression being associated with diabetic kidney disease, which implies that systemic health can also reflect on thyroid health indirectly (Adeshara et al., 2024). Its definition as thyroid glands, thus, needs to include its multi-directional interactions with other systems of the body, demonstrating the central function of its role in ensuring overall homeostasis and health (Figure 3.1).

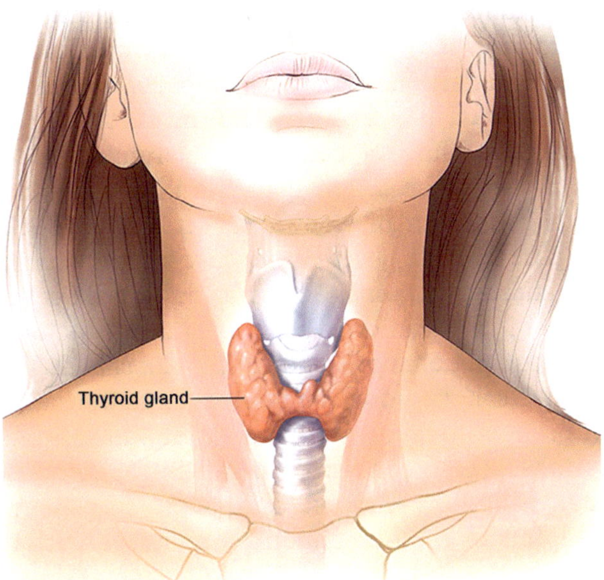

Figure 3.1. Illustration of thyroid gland.

Source: https://endomds.com/wp-content/uploads/2021/03/Thyroid-gland-300x300.jpg.

Importance of the Thyroid Gland in the Endocrine System

The thyroid gland is a key participant in the endocrine system, primarily responsible for secreting thyroid hormones that play a crucial role in various metabolic processes. The butterfly-shaped gland lies in the anterior region of the neck and secretes hormones such as thyroxine (T4) and triiodothyronine (T3), which regulate metabolism, energy consumption, and development. The hormones impact almost all organ systems in the body, from cardiovascular to mental function. Imbalances in thyroid hormone levels may result in severe health issues, such as hypothyroidism and hyperthyroidism, which can arise in a range of symptoms from weight changes and fatigue to anxiety and cardiac issues. Understanding the function of the thyroid gland is crucial in maintaining overall health and addressing metabolic disorders resulting from thyroid dysfunction. Moreover, the interaction between the immune system and thyroid hormones highlights the intricacies of the endocrine system. Thyroid hormones have been involved in various immune responses and have a role in modulating inflammation and autoimmunity. The intricate interaction between the immune system and these hormones suggests that any deviations from thyroid function can initiate or augment autoimmune diseases. Recent evidence has shown that alterations in gut microbiota can influence thyroid hormone metabolism and, consequently, immune function, underscoring the importance of environmental factors in endocrine health. The interaction of the systems attests to the need for a multidisciplinary approach to the treatment of medical afflictions, especially in the context of chronic disease related to thyroid dysfunction. Examining these relationships can reveal new, tailored therapeutic strategies for simultaneously addressing endocrine and immune function (Fern et al., 2021). Moreover, the thyroid gland's importance even transcends to development, more precisely, to brain development. The role of thyroid hormones in embryonic brain development has been a central interest since thyroid hormone deficiency was identified as a cause of severe neurodevelopmental retardation. As the gland develops in pregnancy and child development, it plays a critical role in neurogenesis and the development of brain function. Coordination between thyroid hormones plays a crucial role in processes such as neuronal proliferation, migration, and survival. Endocrine and central nervous system barriers also tightly regulate the delivery of the hormones to achieve optimal developmental outcomes. As science continues to unravel the intricate roles played by thyroid hormones in neurodevelopment, it is increasingly becoming clear that a delicate balance of these hormones is paramount if the brain is to develop properly and function (Barbara et al., 2019).

3.1. Anatomy of the Thyroid Gland

Learning Outcome

1. Discuss the location and physical structure of the thyroid gland;
2. Understand lobes and isthmus of the thyroid;
3. Focus on blood supply and innervation.

Located in the anterior part of the neck, the thyroid gland is an essential part of the endocrine system, mostly for controlling metabolism and growth. This butterfly-like organ consists of two lateral lobes that are joined by an isthmus, which traverses the midline and rests above the upper trachea. The anatomical position of the thyroid is very remarkable since it surrounds the tracheal rings and cricoid cartilage between the level of the fifth cervical vertebra and that of the first thoracic vertebra. Furthermore, the proximity of the glands to vital structures such as the parathyroid glands and the recurrent laryngeal nerves necessitates utmost care during surgical operations. Its anatomy knowledge not only enhances the identification of its physiological processes but also highlights the possibility of complications arising from surgical procedures on the neck area, e.g., incidental damage to adjacent tissues (Smitha et al., 2023). The thyroid gland plays a key role in the attainment of homeostasis by the hormone synthesis of thyroxine (T4) and triiodothyronine (T3) and calcitonin, which helps regulate blood calcium levels. Functional integrity is threatened by a range of disorders, from autoimmune diseases like Graves' disease to the presence of neoplasms such as papillary or follicular carcinoma. The anatomical arrangement of the thyroid forms a foundation upon which these functional operations are carried out. The thyroid is significant in that it sits in the neck's visceral space, which subjects it to some danger of damage during surgery. Such interaction with the parathyroid glands emphasizes again the importance of preserving these glands during thyroid surgery, as damage to them would cause severe conditions such as hypoparathyroidism (Smitha et al., 2023). The importance of meticulous surgery cannot be overemphasized in surgeries for the thyroid. Techniques aimed at preservation of significant structures, such as parathyroid glands, play a central role in the successful management of thyroid disease. Anatomical variation in position and morphology between patients presents additional challenges to surgical procedure and emphasizes the value of preoperative imaging and careful dissection. Indocyanine green fluorescence intraoperative identification is a method that has been adopted to further enhance the preservation of parathyroid glands. Notably, parathyroid autotransplantation techniques also provide therapeutic avenues for incidental damage during thyroidectomies. Lastly, the relationship between the thyroid gland and its surrounding anatomical environment creates a foundation for managing both the clinical relevance of thyroid disease and the complexities that occur when conducting surgical operations (Allen et al., 2019) (Figure 3.2).

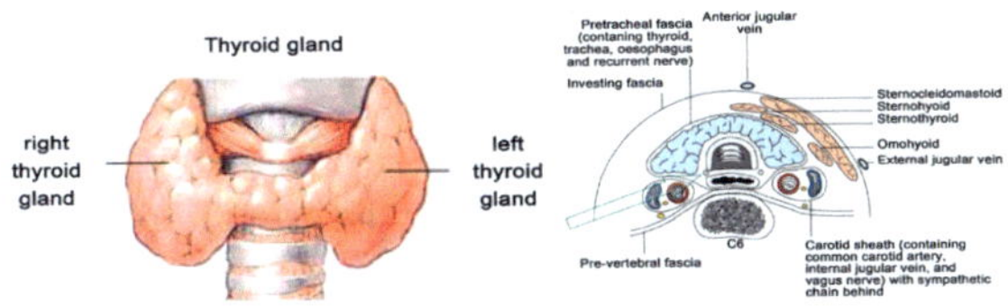

Figure 3.2. The thyroid gland and its anatomic relationships.

Source: https://www.researchgate.net/profile/Rodrigo-Arrangoiz-2/publication/326375395/figure/fig2/AS:647919061442571@1531487350671/The-thyroid-gland-and-its-anatomic-relationships.png.

3.1.1. Location and Physical Structure

The thyroid gland, a vital component of the endocrine system, is strategically positioned in the front of the neck, directly under the larynx. This singular positioning gives it a pivotal function in monitoring metabolism and hormonal balance in the body. The butterfly or bow-like shape of the thyroid gland is composed of two lobes connected by a middle piece of tissue known as the isthmus. This body structure makes it possible for its function in the synthesis and secretion of thyroid hormones, such as thyroxine (T4) and triiodothyronine (T3), which are required for most physiological processes. The closeness of the thyroids to large blood vessels, the carotid arteries, and jugular veins, underscores its significance in vascular mechanisms and the transportation of hormones to the rest of the body. Physically, the thyroid gland is enveloped in a fibrous capsule that provides support as well as shape. Internally, the gland consists of numerous follicular units, spherical structures lined by follicular cells that produce the hormones. Inside the follicles is colloid, a thick watery substance that contains thyroglobulin, the precursor to the thyroid hormones. This organizational structure not only maximizes the surface area for the manufacture of hormones but also allows for the gland's quick response to metabolic demands. The addition of parafollicular cells, or C cells, in the interstitial space also increases the gland's functional range through the manufacture of calcitonin, a hormone involved in the control of calcium homeostasis. This is such a detail of fine structure that it indicates how sophisticated the thyroid's role is in endocrine regulation. The vascularization of the thyroid gland is also impressive, with it being supplied primarily by the superior and inferior thyroid arteries to provide an adequate blood supply necessary for its metabolic functions. Moreover, its ability to accommodate varying physiological conditions, such as pregnancy or growth with the higher requirement of thyroid hormones, highlights the significance of its spatial and physical properties. The thyroid's interaction with the tissues immediately around it—and with its encapsulated environment—emphasizes the gland's intricate function in homeostasis. With its unique position and intricate structural organization, the thyroid gland exemplifies the intricate interplay between anatomy and function in human physiology, solidifying its status as a foundational endocrine organ (Figure 3.3).

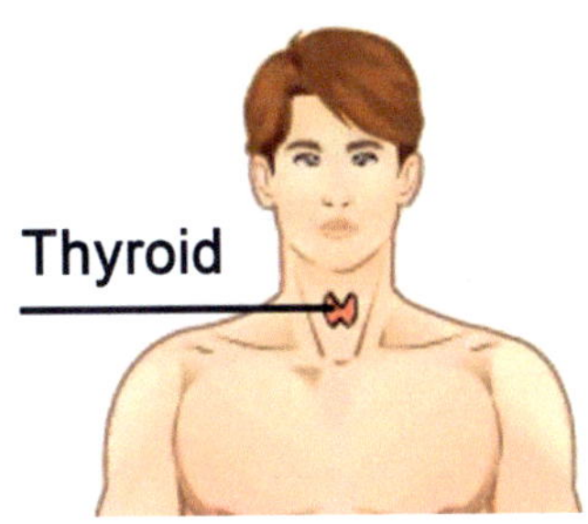

Figure 3.3. The thyroid gland is a butterfly-shaped gland located in the neck, just below the Adam's apple.

Source: https://upload.wikimedia.org/wikipedia/commons/b/b8/Thyroid_dummy.jpg.

3.1.2. Lobes and Isthmus of the Thyroid

Thyroid gland is an endocrine organ in the middle that consists primarily of two lobes—right and left—united by thin isthmus tissue. This type of structural organization enables the gland to efficiently regulate metabolic processes through the secretion of thyroid hormones, affecting nearly every organ in the human body. Both of the butterfly-shaped lobes are crucial to hormone secretion and production. The isthmus itself, typically lying over the trachea, is not only a transitional region but also an area from which vascular supply and nerve innervation originate. There can be differences in the isthmus shape and size, which influence thyroid function and surgical operations for certain illnesses, such as goiter or thyroid nodules, thus presenting the anatomical significance of the structures in clinical practice. Embryological development of the thyroid is key to understanding the anatomical features of its lobes and isthmus. The thyroid gland forms by the union of the medial and lateral thyroid anlagen; defects in this process can result in congenital malformations, like incomplete fusion or the absence of an isthmus. Such developmental variations can lead to dramatic differences in thyroid structure and may influence hormone secretion and metabolism. For instance, incomplete fusion results in abnormal structures such as accessory lobes or ectopic thyroid tissue, making diagnosis and treatment challenging. Knowledge of the variations is crucial for medical professionals, especially radiologists and surgeons, to adequately diagnose and treat thyroid pathologies, as indicated by research in line with the relevance of increased knowledge of these anatomical variations (N/A, 2025). Despite its small size, the thyroid has an important role in overall health, well-marked by research that seeks to create awareness of thyroid illnesses. That information concerning the functions of the thyroid gland, including the function of each of the two lobes and the isthmus, is vital to doctors as well as patients. According to studies, there is a demand for educational initiatives designed to enhance information about thyroid problems. A study conducted in the medical outpatient department revealed variation between the patients' levels of knowledge, which indicated that there are many patients who are not aware of the functions and dysfunctions of the thyroid gland (Rana et al., 2024). Public and professional education about the thyroid's anatomy and physiology can help towards better prevention and treatment outcomes and thus fulfill the utmost need of good-quality healthcare decisions (Figure 3.4).

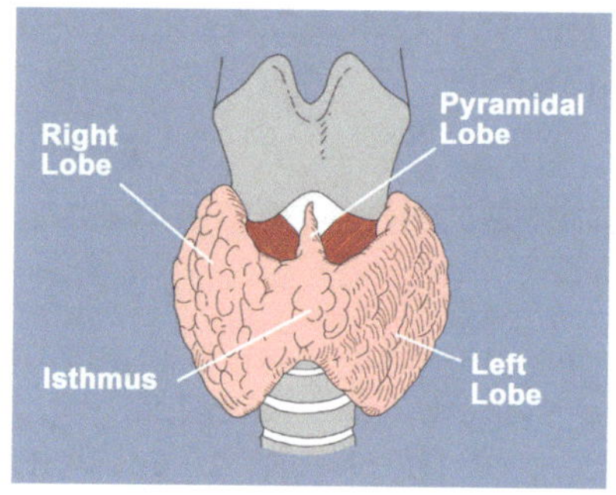

Figure 3.4. The two lobes—right and left—are linked by a narrow band of tissue known as the isthmus.

Source: https://miamiendocrinesurgery.org/wp-content/uploads/2017/10/Thyroid-Surgery-in-Miami-300x241.jpg.

3.1.3. Blood Supply and Innervation

The vascularity of the thyroid glands is critical in supplying their endocrine functions, which is predominantly explained by their requirement for a rich vascular supply to facilitate secretion of the hormones. The thyroid blood supply is mainly derived from the superior thyroid artery, a branch of the external carotid artery, and the inferior thyroid artery, a branch of the thyrocervical trunk. This double-arterial supply gives the gland plenty of oxygen and nutrients and also a route by which thyroid hormone can enter the systemic circulation. Of note is that neural control alters the blood flow; the sympathetic fibers are responsible for the control of the vascular resistance of the gland. Through such mechanisms, the thyroid reaches homeostasis by adjusting the blood supply in proportion to metabolic demand, a role that indicates the importance of familiarity with its vascular anatomy in both physiological and operating states. Autonomic innervation of the thyroid gland is predominant, with the participation of both sympathetic and parasympathetic fibers. Sympathetic nerves originate from cervical sympathetic ganglia, which control blood flow and the gland's functional state in stress conditions. Such fibers are activated during the fight or flight response, controlling the gland's activity and offering a suitable metabolic response. Parasympathetic innervation, on the other hand, is from the recurrent laryngeal nerve, which plays a significant role in the overall functioning of the glands. This intricate innervation affects the gland's sensitivity to regulatory hormones, such as Thyroid-Releasing Hormone (TRH), which controls the hypothalamic-pituitary-thyroid axis (Fekete et al., 2013). A thorough understanding of your neural architecture is necessary in the avoidance of surgical complications with thyroid surgery, such as damage to the recurrent laryngeal nerve, which has the potential to result in severe post-operative morbidity (Mohebati et al., 2011). The relationship between blood supply and innervation places further significance on the anatomical relationship within the thyroid region. Optimal blood supply is crucial in maintaining maximal gland function, allowing for effective hormone synthesis and release. In contrast, precise nerve relationships ensure that the gland responds to metabolic demands, particularly during the situation of physiological stress. The interaction of these systems becomes particularly crucial within the operating room; surgeons need high levels of awareness of what surrounds critical structures to avoid complications due to inadvertent damage to the recurrent laryngeal nerve or surrounding vasculature. Correct surgical procedure based on a correct understanding of the anatomy of the thyroid serves to enhance patient outcomes and lower the risk of serious complications that could have long-term health consequences (Mohebati et al., 2011). The thyroid gland's blood supply and innervation are therefore rudimentary aspects of its anatomy, which must be accorded due attention in the clinic (Figure 3.5).

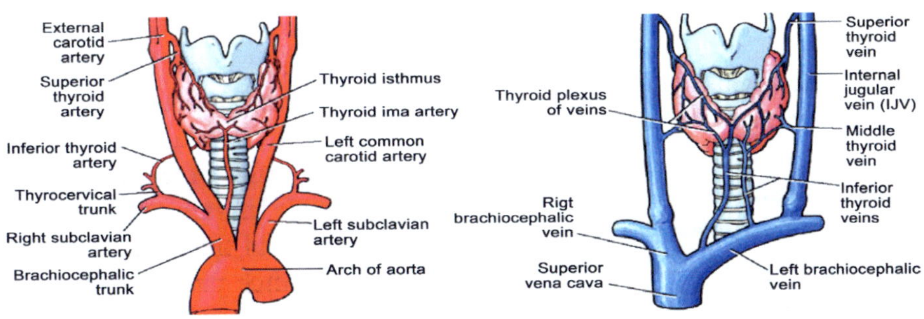

Figure 3.5. Arterial supply to the thyroid gland and venous drainage from the thyroid gland.

Source: https://www.researchgate.net/profile/Rodrigo-Arrangoiz-2/publication/326375395/figure/fig3/AS:647919061458944@1531487350872/Arterial-supply-of-the-thyroid-gland-and-venous-drainage-of-the-thyroid-gland.png.

Test Your Knowledge

1. Where is the thyroid gland located in the neck, and what major anatomical structures is it closely associated with?
2. What are the main anatomical components of the thyroid gland?
3. Which arteries supply blood to the thyroid gland, and from which larger arteries do they originate?

3.2. Functions of the Thyroid Gland

Learning Outcome

1. Deal with the production of the hormones triiodothyronine (T3) and thyroxine (T4);
2. Focus on the regulation of metabolism;
3. Explain how the thyroid gland plays a pivotal role in growth and development throughout various stages of life.

The thyroid gland plays the central role in regulating metabolism, growth, and development of the human body. Its primary function is the generation and secretion of thyroid hormones, i.e., thyroxine (T4) and triiodothyronine (T3), which are crucial for metabolic processes. The hormones facilitate converting food into energy and influence the rate at which the body burns calories and maintains weight. Additionally, thyroid hormones regulate various bodily functions, including heart rate, body temperature regulation, and muscle strength. Metabolic disorders like hypothyroidism and hyperthyroidism result from dysregulation of the production of thyroid hormones, both of which highlight the significance of this gland to ensure metabolic homeostasis. Release of T3 and T4 is regulated by thyroid-stimulating hormone (TSH), which the pituitary gland secretes, so it shows how dependent the endocrine system is and how central thyroid hormones are to overall well-being. Aside from the regulation of metabolism, the thyroid also plays a significant role in growth and development, particularly during infancy and childhood. Proper amounts of thyroid hormones are crucial during the developmental stages since it decides neurological development and physical growth. The absence of these hormones can have extremely deleterious consequences, such as growth retardation and mental handicaps, to presume the gland's critical function in brain development and activity. Research demonstrates that in children, even a slight thyroid deficiency can lead to learning handicaps and delays in motor skills. The significance of iodine, a vital component in the production of thyroid hormone, cannot be overstated. Iodine deficiency remains a significant public health issue in much of the world and leads to goiter and mental impairment, again pointing to the necessity for adequate dietary intake of iodine for maximum thyroid function and health. The role of the thyroid glands also extends into the area of reproductive health and affects fertility and pregnancy outcome. Thyroid hormones have been shown to play a role in ovulation and menstrual cycles of females with both deficiency and excess, impairing fertility. In pregnancy, the function of the thyroid glands is even more prevalent since proper thyroid hormone levels are crucial for the development of the fetus. Impaired thyroid function in pregnancy can lead to complications like premature birth and congenital abnormalities in the fetus. The interaction between thyroid function and reproductive health underscores the need to track thyroid hormone levels in the reproductive-aged population. In addition, the gut microbiota has been found to affect thyroid function by modulating mineral absorption, further adding to the understanding of how different systems in the body work together to maintain endocrine function and general health (Eöhlich et al., 2019; Mojadadi et al., 2021).

3.2.1. Hormone Production: T3 and T4

The thyroid gland, one of the endocrine system's major organs, is primarily responsible for the biosynthesis of the hormone thyroxine (T4) and triiodothyronine (T3). These hormones are both significant in the regulation of the body's metabolism, heart rate, and energy expenditure. T3 and T4 are synthesized from the amino acid tyrosine and from iodine, and the most important function is that of the thyroid follicular cells in synthesizing these. Synthesis begins with the uptake of iodine from the bloodstream, which is incorporated into the thyroglobulin molecule, a precursor protein that is produced within the thyroid gland. The intricacy of this process is meant to underscore the significant role played by the thyroid in maintaining metabolic homeostasis and illustrates how disruption of hormone synthesis will have significant physiological consequences. T3 and T4 secretion is controlled by TSH, which is secreted from the anterior pituitary gland. TSH is the key controller that activates the function of the thyroid glands, both the production and release of T3 and T4 into the circulation. Interestingly, the body's metabolic requirements control the release of TSH through a very sensitive feedback system. For instance, under conditions of low levels of T3 and T4, secretion of TSH is stimulated to force the thyroid to produce increased levels of hormones. In the case of high levels of T3 and T4, they inhibit the secretion of TSH, illustrating the critical function of this hormonal axis in maintaining proper metabolic function. Faulty feedback mechanisms can lead to disease conditions such as hyperthyroidism or hypothyroidism, thus illustrating the importance of T3 and T4 regulation in health. New research has demonstrated the manner in which environmental exposures can affect T3 and T4 production, illustrating the intricate relationship between environmental exposures and thyroid function. To illustrate, exposure to certain chemicals, such as neonicotinoids, can alter thyroid hormone composition and tissue architecture in animal models and affect future generations as well. In research on pregnant mice that were administered the insecticide thiacloprid, there was a significant change in T4 levels, indicating that ancient exposure could induce a shift in thyroid function across generations (Lahmidi et al., 2024). Also, research has illustrated the pathological consequences of congenital infections, for example, Toxoplasma gondii, that resulted in high T3 and T4 levels and also revealed structural changes in the thyroid gland (Elgawad et al., 2025). The evidence is geared toward the susceptibility of the thyroid gland to environmental causes, reiterating the need for more research on this essential area of endocrine health (Figure 3.6).

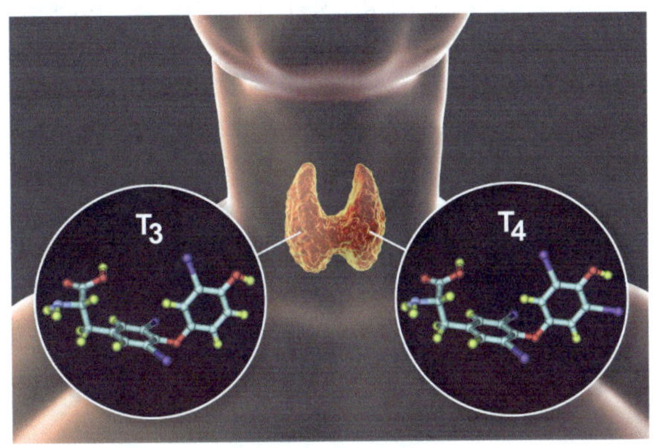

Figure 3.6. Triiodothyronine (T3) and thyroxine (T4).

Source: https://health.selfdecode.com/app/uploads/2019/11/Thyroid-Hormones-T3-T4-Roles-Functions-High-Low-Levels.jpg.

3.2.2. Regulation of Metabolism

The thyroid gland plays the greatest role in metabolic control by secreting thyroxine (T4) and triiodothyronine (T3) hormones. They exert numerous impacts on metabolic processes, including energy production in cells, fat breakdown, and protein synthesis. Thyroid hormone activation is tightly controlled by TSH, which is secreted from the pituitary gland. When the levels of thyroid hormones decrease, TSH release is increased to stimulate the thyroid gland to release more hormones. In turn, a high amount of T4 and T3 gives negative feedback to the pituitary and hypothalamus, thus controlling TSH release. This fine balance is crucial for maintaining metabolic homeostasis and is particularly important during the phases of growth and development (Yu et al., 2024). In addition to their role in hormone synthesis, systemic factors such as homocysteine (Hcy) levels and diet also influence thyroid function and metabolism. Evidence has shown that elevated levels of Hcy induce structural and functional changes within the thyroid gland, particularly among populations exposed to environmental stress factors, such as populations residing near the Chornobyl Nuclear Power Plant (Yu et al., 2024). The relationship between Hcy and thyroid hormones is complex, as Hcy can stimulate the release of TSH, which has an effect on the conversion of T4 to its active metabolite T3. In addition, the nutritional adequacy of such things as vitamins B9 and B12 is important to sustaining the healthy operation of the folate cycle, which is related to the balance of homocysteine levels and, by direct extension, thyroid function (Yu et al., 2024). Besides, the oxidative environment in the thyroid gland strongly affects its metabolic activity. Hydrogen peroxide (H_2O_2) is required for the synthesis of thyroid hormones, as it oxidizes iodide. Retinol Saturase (RetSat), a catalyst, plays a crucial role in maintaining control over oxidative stress in thyrocytes. Thyroid hormone status and nutrition control the expression of RetSat, and therefore, it plays an important role in metabolic regulation of the thyroid gland (Yang et al., 2024). Once RetSat is eliminated in some models, it will impinge on metabolic homeostasis and regulate thyroid morphology, leading to elevated TSH levels and impaired hormone biosynthesis. Thus, the maintenance of RetSat activity is crucial for the persistence of the metabolic processes of the thyroid gland and hence the metabolic well-being of the organism (Yang et al., 2024) (Figure 3.7).

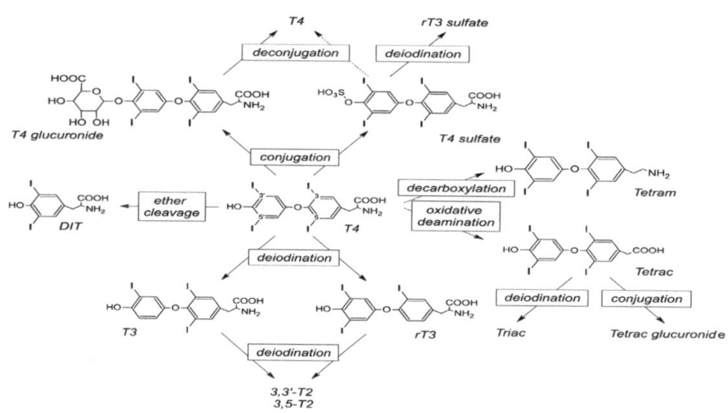

Figure 3.7. Pathways of thyroid hormone metabolism. Here, T4 is chosen as the central metabolite, but most reactions are also applicable to T3 and T2s, respectively.

Source: https://www.researchgate.net/profile/Peter-Klaren/publication/230616230/figure/fig1/AS:654786470891523@1533124668900/Pathways-of-thyroid-hormone-metabolism-adapted-from-Koehrle-et-al-1987-Here-T4-is.png.

3.2.3. Role in Growth and Development

The thyroid gland plays a core role in growth and development throughout various stages of life, particularly in children and adolescents. It releases thyroid hormones, primarily thyroxine (T4) and triiodothyronine (T3), which are vital for metabolic activities and body growth. The hormones influence the growth processes such as cell differentiation, protein synthesis, and energy consumption. During early neurocognitive development, normal thyroid function is required; inadequacies may result in cognitive impairment as well as intellectual growth being stunted. The function of these hormones is particularly evident during periods of augmented growth, since the individual must have their thyroid function tracked carefully among young populations in order to achieve optimal health outcomes (Patrick et al., 2016). To understand the comprehensive role of thyroid hormones in growth patterns, it is critical for medical professionals and highlight the importance of prompt identification and management of any thyroid disease. Moreover, the influence of the thyroid extends beyond physical growth to intellectual and emotional development. Deficient levels of thyroid hormone, as seen in hypothyroidism, will lead to delayed development, characterized by reduced energy levels, lethargy, and impairment of cognitive functions. In contrast, excessive, abnormal levels of such hormones, as in hyperthyroidism, may result in mental impairment, hyperactivity, and anxiety. These conditions further underscore the importance of regular thyroid function screening, particularly in high-risk groups such as children and adolescents, to prevent potential imbalances from adversely affecting growth and development. Literature is also available to relate childhood thyroid disease with developmental issues in later life; hence, early intervention becomes crucial in mitigating such risks and fostering more positive developmental trajectories (Patrick et al., 2016). The role of the thyroid gland in growth and development is also highlighted by the fact that it is required in regulating metabolic processes, which are vital during formative years. The thyroid hormone interaction with growth hormone and insulin-like growth factors is a complex interaction that influences the growth of the body and general health. When the thyroid does not function optimally, the body may not react appropriately to these growth signals, with the potential consequence being disturbed growth or stunted growth. Moreover, since thyroid and environmental factors can impact the health of the thyroid, increased vigilance is required for parents and teachers to identify early the symptoms of thyroid disease. Through the development of an appreciation of thyroid health, interested parties are better placed to assist children and youths to achieve their full physiological and intellectual potential, which is the precursor to long-term health and well-being (Patrick et al., 2016).

Test Your Knowledge

1. Which two main hormones are produced by the thyroid gland, and what element is essential for their synthesis?
2. How do T3 (triiodothyronine) and T4 (thyroxine) influence the body's metabolic rate?
3. What is the role of thyroid hormones in normal growth and development, particularly during childhood?

3.3. Thyroid Hormones and Their Regulation

Learning Outcome

1. Understand the mechanism of hormone release;
2. Explain the role of the hypothalamus and pituitary gland;
3. Discuss feedback loops in hormone regulation.

The regulation of thyroid hormones, primarily thyroxine (T4) and triiodothyronine (T3), is important to most metabolic processes in the human body. Hormones are synthesized in the thyroid gland and secreted into the bloodstream, where they affect almost all organ systems. The production of T4 and T3 is controlled by TSH, which is secreted by the pituitary gland following the reception of hypothalamic release of thyrotropin-releasing hormone (TRH). This feedback process is a paradigm case of an endocrine control model, whereby increased levels of thyroid hormones inhibit the release of TSH to maintain homeostasis. When this regulatory process is disrupted, as in hyperthyroidism or hypothyroidism, most of these physiological deviations are possible, making it imperative to have finely calibrated levels of hormones for metabolic balance and overall health. Thyroid hormones have impacts beyond metabolic regulation; their actions on bone metabolism are significant. T3, in particular, has been shown to stimulate osteoblast activity, thereby facilitating bone formation. This is particularly significant as it contributes to maintaining bone density and strength, thereby supporting skeletal integrity. On the other hand, an overactive level of thyroid hormone can enhance osteoclast activity, inducing abnormally active bone resorption and loss of bone mass. Such a pathological effect has a serious impact on functions like denture retention among edentulous patients, which serves as an example for the subtle interaction between thyroid hormone regulation and skeletal well-being. Understanding these mechanisms emphasizes the need for careful monitoring of thyroid function in at-risk groups for osteoporosis or other skeletal illnesses (Bhanu, 2024). In addition to their role in physiological function, thyroid hormones play important roles in brain development and mental processes. Their regulatory effects also extend to the process of neural circuit formation during critical periods of brain maturation, underscoring their designation as critical signaling molecules in the central nervous system. However, exposure to endocrine-disrupting chemicals (EDCs) is an emerging threat that can adversely affect thyroid function and cause cognitive impairments and disturbances in behavior. It might worsen if nothing is done. Research has revealed that such interferences are by way of mimicking or blocking thyroid hormones, especially at sensitive stages of development. Hence, vigilant responses and stronger controls on EDC exposure must be ensured to protect vulnerable populations, such as pregnant women and infants, from such harmful effects (Dsouki et al., 2024). There is a need to counter such challenges in ensuring proper thyroid and cognitive function throughout the life cycle (Figure 3.8).

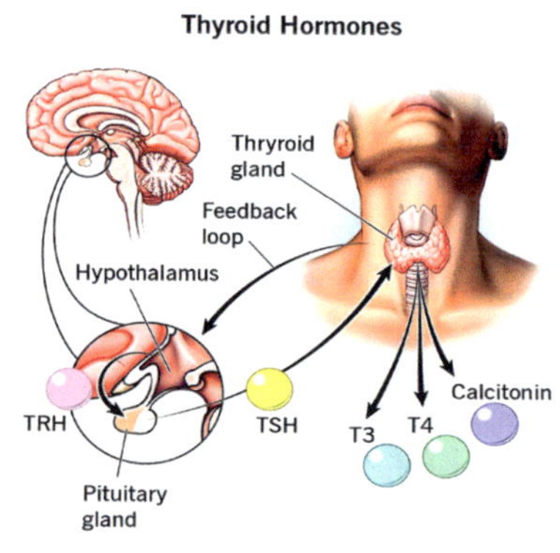

Figure 3.8. Thyroid hormones.

Source: https://my.clevelandclinic.org/-/scassets/images/org/health/articles/22391-thyroid-hormone.

3.3.1. Mechanism of Hormone Release

Thyroid hormone discharge is controlled predominantly by TSH, which is secreted by the pituitary gland. The pituitary secretes TSH into the blood on stimulation by the hypothalamic TRH. TSH attaches to the thyroid follicular cell surface receptors, stimulating a chain of biochemical reactions that result in the synthesis and release of thyroid hormones, with thyroxine (T4) and triiodothyronine (T3) as the primary hormones. This is via a negative feedback mechanism; elevated T4 and T3 inhibit the secretion of TSH and TRH to maintain the balance of hormones and prevent thyroid gland overstimulation. This finely regulated interaction is such that thyroid hormones are released according to the body's metabolic need, reflecting the central role of feedback mechanisms in endocrine function and homeostasis (Sun et al., 2025). Moreover, the release of the hormones is dependent on specific cell transport mechanisms, which permit the transport of thyroid hormones from the thyroid gland to the systemic circulation.

The role of certain plasma membrane transporters, such as monocarboxylate transporter (MCT)8 and MCT10, becomes apparent in this context. These transport proteins have a significant role in the effective uptake of T3 and T4 into target tissues, where their metabolic effects are observed. New knowledge of these transporters shows that ligand binding, like that of thyroxine, induces conformational changes in these proteins so that the transport of hormones through the membrane is facilitated (Tassinari et al., 2024). Their significance is also proved by the fact that mutations of MCT8 have been found to lead to severe neurodevelopmental disorders, proving the significance of hormone transport in physiological function. Besides, the release of the thyroid hormones is not by passive diffusion but involves complex regulatory mechanisms that are sensitive to the physiological status of the body. Disease, stress, and diet can all affect TSH levels and consequently T3 and T4 release. For instance, bad health conditions might result in excessive levels of TRH, hence increasing the secretion of TSH even when the thyroid gland is in perfect condition. Secondly, circulating antibodies that affect the binding of TSH may result in misleading hormone levels, complicating both the diagnosis and treatment processes for thyroid disorders (Sun et al., 2025). Accordingly, it is essential to understand the dynamic processes of hormone secretion to accurately diagnose and manage thyroid pathology, as a demonstration of the intricacy of endocrine functioning in disease and health (Figure 3.9).

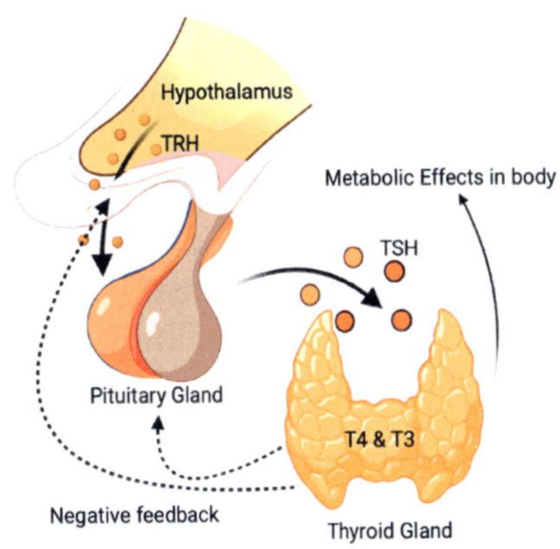

Figure 3.9. Regulation of thyroid hormone secretion by the hypothalamus and anterior pituitary. Thyrotropin-releasing hormone (TRH) from the hypothalamus regulates the secretion of thyrotropin, or thyroid-stimulating hormone (TSH), from the pituitary gland.

Source: https://www.researchgate.net/publication/372399748/figure/fig1/AS:11431281174991735@1689510741716/Regulation-of-thyroid-hormones-secretion-by-the-hypothalamus-and-anterior-pituitary.png.

3.3.2. Role of the Hypothalamus and Pituitary Gland

The hypothalamus and pituitary gland are central components of the endocrine system, controlling the thyroid gland. The hypothalamus is a regulatory center, sensing the metabolic needs of the body and acting by the discharge of TRH. TRH induces the discharge of TSH by the pituitary gland, which directly stimulates the thyroid glands. This pituitary-hypothalamic-thyroid axis is essential to metabolic homeostasis because it precisely regulates the release of thyroid hormones, T3 and T4, which are required for various body functions like metabolism, energy expenditure, and conservation of body temperature. Therefore, interaction among these neuroendocrine tissues underscores the importance of the pituitary and hypothalamus in making thyroid function adaptive as well as responsive to physiological conditions. In addition, the interaction between the hypothalamus and pituitary and other hormonal systems illustrates the intricacy of endocrine control. An example is the effect of zinc on thyroid hormone metabolism, which illustrates how micronutrients may affect this endocrine control loop. Zinc increases thyroid hormone synthesis, action, and controls critical thyroid-metabolizing enzymes. The presence of zinc transporters in the hypothalamus, pituitary, and thyroid suggests a sophisticated relationship where nutrient availability is directly capable of influencing levels and function of hormones. This is particularly pertinent because interference with thyroid function has been found to cause significant health problems, as described in publications discussing the impact of plant-based constituents on endocrine well-being (Khalid et al., 2022). Nutritional status thus becomes one that can potentially alter hormonal balance, revealing the function of the hypothalamus and pituitary in relating metabolic and nutritional states to thyroid gland activity. In conclusion, the pituitary gland and the hypothalamus serve as major regulators of thyroid function through intricate feedback mechanisms. This regulation encompasses not only the initial stimulation of the release of TSH but is extended to the modulation of thyroid hormone availability in relation to nutritional effects, e.g., the role of zinc (Severo et al., 2019). Pathologies due to dysregulation along this axis may present as varied endocrine disorders, thereby illustrating the significance of these brain structures for endocrine health in general. As research continues to explore the interactions between hormone production and micronutrients, it is increasingly clear that understanding these interactions is critical to the treatment of thyroid disease. The hypothalamic-pituitary axis remains, accordingly, a key focus in endocrinology and nutrition, with an ongoing effort to know the long-term implications of these hormonal interactions on human health.

3.3.3. Feedback Loops in Hormone Regulation

Regulation of hormone levels in the body is mostly dependent on intricate feedback mechanisms that ensure homeostasis. In the control of the thyroid gland, the hypothalamic-pituitary-thyroid (HPT) axis demonstrates this concept via an active play between hormonal signals. TRH, released from the hypothalamus, stimulates the anterior pituitary to release TSH. On the other hand, TSH encourages the release and synthesis of thyroid hormones (THs) from the thyroid gland. This is a cycle that is extremely significant, since it allows the body to respond to variations in metabolic demand by adjusting hormone levels appropriately. Surprisingly, when TH levels rise, they inhibit the secretion of both TRH and TSH negatively, hence preventing overproduction of the hormone and maintaining harmony in the HPT axis. Tanycyte activity in the hypothalamus also reflects the complexity of feedback mechanisms in hormone regulation. Tanycytes are glial cells specialized in regulating thyroid hormone transport and metabolism, particularly under conditions of altered energy status. Studies reveal that TSH triggers the transcription of genes responsible for the transport and metabolism of TH by tanycytes, such as Dio2 and Slco1c1, demonstrating that thyroid hormones never act alone. Instead, the TSH stimulation activates specific intracellular pathways that enhance the expression of these gatekeeper genes, highlighting the crucial roles of both the hormones and neural substrates in the regulation of TH homeostasis (Chandrasekar et al., 2023). This commentary highlights the adaptive capability of the feedback loop in terms of the response of tissues to hormonal signals to accommodate adequate TH availability to the central nervous system. In addition to tanycyte regulation, the feedback loop also includes direct TRH neuron control from within the paraventricular nucleus (PVN) of the hypothalamus, which itself significantly regulates TH levels. Activation of such TRH neurons produces a profound effect on TSH and TH levels, demonstrating their pivotal role in regulating the HPT axis. Such neurons are responsive to energy-sensing inputs, e.g., from arcuate nucleus neurons, which can modulate TRH expression during fasting, indicating the feedback mechanism's sensitivity to metabolic status (Costa-e-Sousa et al., 2023). Of special significance, thyroid hormone signaling disturbances may lead to imbalances affecting the overall stability of metabolism, thus demonstrating not only the importance of hormonal feedback processes but also the potential consequences when such systems fail. From appreciation of these feedback processes, researchers are well-placed to identify targets for therapeutic intervention in thyroid dysfunctions.

Test Your Knowledge

1. Which hormone is released by the hypothalamus to stimulate the pituitary gland in the thyroid hormone regulatory pathway?
2. What hormone does the anterior pituitary secrete to act on the thyroid gland, and what does this hormone do?

3.4. Common Thyroid Disorders

Learning Outcome

1. Describe causes and symptoms of hypothyroidism;
2. Understand causes and symptoms of hyperthyroidism;
3. Explain goiter and thyroid nodules.

The thyroid gland is a critical regulator of metabolism and general well-being, and multiple disorders can result from its malfunction. Two of the most common are hypothyroidism and hyperthyroidism, which plague millions of people worldwide. Hypothyroidism is characterized by the gland's inability to secrete adequate amounts of thyroid hormones, causing a lowering of metabolic rates. This condition can manifest itself with a variety of symptoms, ranging from weight gain, depression, and fatigue, and may significantly impact the quality of life. Hyperthyroidism, however, results from overproduction of hormones, most typically secondary to conditions such as Graves' disease. The most frequently noted symptoms are weight loss, tachycardia, and irascibility. It is crucial to recognize these conditions to make an early diagnosis and management since uncomplicated thyroid disease, if left untreated, can lead to severe consequences, including cardiovascular, and even life-threatening crises in advanced cases. Thyroid nodules are also being increasingly discovered in clinical practice, with their incidence differing depending on the method of detection. Such nodules, being mostly benign, may be observed or treated if there are suspicious findings because they could be thyroid cancer in some instances. Development of thyroid nodules is influenced by multifactorial factors, including the consumption of iodine, age, and sex, and in females, more than in males. While most thyroid nodules are not related to symptoms, they may cause uneasiness or even compress surrounding structures if large enough. Evaluation of nodules by clinical examination, ultrasound, and fine-needle aspiration biopsy, if required, is critical for managing potential risks and ensuring appropriate follow-up (Eöhlich et al., 2019). Gut microbiota has also been reported to play a crucial role in regulating thyroid function, particularly in autoimmune thyroid diseases such as Hashimoto's thyroiditis and Graves' disease. Epidemiological evidence further shows that a compromised gut microbiome can further worsen such ailments and further contribute to dysregulation of thyroid metabolism and immune status. The interplay between the microbiota, iodine nutrition, and mineral absorption further adds complexity to thyroid pathophysiology, with dietary and environmental influences now further being regarded as playing an important role in these diseases. New research identifies that therapies on gut health, pre- and probiotics, may be implicated in the treatment of autoimmune thyroid disorders by refreshing microorganisms and improving thyroid function (Eöhlich et al., 2019). An integrated strategy amalgamating the paradigms of endocrine as well as microbiological is thus a requirement for an effective treatment plan of common thyroid disease.

3.4.1. Hypothyroidism: Causes and Symptoms

Hypothyroidism, or underactive thyroid, is the inability of the thyroid gland to produce sufficient thyroid hormones, primarily thyroxine (T4). Hypothyroidism may be due to a variety of reasons, the most common being Hashimoto's thyroiditis, an autoimmune disease in which the immune system of the body attacks the thyroid gland. Iodine deficiency, certain medications, radiation treatment, and thyroid removal are other causes that may lead to hypothyroidism. In addition, subclinical hypothyroidism, i.e., elevated TSH levels with normal free T4 levels, has been the area of interest in elderly as well as younger populations. Though its clinical significance is debatable, findings show that the condition must be treated and monitored in order to avoid further thyroid dysfunction and associated health risks, as has been shown in studies on the overall implications of thyroid hormone therapy among various populations (Bauer et al., 2017). The signs of hypothyroidism are quite variable per person but usually include fatigue, weight gain, intolerance to cold, and depressed moods. The insidious onset of the aforementioned symptoms often leads to delayed diagnosis, especially when they are incorrectly attributed to other diseases or to senility. Moreover, most patients also have a set of other symptoms consisting of skin dryness, hair loss, muscle weakness, and mental impairments, collectively impacting quality of life severely. In other cases, patients may develop subclinical symptoms despite maintaining normal levels of circulating thyroid hormone, complicating diagnosis and treatment even further. Recent research has determined that subclinical thyroid dysfunction is related to cardiovascular morbidity, meaning both symptomatic and asymptomatic patients need to be completely evaluated to intervene properly (Biondi et al., 2008). Therapy for hypothyroidism is typically thyroid hormone replacement, and the most widely prescribed drug is levothyroxine. This man-made hormone is formulated to restore hormone levels to normal, hence improving symptoms and preventing complications such as cardiovascular disease. Factors that influence the efficacy of the treatments, however, include those pertaining to the patient themselves, such as age, comorbidities, and subclinical hypothyroidism. Increasing evidence underscores the importance of close monitoring during treatment, especially in older patients, as they are likely to be at risk for over- and undertreatment of thyroid disease. Clinical trials, such as those evaluating symptomatic benefit with levothyroxine in older adults with subclinical hypothyroidism, are essential for refining treatment algorithms and optimizing management strategies across various patient populations (Bauer et al., 2017) (Figure 3.10).

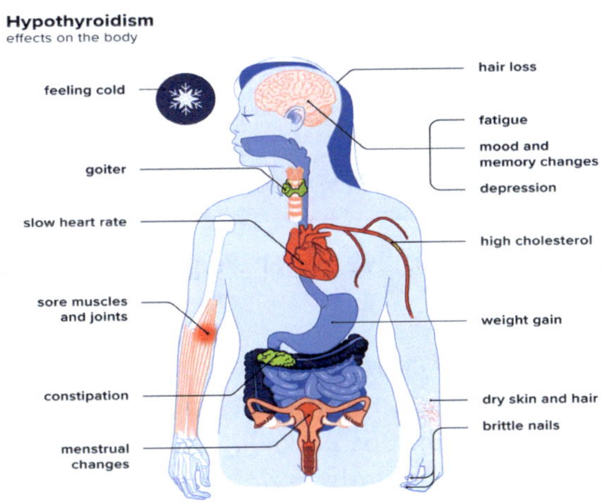

Figure 3.10. Hypothyroidism: Effect on body.

Source: https://media.post.rvohealth.io/wp-content/uploads/sites/3/2025/05/3792894-symptoms-of-hypothyroidism_1296x1317-body.png.

3.4.2. Hyperthyroidism: Causes and Symptoms

Hyperthyroidism, where thyroid hormones are produced in excess, can have several causes, of which the most common is Graves' disease. This is an autoimmune condition that leads to stimulation of the thyroid gland and, in turn, excessive secretion of the hormones thyroxine (T4) and triiodothyronine (T3). Other potential etiologies include toxic adenomas, or benign thyroid tumors independently secreting thyroid hormones, as well as thyroiditis, or thyroid gland inflammation resulting in the release of hormones. Moreover, high dietary intake of iodine can also lead to hyperthyroidism in susceptible patients. It is essential to recognize these origins because etiology has direct implications for management and treatment strategies employed by clinicians. Clinical presentation of hyperthyroidism is varied and has the potential to influence patients' quality of life in a serious manner. Weight loss despite increased appetite, sweating, intolerance to heat, and nervousness or anxiety are some of the frequent symptoms. Palpitations, fatigue, and muscle weakness may also be experienced by patients, which renders their physical status overall poor. Superficially, hyperthyroidism can lead to disturbances in reproductive function, and thus fertility in all genders is affected.

These studies have provided connections between thyroid hormones and reproductive physiology, demonstrating that thyroid dysfunction adversely affects sexual function and sexual health in general. The complexity of such symptoms underlines the need for prolonged evaluation and management by health professionals encompassing both metabolic and reproductive health issues. Hyperthyroidism has particular challenges and concerns in children. Though the incidence of thyroid diseases, such as hyperthyroidism, is relatively low, an awareness of the importance of thyroid function in children is crucial. The surgical options, such as thyroidectomy in the case of malignancy or serious complications, demand an exclusive approach due to the higher risks involved in surgery in children. Expert pediatric thyroid surgeons, as reported in recent literature, recommend a multidisciplinary approach to treating such conditions, involving the collaboration of specialized pediatric endocrinologists, anesthesiologists, and other medical professionals. Such an approach is needed to maximize clinical outcomes and make sure children obtain the best possible treatment, highlighting the intricate relationship between the thyroid gland and pediatric growth and development (Figure 3.11).

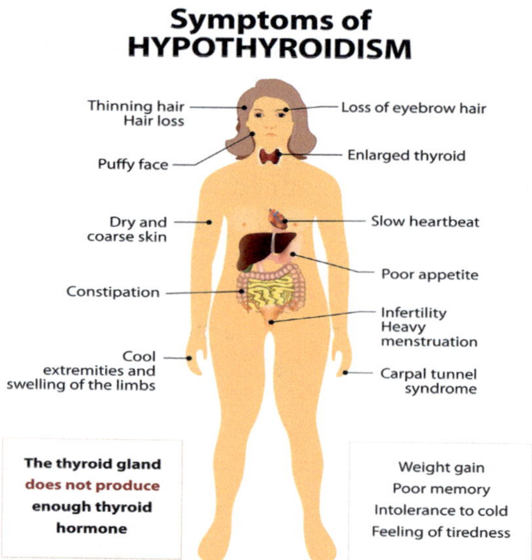

Figure 3.11. Symptoms of hyperthyroidism.

Source: https://www.news-medical.net/image-handler/picture/2016/6/Hyperthyroidism2_shutterstock_344511191.jpg.

3.4.3. Goiter and Thyroid Nodules

Goiter, thyroid gland enlargement, can be caused by numerous underlying etiologies, including iodine deficiency, autoimmune disease, and endocrine disturbances. Goiter is best classified as diffuse and nodular, with nodular goiter consisting of solitary or multiple thyroid nodules, palpable or nonpalpable. Goiter has been found to have an increased incidence directly related to diet and deficiencies in iodine, an essential constituent of thyroid hormone synthesis. Where the ground and water are low in iodine, goiters develop more frequently because the thyroid gland attempts to compensate for its deficiencies. Also, autoimmune disorders such as Hashimoto's thyroiditis and Graves' disease play a significant role in goiter development and in thyroid dysfunction. Both can develop unbalanced hormone levels, yet again obscuring the picture and necessitate a multifaceted approach to diagnosis and treatment (Figure 3.12).

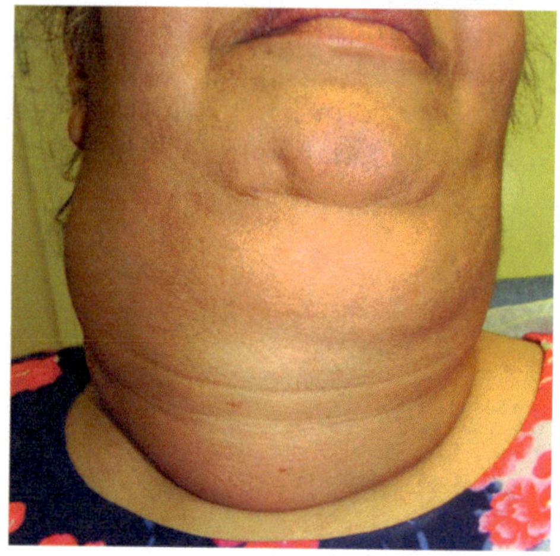

Figure 3.12. Massive goiter weighing more than 800 grams.

Source: https://www.researchgate.net/profile/Norman-Machado/publication/211852346/figure/fig1/AS:305925790420992@1449949800155/Massive-goiter-weighing-more-than-800-grams.png.

Thyroid nodules, although typically benign, can evoke suspicion of underlying malignancy. Studies suggest that the majority of thyroid nodules are nonmalignant but require thorough evaluation to exclude thyroid cancer, particularly in candidates for screening due to high-risk factors. Diagnosis is typically made by ultrasound studies to evaluate the characteristics of the nodule, i.e., size, structure, and vascularity, and then fine-needle aspiration biopsy for cytology if required. Thyroid nodule detection rates have increased due to enhanced imaging modalities, leading to so-called epidemics of overdiagnosis. The implications of such findings are multifaceted; while most nodules are clinically insignificant, the need for intensive monitoring and treatment creates issues with regard to maintaining patient protection and the psychological impact of surveillance. Medical practitioners must handle these complexities with guidelines in place to avoid unnecessary interventions. Additional research shows that lifestyle and environmental influences contribute significantly to goiter and thyroid nodule formation. Iodine intake, a critical element of normal thyroid function, is significant in that both a deficit and a surfeit encourage the manifestation of thyroid disease in the form of goiter and nodular formations. Moreover, thyroid dysfunctions can also be caused by comorbidities such as obesity, which influences hormonal pathways related to thyroid function. Obese individuals can undergo changes in their levels of thyroid hormones, thereby leaving them at an increased risk of the development of thyroid nodules and associated malignancies. In addition, the interplay between genetic susceptibility and environmental factors, such as ionizing radiation or some environmental toxicants, has been the crux of investigation into thyroid abnormalities. As public health interventions persist, management of these interrelated factors will increasingly become important in preventing goiter and thyroid nodules as well as improving patient outcomes (Figure 3.13).

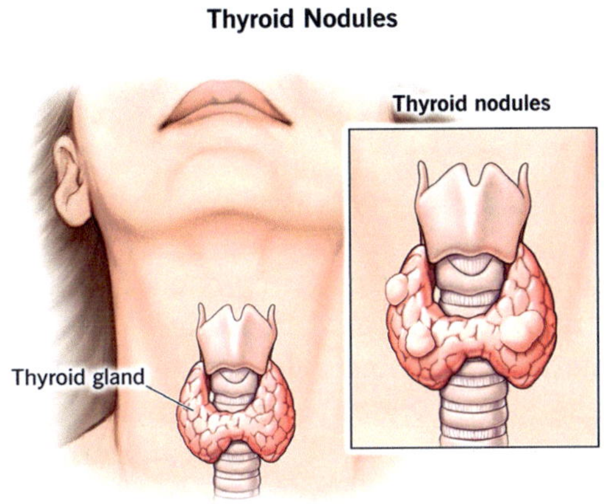

Figure 3.13. Thyroid nodules illustration,

Source: https://my.clevelandclinic.org/-/scassets/images/org/health/articles/13121-thyroid-nodules-illustration.

Test Your Knowledge

1. What are the common causes and symptoms of hypothyroidism?
2. What are the typical causes and symptoms of hyperthyroidism?
3. What is a goiter, and what are its potential causes?

3.5. Diagnosis of Thyroid Disorders

Learning Outcome

1. Explain the importance of blood tests for hormone levels;
2. Describe imaging techniques in the evaluation of the thyroid gland;
3. Describe biopsy procedures for nodules.

Diagnosis of thyroid disorder requires an integrative approach that involves clinical evaluation, biochemical testing, and imaging studies. Initially, physicians review patient history and perform a physical examination with special attention to symptoms indicative of thyroid pathology. Common symptoms include weight loss or gain, intolerance of temperature, and fatigue, which mandate the requirement for additional biochemical evaluation. The most important biomarkers to diagnose thyroid disease are TSH and thyroid hormones like Free T4 and Free T3. Inversely changing levels of TSH typically indicate hypothyroidism, and suppressed levels indicate hyperthyroidism. The presence of thyroid antibodies can also be useful to determine autoimmune diseases like Hashimoto's thyroiditis or Graves' disease, thereby allowing for the diagnosis of thyroid disease based on etiology rather than functional impairment alone. Along with biochemical investigations, imaging studies such as ultrasonography also play a significant part in the diagnosis of thyroid diseases. Ultrasonography can detect structural abnormalities like the presence of nodules, cysts, or goiters in the thyroid gland. It also helps to identify the size and composition of such abnormalities and whether further treatment, such as fine-needle aspiration biopsy for cytological examination, is necessary. For instance, new technological improvements have made the sensitivity and specificity of ultrasound higher, which is able to distinguish between nodules that could potentially require further assessment. In groups where thyroid cancer incidence is on the rise, such as in the United States, where overdiagnosis can be suspected, imaging studies must be applied judiciously so as to balance the harms and benefits of possible overtreatment (Cari et al., 2022). Moreover, emerging evidence indicates the implication of gut microbiota in thyroid function, emphasizing a two-way, multifaceted interplay between the microbiome and thyroid function. Shifts in microbiota composition have been linked to autoimmune thyroid diseases, such as Hashimoto's thyroiditis and Graves' disease, with potential implications for diagnostic purposes in assessing gut health and thyroid disorders. Microbes are a significant regulator of mineral nutrition, particularly of selenium and iodine, both of which play a critical role in the biosynthesis of thyroid hormones. The microbiota and how it interacts with host physiology may be regulated by food intake, obesity, and even sex hormones (Eöhlich et al., 2019). With the addition of microbiota tests to the diagnostic plan, clinicians can possibly reveal even greater information regarding potential underlying pathophysiology of thyroid dysfunction, with applicability to targeted therapy strategies incorporating both endocrine and gastrointestinal function.

3.5.1. Blood Tests for Hormone Levels

Blood tests are critical diagnostic procedures used to identify hormone levels, in particular the health of the thyroid gland. The primary hormones examined are TSH, free thyroxine (FT4) and thyroid peroxidase antibodies (TPO-Ab) that measure thyroid health and function. TSH typically is elevated in hypothyroidism when the thyroid gland is underactive, and FT4 is a direct indicator of thyroid hormone production. The presence of TPO-Ab can be an indicator of autoimmune thyroiditis, suggesting that the immune system is damaging thyroid tissue in error. Regularly monitoring these hormone levels through blood tests can provide very valuable information about an individual's thyroid status and aid in treatment plans as necessary to control diseases such as hypothyroidism and hyperthyroidism. Once baseline hormone levels are established, clinicians will often employ blood tests to guide the treatment of thyroid disease. For instance, in subclinical hypothyroidism (SH), research has shown that treatment efficacy in some instances can be determined by some trace elements in the blood, apart from TSH and FT4 levels. A study of 859 women that reported lowered levels of iodine, selenium, and zinc was associated with the occurrence of SH after adjusting for TPO-Ab levels (Serikbayeva et al., 2024). Documenting such associations aids in comprehending the interrelationship between blood chemistry and thyroid function. Consequently, clinicians can more effectively treat potential deficiencies in these trace elements through diet modification or supplementation and thereby improve overall thyroid function and patient outcomes. In critically ill patients, the prognostic utility of free thyroid hormones has been reported to be of interest, primarily in predicting outcomes in a hospital setting. A recent study reviewed thyroid function in relation to the Acute Physiology and Chronic Health Evaluation II (APACHE II) scoring system and showed significant correlations between free triiodothyronine (FT3) levels and patient survival rates (Swathi et al., 2023). The study indicates that the assessment of these hormone levels can provide valuable prognostic information on mortality risk within intensive care units. Awareness of the interactions between thyroid hormones and patient health as a whole underscores the need for ongoing studies in the area. These investigations point to how sweeping blood screening for thyroid hormones might further evolve, increasing the potential for implementing timely interventions that ultimately lead to a better chance of survival in critically ill patients (Figure 3.14).

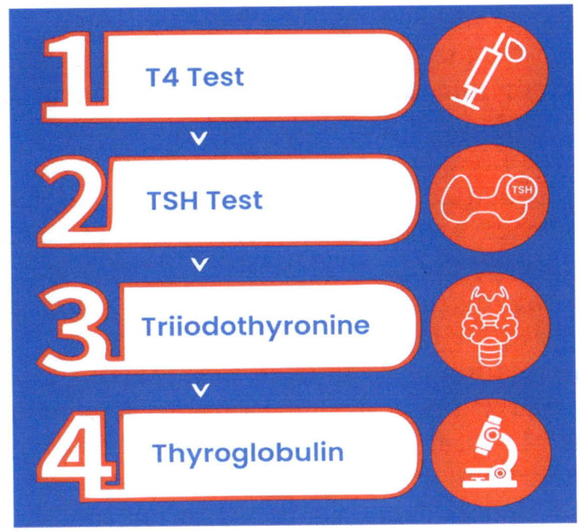

Figure 3.14. Thyroid blood test and types.

Source: https://pathcareindia.com/wp-content/uploads/2022/10/Pathcare_2.jpg.

3.5.2. Imaging Techniques: Ultrasound and Scans

In thyroid gland assessment, imaging modalities prove most important, particularly ultrasound. Ultrasound is non-invasive, providing real-time anatomy images of the thyroids to enable clinicians to assess for abnormalities of the thyroids, including nodules and goiters. Benign versus malignant lesion differentiation is enhanced with this imaging technique. Notably, newer technologies in ultrasound, such as volume sweep imaging (VSI), provide greater access to diagnostic capabilities. The technology is of specific significance in rural communities, where health inequities limit access to skilled radiologists. Research demonstrated that non-expert operators, after receiving just eight hours of instruction, were able to accomplish thyroid ultrasounds with an outstanding 88% image quality score, indicating the strength of tele-diagnostic systems for expanding thyroid assessment across the world. This innovation enables enhanced monitoring and healthcare in thyroid diseases (Thomas et al., 2021). In addition to ultrasound, other imaging studies, such as radioactive iodine uptake scans, play a significant role in the diagnosis of hyperthyroidism and thyroid disease. Hyperthyroidism often provides a complex image, and precise imaging is required to establish the etiology, such as toxic multinodular goiter and Graves' disease. Radioactive iodine scans measure the functional activity of the glands by assessing the capacity of the thyroid to absorb iodine, which is utilized for thyroid hormone production. This information is invaluable because excessive uptake will typically indicate hyperfunctioning thyroid tissue, guiding treatment. Furthermore, integration with radiological examinations and clinical assessments allows for complete care plans tailored to the individual patient. An example is the presence of cardiovascular symptoms in hyperthyroidism cases, which demands early treatment, highlighting the importance of coordinating imaging findings with overall clinical assessment (Amanda et al., 2020). Integration of various imaging modalities fosters an in-depth understanding of thyroid pathology and ultimately more effective patient care. Further advancements of these technologies by the medical fraternity have created a compelling need for effective training and resource planning, especially in remote regions with poor healthcare facilities. Tele-diagnostic ultrasound technology, as noted in literature, appears to be a feasible solution to combat this lack, facilitating local healthcare workers to undertake essential thyroid evaluation. This method not only accelerates diagnostic processes but also enables the timely treatment of thyroid conditions. Moreover, by establishing an expert telediagnostic center, healthcare disparities can be significantly reduced, facilitating better control of conditions such as hyperthyroidism, which, if not treated, can lead to severe complications. While the importance of good imaging techniques is rapidly gaining recognition, the potential for improvement in thyroid management globally remains significant (Thomas et al., 2021) (Figure 3.15).

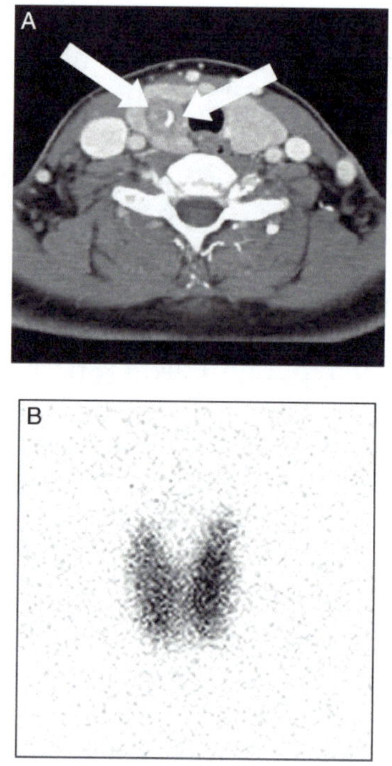

Figure 3.15. Radiologic imaging tests. (A) Enhanced CT shows diffuse enlargement of the thyroid gland and a tumor (arrows) in the right lobe of the thyroid. (B) Thyroidal uptake of radioiodine shows diffuse enlargement of both lobes of the thyroid with homogeneously increased uptake (52.74%).

Source: https://www.researchgate.net/publication/302915320/figure/fig1/AS:621563502137344@1525203695334/Radiologic-imaging-tests-A-Enhanced-CT-showed-diffuse-enlargement-of-the-thyroid-gland.png.

3.5.3. Biopsy Procedures for Nodules

Diagnosis of thyroid nodules often necessitates the use of biopsy methods to assess for possible malignancy. FNAB is widely accepted as the primary technique for thyroid nodule diagnosis since it is less invasive and very diagnostic. The procedure uses a thin needle to penetrate the nodule to harvest cellular material for cytological examination. Studies have shown that the sensitivity of FNAB could be influenced by several factors, such as the characteristics of the nodule, whether its size or composition. Also, the reliability of FNAB results is dependent upon the experience and level of expertise of the physician performing the test. This inconsistency underscores the need for standard protocols and training to enhance reproducibility and consistency of FNAB results in different health facilities so that early detection and intervention become central to patient improvement. Additional biopsy techniques can be employed for indeterminate thyroid nodules to enable proper diagnosis. Molecular testing of aspirated material has emerged as the most important advance, with the ability to identify malignancy-associated genetic markers. The tests are especially helpful in nodules that fall within the category III and IV of Bethesda, where cytologic results remain indefinite. The in-study usefulness of these newer molecular tests best stratifies risk and informs clinical decision-making regarding operation. Yet, implementation of molecular testing in clinical practice must be cautious on cost-effectiveness as well as psychological burden on patients waiting for a diagnosis. Thus, health practitioners must balance the benefits of additional testing against the burden of additional procedures on the patients in a bid to uphold a patient-centered approach to thyroid nodule management. Consequences of the surgical procedure are particularly when the results of FNAB indicate malignancy or high risk. It is in the operating room that FS analysis finds its purpose, where pathologists are enabled to render real-time diagnosis when they carry out thyroid operations. The sensitivity of FS analysis, though generally high, is found to be heterogeneous with regard to certain nodule attributes being examined, such as those with the follicular variant of papillary thyroid carcinoma (fvPTC). Evidence does indicate FS sensitivity to be reduced in certain circumstances, most significantly in the case of MIBI-positive hypofunctional nodules and Bethesda III cases. This correlation favors tailoring biopsy and surgical methods based on each patient's risk factors and nodule characteristics to optimize diagnostic sensitivity and surgical outcomes. The ongoing progressive refinement of biopsy methods and laboratory tests remains essential in the management of the complexity of thyroid nodules as well as in general patient care, as shown by recent studies in the field (Gern et al., 2024; Uysal et al., 2025) (Figure 3.16).

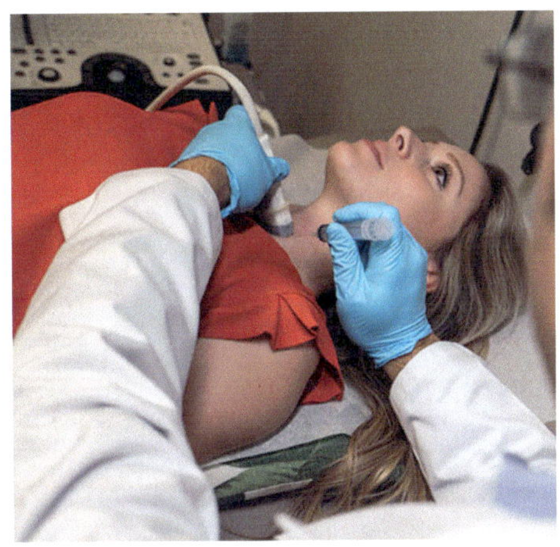

Figure 3.16. Biopsies for thyroid nodules.

Source: https://wp02-media.cdn.ihealthspot.com/wp-content/uploads/sites/469/2019/07/biopsies-content-img.jpg.

Test Your Knowledge

1. Which hormone levels are typically measured in blood tests to assess thyroid function?
2. How is thyroid ultrasound used in diagnosing thyroid disorders?
3. What is the purpose of a radioactive iodine uptake (RAIU) scan in thyroid diagnosis?

3.6. Treatment Options for Thyroid Disorders

Learning Outcome

1. Describe medications for hypothyroidism and hyperthyroidism;
2. Understand radioactive iodine therapy;
3. Deal with surgical interventions for thyroid conditions.

Therapeutic management of thyroid disease varies significantly based on the disease nature and its severity. For hyperthyroidism, a surplus production of thyroid hormones, three basic therapeutic modalities are often employed. Antithyroid drugs such as methimazole inhibit hormone production and are typically the first option, particularly in those who do not wish to undergo surgery or have mild symptoms. Radioiodine therapy, which is highly favored by thyroid specialists in America, involves the killing of excessive thyroid tissue, followed by a gradual decrease in hormone production. Thyroidectomy, i.e., thyroid gland removal through surgery, is reserved for significant indications, for example, giant goiter or suspicious nodules, and also for those individuals with Graves orbitopathy or who express a strong aversion to surgery (Barczy, 2021).

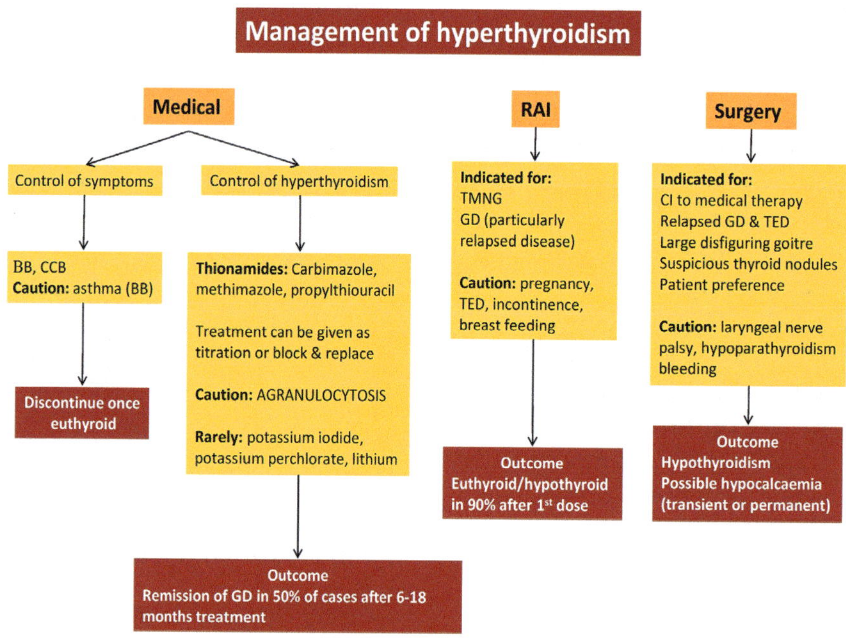

Figure 3.17. Management of hyperthyroidism.

Source: https://www.google.com/url?sa=i&url=https%3A%2F%2Fwww.intechopen.com%2Fchapters%2F31311&psig=AOvVaw05KbtPrhVY_MDA_Nqkdx7&ust=1751279352413000&source=images&cd=vfe&opi=89978449&ved=0CBcQjhxqFwoTCIC9wpK2lo4DFQAAAAAdAAAAABAT.

Each treatment has its advantages and disadvantages, demanding careful consideration in the patient's assessment. The primary treatment for hypothyroidism, a state of insufficient thyroid hormone production, is replacement with hormone. Levothyroxine is the most commonly used medication, a synthetic form of thyroxine (T4), which effectively normalizes the hormone level and alleviates symptoms. It is important for levothyroxine patients to get their TSH checked often to monitor the dosage, which sometimes needs to be altered. And where patients also suffer from other autoimmune thyroid diseases, such as Hashimoto's thyroiditis, other aspects of their health need to be managed because of potential overlap with other diseases. Ideally, a well-balanced TSH level between 0.5 and 2.5 mIU/L is required for normal metabolic function and has the potential to significantly enhance quality of life for those impacted (Poppe, 2021). Thyroid disease also has multidimensional impacts on reproductive health, particularly for women. Thyroid disease correlates with menstrual dysfunction as well as infertility due to its impact on the hypothalamo-pituitary-ovarian axis and reproductive tract. Normalizing thyroid function is necessary, but infertility can remain even after treatment. When assisted reproductive technology (ART) is being considered, it is even more crucial to follow thyroid levels; a single TSH level below 2.5 mIU/L is optimal before being treated with ART to maximize chances of a successful pregnancy. Those presenting with thyroid autoimmunity or who are already on hormone therapy can potentially develop irreversible hypothyroidism and thus need individualized treatment protocols (Poppe, 2021). The interaction between thyroid function and reproductive achievement underlines the importance of integrative care and multidisciplinary approaches in treating thyroid disease effectively (Figure 3.17).

3.6.1. Medications for Hypothyroidism and Hyperthyroidism

Treatment of thyroid disorders such as hypothyroidism and hyperthyroidism often calls for drug regimens towards the re-establishment of endocrine homeostasis. In patients with hypothyroidism, one of the most common treatment procedures involves the prescription of levothyroxine, a man-made substance that mimics the thyroid hormone thyroxine (T4). Levothyroxine works by substituting for the deficient amount of the hormone, eventually eliminating the signs of weakness, weight gain, and depression. Patients typically are given usual monitoring to ensure that the thyroid hormone becomes normal within the range of normal, as inappropriate dosing will result in unwanted side effects. Individualized treatment protocols are strictly necessary as age, weight, and other present medical illnesses can influence the optimal dose of levothyroxine for successful therapy of hypothyroidism (Far et al., 2023). Hyperthyroidism, however, owing to excessive production of thyroid hormone, requires various therapeutic measures. Thionamides, namely methimazole and propylthiouracil, are standard drugs for hyperthyroidism. These inhibit thyroid hormone production, stabilizing the overactive gland. Alternatively, one employs radioactive iodine, which selectively destroys thyroid tissue, ultimately reducing hormone secretion. In critical cases, beta-blockers are commonly prescribed in order to decrease symptoms such as heart palpitations and anxiety prior to the primary therapy taking effect. All of these drugs come with their respective side effects, and monitoring and regulation are thus important. A successful management plan for hyperthyroidism thus centers on a multidisciplinary character with the collaboration of endocrinologists and primary care physicians working together in a manner aimed at optimizing patient outcomes (Cari et al., 2022). Though drug intervention constitutes the bulk of treatment for thyroid dysfunctions, other methods exploring adjunct therapy could prove fruitful in improving patient well-being. New evidence suggests that the addition of antioxidants, such as vitamin C, may prove valuable in enhancing current treatments for certain thyroid disorders. For example, vitamin C has been linked with probable therapeutic value in autoimmune thyroid diseases that tend to coincide with Graves' disease, a cause of hyperthyroidism (Far et al., 2023). However, even as some studies lean towards the effectiveness of vitamin C with combinations involving drug therapies, as yet, there is a paucity of high-quality clinical evidence testifying to this adjunctive role. The study of lifestyle modification and dietetic impacts, as well as medication compliance, offers an integrated framework for understanding the complicated nature of thyroid disease and emphasizes the persistent need for research in this field (Cari et al., 2022).

3.6.2. Radioactive Iodine Therapy

Radioactive iodine therapy (RAI) is today a well-established pillar in the treatment of thyroid diseases, such as hyperthyroidism due to Graves' disease and differentiated thyroid cancers. RAI harnesses the specificity of iodine-131 to selectively target thyroid cells. RAI, once ingested, gets transported by thyroid tissues which leads to excessive or cancerous cells being killed by localized radiation. This method is unique due to its non-surgical nature compared to regular surgical methods and the potential it holds in reducing thyroid hormone production effectively. Clinical guidelines suggest RAI is especially useful in drug-resistant hyperthyroidism as a safe and effective option. Patients receiving RAI are typically required to have thyroid function followed post-therapy in an attempt to assess the success of the therapy and adjust management strategies according to, attaining optimal health outcomes. Effectiveness in RAI is warranted by evidence from research that illustrates its safety and efficacy in suppressing thyroid activity as well as in the management of malignancies. For example, in the case of Graves' disease patients, RAI therapy has indicated promising results in sustaining long-term remission rates and diminishing the frequency of recurrences of hyperthyroidism. Also, recent studies affirm that RAI does not enhance thyroid cancer hazard significantly, substantiating its therapeutic use for the treatment of thyroid disease. Following treatment, most patients are able to transition successfully to a state of hypothyroidism, thus allowing for the institution of thyroid hormone replacement therapy, thus avoiding potential dangers of under-treatment. This type of management is important, given growing incidences of thyroid disease, as supported by USA trends (Cari et al., 2022), implicating RAI as a potential therapy. Although the advantages of RAI are relevant, potential side effects and issues call for meticulous management. For instance, patients may develop transient hypothyroidism and, in some cases, symptoms related to radiation exposure, such as sialadenitis. Healthcare workers must evaluate the risk-benefit ratio for every patient, particularly in vulnerable groups. There would be contraindication in some instances, particularly in patients presenting with active thyroid ophthalmopathy, because it can exacerbate the conditions (George et al., 2018). With the advances made in the field of endocrinology, studies continue to look at how best to optimize RAI therapy, as well as minimize side effects through the use of adjunct therapies, thereby pointing to the importance of customized patient care. Such meticulousness not only fosters efficient management of thyroid diseases but also improves patient safety and quality of life in the long-term treatment of thyroid diseases (Figure 3.18).

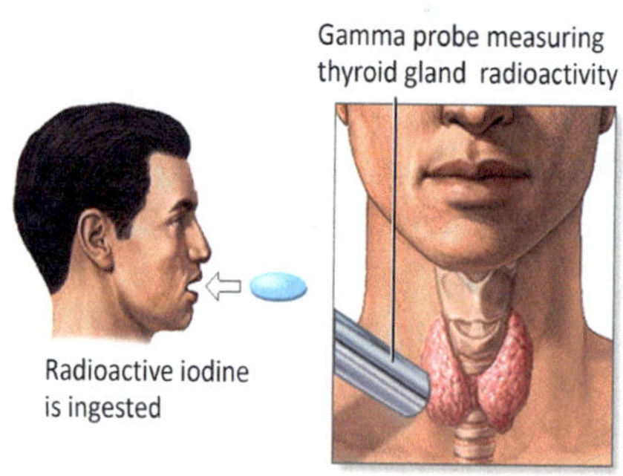

Figure 3.18. Radioactive iodine therapy (RAI) has become a cornerstone in the management of thyroid conditions.

Source: https://ssl.adam.com/graphics/images/en/9806.jpg.

3.6.3. Surgical Interventions

Thyroid surgeries are often necessitated to correct many different disorders, including malignancies and non-malignant tumors like nodules. Partial or total removal of the thyroid gland in a thyroidectomy is one of the most commonly undertaken procedures. This operation is most often suggested in thyroid cancer patients, in whom surgery must be done forthwith to prevent metastasis. Besides, big nodules causing compressive symptoms may also require removal through surgery to alleviate symptoms of swallowing and respiratory distress. Like every surgery, there are risks involved, including bleeding, infection, and potential damage to the surrounding tissues, particularly the recurrent laryngeal nerve and parathyroid glands. Hence, the decision to go ahead with surgery must be balanced thoroughly with the likely benefits and complications, with an immense need for scrupulous preoperative assessment. The evolution of complications as a result of delayed surgery has been particularly astonishing in recent medical literature. Data from studies have shown that the COVID-19 pandemic resulted in decreased rates for elective surgery, including for thyroid disorders. The lateness of these interventions not only accounted for poor clinical outcomes for the patients but also for increased future surgical complexity. Particularly, increased incidence rates of thyroid pathology in this period have been noted, with prompt control being essential. As indicated by ongoing multicenter studies, delaying surgery can have significant consequences, necessitating the prompt reconsideration of surgical schedules in the setting of public health crises. This situation highlights the key role of surgical treatment in managing thyroid diseases efficiently and effectively. In exceptional cases, where surgery initially seems to be unavoidable, a patient's diagnostic workup could lead to alternative forms of therapy. For example, tuberculosis of the thyroid gland, although extremely rare, presents symptoms that may mimic other, more common thyroid pathologies, so that diagnosis is challenging. In two reported cases of thyroid tuberculosis, imaging techniques such as ultrasonography and contrast-enhanced computed tomography (CECT) were of paramount value in proper diagnosis. Fine-needle aspiration cytology (FNAC) with molecular examination confirmed the presence of Mycobacterium tuberculosis and provided an option for successful medical cure with anti-tubercular therapy. These instances show how new developments in diagnostic imaging and minimally invasive techniques can reduce the need for surgical operations and provide quicker and efficient therapies. Recognizing such complications is important in delivering the best patient care for thyroid gland pathology, so much so that individualized treatment to each patient's clinical status is necessary.

Test Your Knowledge

1. What is the standard medication used to treat hypothyroidism, and how does it work?
2. What medications are commonly used to treat hyperthyroidism, and what are their functions?

SUMMARY

The thyroid gland regulates many of the metabolic processes, growth, and health, and its role is worth valuing, especially in relation to modern health challenges. The intricate relationship between thyroid hormone and weight, as highlighted in many research papers, underscores the significance of maintaining thyroid functions in order to prevent metabolic disorders. With consistent rises in obesity globally, the correlation between thyroid impairment is increasingly relevant, particularly among those populations suffering. Research is quoted as showing a high percentage of those with thyroid disease are presented with spectacular fluctuations in metabolic activity and hence are faced with more complicated management of health outcomes. Therefore, thyroid health must be a priority as a subject of discussion and intervention in public health for obesity and other metabolic syndromes, as argued in research on the relationship between hormonal balance and body index readings (Syal et al., 2024). Also, the COVID-19 pandemic has provided new aspects to thyroid disorder management, implying that the long-term viral infection effects might be more comprehensive than the short-term respiratory effects. Evidence suggests that about 15% of patients who have COVID-19 may develop thyroid dysfunction, and it may also manifest in different presentations like hypothyroidism and inflammatory thyroiditis (Syal et al., 2024). This discovery necessitates active monitoring and management of patients, which underscores the value of longitudinal studies to provide an integral level of knowledge regarding the implications of such viral infections on thyroid function. Ongoing assessment of thyroid health within the framework of COVID-19 is significant because it informs treatment strategies and aids in the development of therapeutic interventions with consideration of the unique challenges of preexisting as well as emerging thyroid conditions. Lastly, continued research into the intricacy of the thyroid glands will provide incalculable insight into endocrine disorders, their interdependence with systemic health, and potential therapy. The dynamic nature of thyroid physiology, given its significant influence by diet, environment, and disease, necessitates a comprehensive understanding of thyroid pathologies and their contribution to systemic health. As healthcare professionals strive for better treatments, collaboration between endocrinologists and primary care doctors will be the key to constructing a total picture of the patient. Finally, increased awareness of the thyroid glands crucial role in body function makes way for better public health results as well as quality of life for thyroid disease and related metabolic disorders (Beadini et al., 2024).

When discussing the significance of the thyroid gland, it is essential to note that it plays a crucial role in regulating metabolic processes and maintaining overall hormonal balance within the body. The thyroid gland is responsible for producing vital hormones in the guise of thyroxine (T4) and triiodothyronine (T3), which influence basal metabolic rate, heart rate, and temperature in the body, among other functions within the body. Thyroid hormone disruption can lead to a wide variety of health issues, from hypothyroidism to hyperthyroidism, each with its specific difficulties to health. The preservation of health in the thyroid is necessary for maintaining metabolic vitality and preventing complex diseases involving disparate organ systems, such as the cardiovascular and nervous systems. The effects of the thyroid glands extend beyond basic metabolic regulation; their deficiency has been linked to many life-threatening diseases, including thyroid cancer and other consequences. A considerable increase in thyroid cancer has been reported, drawing attention to the gland's function as an endocrine gland exposed to emerging health issues (Sunavala, 2018). In addition, the therapy of thyroid cancer frequently requires procedures to compromise normal gland function, including thyroidectomy or radioactive iodine ablation. These therapies not only eliminate or destroy neoplastic tissue but also threaten the adjacent salivary glands, resulting in xerostomia and, more generally, a considerable reduction in quality of life in patients. Therefore, it is essential to consider the therapeutic approaches employed in thyroid disease management to fully understand the broader implications of thyroid disease and its impact on overall health. Emerging research also indicates an evocative relationship between endocrine conditions and thyroid dysfunction, as in studies linking gallbladder mucocele development to hypothyroidism and hyperadrenocorticism (Kathleen et al., 2019). This exchange results in a recommendation that thyroid gland performance may affect and be affected by digestive status and adrenal function. The excessive occurrence of hypothyroidism among some groups of animals with the presence of deranged thyroid hormone metabolism further results in the necessity of close observation and effective management of thyroid performance. The complex relationships between the thyroid and the rest of the endocrine glands emphasize the role of the thyroid as an essential member of the endocrine system and its critical role in maintaining overall physiological balance.

KEY TERMS FROM THIS CHAPTER

- Autoimmunity
- Calcium balance
- Cytological examination
- Diagnostic sensitivity
- Endocrine organ
- Environmental influences
- Fine-needle aspiration biopsy
- Goiter development
- Gut microbiota
- Biopsy techniques
- Central nervous system
- Diagnostic capabilities
- Ectopic thyroid tissue
- Energy consumption
- Fibrous capsule
- Glyoxalase 1 expression
- Graves' disease
- Hormonal pathways

CRITICAL THINKING QUESTIONS

1. **Which of the following best describes the anatomical location of the thyroid gland?**
   a. Posterior to the trachea and inferior to the larynx
   b. Anterior to the trachea and inferior to the larynx
   c. Superior to the larynx and anterior to the esophagus
   d. Lateral to the trachea and inferior to the clavicles
2. **The primary function of the thyroid gland is to:**
   a. Produce insulin and regulate blood glucose
   b. Store calcium and phosphorus
   c. Secrete hormones that regulate metabolism
   d. Stimulate red blood cell production
3. **Which hormone from the pituitary gland regulates thyroid hormone production?**
   a. TSH
   b. ACTH
   c. LH
   d. FSH
4. **Which of the following is a symptom of hypothyroidism?**
   a. Rapid heartbeat and weight loss
   b. Tremors and sweating
   c. Fatigue and weight gain
   d. Heat intolerance and increased appetite
5. **What is the most commonly used treatment for hyperthyroidism?**
   a. Levothyroxine
   b. Calcium supplements
   c. Insulin injections
   d. Radioactive iodine therapy

Short Answer Questions

1. Where is the thyroid gland located, and what is its anatomical structure?
2. What are the primary functions of the thyroid gland?
3. What are the main thyroid hormones, and how are they regulated?
4. What is the role of iodine in thyroid hormone production?
5. What are the common symptoms and causes of hypothyroidism?
6. What are common symptoms and causes of hyperthyroidism?
7. How are thyroid disorders diagnosed through blood tests?
8. What imaging techniques are used to assess thyroid structure and function?
9. When is a thyroid nodule biopsy necessary, and how is it done?
10. What are the main treatment options for thyroid disorders?

Answers to Critical Thinking Questions

1. (b); 2. (c); 3. (a); 4. (c); 5. (d)

REFERENCES

1. Abd Elgawad, H., Elmehankar, M., Nabih, N., Sheta, H., & Awad, S. (2025). Impact of experimental congenital toxoplasmosis on the thyroid gland: Histopathological and immunobiochemical indices assessment. *Acta Parasitological, 70*. https://www.semanticscholar.org/paper/717d64922add265541bb8da4bfb6e752906392de (accessed on 22nd July 2025).
2. Adeshara, K., Dahlstrom, E., Lehto, M., Groop, P., Sandholm, N., On Behalf of The Finn Diane Study Group. (2024). 7-OR: Causal associations between glyoxalase 1 expression and kidney disease in type 1 diabetes. *Diabetes*. https://www.semanticscholar.org/paper/c4d36891df98debbcd8fe2541e3a708ba231774e (accessed on 22nd July 2025).
3. Aicher, K. M., Cullen, J. M., Seiler, G. S., Lunn, K. F., Mathews, K. G., & Gookin, J. L. (2019). Investigation of adrenal and thyroid gland dysfunction in dogs with ultrasonographic diagnosis of gallbladder mucocele formation. *PLoS ONE, 14*, e0212638–e0212638. https://doi.org/10.1371/journal.pone.0212638 (accessed on 22nd July 2025).
4. Allen, E., & Fingeret, A. (2019). Anatomy, head and neck, thyroid. *StatPearls Publishing eBooks*. (accessed on 22nd July 2025).
5. Bandazhevskyi, Y. I., & Dubova, N. (2024). Participation of homocysteine in the regulation of thyroid hormone metabolism in children living near the Chornobyl nuclear power plant. *Environment & Health*. https://www.semanticscholar.org/paper/c23844b0aeec3ba80c9e66695415e7861ba82241 (accessed on 22nd July 2025).
6. Barczyński, M. (2021). Current approach to surgical management of hyperthyroidism. *The Quarterly Journal of Nuclear Medicine and Molecular Imaging, 65*. https://doi.org/10.23736/s1824-4785.21.03330-6 (accessed on 22nd July 2025).
7. Bauer, D., Blum, M., Browne, J., Byrne, D., et al. (2017). Study protocol; thyroid hormone replacement for untreated older adults with subclinical hypothyroidism–a randomized placebo controlled trial (TRUST). https://core.ac.uk/download/80696861.pdf (accessed on 22nd July 2025).
8. Beadini, A., Ameti, I., Elezi, A., Beadini, A., Nazifi, A., & Ziberi, E. (2024). Correlation between the disorder of the thyroid gland, obesity and overweight in the female gender. *International Journal of Medical Sciences–Acta Medica Balkanica*. https://www.semanticscholar.org/paper/a2fc0edf530dc2d7a81236c044e29c5d06c145d3 (accessed on 22nd July 2025).
9. Bhanu, U. K. (2024). The role of thyroid & parathyroid hormones in prosthodontic treatment–A narrative review. *International Journal of Scientific Research in Engineering and Management*. https://www.semanticscholar.org/paper/3fd63c34e5e8dfb8cfa7ed72c8d9f9f0ce539ac9 (accessed on 22nd July 2025).
10. Biondi, B., & Cooper, D. S. (2008). The clinical significance of subclinical thyroid dysfunction. https://core.ac.uk/download/54955329.pdf (accessed on 22nd July 2025).
11. Bray, F., Ferlay, J., Soerjomataram, I., Siegel, R. L., Torre, L. A., & Jemal, A. (2018). Global cancer statistics 2018: GLOBOCAN estimates of incidence and mortality worldwide for 36 cancers in 185 countries. *CA: A Cancer Journal for Clinicians, 68*, 394–424. https://doi.org/10.3322/caac.21492 (accessed on 22nd July 2025).
12. Breuer, C., Solomon, D., Sosa, J. A., Tuggle, C., et al. (2013). Pediatric thyroid disease: When

is surgery necessary, and who should be operating on our children? https://core.ac.uk/download/323075246.pdf (accessed on 22nd July 2025).

13. Carosa, E., Jannini, E. A., & Lenzi, A. (2018). Thyroid hormone receptors and ligand, tissue distribution and sexual behavior. https://core.ac.uk/download/160052696.pdf (accessed on 22nd July 2025).

14. Castillo-Armengol, J., Fajas, L., & López-Mejía, I. C. (2019). Inter-organ communication: A gatekeeper for metabolic health. *EMBO Reports, 20*. https://doi.org/10.15252/embr.201947903 (accessed on 22nd July 2025).

15. Chandrasekar, A., Schmidtlein, P. M., Neve, V., Rivagorda, M., Spiecker, F., Gauthier, K., Prevot, V., et al. (2023). Regulation of thyroid hormone gatekeepers by TSH in tanycytes. *Thyroid: Official Journal of the American Thyroid Association*. https://www.semanticscholar.org/paper/aa1e0831c0742ce48b763d8a075cfe52bbc7720d (accessed on 22nd July 2025).

16. Costa-e-Sousa, R. H., Rorato, R., Hollenberg, A., & Vella, K. (2023). Regulation of thyroid hormone levels by hypothalamic TRH (thyrotropin-releasing hormone) neurons. *Thyroid: Official Journal of the American Thyroid Association*. https://www.semanticscholar.org/paper/1650acaae67a7bc97009f98ee6d7329cab6f0e20 (accessed on 22nd July 2025).

17. Doubleday, A. R., & Sippel, R. S. (2020). Hyperthyroidism. *Gland Surgery, 9*, 124–135. https://doi.org/10.21037/gs.2019.11.01 (accessed on 22nd July 2025).

18. Dsouki, N. A., Pereira, B. F., da Silva, R. G., Rodrigues, V. G., Brito, R. S., Kizys, M. M., Chiamolera, M., et al. (2024). The interplay of the mammalian brain and thyroid hormones, and the threat of endocrine-disrupting chemicals. *Endocrines*. https://www.semanticscholar.org/paper/edb3146060a029023d95cb92a0867f847f30443f (accessed on 22nd July 2025).

19. Farasati Far, B., Behnoush, A. H., Ghondaghsaz, E., Habibi, M. A., & Khalaji, A. (2023). The interplay between vitamin C and thyroid. *Endocrinology Diabetes & Metabolism, 6*. https://doi.org/10.1002/edm2.432 (accessed on 22nd July 2025).

20. Fekete, C., & Lechan, R. M. (2013). Central regulation of hypothalamic-pituitary-thyroid axis under physiological and pathophysiological conditions. *Endocrine Reviews, 35*, 159–194. https://doi.org/10.1210/er.2013-1087 (accessed on 22nd July 2025).

21. Fernández-García, V., González-Ramos, S., Martín-Sanz, P., Laparra, J. M., & Boscá, L. (2021). Beyond classic concepts in thyroid homeostasis: Immune system and microbiota. *Molecular and Cellular Endocrinology, 533*, 111333–111333. https://doi.org/10.1016/j.mce.2021.111333 (accessed on 22nd July 2025).

22. Fröhlich, E., & Wahl, R. (2019). Microbiota and thyroid interaction in health and disease. *Trends in Endocrinology and Metabolism, 30*, 479–490. https://doi.org/10.1016/j.tem.2019.05.008 (accessed on 22nd July 2025).

23. Gern, J., Arbogast, M., Alakus, H., Brunner, S., Schmidt, M., Faust, M., Bruns, C., et al. (2024). Intraoperative thyroid frozen section: Indications, results and consequences. *Gland Surgery, 13*, 630–639. https://www.semanticscholar.org/paper/b0471aa4fbc00182be6c3a74c3e7821c722f9c07 (accessed on 22nd July 2025).

24. Hanley, P. C., Lord, K., & Bauer, A. J. (2016). Thyroid disorders in children and adolescents. *JAMA Pediatrics, 170*, 1008–1008. https://doi.org/10.1001/jamapediatrics.2016.0486 (accessed on 22nd July 2025).

25. Kahaly, G. J., Bartalena, L., Hegedüs, L., Leenhardt, L., Poppe, K., & Pearce, S. H. S. (2018). 2018 European Thyroid Association guideline for the management of Graves' hyperthyroidism. *European Thyroid Journal, 7*, 167–186. https://doi.org/10.1159/000490384 (accessed on 22nd July 2025).

26. Karcioglu, A. S., Triponez, F., Solórzano, C., Iwata, A. J., Abdelhamid Ahmed, A. A., Almquist, M., Angelos, P., et al. (2023). Emerging imaging technologies for parathyroid gland identification and vascular assessment in thyroid surgery: A review from the American Head and Neck Society Endocrine Surgery Section. *JAMA Otolaryngology–Head & Neck Surgery*. https://www.semanticscholar.org/paper/992f68d79f1e88af9e84b8f1ba34f7211cd60960 (accessed on 22nd July 2025).

27. Khabarov, O. R., Zima, D. V., Bezrukov, O. F., & Yu Zyablitskaya, E. (2024). Consequences of the COVID-19 pandemic on the structure of surgical pathology of the thyroid gland. *Cardiometry*. https://www.semanticscholar.org/paper/4b2fa60f4d0a02a7350a57e2ef643ba0606af1ed (accessed on 22nd July 2025).

28. Khalid, W., Maqbool, Z., Arshad, M. S., Kousar, S., Akram, R., Siddeeg, A., Ali, A., et al. (2022). Plant-derived functional components: Prevent from various disorders by regulating the endocrine glands. *International Journal of Food Properties, 25*, 976–995. https://doi.org/10.1080/10942912.2022.2070643 (accessed on 22nd July 2025).

29. Kitahara, C. M., & Schneider, A. B. (2022). Epidemiology of thyroid cancer. *Cancer Epidemiology Biomarkers & Prevention, 31*, 1284–1297. https://doi.org/10.1158/1055-9965.epi-21-1440 (accessed on 22nd July 2025).

30. Lahmidi, M. D., Le Noc, M., Dali, O., Kernanec, P. Y., Merret, P. E., Jaulin, C., & Smagulova, F. (2024). Sex-specific transgenerational effects on murine thyroid gland imposed by ancestral exposure to neonicotinoid thiacloprid. *Scientific Reports, 14*. https://www.semanticscholar.org/paper/bc02f8078152ba5647ab38a81e21a49a55d585ba (accessed on 22nd July 2025).

31. Mariani, G., Tonacchera, M., Grosso, M., Orsolini, F., Vitti, P., & Strauss, H. W. (2020). The role of nuclear medicine in the clinical management of benign thyroid disorders, part 1: Hyperthyroidism. *Journal of Nuclear Medicine, 62*, 304–312. https://doi.org/10.2967/jnumed.120.243170 (accessed on 22nd July 2025).

32. Marini, T. J., Weiss, S. L., Gupta, A., Zhao, Y., Baran, T. M., Garra, B. S., Shafiq, I., et al. (2021). Testing telediagnostic thyroid ultrasound in Peru: A new horizon in expanding access to imaging in rural and underserved areas. *Journal of Endocrinological Investigation, 44*, 2699–2708. https://doi.org/10.1007/s40618-021-01584-7 (accessed on 22nd July 2025).

33. Mohebati, A., & Shaha, A. R. (2011). Anatomy of thyroid and parathyroid glands and neurovascular relations. *Clinical Anatomy, 25*, 19–31. https://doi.org/10.1002/ca.21220 (accessed on 22nd July 2025).

34. Mojadadi, A., Au, A. L. S., Salah, W., Witting, P. K., & Ahmad, G. (2021). Role for selenium in metabolic homeostasis and human reproduction. *Nutrients, 13*, 3256–3256. https://doi.org/10.3390/nu13093256 (accessed on 22nd July 2025).

35. N/A. (2007). *Focal Spot, Summer/Fall 2007*. https://core.ac.uk/download/129069359.pdf (accessed on 22nd July 2025).

36. N/A. (2008). *Focal Spot, Spring 2008*. https://core.ac.uk/download/129069364.pdf (accessed on 22nd July 2025).

37. Pachipala, M. S., & Aiyappan, S. (2024). Two interesting cases of thyroid gland tuberculosis. *Cureus, 16*. https://www.semanticscholar.org/paper/cbfce0d0dbe380a53a5c70742945b9315dd2a89e (accessed on 22nd July 2025).

38. Poppe, K. (2021). Management of endocrine disease: Thyroid and female infertility: More questions than answers?! *European Journal of Endocrinology, 184*, R123–R135. https://doi.org/10.1530/eje-20-1284 (accessed on 22nd July 2025).

39. Rana, S., Sati, R., Thapa, T., Rana, P., Joshi, M., Praveen, S., Pundir, N., et al. (2024). Assess the knowledge regarding thyroid disorders among patients attending medical OPD. *International Journal of Community Medicine and Public Health*. https://www.semanticscholar.org/paper/05d1f1bf3fbc5fd7b83c172f2293dc82d8423789 (accessed on 22nd July 2025).

40. Rao, S. S., Rao, H. K., Moinuddin, Z., Rozario, A. P., & Augustine, T. (2023). Preservation of parathyroid glands during thyroid and neck surgery. *Frontiers in Endocrinology, 14*. https://doi.org/10.3389/fendo.2023.1173950 (accessed on 22nd July 2025).

41. Ribas, A., & Wolchok, J. D. (2018). Cancer immunotherapy using checkpoint blockade. *Science, 359*, 1350–1355. https://doi.org/10.1126/science.aar4060 (accessed on 22nd July 2025).

42. Serikbayeva, A., Rymar, O., Shcherbakova, L. V., & Tauesheva, Z. B. (2024). Hormonal, biochemical parameters and blood microelement levels in young women with subclinical hypothyroidism combined with thyroid peroxidase antibody positivity. *Therapist's Bulletin*. https://www.semanticscholar.org/paper/4fd67703740c4b58146866da2d340a7a90925ed8 (accessed on 22nd July 2025).

43. Severo, J. S., Morais, J. B. S., de Freitas, T. E. C., Andrade, A. L. P., Feitosa, M. M., Fontenelle, L. C., de Oliveira, A. R. S., et al. (2019). The role of zinc in thyroid hormones metabolism. *International Journal for Vitamin and Nutrition Research, 89*, 80–88. https://doi.org/10.1024/0300-9831/a000262 (accessed on 22nd July 2025).

44. Stepien, B. K., & Huttner, W. B. (2019). Transport, metabolism, and function of thyroid hormones in the developing mammalian brain. *Frontiers in Endocrinology, 10*. https://doi.org/10.3389/fendo.2019.00209 (accessed on 22nd July 2025).

45. Sun, H. G., & He, L. Q. (2025). Macro-TSH interference in thyroid function testing: A case report and literature review. *Clinical Laboratory, 71*(4). https://www.semanticscholar.org/paper/55283f2b4af191c6e9ffb870c260705537731855a (accessed on 22nd July 2025).

46. Sunavala-Dossabhoy, G. (2018). Radioactive iodine: An unappreciated threat to salivary gland function. *Oral Diseases, 24*, 198–201. https://doi.org/10.1111/odi.12774 (accessed on 22nd July 2025).

47. Swathi, P. K., S. N., S. L., & Anil, A. (2023). Thyroid hormone levels and its relation to outcomes in ICU patients. *Global Journal for Research Analysis*. https://www.semanticscholar.org/paper/fa06756dff9f5a222bf0c4072685e2e1452ebe73 (accessed on 22nd July 2025).

48. Syal, R., Kaur, J., Siddiqui, M., Amatul-Raheem, H., Suarez, C., Avinash Bojanki, N. L. S. V., Kapadia, S. D., et al. (2024). Long-term impacts of COVID-19 on thyroid health: Insights from clinical studies. *Cureus, 16*. https://www.semanticscholar.org/paper/939265ea81bc77aac1e20b6357a4776c76fad2bc (accessed on 22nd July 2025).

49. Tassinari, M., Tanzi, G., Maggiore, F., Groeneweg, S., van Geest, F. S., Freund, M. E. T., Stavast, C. J., et al. (2024). Molecular mechanism of thyroxine transport by monocarboxylate transporters.

Nature Communications, 16. https://www.semanticscholar.org/paper/007ef2aa8cf44fffe91db52ed369c8f60c99cf69 (accessed on 22nd July 2025).

50. Uysal, E., Yangoz, B., Sagan, M., Duman, I., & Alparslan, A. S. (2025). An interobserver comparison of the ultrasound lexicon classification of thyroid nodules: A single-center prospective validation study. *Journal of Clinical Medicine, 14*. https://www.semanticscholar.org/paper/29b984f9cc17aaab8be76822fbd02c2169bc3a2d (accessed on 22nd July 2025).

51. Yang, N., Wessoly, L., Meng, Y., Kiefer, M. F., Chen, Y., Vahrenbrink, M., Wulff, S., et al. (2024). The oxidoreductase retinol saturase in thyroid gland is regulated by hypothyroidism and iodide overload and its deletion impairs metabolic homeostasis in mice. *Antioxidants & Redox Signaling*. https://www.semanticscholar.org/paper/ec29f6db6609d7e373a98d5eefe5760c6e157969 (accessed on 22nd July 2025).

ADRENAL GLAND

4

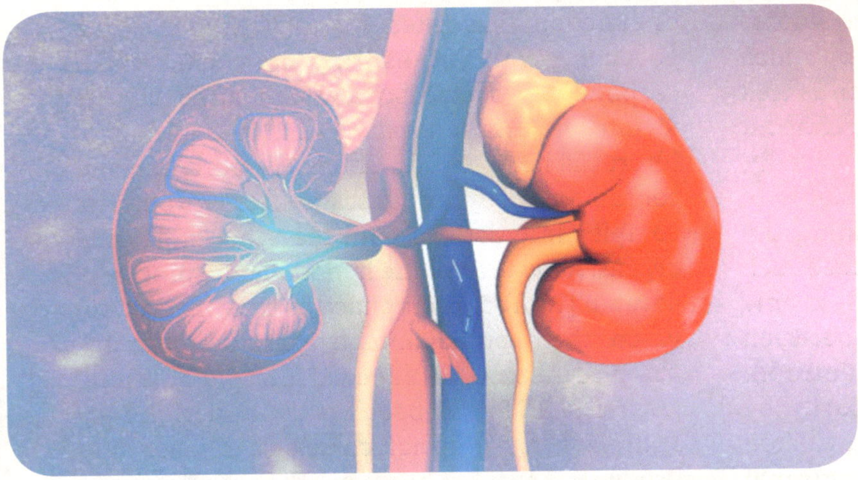

Introduction

The adrenal gland, the prime organ of the endocrine system, is responsible for the body's response to stress, metabolism, and general hormonal balance. Positioned on top of each kidney, the glands are divided into an outer cortex and an inner medulla that each release various hormones essential for varying physiological processes. The adrenal cortex also secretes corticosteroids, such as cortisol, which regulate metabolism, immune responses, and stress, while the adrenal medulla produces catecholamines such as adrenaline and norepinephrine, which influence blood pressure and heart rate in the case of stress (cortisol and catecholamines). It is essential to realize the complex relationship of these hormones and how they affect bodily functions to realize the larger significance of adrenal health, as imbalances can lead to severe disorders, including adrenal insufficiency and Cushing's syndrome. There has been growing interest in the last few years in challenging the effect drugs have on the adrenal activity, in particular,

LEARNING OBJECTIVES

After studying this chapter, you will be able to:

1. Understand the anatomy of the adrenal gland;
2. Discuss hormones produced by the adrenal gland;
3. Explain the functions of the adrenal gland;
4. Describe the disorders of the adrenal gland;
5. Define diagnostic methods for adrenal gland disorders;
6. Focus on treatment options for adrenal gland disorders.

atypical antipsychotics. For instance, the use of paliperidone — an atypical antipsychotic — has been linked to cases of central adrenal insufficiency, demonstrating the efficacy of the drug in impacting adrenal hormone release (paliperidone). A case report from a patient with schizoaffective disorder demonstrates the mechanism by which paliperidone might have contributed to adrenal insufficiency, demonstrating the responsibility of clinicians to understand the risks of long-term antipsychotic use. These findings necessitate further studies to account for the specific mechanisms by which some drugs can disturb adrenal function, as well as the ensuing implications for patient treatment and management in psychiatric therapy. Finally, the addition of hormonal tests and states of body metabolism is crucial in elucidating the role of the adrenal gland in health diseases such as obesity and endocrine dysfunction. It is now established that there are correlations between the body mass index (BMI) and gonadotropin hormones, which are regulated primarily by the pituitary gland and secondarily regulated by the hormone production of the adrenal gland (gonadotropins). The correlations may provide an explanation for the disturbances in metabolism observed among certain populations, particularly females. With the adrenal gland at the hub of regulation of hormones, disruption of its function can have implications beyond direct impact on the adrenal itself, extending to more generalized endocrine processes and contributing to such complications as polycystic ovary syndrome and infertility. The adrenal gland remains, therefore, central in the search to elucidate the complex interdependencies of endocrine function and their expression in health and disease.

Definition of the Adrenal Gland

The adrenal glands are two small triangular endocrine glands located at the top of each kidney and play a vital role in the regulation of hormones in the body's system. The two most prominent parts of each gland are the adrenal cortex and the adrenal medulla. The adrenal cortex produces vital steroid hormones, including cortisol, aldosterone, and sex hormones, that the body utilizes for various physiological functions, such as metabolism, immunity, and the regulation of blood pressure. Conversely, the adrenal medulla secretes catecholamines, such as adrenaline and noradrenaline, necessary for the fight-or-flight response of the body. This segmentation of function illustrates the overall role of the adrenal glands in ensuring homeostasis and responding to stressors, again affirming its significance in general health. In addition to its crucial hormonal functions, the adrenal gland coordinates body responses to stress through its complex interactions with the other endocrine organs. Activation of the hypothalamic-pituitary-adrenal (HPA) axis emphasizes this interaction, where the hypothalamus triggers the pituitary gland to release adrenocorticotropic hormone (ACTH). ACTH subsequently functions to stimulate the adrenal cortex to release and produce cortisol, a hormone that regulates not only metabolism but also modulates immune response and inflammation. The interaction between the elements is typical of the adrenal glands' facilitative role in adaptive responses to acute and chronic stress, reaffirming its significance as part of a bigger endocrine system. Understanding the functionality of the adrenal glands is crucial because dysfunction in this gland can lead to serious health problems. Conditions such as Addison's disease, with a deficiency of hormone secretion, and Cushing's syndrome, due to an oversecretion of cortisol, exemplify the importance of health monitoring as it pertains to adrenal function. The potential outcomes of adrenal disease can range from fatigue, weakness in the muscles, and weight alteration to infection susceptibility and cardiovascular compromise. Thus, studying the adrenal gland's definition and function becomes crucial in determining its critical role in preserving health, demonstrating the fine-tuned balance that must be achieved in the endocrine system to provide physiological homeostasis and to resist external stress (Kling et al., 1939; Matthew et al., 1981) (Figure 4.1).

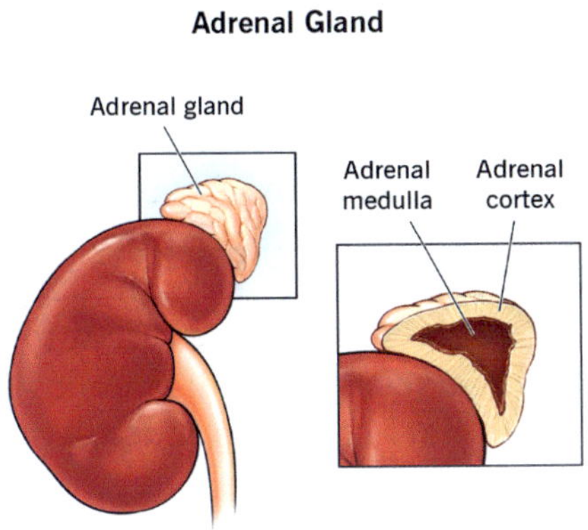

Figure 4.1. Illustration of the adrenal gland.

Source: https://my.clevelandclinic.org/-/scassets/images/org/health/articles/23005-adrenal-gland.

Importance of the Adrenal Gland in the Endocrine System

The adrenal gland is crucial in the endocrine system, mainly through its hormone production, which is critical to metabolic activity and physiological regulation. The two principal components of the adrenal gland—the adrenal cortex and the adrenal medulla—both function to produce diverse hormones that all affect numerous body functions. The adrenal cortex secretes corticosteroids such as cortisol and aldosterone, which are essential for stress reaction, immune function, and maintaining blood pressure and electrolyte balance. The adrenal medulla, however, secretes catecholamines such as adrenaline and noradrenaline, which play a pivotal role in the fight or flight response, which prepares the body to react against stress. This intricate hormonal interaction indicates the function of the adrenal glands in maintaining homeostasis and responding to environmental change. Research has established that dysfunction within the hypothalamic-pituitary-adrenal (HPA) axis, to which the adrenal gland belongs, can result in severe health disorders. For instance, disturbance of this axis might result in disease in the form of Addison's disease or Cushing's syndrome and highlights the significance of hormonal balance and glandular function. This axis is crucial not only for individual responses to stress, but also for overall endocrine health, as the hormones released by the adrenal gland have functions that impact other endocrine glands and, in turn, influence bodily functions such as growth, metabolism, and reproductive function. The seamless function of the HPA axis is particularly critical during the preterm developmental stages, as its dysfunction has been linked with adverse effects, which illustrate vividly how health and adrenal function are intertwined in the overall context of endocrine balance (Göransson et al., 2013). Additionally, the mechanisms of control that operate on the adrenal gland are directly connected to circadian rhythms, which serve to emphasize its role as one of the body's internal clocks controlling a number of its physiological and metabolic processes. Modern studies have unveiled the intricate molecular machinery that governs the biological clocks with significant bearings on our understanding of hormonal and metabolic homeostasis. Disturbances of circadian biology are now well-documented as underlying factors for many endocrine pathologies, thus illustrating the necessity of comprehensive health management, including evaluation of both adrenal function and synchronization of circadian rhythms. As our knowledge of such interrelations progresses, it creates possibilities for novel therapeutic approaches to cure endocrine disorders by fixing not only hormonal imbalances but also their underlying circadian abnormalities (Bruscalupi et al., 2017).

4.1. Anatomy of the Adrenal Gland

Learning Outcome

1. Discuss the location and structure of the adrenal glands;
2. Describe the cortex and medulla;
3. Understand the concept of blood supply and innervation.

The adrenal glands, which lie over the kidneys, are vital components of the endocrine system that undergo a complex balance of hormone production and secretion required for the regulation of various physiological events. Both glands have two major components: the adrenal cortex and the adrenal medulla. The adrenal cortex is further divided into three separate layers: zona glomerulosa, zona fasciculata, and zona reticularis, each of which secretes specific hormones. The zona glomerulosa produces primarily mineralocorticoids, responsible for the regulation of electrolyte balance and blood pressure, and the zona fasciculata synthesizes glucocorticoids, like cortisol, used in metabolism and stress. The zona reticularis synthesizes androgens, which are precursors to sex hormones. An understanding of the structure and function of these layers is essential to comprehend the fundamental importance of adrenal gland function in overall health and disease states. The adrenal medulla, the medullary portion of the adrenal gland, is centrally located in the body's fight-or-flight reaction. It is the source of the release and synthesis of catecholamines, such as adrenaline and norepinephrine, which are central to preparing to respond to stress. Upon stimulation by the sympathetic nervous system, the adrenal medulla releases these hormones into the circulatory system, resulting in an accelerated heartbeat, heightened alertness, and improved supply of energy. Interesting to note is that the functionality of the adrenal medulla is directly related to the response of stress, enabling the body to quickly react to danger. Moreover, neurochemical mechanisms that utilize such catecholamines are controlled by the interactions between the limbic system, in charge of emotion and memory, and the adrenal gland (Kohl et al., 2025). This interaction reveals the broader significance of the adrenal medulla in psychological and physiological contexts. Emerging research indicates how pituitary gland functional connectivity contributes to BMI, exemplifying the intricate relationship between metabolic function and hormonal regulation. While the primary role of the pituitary gland is to regulate the secretion of hormones in other glands, like the adrenal glands, connectivity patterns provide insights into obesity and body weight regulation. Research involving resting-state functional Magnetic Resonance Imaging (rsfMRI) has identified BMI to be strongly correlated with the functional connectivity of the pituitary gland with other brain regions, such as the hippocampus and orbitofrontal cortex, both regions linked to eating behavior and weight control (Rucker et al., 2017). This highlights how imbalances in the endocrine system, particularly involving adrenal hormones like cortisol, may contribute to metabolic disorders, illustrating the importance of the adrenal glands' anatomical and functional integrity in maintaining homeostasis (Figure 4.2).

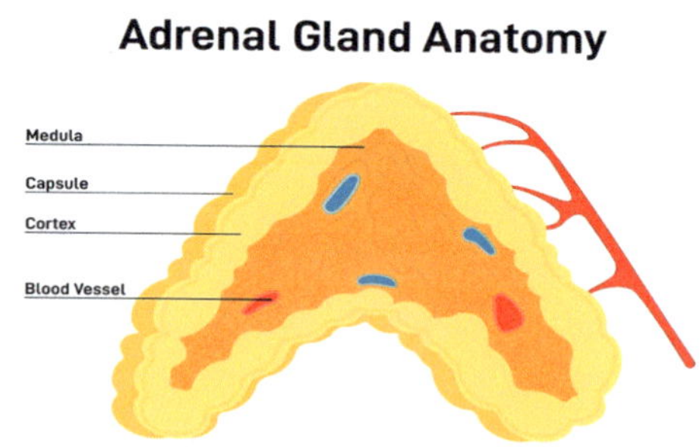

Figure 4.2. Adrenal gland anatomy.

Source: https://acesurgery.sg/wp-content/uploads/2023/11/image-41-1024x748.jpeg.

4.1.1. Location and Structure of the Adrenal Glands

Adrenal glands, which are also key components of the endocrine system, are positioned hopefully on the top surface of the kidneys in the retroperitoneal space. The proximity to the kidneys allows for smooth interaction of hormones, particularly during a situation of stress. The two primary zones of each gland include the outer cortex and the inner medulla. The cortex is also responsible for the secretion of steroid hormones, including glucocorticoids and mineralocorticoids, to regulate metabolism and electrolyte balance. The medulla, however, secretes catecholamines like epinephrine and norepinephrine, which cause the body's fight-or-flight response. Understanding the anatomy and location of the adrenal glands is important to appreciate their active participation in homeostasis and response to physiological stressors. Interestingly, structural and positional abnormalities of the adrenal glands also occur. Ectopic adrenal tissue, in certain instances, results from defective migration of the mesodermal cells during the development process. In a study of adrenal ectopias in adult rats, 27.90% of the occurrences presented with abnormal adrenal positions, which were categorized as intracapsular, extracapsular, and extraorganic types. In spite of such differences, the basic organization remains a mixture of cortex and medulla with discrete functional areas of different physiological functions. Histological distinction of ectopic adrenal tissue can yield knowledge regarding varied morphological adaptive changes of adrenal glands in various species, which could be used to understand their evolutionary significance in different organisms, e.g., birds whose adrenal organization varies considerably between them (Morozov, 2024). Furthermore, the morphology of the adrenal gland differs considerably from one animal species to another in sync with their distinct environmental and physiological needs. In birds, for example, adrenal glands differ in shape, such as oval, triangular, and pyramidal shapes, corresponding to the species type. Histologically, the cortex is made up of steroid-producing acidophilic cells, while the medulla is made up of catecholamine-synthesizing basophilic cells. The morphological characteristics of bird adrenal glands are inhomogeneous and exhibit great differences in size and cell composition based on age as well as sexual activity. Studies have outlined the intricate relationship among these variables, giving insight into how poultry adrenal glands are pivotal with regard to development, stress, and metabolic processes (Kot et al., 2023). Understanding these differences makes us more knowledgeable about the roles and significance of the adrenal glands between diverse species (Figure 4.3).

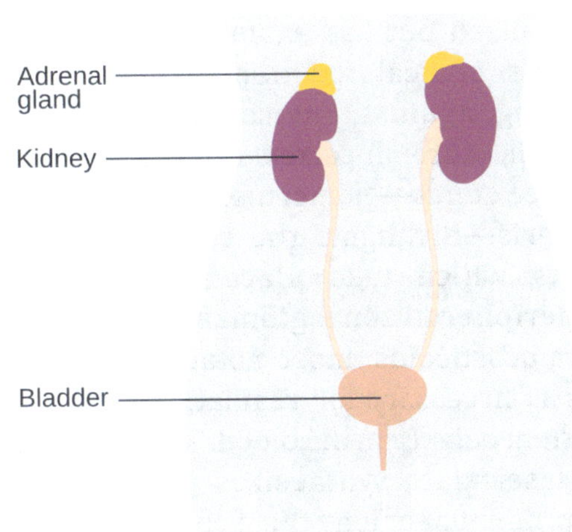

Figure 4.3. Diagram showing the position of the adrenal glands.

Source: https://upload.wikimedia.org/wikipedia/commons/thumb/8/8e/Diagram_showing_the_position_of_the_adrenal_glands_CRUK_343.svg/1024px-Diagram_showing_the_position_of_the_adrenal_glands_CRUK_343.svg.png.

4.1.2. Division into Cortex and Medulla

The adrenal gland, being an essential endocrine organ, possesses a special structural organization into two primary regions: the cortex and the medulla. The adrenal cortex secretes various steroid hormones, including glucocorticoids, mineralocorticoids, and androgens. These hormones play very significant roles in regulating metabolism, immune function, and electrolyte balance. For instance, cortisol, the primary glucocorticoid, facilitates the body's response to stress by influencing glucose metabolism and inflammation. The adrenal medulla, being of neuroectodermal derivation, also has a primarily secretory function, that of catecholamines, such as epinephrine and norepinephrine, which are crucial in initiating the fight-or-flight response. Hence, each component of the adrenal gland is specialized but has analogous physiological functions critical for homeostasis and for defending against environmental stresses. Within the adrenal cortex, further subdivision into three zones—glomerulosa, fasciculata, and reticularis—highlights the complex hormone outputs which take place in this region. The peripheral zona glomerulosa produces mineralocorticoids, most notably aldosterone, which is necessary for regulating sodium and potassium balance in the blood. The intermediate zona fasciculata synthesizes glucocorticoids, most prominent among them cortisol, utilized to support metabolic processes and help respond to acute stressors. Concurrently, the inner zona reticularis secretes adrenal androgens, which contribute to the development of secondary sex characteristics and other metabolic functions. The intricate control of hormone release by the zones is influenced by the renin-angiotensin system and adrenocorticotropic hormone (ACTH) released by the pituitary gland. This sophisticated system of regulation emphasizes the complexity of adrenal function, particularly in the interplay between different zones of the cortex and between cortex and medulla. Conversely, the adrenal medulla is best suited to produce a rapid response to stress by virtue of its quick release of catecholamines. This response is critical in preconditioning the body for strenuous exercise by increasing heart rate, blood pressure, and energy stores. Medulla's release of epinephrine and norepinephrine is carefully regulated through the sympathetic nervous system to allow quick adaptation to environmental stress. Awareness of the role of both cortex and medulla in stress reactions explains their combined effect on overall health and well-being. Further, pathologies of hormone secretion and production from these two regions can lead to numerous disorders like Cushing's syndrome or Addison's disease. Therefore, demarcation into cortex and medulla not only reveals the intricate functional organization of adrenal glands but also informs us about clinical perception of endocrine health and disease therapy (Figure 4.4).

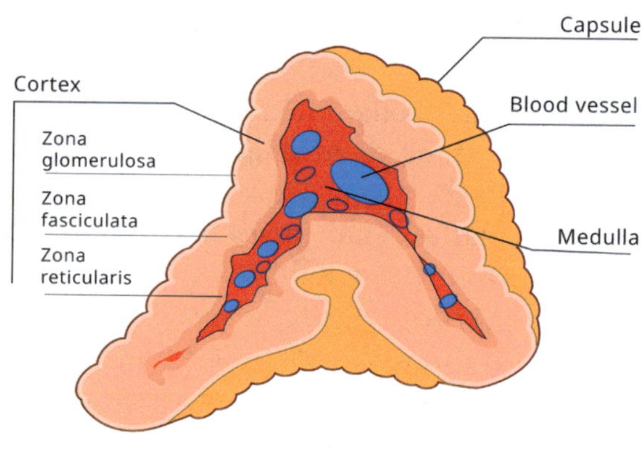

Figure 4.4. The adrenal gland is divided into two primary regions – the cortex and the medulla.

Source: https://upload.wikimedia.org/wikipedia/commons/thumb/5/5c/Adrenal_gland_hariadhi.svg/1024px-Adrenal_gland_hariadhi.svg.png.

4.1.3. Blood Supply and Innervation

The adrenal gland, an important endocrine organ, relies considerably on a robust blood supply to facilitate its diversified functions, including the release of hormones. The gland is perfused with blood through the adrenal arteries, which arise directly from major vessels such as the aorta and the renal arteries. The arteries form a rich vascular bed, which ensures the suitable delivery of nutrients and oxygen, necessary in the production of hormones such as cortisol and adrenaline. The arterial structure includes a unique arrangement that allows for both central and peripheral circulation, paving the way for instantaneous hormonal release relative to physiological demand. Such a sophisticated blood supply has extensive implications on adrenal activity and overall health, as it serves as a central interface between systemic circulation and adrenal activity. The innervation of the adrenal gland reinforces its blood supply, playing a critical role in the gland's function. The adrenal medulla contains sympathetic nerve terminals that respond to stimuli for stress and elicit the release of catecholamines like epinephrine and norepinephrine. The sympathetic innervation allows the body to respond quickly to acute stress situations and coordinate the physiological changes necessary to support the fight-or-flight response. The action of these neurotransmitters plays a significant role in the modulation of cardiovascular function, metabolic processes, and other systemic responses. Interestingly, the coaction of blood supply and innervation emphasizes the ability of the adrenal glands to dynamically respond to shifting physiological demands, thus further demonstrating their crucial function in maintaining homeostasis. In studies exploring the mechanisms of adrenal physiology, the coaction of the release of hormones and blood supply has gained increased interest. Experiments show that certain secretagogues, including adrenaline, may produce a localized effect on the vascular regulation of adrenal glands, and hence enhance the flow of blood in instances of heightened adrenal function. This is noteworthy against the background of wider implications of adrenal well-being, including the effects of chronic stress and other disease processes. Additionally, histopathological examination of adrenal tissue reveals that nerve fibers and blood vessels are closely intertwined, highlighting the importance of their interaction in maintaining a normal function of the adrenal gland. Besides their participation in hormonal regulation, this entangled network offers insight into potential targets for the treatment of diseases accompanying adrenal failure (Bobr et al., 2005; Parker et al., 1938) (Figure 4.5).

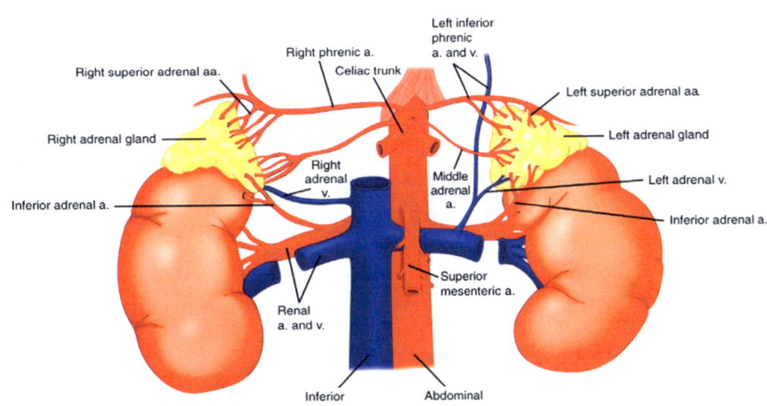

Figure 4.5. Adrenal gland blood supply.

Source: https://www.researchgate.net/profile/Volodymyr-Chernylovskyi/publication/346652964/figure/fig1/AS:1001166699769860@1615708150591/Adrenal-Gland-Blood-Supply.png.

Test Your Knowledge

1. Where are the adrenal glands located in the human body?
2. What are the three zones of the adrenal cortex, and what does each secrete?
3. How are the adrenal glands innervated?

4.2. Hormones Produced by the Adrenal Gland

Learning Outcome

1. Describe corticosteroids and their functions;
2. Explain catecholamines and their effects on the body;
3. Discuss the role of adrenal hormones in stress response.

The adrenal gland is a critical endocrine gland that secretes some of the crucial hormones that play a role in metabolizing stress and maintaining homeostasis. Among the most critical groups of hormones secreted by the adrenal cortex are the glucocorticoids, of which cortisol is the most significant. Cortisol has been referred to as the stress hormone due to its pivotal position in the response of the body to stress and regulation of carbohydrate, fat, and protein metabolism. Cortisol release is controlled by adrenocorticotropic hormone (ACTH), which is released from the pituitary gland in response to stressors. Increased cortisol secretion encourages gluconeogenesis in the liver, glycogen storage, and inflammatory responses, and thus plays crucial protective roles under different physiological conditions. Elucidation of the intricacies of cortisol and its actions remains crucial to understanding adrenal gland function. A second significant role in the production of adrenal hormones is that of mineralocorticoid synthesis, and the most prominent of these is aldosterone. Aldosterone regulates sodium and potassium balance, thereby directly influencing blood pressure regulation. Its secretion is primarily stimulated by the renin-angiotensin-aldosterone system (RAAS) on the detection of decreased renal blood flow. Increased aldosterone stimulates sodium reabsorption by renal tubules, producing increased water retention, resulting in an increase in blood volume and pressure. This extremely sensitive cascade of hormones emphasizes the role of the adrenal gland in cardiovascular and fluid regulation. Furthermore, dysfunction of the production of aldosterone can lead to hypertension and electrolyte disturbance, further emphasizing the gland's role in maintaining physiological homeostasis. The adrenal medulla, the internal part of the adrenal gland, releases catecholamines, namely epinephrine and norepinephrine.

These hormones play a key role in the body's fight or flight response, rapidly mobilizing the body to react to threatening situations. Epinephrine increases heart rate, dilates air passages in the lungs, and releases energy stores, and norepinephrine is essentially a neurotransmitter in the central nervous system and affects the narrowing of blood vessels. Importantly, however, more recent studies have begun to explore sexual dimorphism underlying adrenal function and, via this, hypothesized that factors like testosterone might play a role in hormone secretion and sensitivity. Sexual dimorphisms in glucocorticoid production, for instance, reflect the intricate interdependence of sex-specific physiological responses to stressors and adrenal hormones, making plain the importance of understanding how these hormones operate within the physiology of males and females (Evans et al., 2016; Hiraki et al., 1959).

4.2.1. Corticosteroids and Their Functions

Corticosteroids, derived from the adrenal cortex, play a crucial role in the body's response to stress and homeostatic regulation. Steroid hormones are primarily classified into glucocorticoids and mineralocorticoids, both of which influence diverse physiological functions. Glucocorticoids, such as cortisol, play a vital role in sustaining metabolism, immune function, and adaptation to stress. They suppress the inflammatory pathways while stimulating gluconeogenesis, underscoring their key role in regulating the body's stress response to stressors.

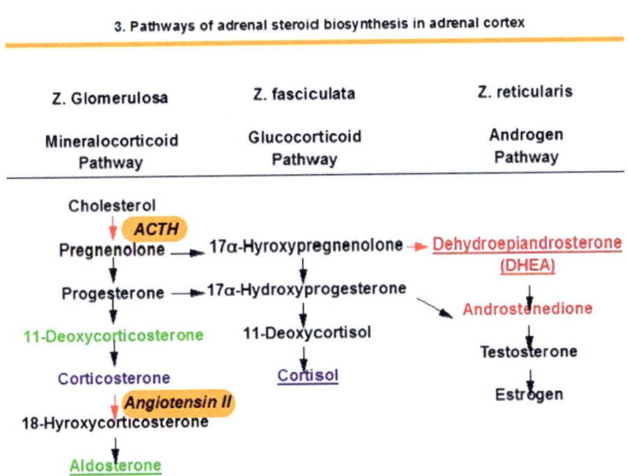

Figure 4.6. Pathways of adrenal corticosteroid biosynthesis in the adrenal cortex.

Source: https://www.researchgate.net/profile/Joseph-Hageman/publication/280576904/figure/fig2/AS:284629165723658@1444872290048/Pathways-of-adrenal-corticosteroid-biosynthesis-in-the-adrenal-cortex-ACTH.png.

Cortisol regulation is particularly significant in cases of prolonged emotional stress, in which the hormonal synthesis can be contingent upon the subjects' adapting capacity and the nature of the stress encountered. This dynamic hormonal release highlights the delicate balance the adrenal gland attains concerning physical and psychological stress, showing the complexity of corticosteroid activities in human disease (Amiragova et al., 2025).

During disease conditions, corticosteroids become significant as they control the response of the immune system. For instance, during infectious diseases like malaria, the activation of the hypothalamic-pituitary-adrenal (HPA) axis leads to increased glucocorticoid levels. Such glucocorticoids are not only crucial for systemic regulation but also for maximal immune defense and vascular integrity during disease. The lesser-recognized spectrum of glucocorticoids in modulating disease tolerance indicates their capacity to serve beyond mere stress adaptation. The neglect of glucocorticoids in medical practice, even when they would be beneficial in disease treatment, such as malaria, indicates a lack of understanding of their diverse functions, calling for more comprehensive research on the roles of these hormones across various disease stages (Bosscher et al., 2019). Not only are corticosteroids, but also to a very large degree, concerned with mineral balance, particularly through the activity of mineralocorticoids, i.e., aldosterone. This category of steroid hormone is important in the control of body sodium and potassium levels, hence total fluid balance and blood pressure. Aldosterone causes reabsorption of sodium and potassium by stimulating the kidneys to enable homeostatic regulation in response to physiological stress. The close relationship between glucocorticoids and mineralocorticoids is important in that their actions overlap in bringing about metabolic processes and cardiovascular functions. Thus, the secretion of corticosteroids by the adrenal glands not only supports the short-term physiological requirements but also has a foundation in long-term health repercussions. This realization of the dualistic aspect of corticosteroids speaks to their utility in health as well as illness, demanding that the function of the adrenal glands in creating a sense of well-being remains paramount (Amiragova et al., 2025; Bosscher et al., 2019) (Figure 4.6).

4.2.2. Catecholamines and Their Effects on the Body

Catecholamines, mainly adrenaline and noradrenaline, are the key players in the body's stress response system, affecting a variety of physiological responses in states of stress. Released by the adrenal medulla, these hormones are vital for the initiation of the fight-or-flight response. When provoked, catecholamines rapidly prepare the body to react to danger by increasing heart rate, providing increased blood flow to the muscles, and increasing blood sugar levels for immediate utilization. This hormonal reaction plays a vital role in survival by allowing rapid decision-making and physical reaction during a crisis. Nonetheless, prolonged availability of elevated levels of catecholamines has negative impacts on health, including enhanced risks of cardiovascular diseases, anxiety disorders, and metabolic disturbances. Thus, the necessity arises to understand the two-sided aspect of catecholamines, both on the positive and the negative side, while conducting research on the cumulative effect of adrenal gland activity on body health. Research has shown that lifestyle factors, including stress and diet, affect the levels of catecholamines and their subsequent impact on the body. Sucrose intake, for instance, has been found to alter catecholamine dynamics and enhance aggression, with impaired metabolic functions. In one of the studies on BALB/c mice, it was found that the high-sucrose-fed animals contained very high levels of noradrenaline and adrenaline with enhanced aggressive behavior and adrenal weight, clearly establishing the relationship between diet, stress response, and catecholamine production (Miyata et al., 2025). These findings underscore the importance of diet and its interaction with hormonal regulation, suggesting that excessive sugar consumption might enhance stress-induced hormone responses, potentially leading to more widespread conditions like obesity and metabolic syndromes. In older age, the function of the adrenal gland, specifically in catecholamine synthesis, is characterized by notable changes. Aging has been linked to increased cortisol release and decreased androgen release within the adrenal cortex, thereby impacting catecholamine secretion (Nejat et al., 2024). This alteration in hormone production can have various physical and psychological effects, such as decreased stress resistance and susceptibility to metabolic disorders.

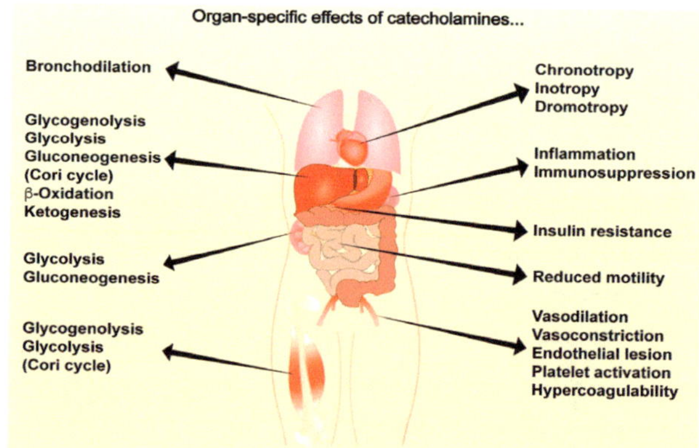

Figure 4.7. Organ-specific effects of catecholamines.

Source: https://www.researchgate.net/profile/Clair-Hartmann/publication/316052992/figure/fig3/AS:729203288854536@1550867020865/Organ-specific-effects-of-catecholamines-Simplified-scheme-of-organ-specific-effects-of.ppm.

Further, the disappearance of endothelial cells within the adrenal glands as a result of ageing has additional risks for hormonal balance and cardiovascular health. These changes associated with age underscore the important role of the adrenal glands in maintaining homeostasis and the importance of further research on how these hormonal changes contribute to the overall process of ageing and the consequent health issues that arise (Figure 4.7).

4.2.3. Role of Adrenal Hormones in Stress Response

The adrenal glands are a key component of the stress response at the physiological level, most notably through the release of glucocorticoids, mainly cortisol. Glucocorticoids are vital for regulating many functions of the body, such as metabolism, immune function, and blood pressure. When a stressor is perceived by an individual, the hypothalamic-pituitary-adrenal (HPA) axis is stimulated, resulting in the enhanced release of adrenocorticotropic hormone (ACTH) from the pituitary gland. ACTH then acts on the adrenal cortex to cause the release of glucocorticoids. The cascade of hormones enables the body to mobilize stored energy, become more alert, and survive in acute stress. Glucocorticoids have also been discovered to influence the activity of immune cells, thereby providing a pathway by which the body can adapt to both physical and psychological stress through complex feedback mechanisms. The role of macrophages within the adrenal gland also illustrates the intricacies of the stress response. Recent studies indicate that such immune cells are not just along for the ride but actively contribute to the regulation of adrenal hormone production. Specifically, macrophages in the adrenal gland possess a dynamic response to acute and chronic stressors and exhibit polarization to an inflammatory phenotype. This reprogramming is associated with the augmentation of inflammatory cytokines and lipid uptake factors, such as Trem2. Trem2 involvement is particularly intriguing, as its disruption has been shown to increase the release of glucocorticoids upon stress. This suggests that adrenal macrophages play a protective role in maintaining homeostasis by modulating steroidogenesis, thereby affecting the general stress response and also potentially guiding therapeutic strategies in stress conditions (Xu et al., 2022, 2024). In addition, the systemic implications of disrupted adrenal hormone levels extend beyond acute physiological adaptations to encompass broader health implications. Increased glucocorticoid secretion in chronic stress correlates with inflammatory diseases and metabolic disturbances, including cardiovascular disease and obesity. This highlights the importance of comprehending stress response homeostasis, as the dysregulation under chronic conditions could lead to significant complications in health. Following the results from recent studies on adrenal macrophages, scientists expect to investigate novel immunotherapeutic interventions for addressing the negative effects of long-term hormonal imbalance. With the clarification of how the immune system and adrenal hormones interact, researchers can enhance the control of the issues produced by long-term stress, ultimately toward improved health and well-being (Xu et al., 2022, 2024).

Test Your Knowledge

1. What are the main corticosteroids produced by the adrenal cortex?
2. What hormones are produced by the adrenal medulla, and how do they affect the body?
3. How does cortisol help the body respond to stress?

4.3. Functions of the Adrenal Gland

Learning Outcome

1. Understand the function of the adrenal gland in regulation of metabolism;
2. Explain how adrenal gland maintain blood pressure;
3. Explain the role of adrenal gland in regulating the immune response.

The adrenal gland plays an essential role in the human body in the synthesis of a series of hormones that are essential in maintaining homeostasis regulation. Situated above every kidney, the gland has two major zones: the outer cortex and the inner medulla. The adrenal cortex produces glucocorticoids, mineralocorticoids, and androgens. Glucocorticoids, such as cortisol, regulate metabolism, immunity, and adaptation to stress, while mineralocorticoids, such as aldosterone, regulate blood pressure and electrolyte balance. Knowledge of these hormonal products is not only relevant to the understanding of normal physiological function but also to the diagnosis of disorders of adrenal abnormality. For example, derangements of cortisol production lead to the establishment of disease states such as Cushing's syndrome or adrenal insufficiency, highlighting the importance of the regulatory function of the adrenal gland in promoting health. Within the adrenal medulla, catecholamine production—predominantly epinephrine and norepinephrine—occurs in response to acute stress stimuli. Hormones play a critical role in the body's fight-or-flight response, initiating rapid physiological changes that prepare the organism for immediate action. When released, catecholamines raise heart rate, increase respiratory rate, and mobilize glucose from energy storage sites, hence acting as an instant source of energy. Recent research shows that the expression of the adrenal β2-adrenergic receptor (β2-AR) was different depending on the cause of death, suggesting its activity in the adrenal cortex's hormonal stimulation. This variant expression of the receptor in the varied zones of the adrenal gland points to the complexity of the gland's functioning in stress and physiological adaptation, revealing its role not just in emergency but in the daily homeostatic balance as well (Alibrandi et al., 2019). Moreover, the action of the adrenal cortex on various signaling molecules once again reveals the complex nature of the functioning of this gland. Melanocortin-2-receptor (MC2R) and its partner protein MRAP form a critical complex that facilitates glucocorticoid synthesis. Abnormalities in the proteins can cause familial glucocorticoid deficiency, demonstrating the critical interdependence of adrenal hormone synthesis. Research has shown that while MRAP and MC2R are strongly expressed within the zona fasciculata, another isoform referred to as MRAP2 has a distinct expression pattern within the adrenal cortex. This differential localization hints at a complex regulatory process in the synthesis of hormones and suggests that ACTH plays a significant role to play in the differentiation of cells and in the maintenance of the adrenal gland (Chan et al., 2011). Elucidation of such molecular interactions is important for therapeutic intervention design for diseases resulting from adrenal dysfunction.

4.3.1. Regulation of Metabolism

The control of metabolism is directly related to the functioning of the adrenal gland to control the homeostasis of the body. The gland releases various hormones, predominantly glucocorticoids, which participate in metabolic functions. Cortisol is a primary glucocorticoid that influences glucose metabolism by gluconeogenesis in the liver and thus elevates blood sugar to meet the energy demand of the body during stress or fasting. Besides this, cortisol helps to regulate protein and fat metabolism in a way that an equilibrated supply of substrates for energy is presented. This role of cortisol in homeostasis points to the general function of the adrenal gland in metabolic health, since dysregulation will lead to metabolic illness like obesity and diabetes, where metabolic pathways are disrupted and energy expenditure by hormonal derangements. Follow-up research has made clear the intricate interaction between circadian rhythms and adrenal hormone production, demonstrating a complex interplay affecting control of metabolism. The internal clock of the body regulates the secretion of the adrenal hormones, such as cortisol, in a manner dependent on physiological daily requirements. Disrupting circadian rhythms can have detrimental effects on metabolic activity, thereby increasing the risk of increased cardiovascular disease and metabolic syndrome. As a result, understanding the molecular basis of the circadian system teaches us about the importance of the timing of hormone release and the consequent impact on metabolic homeostasis. Recent research emphasizes the significance of this circadian regulation not only in the control of metabolism but also in coordinating endocrine functions and their contribution to general well-being, as discussed in recent papers on this new area (Bruscalupi et al., 2017). Their activity is not confined to metabolism regulation; they also play an important role in the regulation of the immune response and the vascular system, particularly during stressful conditions. HPA axis activation elevates the levels of glucocorticoids during diseases such as malaria, which, in turn, regulate the response of the body to infection. Glucocorticoids are a double-edged sword: they exert protective effects against overinflammation and stabilize metabolic homeostasis, but can simultaneously destroy both metabolic and immune health if dysregulated. This reflects directly the central role that glucocorticoids have in systemic metabolic control and highlights the need to endeavor towards an understanding of their functions in disease pathology. Clarifying these interactions can yield novel therapeutic approaches to treating metabolic and endocrine diseases, especially in light of the expanding understanding of the multifaceted role of glucocorticoids in stress disorders, such as malaria (Bosscher et al., 2019) (Figure 4.8).

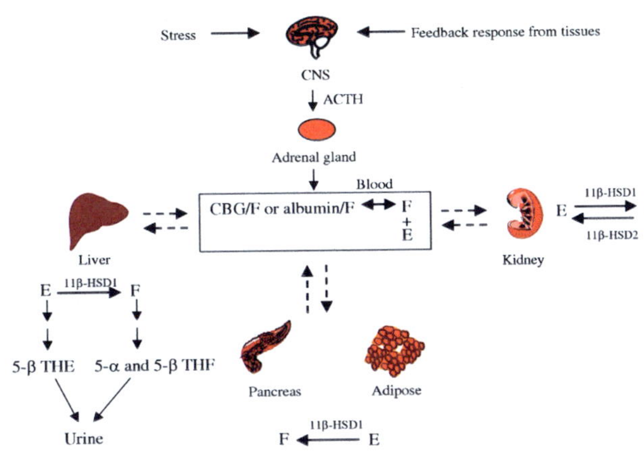

Figure 4.8. Glucocorticoid metabolism. The secretion of glucocorticoids by the adrenal gland is regulated by the HPA axis via the secretion of ACTH. The main plasma cortisol (F) is protein-bound, with a 4–5% free fraction.

Source: https://www.researchgate.net/publication/8043782/figure/fig1/AS:281137504112653@1444039812640/Glucocorticoid-metabolism-The-secretion-of-glucocorticoids-by-the-adrenal-gland-is.png.

4.3.2. Maintenance of Blood Pressure

Blood pressure regulation is a critical physiological function under the control of a number of neuroendocrine elements, with the central role being played by the adrenal gland. Through hormone secretion, such as cortisol and catecholamines, the gland supports the body's stress response by regulating fluid balance and blood vessel tone. The adrenal gland stimulates the activation of the hypothalamic-pituitary-adrenal axis in response to stress, leading to increased glucocorticoid levels. These hormones contribute to enhancing the availability of energy and the regulation of blood pressure through direct effects on vascular smooth muscle and the kidneys, wherein they manage sodium retention. Such intricate interaction helps provide optimal blood pressure under conditions of physiological stress, ensuring essential organs an adequate supply of blood and nutrients. Thus, the stress response of the adrenal gland not only acts to regulate acute health threats but also has a more chronic role to maintain cardiovascular homeostasis. Furthermore, mechanisms whereby the adrenal gland facilitates regulation of blood pressure are interconnected with the renin-angiotensin system (RAS). Stimulation of the RAS leads to the release of angiotensin II, a potent vasoconstrictor, which increases blood pressure and is necessary for stress responses. Evidence that overactivity of glucocorticoids can stimulate overactivity of the RAS and promote conditions like hypertension. For instance, studies have demonstrated that mice with increased expression of 11β-hydroxysteroid dehydrogenase type 1 in adipose tissue develop salt-sensitive hypertension characterized by increased plasma levels of angiotensinogen, angiotensin II, and aldosterone. This interaction is important in pointing out the role of adrenal gland hormonal production in the onset of hypertension and determines that dysregulation in such a feedback mechanism is capable of significantly deranging blood pressure homeostasis (Aubert et al., 2003). Moreover, the response of the adrenal glands is not limited to acute stress but extends to chronic stress as well as blood pressure regulation. Processes such as metabolic syndrome and obesity are expressed as increased demand for stress on the adrenal gland to secrete glucocorticoids to meet chronic stress. The adaptations result in sustained hypertension, as observed in certain conditions where regulation of adrenal hormone secretion becomes altered from central to local control. Even in critically ill patients, whose pituitary hormone levels are low, the levels of glucocorticoids remain elevated, indicating altered stress responses. This dysregulation is significant because it has the potential to cause long-term cardiovascular morbidity. The interaction between adrenal function and blood pressure regulation, therefore, illuminates therapeutic targets for treating hypertension and related disorders (Bornstein et al., 2016).

4.3.3. Influence on Immune Response

Adrenal gland plays a significant role in controlling the immune response, and this is by the release of hormones such as cortisol. Cortisol, released during stress, is a hormone that can control the immune function. It contains powerful anti-inflammatory actions, which are capable of suppressing excessive immune responses that would lead to tissue damage. Under chronic stress situations, the steady increase in cortisol levels can lead to immune dysregulation and, as a direct result, enhanced vulnerability to infections and reduced vaccine effectiveness. This all-around role of cortisol highlights the importance of maintaining homeostasis within the adrenal gland, as hyper- and hypo-functioning of adrenal function can have a negative impact on immune function. This underscores the subtle dynamics between hormones and immune systems that determine overall health. In addition, the interplay of the adrenal gland and cytokine activity is significant in highlighting the way stress influences the immune system. Research indicates that inflammatory cytokines can influence the secretion of adrenal hormones, thereby creating a two-way process that influences stress as well as immunity. Inflammation can trigger the hypothalamic-pituitary-adrenal axis, leading to an increase in cortisol production. In contrast, elevated levels of cortisol have been demonstrated to reduce pro-inflammatory cytokine production and thus modulate the immune response. A balance between the processes is crucial, as inflammation caused by stress over the long term could make illnesses like depression and anxiety worse, which may, in turn, impair the immune response. That these systems interact makes it critical that the adrenal gland be explored in relation to immune response. Furthermore, dietary treatment and the influence of immune response introduce another aspect of complexity that is linked with adrenal function. Dietary substances such as quercetin, a flavonoid occurring naturally in the body, have been shown to enhance immune responses, and this might mean that proper nutrition can positively influence the health of the adrenal glands. Evidence indicates that quercetin supplementation is able to induce significant increases in immunoglobulin levels and immune gene function changes, which subsequently can increase the general resilience of the immune system. The immune-enhancing action of these dietary constituents hints at therapeutic strategies that could prevent stress-induced immune compromise. With continued findings that unveil the intricate dynamics between diet, adrenal hormone release, and immunity, it becomes more obvious that integrative treatments can enhance immunocompetence, particularly in persons who are experiencing ongoing stress (Hole et al., 2025; Wei et al., 2025) (Figure 4.9).

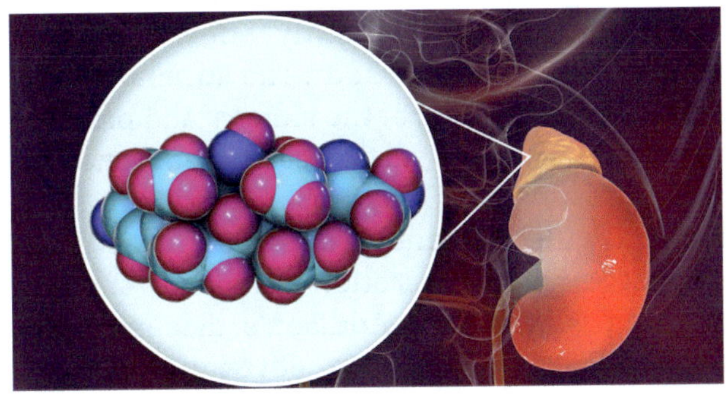

Figure 4.9. The adrenal gland plays a pivotal role in regulating the immune response.

Source: https://www.endocrine.org/-/media/endocrine/images/patient-engagement-webpage/condition-page-images/hormones/hormones_adrenal_1796x943.jpg.

Test Your Knowledge

1. How does cortisol from the adrenal cortex regulate metabolism?
2. What is the role of aldosterone in maintaining blood pressure?
3. What happens when adrenal function is impaired in relation to metabolism and immunity?

4.4. Disorders of the Adrenal Gland

Learning Outcome

1. Describe Addison's disease and its symptoms;
2. Define Cushing's syndrome and its causes;
3. Understand adrenal tumors and their implications.

Adrenal gland disease involves a range of conditions that significantly affect hormone equilibrium within the body. The adrenal glands are positioned on top of the kidneys and produce essential hormones such as cortisol, adrenaline, and aldosterone. Disorders may result from adrenal insufficiency, such as Addison's disease, or hypersecretion disorders such as Cushing's syndrome. Addison's disease leads to insufficient secretion of adrenal hormones, with the consequences being weakness, weight loss, and low blood pressure. Cushing's syndrome, a condition resulting from excess production of cortisol, has symptoms such as obesity, elevated blood pressure, and changes in mood. These conditions highlight the delicate balance that exists between adrenal hormones in physiological function, underscoring the importance of accurate diagnosis and effective management of adrenal disorders, which can have a profound impact on an individual's health and well-being. Diagnosis of adrenal disorders typically involves combining clinical evaluation with laboratory evaluation. Physicians assess the symptoms in detail and may suggest specific tests to measure hormone levels in urine or blood. For instance, elevated cortisol levels typically indicate Cushing's syndrome, and low cortisol levels can be used to diagnose Addison's disease. Imaging diagnostic procedures, such as CT or MRI scans, may be employed to identify abnormalities in the adrenal glands, such as tumors or enlargement, which may help expedite the proper diagnosis. In addition, the relationship between primary adrenal disease and secondary disease, such as pituitary tumors on the level of adrenocorticotropic hormone (ACTH), must be approached in an integrated manner. Following diagnosis, treatment can vary from replacement therapy for adrenal insufficiency to surgical treatment for tumors, emphasizing the multifaceted approaches to successful treatment of these disorders. Recent reports emphasize the systemic impact of adrenal gland disorders beyond hormonal dysregulation. For instance, research has indicated that primary hyperparathyroidism, which is often found incidentally, can exhibit interactions with adrenal function to ascertain that the chronic stress of such conditions might result in hypercortisolism and pose risks for a variety of complications (Armanini et al., 2015). The effects of aging on adrenal disorders have also been in focus, where aging individuals can present with a greater variety of symptoms and comorbidities. Increased rates of these conditions necessitate the development of specialized guidelines for optimal management, particularly in older patients who are at a higher risk of complications and more complex healthcare needs. Taking a holistic approach, healthcare workers will be more sensitive to managing the complexity that accompanies adrenal gland disorders, ultimately promoting improved patient outcomes and quality of life (Birrell et al., 1924).

4.4.1. Addison's Disease and Its Symptoms

Addisons disease, also referred to as primary adrenal insufficiency, is characterized by a failure to synthesize necessary hormones, primarily cortisol and aldosterone, produced by the adrenal gland. The condition is more likely to be a result of autoimmune destruction of the adrenal cortex, but can be brought about by infection, congenital abnormalities, or conditions such as tuberculosis. The failure to secrete adequate cortisol leads to a cascade of symptoms that have a significant impact on the quality of life. Patients may have weakness, weight loss, and hypotension, often with gastrointestinal distress. In addition, the hormonal imbalance is not solely for physical symptoms; subjects may also experience psychological effects, such as depression or irritability. Understanding such intricate symptoms is critical for accurate diagnosis and management since timely treatment will increase patient outcome and mental status, underlining the importance of adrenal health in general well-being (Van't Westeinde et al., 2023). Clinical presentation of Addison's disease usually happens insidiously, which may result in an adrenal crisis if not treated. Symptoms of the sudden onset are severe weakness, hypotension, and even loss of consciousness, which could be lethal. Symptoms of hyperpigmentation of the skin due to increased adrenocorticotropic hormone (ACTH) levels, to overcome low cortisol levels, can also be reported by patients. Interestingly, while the vast majority of patients with Addison's disease will test with normal cognition on clinical examination, in everyday life, they report executive functioning deficits exacerbated by mental fatigue. Recent studies show that the interaction between the adrenal hormones and cognition is a field deserving further research, as the implications for brain structure and function are significant. These findings affirm that not only is Addison's disease an endocrine illness, but it has profound impacts on a patient's mental health and cognitive function (Van't Westeinde et al., 2023). Management of Addison's disease typically involves lifelong hormone replacement therapy, which is meant to restore cortisol and aldosterone levels and therefore alleviate symptoms. But the challenge is that it is difficult to replicate the physiological cycles of cortisol secretion with drugs alone. Further, more recent research focuses on learning how various impacts on cognitive function from adrenal hormone deficiency are between conditions such as Addison's disease and congenital adrenal hyperplasia. While patients with adrenal insufficiency may have abnormalities in brain structure, as suggested by studies that cited differences in brain volume and connectivity, the general cognitive impact of Addison's disease requires more studies and tailored treatment approaches. It is crucial for healthcare professionals to be on the lookout for the physiological and psychological management in this condition so that better care can be provided to affected individuals (Figure 4.10).

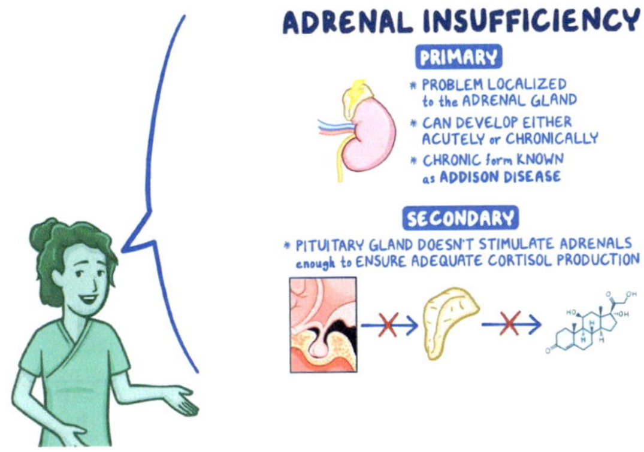

Figure 4.10. Addisons disease (primary adrenal insufficiency).

Source: https://www.osmosis.org/_next/image?url=https%3A%2F%2Fd16qt3wv6xm098.cloudfront.net%2FI92AfK9qTRWMtXMh9RNsUx5sQAesNccH%2F_.jpg&w=3840&q=75.

4.4.2. Cushing's Syndrome and Its Causes

Cushing's syndrome with hypercortisolism can occur following diverse etiologies, the most significant being adrenal gland disease and ectopic ACTH production. The adrenal glands, which play critical roles in stress response regulation and metabolism, can have benign tumors such as adrenal adenomas that lead to excess cortisol production. Cushing's syndrome can also occur from pituitary adenomas secreting Cushing's disease, resulting from adrenocorticotropic hormone (ACTH), which stimulates the adrenal glands to secrete excess cortisol. Furthermore, ectopic ACTH secretion by tumors other than pituitary tumors, such as lung carcinoma, contributes to the clinical nuance. Thus, an understanding of these pathogenetic mechanisms of Cushing's syndrome serves to emphasize the function of the adrenal glands, their endocrine secretions, and the systemic impact of dyscorticism on body function. The clinical manifestation of Cushing's syndrome demonstrates the far-reaching systemic effects of long-standing cortisol overproduction. The patient normally presents with signs of weight gain, hypertension, and cutaneous changes like bruising and striae. In addition, the syndrome is particularly concerning since it has been associated with severe morbidity, such as increased risk of cardiovascular disease and infection despite treatment. In a retrospective look, outcomes showed that patients, despite having remitted from Cushing's syndrome, were yet at risk of such factors as cognitive impairment, mental fatigue, and a higher incidence of conditions such as stroke and thromboembolism. These adverse effects mandate the early identification and proper treatment of Cushing's syndrome, and this requires a solid understanding of its causes and medical risks, especially the role of the adrenal glands. Current studies emphasize the complexities of the diagnosis and treatment of Cushing's syndrome. For instance, in a patient who was 64 years old and a male, it was demonstrated that traditional techniques of diagnosis, like the dexamethasone suppression test, can fail when there is ectopic ACTH, as was true in this patient with neurofibromatosis. The aforementioned research illustrated the effect of ectopic ACTH secretion on therapeutic guidelines, creating the demand for new diagnostic procedures to include adrenal venous sampling. The patients' initial response to imatinib treatment further illustrates the evolving face of interventions critical to the success of Cushing's syndrome therapy. The intricate interaction between adrenal gland function and overall well-being, along with potential interventions, provides a holistic framework for understanding and treating the complex dynamics of Cushing's syndrome (Bano et al., 2013; Papakokkinou et al., 2022) (Figure 4.11).

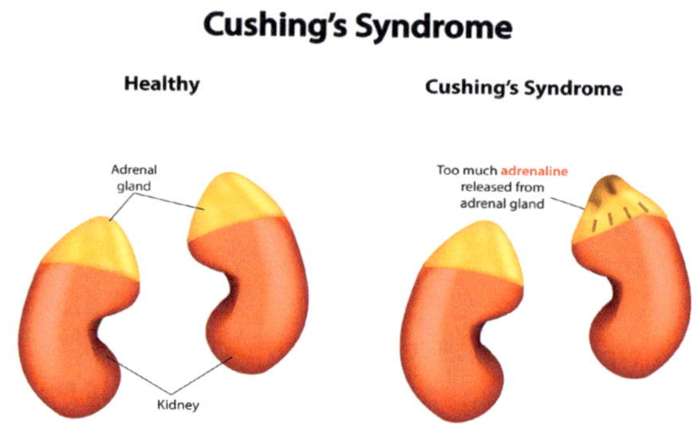

Figure 4.11. Illustration of Addison's disease.

Source: https://www.news-medical.net/image-handler/picture/2016/8/Cushing%27s_Syndrome_shutterstock_205972057.jpg.

4.4.3. Adrenal Tumors and Their Implications

The presence of adrenal tumors has a significant impact on the functioning of the adrenal glands and can have a wide variety of health problems. The benign or malignant tumors can interfere with hormone production and cause varied endocrine disorders. As an example, pheochromocytomas, which are one of the adrenal tumors, overproduce catecholamines, which can cause hypertension, palpitations, and excessive anxiety. The medical implications of such disturbances are enormous in that they are likely to require a diagnostic process involving biochemical assessment and imaging studies to ascertain the extent and type of the tumor. Moreover, adrenal tumors like adrenal cortical carcinoma have the potential to metastasize and require serious therapeutic interventions, hence necessitating early diagnosis and treatment in order to contain adverse health effects. Another recent focus of investigation in adrenal tumors is their endocrine interaction and influence on neighboring endocrine systems. Androgen receptor expression, particularly in tumors, plays a crucial role in the mediation of growth and development in various cancers. As explained in recent reviews, these androgen receptors can be targeted therapeutically in prostate cancer and other cancers potentially associated with adrenal hormone imbalance. By knowing the hormonal context surrounding adrenal tumors, researchers are able to create targeted treatments that could enhance patient care. This indicates the interconnected nature of hormone pathways, implying that treatment of adrenal tumors is a multidisciplinary field that incorporates endocrinology, oncology, and surgery so that treatments can be appropriately tailored. In addition to the direct medical ramifications, adrenal tumors also play a role in larger health dynamics, such as metabolic function and mental health. Steroid hormones produced in the adrenal cortex, such as cortisol and aldosterone, have a key role in metabolic regulation, controlling glucose metabolism and electrolyte balance. When these are interfered with by cancer cells, thus, conditions like Cushing's syndrome or primary hyperaldosteronism result, both of which have negative health effects, such as cardiovascular disease. Moreover, hormonal changes induced by adrenal tumors can affect brain function and mood, providing evidence that supports the association between levels of steroid hormones and mental health. Thus, the treatment of adrenal tumors requires a comprehensive understanding of their multidimensional aspects, which impact both physical and psychological health, thereby necessitating holistic therapies, as reflected in existing research on the neuroendocrine axes (Deniselle et al., 2016; Kurzrock et al., 2014) (Figure 4.12).

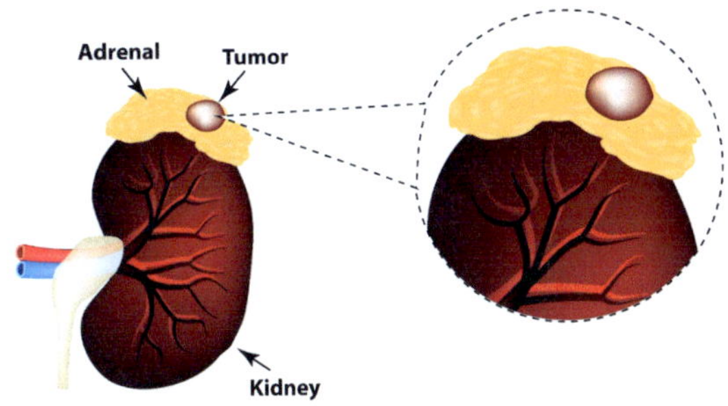

Figure 4.12. The tumor of adrenal grand.

Source: https://medanta.s3.ap-south-1.amazonaws.com/blogs/July2024/q1lzRwK8B6ukAceDAnkzkEeWPBv6K8-metaQ3JhY2tpbmcgdGhlIEhhY2sgb2YgQWRyZW5hbCBHbGFuZCBUdW1vcnMgQmVpbmcgQ2FuY2Vyb3VzIG9yIE5vdC5qcGc=-.jpg.

Test Your Knowledge

1. What is Addison's disease, and what are its primary symptoms?
2. What is Cushing's syndrome, and what causes it?
3. What are adrenal tumors, and how can they affect health?

4.5. Diagnostic Methods for Adrenal Gland Disorders

Learning Outcome

1. Discuss the importance of blood tests for hormone levels;
2. Describe imaging techniques (CT, MRI);
3. Explain biopsy procedures and their significance.

Adrenal glands are vital endocrine organs that supply hormones needed to regulate metabolism, immune processes, and stress management. Malfunctions of these glands must be detected through a multimodal process that involves both clinical assessment and advanced imaging techniques. Preliminary testing can include biochemical testing in the form of serum cortisol and adrenocorticotropic hormone (ACTH) assay to determine if the hormone levels are normal. Furthermore, such biochemical markers can be utilized to diagnose diseases such as Cushing's syndrome and Addison's disease, which entail a significant alteration in the secretion of hormones. These levels must be interpreted to guide further diagnostic tests and treatments. Therefore, a clear understanding of such biochemical tests is essential in the proper diagnosis of adrenal gland pathologies. Following biochemical testing, imaging tests are an important part of the diagnosis. Imaging modalities such as computed tomography (CT) and magnetic resonance imaging (MRI) are commonly employed to define the adrenal glands so that tumors, hyperplasia, or other structural lesions are recognized. These imaging modalities provide high-resolution images that allow clinicians to confirm the existence of lesions and their size and impact on neighboring structures. Furthermore, these imaging modalities can differentiate between benign and malignant tumors by providing useful information regarding vascularity and other physical characteristics. The utilization of these imaging modalities not only enhances diagnostic precision but also influences treatment planning and prognosis. Imaging tests therefore supplement biochemical tests by creating a visual image of adrenal pathology and health. Ultrasonography is increasingly becoming part of the numerous useful, non-invasive diagnostic instruments employed in adrenal gland pathology assessment. Its applicability makes it possible to image adrenal organs in real time, providing information on their shape and possible dysfunction. Ultrasonography has been proven by current research to demonstrate both adrenal glands clearly, thereby assisting in the diagnosis of endocrine pathology in the majority of animals, including domesticated pets (Cerquetella et al., 2016). Its advantages are that it is available and non-ionizing, thus becoming the option for first consults and follow-up visits. Besides, its dynamic ability enables clinicians to measure blood flow as well as diagnose such disorders as adrenal tumors with ease. As ultrasonography advances as a science, it may increasingly cement its place as an essential component of the diagnostic algorithms for adrenal gland disease, providing additional layers of information to enhance sound clinical decision-making.

4.5.1. Blood Tests for Hormone Levels

Hormone level blood tests are a significant diagnostic tool in assessing adrenal gland function and diagnosing potential disorders. The adrenal glands produce a variety of hormones, such as cortisol, aldosterone, and catecholamines, that play a role in significant metabolic regulatory functions, the regulation of blood pressure, and stress responses. A deviation of these hormone levels can lead to Cushing's syndrome, Addison's disease, and hyperaldosteronism. Detection of such abnormalities is often preceded by blood tests measuring levels of hormones at a specific moment of the day as the concentration of certain hormones exhibits a circadian rhythm.

Tests not only establish the diagnosis but can also guide treatment interventions towards normalizing hormonal function in order to finally exert a positive influence on patient outcome. Apart from its diagnostic purpose, blood tests are useful in clinical applications to monitor therapeutic response, particularly in cases with adrenal incidentalomas or hormone-secreting tumors. For instance, in patients undergoing laparoscopic resection of adrenal tumors, studies established that hormonal levels were significantly linked with postoperative recovery, such as the disappearance of hypertension (Wang et al., 2022).

Through the evaluation of factors such as aldosterone and plasma renin activity ratio, clinicians are able to establish which patients can expect favorable recovery courses after surgery. Such findings highlight the value of continuing hormonal monitoring, not only on initial assessment but also during follow-up treatment, allowing for an individualized therapeutic strategy that addresses each patient's unique hormonal level. Additionally, disease conditions such as adrenal insufficiency, which can arise particularly in corticosteroid-treated patients, highlight the role of blood tests in evaluating adrenal function. For example, research indicated that a significant portion of patients had regular adrenocorticotropic hormone (ACTH) levels even in the case of prolonged use of corticosteroids (Salehi et al., 2022). This shows that, with proper dosing, the risk of adrenal insufficiency is likely to be low. Regular hormone level tests provide healthcare practitioners with the means to assess adrenal function stability in patient groups under risk through the influence of medication, hence enhancing care for those with chronic conditions requiring endocrine therapy. Blood hormone tests are thus pivotal in diagnosing and treating health issues related to adrenal glands (Figure 4.13).

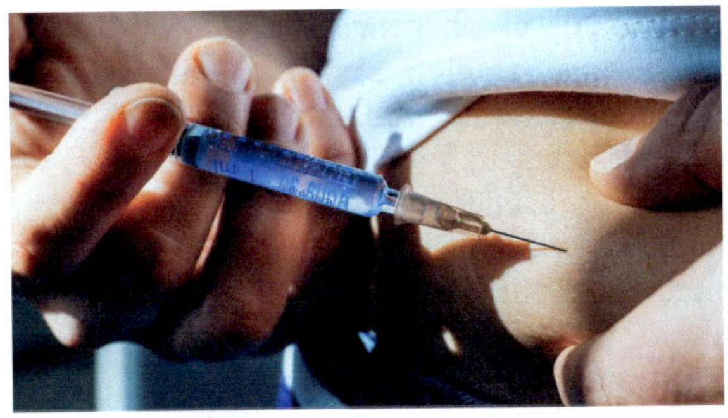

Figure 4.13. Blood tests for hormone levels.

Source: https://dims.healthgrades.com/dims3/MMH/c210112/2147483647/strip/true/crop/7360x4112+0+249/resize/800x447!/quality/75/?url=https%3A%2F%2Fucmscdn.healthgrades.com%2F53%2F78%2F184cc265416db75d05e4acfcefe9%2Fgettyimages-926358710.jpg.

4.5.2. Imaging Techniques (CT, MRI)

The evaluation of adrenal masses is crucial in clinical practice, where it is necessary for accurate imaging techniques so that correct diagnoses can be achieved. Computed Tomography (CT) and Magnetic Resonance Imaging (MRI) are the imaging modalities of choice in this scenario. CT is particularly beneficial since it is highly sensitive for the identification of small adrenal neoplasms and adrenal hyperplasia, as reflected by comparative studies using both imaging techniques. In lesions greater than 2 cm, CT and other MRI techniques can effectively depict such masses and are therefore excellent choices for initial evaluation and characterization. However, as explained in literature, some small adrenal masses with low Hounsfield units are challenging to interpret on the basis of unenhanced CT, but MRI is superior for characterization in those situations (Hrabak-Paar et al., 2015). Therefore, combining both imaging modalities may maximize diagnostic precision when assessing adrenal disease. MRIs value is discerned when characterizing adrenal masses that are still indeterminate through CT imaging. Characterization is especially essential in instances of pheochromocytomas, a tumor in the adrenal glands, which can result in extreme hormonal imbalances. A case report demonstrated that, while an adrenal mass was firstly diagnosed by the assistance of CT, further evaluation with MRI provided useful information concerning the nature of the tumor, which guided the following management strategy. Catecholamine increases were recognized along with imaging Findings, which prompted a detailed assessment culminating in confirming the diagnosis of pheochromocytoma. Hence, the role of MRI in fine-tuning the diagnostic process and clarification of adrenal masses is invaluable, especially where usual imaging studies yield inconclusive findings (Letizia et al., 2015).

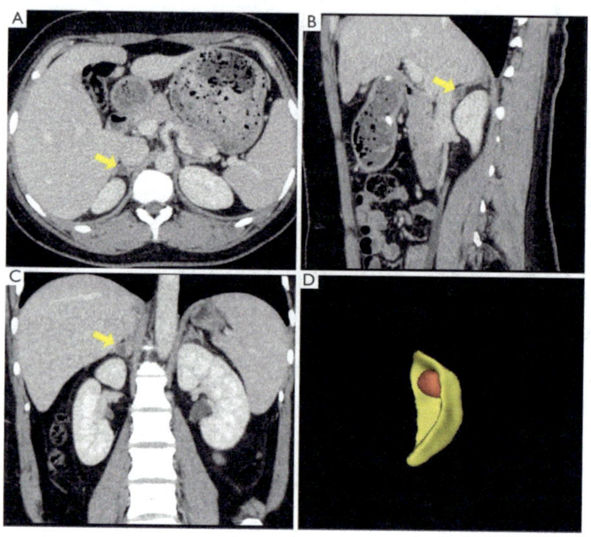

Figure 4.14. Adrenal glands in enhanced computed tomography scan. (A) Horizontal position; (B) sagittal position; (C) coronal position. The yellow arrow indicates an adenoma on the right adrenal gland. (D) 3D reconstructed image of the right adrenal gland and an adrenal adenoma, rendered using 3D slicer.

Source: https://www.researchgate.net/publication/357741314/figure/fig1/AS:1111043950546945@1641904928365/Adrenal-glands-in-enhanced-computed-tomography-scan-A-Horizontal-position-B.png.

Overall, the complementary role of CT and MRI in adrenal gland imaging emphasizes the unique strengths and limitations of each modality. CT is the imaging modality of choice due to the rapid acquisition time and high sensitivity for the detection of large adrenal masses. However, MRI is invaluable in the subtle determination of indeterminate masses, particularly in suspected pheochromocytomas, since high-resolution imaging provides critical diagnostic information. Therefore, a dual-modality approach optimizes patient management through accurate detection and best treatment of adrenal abnormalities. This strategy not only facilitates acute diagnosis but also directs the treatment decisions that play a significant role in patient outcomes and quality of life (Figure 4.14).

4.5.3. Biopsy Procedures and Their Significance

Biopsy techniques play a significant role in the diagnosis and management of adrenal gland abnormalities, particularly in the differentiation between benign and malignant lesions. The significance of these techniques is evidenced by the use of endoscopic ultrasound fine-needle aspiration (EUS-FNA), where it is feasible to selectively biopsy tissue from adrenal masses that, in the majority of instances, are difficult to evaluate based on non-invasive imaging alone. With 86% sensitivity and 97% specificity for malignancy diagnosis, EUS-FNA is a highly sensitive diagnostic tool. It is this sensitivity that is of importance to clinicians as it will influence treatment, apart from providing information on the nature of adrenal masses, whether they are primary tumors or metastatic lesions, thereby directing further diagnostic and therapeutic interventions (Al-Haddad et al., 2014). The implications of carrying out biopsies on adrenal tumors go beyond simple diagnosis; they also have a profound influence on the management strategies adopted for involved patients. Timely cytological assessment from

EUS-FNA has the potential to result in resultant treatment planning, whether surgery or pharmacotherapy. For example, a clear diagnosis of benign masses can favor a conservative management strategy, but a malignant diagnosis becomes imperative for aggressive treatment regimens. In addition, the ability to precisely differentiate between adrenal masses will avoid unnecessary surgeries and, hence, maintain patient safety and resources. Biopsy-based diagnosis is also able to determine or rule out metastasis of primary tumors, which is crucial for determining the prognosis of a patient and the best oncological treatment strategy (Al-Haddad et al., 2014). Aside from their clinical significance, biopsy procedures have a crucial role in broadening our understanding of the pathology of the adrenal glands at the cellular level. By studying tissue samples, researchers are able to review the effectiveness of existing therapeutic interventions and assist in devising new ones. The biopsied tissue contributes to the description not only of the tumor itself, but also of its microenvironment, possibly with regard to such factors as hormone secretion and interaction with adjacent tissue. This may illuminate complicated physiological questions about the interaction of hormones, for instance, insulin and glucagon, which are central to the regulation of metabolism. Overall, the information unveiled by biopsy techniques is invaluable, and it optimizes our knowledge of adrenal diseases in addition to maximizing clinical outcomes via personalized therapeutic interventions (Figure 4.15).

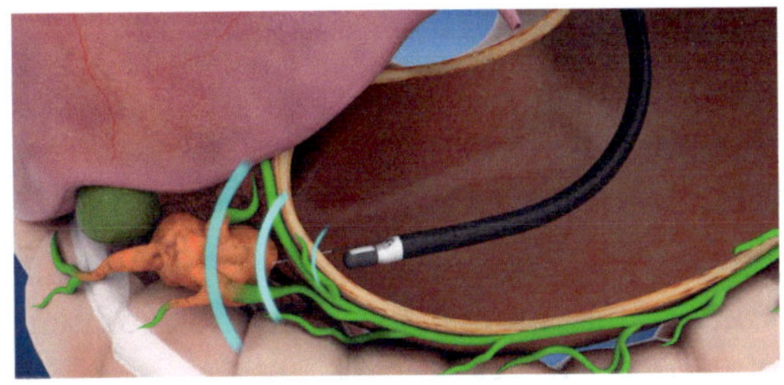

Figure 4.15. Illustration of endoscopic ultrasound-guided fine needle aspiration (EUS-FNA).

Source: https://i.vimeocdn.com/video/1413959619-3cef9b3e8ba0b1f0476bc7961013f0d4ff00c3807a462bc73f2f2e4b5091889d-d?f=webp.

Test Your Knowledge

1. Which blood tests are commonly used to diagnose adrenal gland disorders?
2. How are CT scans used in evaluating adrenal gland disorders?
3. When is a biopsy of the adrenal gland performed, and what is its significance?

4.6. Treatment Options for Adrenal Gland Disorders

Learning Outcome

1. Describe hormone replacement therapy for adrenal gland disorders;
2. Explain how surgical interventions play a crucial role in the management of disorders affecting the adrenal gland;
3. Discuss about lifestyle modifications and their importance in the management of adrenal gland disorders.

Disorders of the adrenal gland refer to a range of conditions that disrupt hormone production and control, necessitating unique treatment modalities for successful management. One of the principal techniques for restoring homeostasis is the administration of glucocorticoids, which are synthetic analogs of cortisol. Treatment is most applicable in patients with adrenal insufficiency, such as patients with Addison's disease. The effectiveness of glucocorticoids results from their ability to bind to the glucocorticoid receptor (GR), thereby initiating cellular responses that modify metabolism and stress response in various tissues, including the liver and adipose tissue. Current research highlights the intricacies of GR signaling pathways and the importance of the "brain-fat axis" here, as these pathways may illuminate novel avenues for modulating glucocorticoid therapy and managing metabolic side effects of adrenal disease (Garabedian et al., 2017). Therapy for hormone overproduction diseases, such as Cushing's syndrome or hyperaldosteronism, is usually surgery or anti-hormone drugs that inhibit hormone synthesis. In hypercortisolism, transsphenoidal removal of pituitary tumors can be utilized to restore cortisol levels. However, in the case where surgery cannot be done, ketoconazole or metyrapone may be employed as alternatives to inhibit adrenal steroidogenesis. Similarly, treatment of hyperaldosteronism typically involves spironolactone, an antagonist of aldosterone, which can correct hypertension and the accompanying electrolyte imbalance. These pharmacological interventions must be carefully watched, as they may have varying actions in different patients, which can be indicative of underlying genetic effects on drug metabolism and on receptor action, and demonstrate the need for an individually tailored treatment regimen in endocrinological practice (Barrese et al., 2014). Changes in lifestyle must also play a significant complementary role in the treatment of adrenal gland disorders. They are typically urged to adhere to healthier nutrition, consistent exercise, and stress management, all of which can be beneficial in maintaining a general state of health and endocrine balance. These steps are particularly important in the instance of patients battling the metabolic effects of hormone imbalance related to the disorder. It is increasingly evident that patient awareness of interactions between lifestyle factors and hormonal therapy can have an influential impact on patient outcomes. With increasing research, a multimodal approach that includes medical treatment with lifestyle modification must be accorded significance in developing efficient management programs for adrenal gland disorders. This integrated perspective, besides addressing the physiological aspect, also encourages improved biological and behavioral health understanding, which is essential in achieving long-term wellness and recovery.

4.6.1. Hormone Replacement Therapy

Hormone replacement therapy (HRT) has become an essential therapy for the treatment of disorders related to adrenal gland malfunction, particularly in adrenal insufficiency. Adrenal glands release critical hormones such as cortisol, aldosterone, and adrenal androgens that are involved in maintaining homeostasis and responding to stress. In instances where these glands are not capable of secreting sufficient hormones due to conditions like Addison's disease or following adrenalectomy, HRT becomes necessary. Replacement with glucocorticoids restores the level of endogenous production of cortisol, alleviating symptoms such as weakness, weakness of muscles, and hypotension. Replacement with mineralocorticoids like fludrocortisone can also be employed to manage electrolyte balance and blood volume and thus maintain cardiovascular integrity. The optimally individualized standardized HRT protocols enhance not only the quality of life of the patients but also normalize physiological function, underscoring its essential role in the regulation of adrenal hormones. The administration of HRT should be done with attention to specificity, taking into account individual differences and special health needs. The factors of age, sex, basic disease, and level of adrenal gland dysfunction may affect the effectiveness and safety of treatment. Close monitoring and adjustment of replacement hormone dosage is necessary to prevent side effects such as weight gain, hypertension, and alterations in glucose metabolism. Such risks must be scrutinized cautiously, particularly in patients with prior comorbidities. Through studies, it has been determined that with close monitoring and appropriate lifestyle modifications, most patients receiving HRT are able to successfully manage their symptoms and remain extremely functional. Hence, regular consultation between endocrinologists and the patients is most important to maximize the treatment regimes and achieve the best results with the least side effects. In children, the situation of HRT becomes challenging due to concerns for growth and development. Children who have conditions such as congenital adrenal hyperplasia or adrenalectomies may need continuous hormone replacement to enhance normal physiological growth and prevent adrenal crises. The unique physiological demands of developing bodies lead to pediatric patients often requiring individualized HRT regimens to adapt to their growth patterns. For instance, as developing patients mature, physicians must be especially responsive to fine-tuning hormone doses in synchrony with changing body dimensions and hormonal demands. This delicate balancing act serves to underscore the importance of sophisticated medical skills in pediatric endocrinology. As showcased in case series, the success of laparoscopic adrenal-sparing surgery also demonstrates potential for favorable results, allowing for improved quality of life and potentially precluding future HRT needs in certain groups (Bartsch et al., 2000). The intersection of HRT and adrenals is then a constantly evolving field that is updated regularly to address evolving patient needs (Allen et al., 2015) (Figure 4.16).

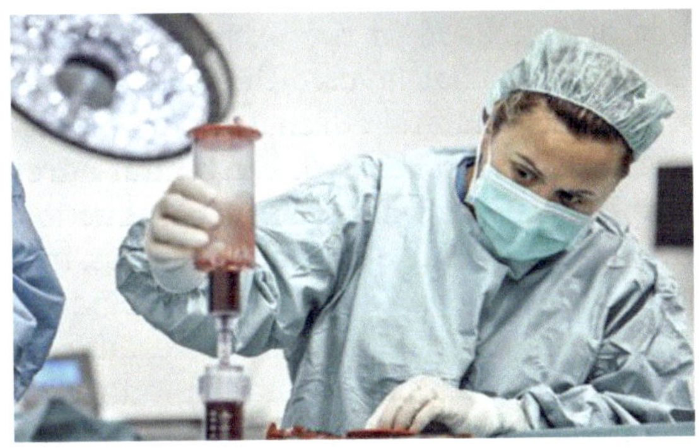

Figure 4.16. Hormone replacement therapy (HRT) has emerged as a critical intervention for managing disorders associated with adrenal gland dysfunction.

Source: https://www.verywellhealth.com/thmb/mXqS5aFvrl0868Gi0mciOneOSm4=/400x250/filters:no_upscale():max_bytes(150000):strip_icc()/GettyImages-1010678628-864f7c97f66d4f51b139ceea2eb938bd.jpg.

4.6.2. Surgical Interventions

Surgery plays a critical role in treating conditions of the adrenal gland, particularly when they are due to adrenal tumors and hyperfunctioning lesions. Adrenalectomy, or surgical excision of one or both adrenal glands, is the primary operation applied. The operation is indicated in those cases where the adrenal gland contains tumors that are either benign, such as adenomas, or malignant, such as adrenocortical carcinoma. In addition, adrenalectomy is required for the management of disorders that cause excessive hormone production, such as Cushing's syndrome. Although it is effective, the risk associated with surgery, such as post-operative infection and hemorrhage, necessitates careful patient selection and preoperative assessment. In addition, the evolution of minimally invasive techniques, for example, laparoscopic adrenalectomy, has decreased recovery times and lowered the physical exhaustion of the procedure, hence the quality of care provided to patients who undergo surgical intervention for adrenal disorders. In addition, surgical treatment is not only needed in the excision of tumors in some cases that involve the adrenal gland. For instance, bilateral adrenalectomy might be performed in patients with congenital adrenal hyperplasia (CAH), where the overproduction of hormones creates huge clinical challenges. In this instance, the removal of both glands would serve to resolve hormonal imbalances, establishing a more stable endocrine state. Additionally, certain surgical procedures can be performed to mitigate symptoms of adrenal crises. These crises are caused by the lack of cortisol production and must be resolved immediately. Surgical procedures, therefore, become central not only in the management of tumors but also in the treatment of life-threatening complications because of adrenal insufficiency. This facet is an indication of the importance of surgical interventions in the overall context of managing adrenal disorders, as indicated in debates on relevant endocrine dysfunctions (Tilvawala et al., 2019). The evolution of surgical technique and adrenal pathology understanding keeps offering supportive innovative treatment plans for enhancing outcomes in patients. Current trends in surgical management include the establishment of robotic-assisted adrenalectomy with enhanced precision and less postoperative pain. Finally, there is an immediate need for a multidisciplinary approach, which includes surgical, medical, and radiological input to enhance the optimization of adrenal gland disorders management. New technologies in imaging modalities also enable more accurate localization of adrenal masses to aid in targeted surgical planning. Lastly, the combination of new surgical techniques with comprehensive patient management emphasizes ongoing research and development in the field of adrenal surgery. As medical science continues to evolve, future studies on less invasive methods and adjuvant therapy will surely transform the management of adrenal gland disorders further entrenching the place of surgery in this vital area of endocrine health (Burity et al., 2014).

4.6.3. Lifestyle Modifications and Their Importance

Lifestyle modifications are increasingly being recognized as essential for maintaining good health and optimal adrenal gland function, integral to the body's stress response. The hormones cortisol, among others, produced by the adrenal glands, helps to modulate metabolism, the immune response, and stress management. As individuals adopt healthier lifestyle choices—such as consistent exercise, improved diet, and mental health—they can enhance the adaptive ability of their adrenal glands. Incorporating stress-reduction techniques, such as yoga or meditation, can also reverse the physical impact of chronic stress on the body, ultimately impacting the hormonal balance required to maintain healthy adrenal glands. Lastly, these changes are a proactive measure against adrenal fatigue and overall hormonal balance, highlighting the need for more awareness and implementation of lifestyle changes among the populace. The incorporation of nutritious foods in one's diet and fluid intake is also a key element of lifestyle changes that can have a significant influence on adrenal function. A diet high in nutrient foods such as whole grains, lean protein, healthy fats, and fruits and vegetables gives the body the vitamins and minerals that support adrenal function and hormone secretion. For example, vitamin C, which is found in citrus fruits and green leafy vegetables, is essential for cortisol production. Proper fluid balance is also critical in maintaining optimal blood supply and nutrient delivery to the adrenal glands. When one neglects dietary lifestyles and hydration, one compounds the risk of disturbed adrenal function and hormonal balance, underscoring the imperative for integral lifestyle changes in preserving health, proper adrenal function, and well-being. Moreover, the interconnection between stress control and adrenal health cannot be understated, particularly regarding lifestyle change. Chronic stress raises cortisol levels, which may lead to a variety of problems with one's health, including anxiety, depression, and metabolic disease. It has been found that environmental and lifestyle variables are a primary determinant for how an individual responds to stress, and therefore, there is a need for an overall approach to well-being. Expanding the scope from the purely physiological level to an integrative model can enable people to take care of themselves in an integrated way. Both stress management techniques and positive social environments form part of living in harmony, and they ensure that the adrenal glands function effectively to counter the challenges of life. As affirmed by available research, addressing the interaction between lifestyle, stress, and adrenal well-being is most essential in building up resilience and long-term health (Cannizzaro et al., 2019; Estrine et al., 2006).

Test Your Knowledge

1. What is hormone replacement therapy in the treatment of adrenal insufficiency?
2. What lifestyle modifications can support treatment and improve outcomes in patients with adrenal disorders?

SUMMARY

The adrenal gland plays a vital role in the maintenance of homeostasis by its several hormone products, primarily glucocorticoids, mineralocorticoids, and adrenal androgens. The hormones are required for the regulation of metabolism, immune responses, and the body's reaction to stress, highlighting the importance of the gland in both physiology and disease. An improved understanding of the role of the adrenal glands provides insight into a number of disparate disorders, including adrenal insufficiency and hypercortisolism, that may have profound impacts on overall health. This intricate interaction warrants continued research into the adrenal axis and its influence on physical and mental health, particularly with new evidence supporting adrenal dysfunction as a correlate of stress-related disorders, as thoroughly explored in current literature for associated pathologies. Furthermore, the relationship between the adrenal gland and the hypothalamic-pituitary-adrenal (HPA) axis cannot be overemphasized. The axis is the primary stress response regulator, implying that any breakdown has the potential to result in extreme physiological distress. Stress processes have been shown to be associated with psychiatric illness, examining the increasingly complex relationship between psychological well-being and adrenal function. Studies of the consequences of environmental stressors during such periodized times of development reveal potential long-term significance for offspring's mental health, thus essentially calling for more advanced explorations into these connections. Profiling the nuance of how indicators of stress, such as cortisol, impact development will be essential in the further articulation of our approaches towards prevention and intervention protocols in clinical settings, particularly in those identified as at risk based on familial and environmental histories. To really understand the importance of the adrenal gland, it is essential to appreciate its holistic effects on not only the health of a person but also its overall implications on public health. The differences in the function of the adrenal and consequent hormonal levels could be accountable for the rising prevalence of concerned disorders in certain populations and require specific health policies. Additionally, integrating knowledge from genetic studies, such as those involving mutations outlined by Aarskog et al. (2009), can lead to advancements in diagnosing and treating conditions stemming from adrenal dysregulation. As our understanding of the adrenal gland expands, so too does the opportunity for better health outcomes through innovative therapeutic strategies. Ultimately, further research into the roles of the adrenal glands is crucial for demystifying the complexities of human disease and health, as noted in the rationale behind the factors that govern HPA axis effectiveness under stress, as reported by Barbazanges et al. (2017).

The adrenal gland plays a pivotal role in the endocrine system of the body, regulating all sorts of critical body functions by secreting hormones. Situated at the top of the kidneys, the adrenal glands are formed of two distinct layers: the adrenal cortex and the adrenal medulla, which secrete various hormones. The cortex secretes glucocorticoids, mineralocorticoids, and androgens, which play a critical role in carbohydrate metabolism, blood pressure, and reproduction. The medulla, however, releases catecholamines like adrenaline that enhance the body's ability to adapt to stressors. By integrating these various hormonal processes, the adrenal gland plays a crucial role in maintaining homeostasis, particularly in response to physical and psychological stress, underscoring its importance as a vital adaptive process of the body. Among the leading research topics is the communication between the adrenal gland and the gut-brain axis, which has become a center of interest in the research of various health conditions. Recent studies have shown that stress can disrupt the balance of the gut microbiome, thereby influencing the hormonal secretion from the adrenal glands. Stressors throughout the course of one's life, such as infections, diet, and lifestyle, can alter microbiota composition, and that in turn could affect the activity of the adrenal glands. The implications of this interaction extend to anxiety, obesity, and neurodegenerative disorders, the interconnectedness of these systems being emphasized. With ongoing research, unravelling the complexities of the microbiota-gut-brain axis will probably steer novel treatment strategies to avoid adrenal disorder and related health conditions, more precisely to cure symptoms of stress (John et al., 2019). Furthermore, melatonin synthesis and its duration, a hormone primarily secreted by the pineal gland, shares communion with adrenal activity and overall health. Melatonin production is controlled by the light-dark cycle, supporting the body's circadian rhythms and modulating physiological reactions. Importantly, melatonin has a protective role in modulating stress and adrenal response regulation, particularly through interaction with cortisol, the primary stress hormone released from the adrenal cortex. This interaction is most important in how the body reacts to environmental changes because prolonged exposure to stress has the potential to lead to dysregulation of the adrenal glands and imbalance of melatonin. Consequently, the understanding of such interactions not only secures the significance of melatonin in metabolic as well as neuroendocrine processes, but also points towards likely therapeutic answers for restoring balance in adrenal activity, namely through particular melatonin therapies (José et al., 2018).

KEY TERMS FROM THIS CHAPTER

- Adaptive responses
- Adrenal failure
- Adrenal hormone deficiency
- Adrenal insufficiency
- Adrenalectomy
- Blood pressure homeostasis,
- Chronic stress
- Circadian regulation
- Corticosteroids
- Adrenal disease
- Adrenal gland
- Adrenal hormone production
- Adrenal macrophages
- Adrenaline
- Body mass index (BMI)
- Circadian biology
- Computed tomography (CT)
- Cushing's syndrome

CRITICAL THINKING QUESTIONS

1. Which of the following correctly describes the layers of the adrenal cortex?

a. Zona glomerulosa, Zona fasciculata, Zona reticularis

b. Zona fasciculata, Zona reticularis, Zona medullaris

c. Zona medullaris, Zona glomerulosa, Zona fasciculata

d. Zona reticularis, Zona fasciculata, Zona glomerulosa

2. Which hormone is primarily secreted by the adrenal medulla?

a. Cortisol

b. Aldosterone

c. Epinephrine

d. Androgens

3. Which of the following is NOT a function of cortisol?

a. Regulation of metabolism

b. Anti-inflammatory effects

c. Stress response

d. Regulation of sodium balance

4. Which condition is characterized by excessive production of cortisol?

a. Addison's disease

b. Cushing's syndrome

c. Pheochromocytoma

d. Conn's syndrome

5. Which of the following tests is commonly used to diagnose adrenal insufficiency?

a. Dexamethasone suppression test

b. Serum calcium test

c. ACTH stimulation test

d. Oral glucose tolerance test

Short Answer Questions

1. What are the two main parts of the adrenal gland, and how do they differ in structure and function?
2. Which hormones are secreted by the adrenal cortex, and what are their primary functions?
3. What hormones does the adrenal medulla produce, and how do they affect the body?
4. How does the release of aldosterone from the adrenal gland regulate blood pressure?
5. How does cortisol help the body respond to stress?
6. What role does adrenaline (epinephrine) play in the "fight or flight" response?
7. How does the adrenal gland contribute to maintaining electrolyte balance in the body?
8. What laboratory tests are used to diagnose adrenal gland disorders?
9. How can imaging techniques such as CT or MRI help in assessing adrenal gland abnormalities?
10. What are the typical treatment approaches for managing adrenal insufficiency or adrenal tumors?

Answers to Critical Thinking Questions

1. (a); 2. (c); 3. (d); 4. (b); 5. (c)

REFERENCES

1. Aarskog, D., Acampora, D., Agarwal, V., Aijaz, A., Alba, M., Ambrosetti, D., Ambrosetti, E., et al. (2009). Genetic regulation of pituitary gland development in human and mouse. https://core.ac.uk/download/1688593.pdf (accessed on 22nd July 2025).
2. Al-Haddad, M., DeWitt, J., LeBlanc, J., et al. (2014). Role of endoscopic ultrasound fine-needle aspiration evaluating adrenal gland enlargement or mass. https://core.ac.uk/download/46961073.pdf (accessed on 22nd July 2025).
3. Alibrandi, A., Asmundo, A., Baldino, G., Cardia, L., Macaione, V., Malta, C., Micali, A., et al. (2019). Post-mortem immunohistochemical evidence of β2-adrenergic receptor expression in the adrenal gland. https://core.ac.uk/download/224993589.pdf (accessed on 22nd July 2025).
4. Allen, A. M., Allende, D. S., Badylak, S. F., Bancos, I., Berkes, J. L., Birke, S. J., Buaas, F. W., et al. (2015). New directions for the treatment of adrenal insufficiency. https://core.ac.uk/download/30697715.pdf (accessed on 22nd July 2025).
5. Amiragova, M. G., Stulnikov, B. V., & Svirskaya, R. I. (2025). Hormone supply of the organism in prolonged emotional stress. https://core.ac.uk/download/pdf/42865972.pdf (accessed on 22nd July 2025).
6. Armanini, D., Bordin, L., Camozzi, V., et al. (2015). Transient hypercortisolism and symptomatic hyperthyroidism associated to primary hyperparathyroidism in an elderly patient: Case report and literature review. https://core.ac.uk/download/53518371.pdf (accessed on 22nd July 2025).
7. Aubert, J., Busetto, G., Butz, H., Kenyon, C. J., Contreras, A., Cowley, M. A., De la Sierra, A., et al. (2003). Transgenic amplification of glucocorticoid action in adipose tissue causes high blood pressure in mice. https://core.ac.uk/download/20448745.pdf (accessed on 22nd July 2025).
8. Bano, G., Beharry, N., Hodgson, S., et al. (2013). A novel medical treatment of Cushing's due to ectopic ACTH in a patient with neurofibromatosis type 1. https://core.ac.uk/download/18302186.pdf (accessed on 22nd July 2025).
9. Barbazanges, A., Harris, A., Kalueff, A. V., Stewart, A., Rodgers, A. B., Vaage, A. B., Arrant, A. E., et al. (2017). Long-term effects of the periconception period on embryo epigenetic profile and phenotype: The role of stress and how this effect is mediated. https://core.ac.uk/download/96767402.pdf (accessed on 22nd July 2025).
10. Barrese, V., Femminella, G. D., Ferrara, N., et al. (2014). Tailoring therapy for heart failure: The pharmacogenomics of adrenergic receptor signaling. https://core.ac.uk/download/29469447.pdf (accessed on 22nd July 2025).
11. Bartsch, G., Elsner, R., Janetschek, G., et al. (2000). Laparoscopic partial adrenalectomy for bilateral pheochromocytomas in a boy with von Hippel-Lindau disease. https://core.ac.uk/download/16432643.pdf (accessed on 22nd July 2025).
12. Berger, J., & Gärtner, J. (2006). X-linked adrenoleukodystrophy: Clinical, biochemical and pathogenetic aspects. https://core.ac.uk/download/pdf/82341248.pdf (accessed on 22nd July 2025).
13. Birrell, E. J. (1924). Interrelations of the endocrine organs. https://open.bu.edu/bitstream/2144/5466/1/Birrell_Ethel_1924_web.pdf (accessed on 22nd July 2025).

14. Bishir, M., Bhat, A., Essa, M. M., Ekpo, O. E., Ihunwo, A. O., Veeraraghavan, V. P., Surapaneni, K. M., et al. (2020). Sleep deprivation and neurological disorders. *BioMed Research International, 2020*, 1–19. https://doi.org/10.1155/2020/5764017 (accessed on 22nd July 2025).

15. Bjørgen, H., & Koppang, E. O. (2021). Anatomy of teleost fish immune structures and organs. *Immunogenetics, 73*, 53–63. https://doi.org/10.1007/s00251-020-01196-0 (accessed on 22nd July 2025).

16. Bobr, A. A., & Miadzelets, A. D. (2005). *Selected themes of histology, cytology and embryology core*. https://core.ac.uk/download/80150430.pdf (accessed on 22nd July 2025).

17. Bornstein, S. R., Kanczkowski, W., & Sue, M. (2016). Adrenal gland microenvironment and its involvement in the regulation of stress-induced hormone secretion during sepsis. https://www.zora.uzh.ch/id/eprint/208323/1/fendo-07-00156.pdf (accessed on 22nd July 2025).

18. Brown, T. H., Francavilla, A., Francavilla, F. R., et al. (1973). The origin, hormonal nature, and action of hepatotrophic substances in portal venous blood. https://core.ac.uk/download/12203718.pdf (accessed on 22nd July 2025).

19. Bruscalupi, G., & Gnocchi, D. (2017). Circadian rhythms and hormonal homeostasis: Pathophysiological implications. https://core.ac.uk/download/98342817.pdf (accessed on 22nd July 2025).

20. Burity, J., da Fonte, I. B., & de Melo, P. B. (2014). Radiological Society of North America (RSNA) 3D printing Special Interest Group (SIG): Guidelines for medical 3D printing and appropriateness for clinical scenarios. https://core.ac.uk/download/212867900.pdf (accessed on 22nd July 2025).

21. Cannizzaro, E., Plescia, F., Cirrincione, L., & Ramaci, T. (2019). Work-related stress, physio-pathological mechanisms, and the influence of environmental genetic factors. https://core.ac.uk/download/287859255.pdf (accessed on 22nd July 2025).

22. Cerquetella, M., Faillace, V., Fruganti, A., et al. (2016). Transrectal ultrasonography of the adrenal glands in donkeys (*Equus asinus*). https://core.ac.uk/download/201725257.pdf (accessed on 22nd July 2025).

23. Chan, L. F., Clark, A. J., Gorrigan, R. J., et al. (2011). Localization of the melanocortin-2-receptor and its accessory proteins in the developing and adult adrenal gland. https://core.ac.uk/download/10674788.pdf (accessed on 22nd July 2025).

24. Cipolla-Neto, J., & do Amaral, F. G. (2018). Melatonin as a hormone: New physiological and clinical insights. *Endocrine Reviews, 39*, 990–1028. https://doi.org/10.1210/er.2018-00084 (accessed on 22nd July 2025).

25. Cryan, J. F., O'Riordan, K. J., Cowan, C. S. M., Sandhu, K. V., Bastiaanssen, T. F. S., Boehme, M., Codagnone, M. G., et al. (2019). The microbiota-gut-brain axis. *Physiological Reviews, 99*, 1877–2013. https://doi.org/10.1152/physrev.00018.2018 (accessed on 22nd July 2025).

26. De Bosscher, K., Opdenakker, G., Van den Steen, P. E., et al. (2019). Critical roles of endogenous glucocorticoids for disease tolerance in malaria. https://core.ac.uk/download/159422440.pdf (accessed on 22nd July 2025).

27. Elezi, A., Beadini, S., Kostovska, I., & Ziberi, E. (2024). Correlation between BMI and gonadotropin hormones in the female gender. *International Journal of Medical Sciences–ACTA MEDICA BALKANICA*. https://www.semanticscholar.org/paper/b2258c99381965ebaf7707b22af4927506703a66 (accessed on 22nd July 2025).

28. Estrine, J., & DeLisle, L. (2006). Stress: Putting the brain back into medicine. https://core.ac.uk/download/71356692.pdf (accessed on 22nd July 2025).

29. Evans, J. A., Gasser, P. J., Klement, C., et al. (2016). Sexual differentiation of circadian clock function in the adrenal gland. https://core.ac.uk/download/213057608.pdf (accessed on 22nd July 2025).

30. Garabedian, M. J., Harris, C. A., & Jeanneteau, F. (2017). Glucocorticoid receptor action in metabolic and neuronal function [version 1; referees: 3 approved]. https://core.ac.uk/download/129069043.pdf (accessed on 22nd July 2025).

31. Gonzalez Deniselle, M. C., Lara, H. E., Recabarren, S. E., et al. (2016). Developmental and functional effects of steroid hormones on the neuroendocrine axis and spinal cord. https://core.ac.uk/download/159294623.pdf (accessed on 22nd July 2025).

32. Göransson, L. (2013). Hypotalamus-hypofys-binjurebarksaxeln och perinatal behandling av prematurföl. https://core.ac.uk/download/11989850.pdf (accessed on 22nd July 2025).

33. Hiraki, K., Nishishita, H., & Sunami, H. (1959). Influences of various hormones on the megakaryocyte in bone-marrow tissue culture. https://core.ac.uk/download/12548128.pdf (accessed on 22nd July 2025).

34. Hole, C., Dhamsania, A., Brown, C., & Ryznar, R. (2025). Immune dysregulation in depression and anxiety: A review of the immune response in disease and treatment. *Cells, 14*. https://www.semanticscholar.org/paper/99ceef2dac0c93551f239269530e14b789b6091d (accessed on 22nd July 2025).

35. Hrabak-Paar, M., Đido, V., & Štern-Padovan, R. (2015). Should we use CT or MRI for detection and characterization of benign adrenal lesions? https://core.ac.uk/download/132303645.pdf (accessed on 22nd July 2025).

36. Kling, I. H. (1939). The hormones of invertebrates. https://open.bu.edu/bitstream/2144/4470/1/Kling_1939_web.pdf (accessed on 22nd July 2025).

37. Kohl, R. L., & Odell, S. (2025). Neurophysiological responses to stressful motion and anti-motion sickness drugs as mediated by the limbic system. https://core.ac.uk/download/pdf/42853678.pdf (accessed on 22nd July 2025).

38. Kot, T., Tkachuk, S., Usenko, S., & Prokopenko, V. (2023). Adrenal gland of poultry: Anatomy, microscopy, morphometry, and histochemistry. *Journal of World's Poultry Research*. https://www.semanticscholar.org/paper/d560b1f0ef542e95ba1bcf2681bb7a2685c18915 (accessed on 22nd July 2025).

39. Kurzrock, R., Munoz, J., & Wheler, J. J. (2014). Androgen receptors beyond prostate cancer: An old marker as a new target. https://core.ac.uk/download/323066033.pdf (accessed on 22nd July 2025).

40. Letizia, C., Concistrè, A., De Vincentis, G., Iannucci, G., Piernatale, L., Petramala, L., Marinelli, C., et al. (2015). Adrenal pheochromocytoma incidentally discovered in a patient with parkinsonism. https://core.ac.uk/download/54525674.pdf (accessed on 22nd July 2025).

41. Matthew, W. D., Reichardt, L. F., & Tsavaler, L. (1981). Identification of a synaptic vesicle-specific membrane protein with a wide distribution in neuronal and neurosecretory tissue. https://core.ac.uk/download/323072860.pdf (accessed on 22nd July 2025).

42. Miara, A. (2013). Differences in sympathetic nervous response due to gender. https://open.bu.edu/bitstream/2144/12160/6/Miara_Amy_2013_nosig_nocv.pdf (accessed on 22nd July 2025).

43. Miyata, T., Nojima, E., & Minai, Y. (2025). Effects of excessive sucrose intake on aggressive behavior and peripheral stress-related hormone and catecholamines in BALB/c mice during adolescent development. *Journal of Nutritional Science and Vitaminology, 71*(1), 16–24. https://www.semanticscholar.org/paper/a0aae9255ba9c0d1791574323d9a33c1f26955ef (accessed on 22nd July 2025).

44. Morozov, V. N. (2024). Classification of adrenal ectopias and their frequency in rats. *Journal of Medical and Biological Research*. https://www.semanticscholar.org/paper/c2cc8550d1e18c2be5bbbdb2aa424c72991344e3 (accessed on 22nd July 2025).

45. Papakokkinou, E. (2022). Clinical challenges in Cushing's syndrome. https://core.ac.uk/download/491189992.pdf (accessed on 22nd July 2025).

46. Parker, G. H. (1938). The color changes in lizards, particularly in *Phrynosoma*. https://core.ac.uk/download/4879095.pdf (accessed on 22nd July 2025).

47. Rucker, E. P. (2017). Pituitary gland functional connectivity and BMI. https://core.ac.uk/download/148695960.pdf (accessed on 22nd July 2025).

48. Salehi, M., Shahmoradi, Z., Razavi, S. M., Lali, I., & Faghihian, E. (2022). Adrenocorticotropic hormone (ACTH) level and adrenal deficiency in patients with mucocutaneous pemphigus. *Hormone Molecular Biology and Clinical Investigation, 43*, 437–440. https://www.semanticscholar.org/paper/98927bd7578df915fd77504f19391b155411f07c (accessed on 22nd July 2025).

49. Shevtsova, I., & Gerstner, S. J. (2024). 7705 Paliperidone induced central adrenal insufficiency: A case report. *Journal of the Endocrine Society, 8*. https://www.semanticscholar.org/paper/25c2f5ae3db216c68b3c8ed0e110e58e9672f8b8 (accessed on 22nd July 2025).

50. Tilvawala, M. (2019). Acromegaly: Pathogenesis & treatment. https://open.bu.edu/bitstream/2144/36629/7/Tilvawala_bu_0017N_14523.pdf (accessed on 22nd July 2025).

51. Ünlükal, N., & Şentürk, A. (2024). Ultrastructural changes in the adrenal gland in terms of age and gender-related. *Turkish Journal of Veterinary Research*. https://www.semanticscholar.org/paper/435175f6cbbfb9e100a5fea1e130d9846ea14395 (accessed on 22nd July 2025).

52. van't Westeinde, A. (2023). Brain structure and function in primary adrenal insufficiency. https://core.ac.uk/download/555550394.pdf (accessed on 22nd July 2025).

53. Wang, J., Zhu, Y., Wang, Z., Liu, C., Liu, S., Li, X., Chen, R., et al. (2022). Hypertension resolution after laparoscopic adrenal tumor resection in patients of adrenal incidentaloma with normal hormone levels. *Urologia Internationalis, 107*, 193–201. https://www.semanticscholar.org/paper/b9e4a359146984acfcec42f04743da4b5c9b7509 (accessed on 22nd July 2025).

54. Wei, Y., Liu, Y., Lei, J., Jiang, Q., Geng, X., Guo, Y., & Zhang, B. (2025). Quercetin-based treatment improves eggshell quality in aged laying hens by modulating immune response, eggshell gland health and serum metabolome. *Journal of the Science of Food and Agriculture*. https://www.semanticscholar.org/paper/efeb259c5d21e383e6d8f4e1623653e190d4dc2d (accessed on 22nd July 2025).

55. Xu, Y., Gallerand, A., Dolfi, B., Zhu, A., Schrank, P. R., Patterson, M. T., Acharya, N. R., et al. (2022). Profiling adrenal gland resident macrophage response to acute and chronic stress. *The Journal of Immunology*. https://www.semanticscholar.org/paper/ecca793237a31b802d7ae8c75af200c008f1dae2 (accessed on 22nd July 2025).

56. Xu, Y., Patterson, M. T., Dolfi, B., Zhu, A., Bertola, A., Schrank, P. R., Gallerand, A., et al. (2024). Adrenal gland macrophages regulate glucocorticoid production through Trem2 and TGF-β. *JCI Insight, 9*. https://www.semanticscholar.org/paper/36a64e9ecb4c7d260d4a86a10552a70602c550cf (accessed on 22nd July 2025).

ENDOCRINE PANCREAS AND DIABETES MELLITUS

5

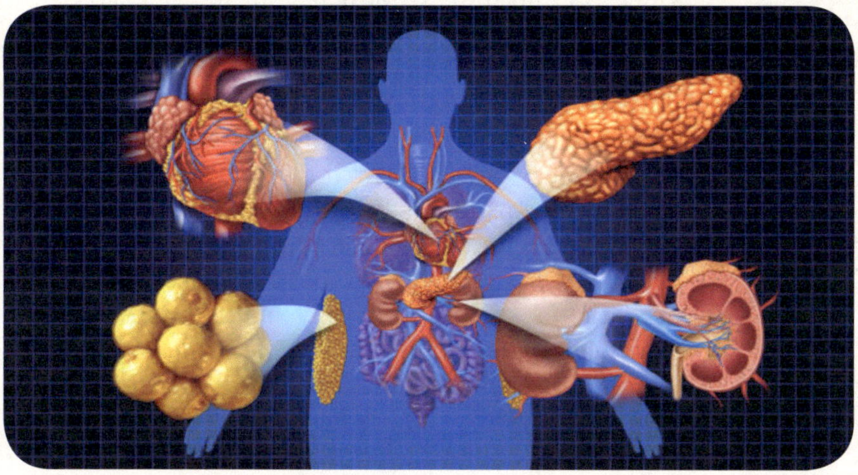

Introduction

The relationship between the endocrine pancreas and diabetes mellitus is a significant area of study in establishing the pathophysiology of metabolic disease. The pancreas is a significant organ responsible for secreting hormones, including insulin, which regulates blood glucose levels. Dysfunctions in this endocrine process could lead to numerous forms of diabetes, primarily type 1 and type 2 diabetes, and these two have distinct mechanisms of dysfunctions. Although type 1 diabetes is a result of autoimmune beta-cell loss that results in insulin deficiency, type 2 diabetes usually has its origin in insulin resistance accompanied by an inappropriately augmented insulin secretion. Given that diabetes is on the rise globally, understanding the intricacies of pancreatic endocrine function is essential to developing targeted interventions to combat this epidemic in public health. Furthermore, the economic burden of diabetes underscores the importance of examining treatment strategies according to pancreatic function and cellular processes. The contribution of pancreatic endocrine cell plasticity to diabetic

LEARNING OBJECTIVES

After studying this chapter, you will be able to:

1. Discuss the anatomy of the endocrine pancreas;
2. Describe the mechanism of insulin secretion;
3. Explain the types of diabetes mellitus;
4. State pathophysiology of diabetes mellitus;
5. Deal with the diagnosis of diabetes mellitus;
6. Focus on management and treatment options for diabetes mellitus.

mellitus pathophysiology has come to be more underscored by studies. Islets of Langerhans, which produce insulin and other hormones, exhibit a multidirectional response to metabolic change, and it will either relieve or worsen diabetic symptoms. In type 2 diabetes, loss of beta-cell function is frequently associated with increasing insulin resistance as a mechanism for chronic hyperglycemia. Also, diseases such as gestational diabetes are the multifaceted expression of endocrine disturbance under conditions of metabolic stress, potentially influencing glucose regulation over time after pregnancy. The examination of endocrine cell adaptation mechanisms and the outcome of these adaptations may help elucidate potential therapeutic avenues. By understanding the cellular responses, researchers can attempt to reverse the signs of deficiency in beta-cells and normalize glucose metabolism in the afflicted individuals, and thus pave the way for new treatments in diabetes care. In an attempt to cope with the increasing menace of diabetes mellitus in an efficient manner, there is a need to study the biomarkers that signify the functioning of the pancreas, both endocrine and exocrine. Their association with diabetes can explain subsequent diagnostic and therapeutic choices. For instance, studies have indicated that some enzymes, such as amylase and lipase levels, are associated with the pancreas function in diabetic patients. Additionally, specific markers such as retinol-binding protein 4 have been associated with insulin resistance and the pathogenesis of type 2 diabetes. Clarification of these interactions will be essential for enhancing diabetic diagnostic criteria and developing novel management strategies, with both the exocrine and endocrine roles of the pancreas in mind. Bridging gaps in existing research regarding pancreatic biomarkers will not only enhance our insight into diabetes pathology but also pave the way for further breakthroughs in treatment and prevention modalities directed against this significant health concern.

Definition of the Endocrine Pancreas

The endocrine pancreas is a significant component of the human system with a crucial role to play in regulating glucose metabolism in the form of the secretion of hormones. Unlike its exocrine counterpart, which secretes digestive enzymes, the endocrine component consists of clusters of cells known as the islets of Langerhans. These islets play a role in the secretion of significant hormones like insulin, glucagon, and somatostatin. Insulin and glucagon work in conjunction to maintain the blood sugar level within balance; insulin lowers blood glucose by stimulating cellular uptake, while glucagon increases blood sugar by stimulating the release of glucose from the stored state in the liver. This coordinated cooperation is crucial for homeostasis, and any discrepancy in hormone secretion can lead to metabolic diseases, such as diabetes mellitus, thereby highlighting the significant role of the endocrine pancreas in overall health. The function of the endocrine pancreas is not just mere hormone secretion; it is most closely related to the pathophysiology of Type II Diabetes Mellitus. The fine balance of insulin and glucagon is most often disturbed in patients with this condition. As Type II Diabetes has been described as a heterogeneous disease controlled by environmental and genetic factors, understanding the intricacy of regulation of the pancreas is instrumental to effective treatment and intervention. In the last few decades, rates of pediatric Type II Diabetes have soared, hastening an immediate investigation into its etiology and long-term health implications of early onset (Kapke et al., 2015). The endocrine pancreas, therefore, plays a central role in not only the acute management of diabetes but also in coping with its overall impact on the public health. Categorization and diagnosis of diabetes based on its fundamental etiology are crucial in the understanding of the multi-aspect presentations of this syndrome. The confirmation of an etiology-based classification system in diabetes studies is a paradigm shift in addressing the complexities regarding the illness (Abdul-Rasoul et al., 2016). Such classifications help one identify between Type I and Type II diabetes, as well as other forms resulting from exocrine pancreatic disease or secondary endocrine disorders. This identification is important in developing focused treatment strategies that can lead to improved results among patients. By gaining an appreciation for the resulting specific deficiencies of hormones that occur from endocrine pancreatic dysfunction, physicians are able to devise tailor-made treatments that not only target blood glucose, but also target the resulting underlying hormonal balances required for long-term health and well-being in diabetic patients (Figure 5.1).

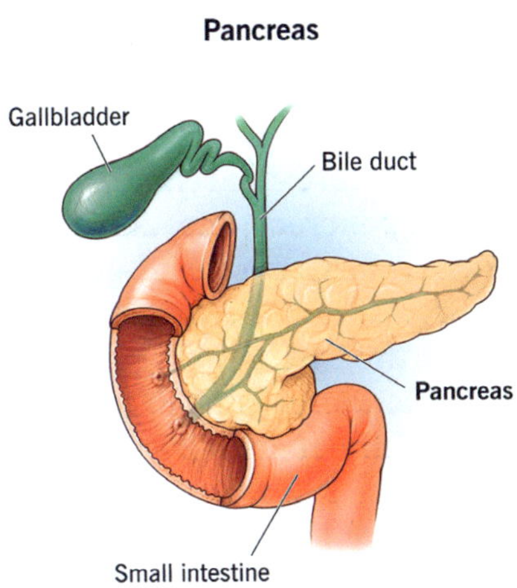

Figure 5.1. Pancreas illustration.

Source: https://my.clevelandclinic.org/-/scassets/images/org/health/articles/21743-pancreas.jpg.

Overview of Diabetes Mellitus

Diabetes mellitus refers to a group of metabolic disorders that are largely characterized by chronic hyperglycemia that results from defects in insulin secretion, action, or both. The two major forms of diabetes, Type 1 and Type 2, have distinct mechanisms of pathophysiology. Type 1 diabetes is predominantly an autoimmune disorder leading to the destruction of insulin-secreting beta cells of the pancreas. This results in absolute insulin deficiency, necessitating lifelong insulin replacement in affected patients. Type 2 diabetes is more prevalent and occurs with insulin resistance and relative insulin deficiency, which can be attributed to lifestyle-related factors such as obesity and physical inactivity. The high global prevalence of diabetes emphasizes the success of management, as untreated and undiagnosed diabetes carries a potential for severe complications like cardiovascular disease, neuropathy, and nephropathy, whose impact on quality of life and healthcare expenditure is high. A key subtype in the diabetes spectrum is fibrocalculous pancreatic diabetes (FCPD), widely placed under malnutrition-related diabetes mellitus (MRDM). This is predominantly found in regions of high malnutrition prevalence, particularly in the tropics. These patients usually present with complications of chronic pancreatitis, a disease that results from dietary deficiency and exposure to toxic substances like cyanogenic compounds in cassava. In research, both micronutrient deficiencies and oxidative stress have been shown to play a role in the pathogenesis of this variant, leading to high morbidity in such individuals. Despite increased mortality rates among youths with FCPD, improved healthcare and conditions of the environment have been shown to enhance survival and alter the disease's clinical presentation, thus underscoring the role of certain healthcare interventions among high-risk groups (Chowdhury et al., 1994). Type 1 diabetes continues to be a complex interaction of environmental, immunological, and genetic determinants. The most recent advances in disease knowledge have disclosed numerous aspects, from the genetic predispositions that modulate susceptibility to the immune processes of beta-cell death. Various gene variants have been discovered with Type 1 diabetes by studies, while innovation in immunotherapy has offered the promise of disease-altering therapy. Severe issues, however, still linger in harmonizing clinical practice, managing complications, and fully characterizing the diseases' mechanisms. Current clinical management is based on tight glycemic control in an effort to minimize long-term complications, which demands a multidimensional system of education, lifestyle modification, and continuous support for the patient (DiMeglio et al., 2018). With continuous advancements in research, the ultimate goal remains the improvement of outcomes for individuals with Type 1 diabetes and the development of prevention and management strategies.

Importance of Understanding the Relationship Between the Two

It is imperative to understand the intricate association of the endocrine pancreas with diabetes mellitus in a bid to improve therapy options and patient prognosis. The endocrine pancreas plays the key role in glucose homeostasis by virtue of the secretion of insulin and glucagon, the hormones that are pivotal in regulating blood glucose concentrations. Derangement or deficiency of insulin secretion equates to type 1 diabetes mellitus, while insulin resistance represents the characteristic feature of type 2 diabetes mellitus. Understanding how these imbalances in hormones interact with metabolic processes is important for devising targeted treatments. In addition, understanding the mechanisms of pathophysiology behind these diseases can allow early intervention strategies to become effective and thus prevent the development of severe metabolic disease and its complications. Healthcare professionals require knowledge to manage diabetes well and educate patients regarding lifestyle modifications that can manage their condition and improve quality of life. The implications of the interaction between the endocrine pancreas and diabetes extend to the broad category of metabolic disorders, including non-alcoholic fatty liver disease (NAFLD). Epidemiologic studies have documented a very high correlation between NAFLD and diabetes, and an overlapping strength in the pathogenesis of the two diseases. Diabetic patients are, in fact, at very high risk of developing NAFLD, which in turn can augment insulin resistance. Physicians should recognize this association since complete management, including the pancreatic derangement as well as the associated liver disease, can lead to improved metabolic control. Liver function testing and control of dyslipidemia, hypertension, and other components of the metabolic syndrome are essential components of an integrated regimen for the control of diabetes. Reducing the burden of diabetes and NAFLD needs interprofessional coordination among healthcare providers, reinforcing the need to understand the interaction of these two entities with one another. Furthermore, the relationship between the endocrine pancreas and diabetes mellitus indicates the potential role of gut microbiota in the general metabolic well-being. Current research puts the microbiota-gut-brain axis at the center of maintaining metabolic homeostasis, influencing insulin sensitivity, and modulating the endocrine function of the pancreas. Diet, stress, and the use of antibiotics may influence this microbial balance to produce metabolic disorders, such as diabetes. Appreciation of these interactions emphasizes the need for investigation of diet-induced interventions and probiotic therapies to optimize metabolic benefits. In addition, as knowledge of the gut-brain interaction advances, it may set the stage for therapeutic strategies directed not just at diabetes but also at its related illnesses like obesity and NAFLD. Deep strategies considering this intricate interaction are unavoidable in planning effective interventions to manage diabetes mellitus deeply and effectively (John et al., 2019; Mary et al., 2023).

5.1. Anatomy of the Endocrine Pancreas

Learning Outcome

1. Describe the structure and function of pancreatic islets;
2. Explain the types of cells in the islets of Langerhans;
3. Understand the hormones produced by the endocrine pancreas.

The anatomy of the endocrine pancreas is critical to the manner in which it operates in glucose metabolism and in regulating the entire endocrine system. Composed largely of clusters known as islets of Langerhans, the endocrine pancreas secretes important hormones including insulin, glucagon, and somatostatin. The hormones function collectively to maintain glucose homeostasis in the body. Insulin, released by the beta cells, results in the absorption of glucose by cells, while glucagon, secreted by alpha cells, stimulates the release of glucose into the bloodstream as and when needed. The fine control of these hormones indicates the significance of the endocrine pancreas in metabolism. Ineffective hormone production or dysregulation of pathways signaling in this organ could lead to metabolic illness, that is, Diabetes Mellitus, where insulin resistance or deficiency leads to profound biochemical derangements. The pathology of Diabetes Mellitus underscores the importance of understanding the structure and function of the endocrine pancreas. Autoimmune destruction of pancreatic beta cells in Type 1 diabetes leads to suboptimal insulin secretion, resulting in immediate hyperglycemic consequences. Conversely, Type 2 diabetes is not only characterized by insulin resistance but also by a resultant beta-cell loss. It has been proven that hyperglycemia, when chronic, triggers oxidative stress and inflammatory responses, which can cause additional pancreatic tissue damage (Zhao et al., 2023). The Langerhans islets exhibit diabetes-induced structural alterations in their mitochondria, such as amyloid deposition and alterations in cell composition, to their α- and β-cell function and ability to secrete hormones. To create useful therapeutic interventions to re-establish pancreatic function and regulate blood glucose levels efficiently, it is essential to know these anatomical and pathologic changes. Moreover, the interaction between early-life environmental factors and the anatomy of the endocrine pancreas has significant implications for metabolic disease emergence. Evidence indicates that the intrauterine environment, as well as maternal health during pregnancy, can program the offspring's metabolic system and make people susceptible to having diabetes in adult life (Luís et al., 2021). Such evidence highlights the role of the endocrine pancreas not only in the regulation of short-term metabolism but also in the etiology of health and disease during development. Through understanding the anatomical form and function of the pancreas and its developmental determinants, researchers are in a better position to appreciate the holistic measures called for in preventing and managing diabetes mellitus, ensuring interprofessional collaboration in healthcare (Figure 5.2).

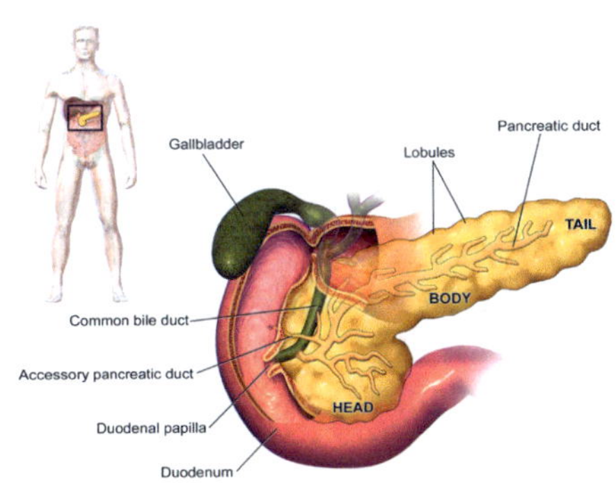

Figure 5.2. Anatomy of the human pancreas.

Source: https://upload.wikimedia.org/wikipedia/commons/thumb/7/7e/Blausen_0699_PancreasAnatomy2.png/1024px-Blausen_0699_PancreasAnatomy2.png.

5.1.1. Structure and Function of Pancreatic Islets

Langerhans' islets, or pancreatic islets, play a key role in the endocrine function of the pancreas, secreting hormones that are responsible for glucose metabolism regulation and homeostasis maintenance. These cell groups account for approximately 1–2% of the pancreas's mass and are primarily organized into four distinct cell types: alpha, beta, delta, and PP (pancreatic polypeptide) cells. All cell types secrete specific hormones, with beta cells playing the leading role, secreting insulin when the blood glucose level is high. It is such a finely regulated mechanism that is crucial for metabolic processes, pointing to the importance of islet structure and function in maintaining glucose homeostasis. In addition, the structural arrangement of these cells in the islets is optimized to facilitate maximal intercellular communication so that they can promptly respond to metabolic alterations. The complex functions of pancreatic islets extend beyond hormone secretion; they involve high-level interactions with the cellular and extracellular microenvironments that surround them. The organization of the extracellular matrix (ECM) within and around the islets provides structural integrity but also plays a critical role in governing cell behavior and function. For instance, ECM defines β-cell survival, function, and responsiveness to stimuli such as glucose. Improved *in vitro* methods have led to new platforms being introduced that can mimic the native microphysiological pancreas islet environment. These systems enable researchers to study the kinetics of insulin secretion in real time and quantify dynamic responses to glucose stimulation and thereby to expose the physiological and pathological processes accountable for diabetes mellitus. The ability to simulate the islet microenvironment provides promising avenues for working out better treatment of diabetes, highlighting the value of understanding islet structure and function in this respect (Schl Künder et al., 2024). The history of our understanding of pancreatic islets is punctuated by significant milestones, from the initial descriptions of islet morphology to breakthroughs in diabetes treatment. The early work of Langerhans laid the foundation for the recognition of the endocrine function of the pancreas, ultimately leading to the isolation of insulin and the transformation of the treatment of diabetes. Since the purification of isletin in the early 1920s, the field has progressed significantly, enabling the synthesis of modified insulin and the development of CGM devices. Despite these advancements, challenges persist, particularly in addressing the underlying pathophysiology of diabetes mellitus types. Research continues today on correcting biochemical defects in type 2 diabetes and fixing islet function in type 1 diabetes. The complexities of pancreatic islet structure and function remain to the fore in these efforts, shaping new therapy development and enhancing our understanding of diabetes mellitus (Christine et al., 2022) (Figure 5.3).

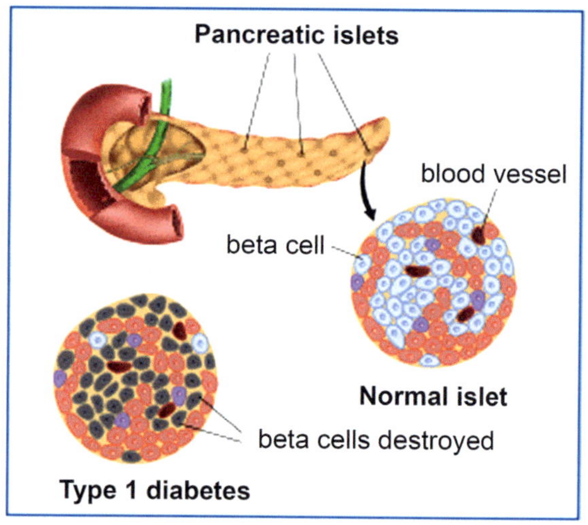

Figure 5.3. Pancreatic islets.

Source: https://www.niddk.nih.gov/-/media/Images/Health-Information/Diabetes/Pancreatic_Islets_02-compressor.png?h=266&w=300&hash=7350D821102B77A9BCBC2DE41B993984.

5.1.2. Types of Cells in the Islets of Langerhans

The islets of Langerhans are a cluster of cells located in the pancreas and are the main actors in the modulation of glucose metabolism and endocrine function. The islets consist predominantly of five distinct types of cells. These islets are involved in multiple roles in the maintenance of homeostasis. The most common among them is the beta (β) cell responsible for insulin release. Insulin is crucial in regulating blood glucose levels, and its impairment or deficiency is a leading cause of diabetes mellitus. Alpha (α) cells, on the other hand, release glucagon, a hormone which acts in the opposite direction to insulin. It triggers glycemic effects in the liver. This delicate equilibrium between the beta and alpha cells represents the complexity of the islets function, and the necessity of knowing both cell types of roles in disease conditions such as diabetes mellitus (Xavier et al., 2018).

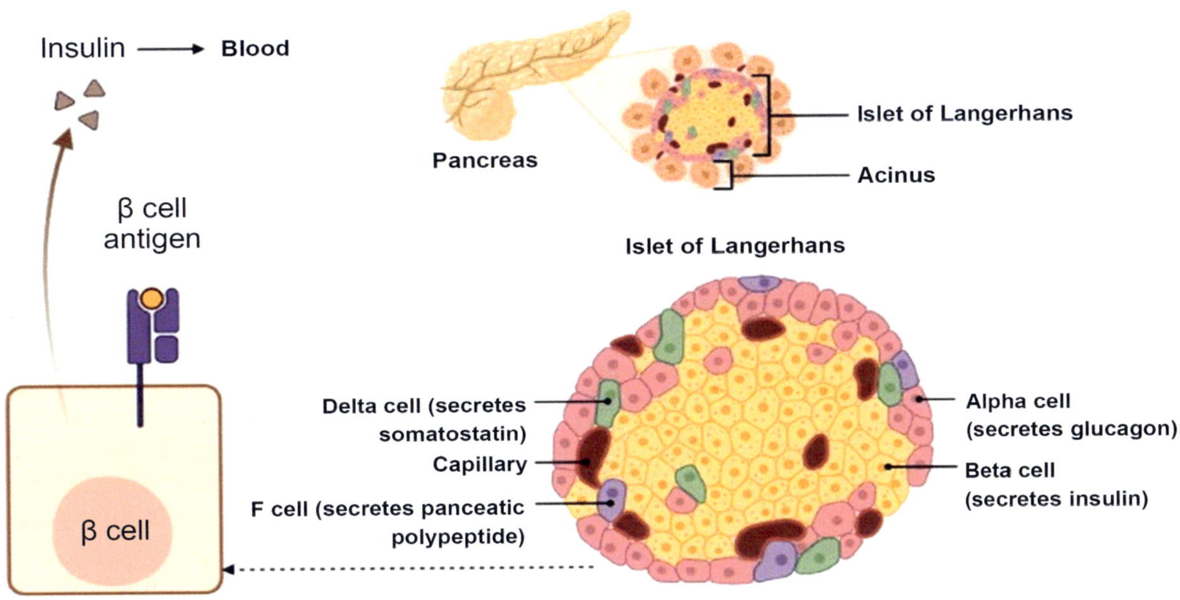

Figure 5.4. Insulin-secreting cells located in the pancreatic islets of Langerhans.

Source: https://www.researchgate.net/publication/361448018/figure/fig2/AS:1176808384937984@1657584391194/Insulin-secreting-cells-located-in-the-pancreatic-islets-of-Langerhans-Type-1.jpg.

The islets also contain delta (δ) cells, which secrete somatostatin, a hormone that has a significant role in regulating the secretion of insulin and glucagon. This negative feedback process is an indication of the endocrine sophistication of the islets and emphasizes the function of δ cells in controlling the overall food consumption and metabolic regulation. Moreover, the pancreatic polypeptide (PP) cells participate in the overall hormonal milieu by releasing PP, which is a modulatory peptide involved in the regulation of appetite and gut functions. While all cell type has specific function, it is their interaction that ultimately controls endocrine balance. With the progression in research, knowledge of such intricate interactions becomes essential while trying to develop therapeutics to maximize islet function and treat such an illness as diabetes mellitus (Xavier et al., 2018). The problems inherent in the therapy of diabetes have once again revived interest in the dynamics of islet cell composition and function. Current research indicates probable ways towards the regeneration of β-cell mass or converting non-β islet cells into insulin-producing cells, which may be substitute treatments to insulin therapy. As greater insight into normal islet cell mass and organization is gained, it becomes increasingly apparent that the preservation of this balance is crucial in energy homeostasis. Furthermore, efforts to investigate islet transplantation as a possibility for type 1 diabetes have brought forth such key challenges as shortage of donor organ and need for post-transplant immunosuppressive treatment. These point out the imperative need for meeting issues with islet cell function and mass to facilitate effective administration and management of diabetes mellitus (Figure 5.4).

5.1.3. Hormones Produced by the Endocrine Pancreas

The endocrine pancreas plays a role in the control of glucose homeostasis through the production and release of several significant hormones, primarily insulin and glucagon. Insulin, produced by the beta cells of the islets of Langerhans, plays a crucial role in reducing blood glucose levels by facilitating glucose entry into the body's cells. On the other hand, glucagon, secreted by the alpha cells, has a counteracting effect to increase blood sugar when they get too low, by promoting glycogenolysis and gluconeogenesis in the liver. This delicate balance between the release of insulin and glucagon is crucial for metabolic balance. Dysfunctions of this regulatory mechanism may lead to the development of diabetes mellitus, whereby the body's ability to produce insulin may be impaired or its action inhibited, resulting in perpetual hyperglycemia and an array of associated complications, including cardiovascular disorders and neuropathy. Apart from insulin and glucagon, other endocrine pancreatic hormones, such as somatostatin and PP, contribute significantly to metabolic control. Somatostatin, secreted from delta cells, plays a critical role in suppressing the release of both insulin and glucagon, thus maintaining the hormonal milieu based on nutrient availability. PP, secreted from PP cells, is said to regulate pancreatic exocrine activity and appetite but is yet incompletely characterized in its metabolic role. These hormones are entangled with crosstalk in other body systems, an indication of the subtle interconnection between the endocrine pancreas and metabolic state. As diabetes becomes more prevalent, understanding the versatile roles of these hormones is crucial in developing improved management strategies and enhancing patient outcomes. The endocrine pancreas plays an even greater role in type 3c diabetes mellitus (T3cDM), which usually develops following pancreatic diseases such as pancreatitis. Here, both endocrine and exocrine structural damages result in a deficiency of hormone secretion and consequent complications that are secondary to malabsorption due to exocrine deficiency. Experiments examining the interaction between insulin, glucagon, and other hormones in T3cDM patients are essential, as they may have to be treated by specialized approaches reacting both to glucose regulation and to feeding (Lokman et al., 2025; Valente et al., 2024). The effect of endocrine pancreas-secreted hormones on the pathophysiologic changes that define diabetes emphasizes the need for a multidimensional treatment approach that takes into consideration the intricate interactions of hormones and their consequence on metabolic health. As our understanding of these interactions continues to advance, it is possible that healthcare workers can further improve treatment schemes and patient quality of life (Figure 5.5).

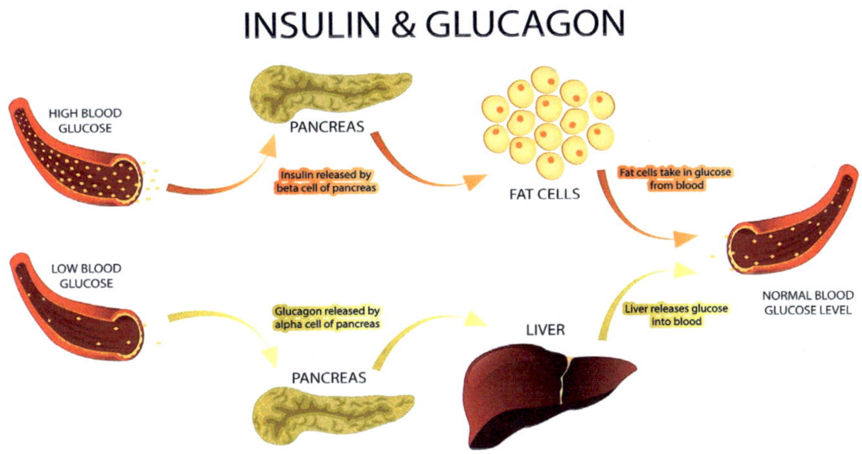

Figure 5.5. Insulin and glucagon.

Source: https://www.news-medical.net/images/Article_Images/ImageForArticle_25538_17322956522701880.jpg.

Test Your Knowledge

1. What is the primary function of the islets of Langerhans in the pancreas?
2. How does insulin regulate blood glucose levels?

5.2. Mechanism of Insulin Secretion

Learning Outcome

1. Explain the role of glucose in insulin release;
2. Discuss the regulation of insulin secretion;
3. Describe the impact of other hormones on insulin release.

The mechanism of insulin secretion by pancreatic beta cells is a strictly controlled process that is provoked by an increase in blood glucose concentrations. Upon their entry into the beta cells, glucose undergoes metabolism by glycolysis and the citric acid cycle, which results in an increase in ATP/ADP ratio. Closure of ATP-sensitive potassium channels due to the resultant increase in ATP provokes depolarization of the membrane. The greater the membrane potential becomes positive, the more voltage-gated calcium channels open, which allow calcium ions to flow into the cell. The calcium entry is critical because it triggers the exocytosis of insulin-containing granules. This illustrates the sophistication of the signaling pathways that connect alterations in metabolism to the physiological response of insulin release, providing evidence of the crucial function beta cells perform in maintaining glucose homeostasis. Circadian rhythms play a significant role in the mechanism of insulin secretion, integrating the endocrine function of the pancreas with the body's internal clock. Disturbances in these rhythms have been found to lead to abnormal regulation of insulin secretion and glucose metabolism, resulting in diabetes mellitus pathogenesis. Pancreatic beta cells contain circadian clocks that regulate their function in synchronization with the central clock in the hypothalamus. Disturbance of such circadian rhythms—by irregular sleep patterns, night shifts, or an imbalanced diet—can cause precipitate circadian desynchronization. Desynchronization is associated with defective insulin release and increased insulin resistance, implicating it in the etiology of diabetes mellitus. As Yu (2023) rightly points out, understanding of such rhythms may be of special importance for the prevention of diabetes, and emphasizes the importance of investigating the molecular mechanism behind such relationships. The genetic and biochemical factors, as well as the regulatory role of glucose and circadian rhythms, are all components of the mechanism of insulin release. A number of genes, including those involved in insulin secretion and production, might have altered expression profiles in such conditions as diabetes mellitus. For example, the Nkx2-1 gene is involved in the pathogenesis of diabetes through its elevated activity in pancreatic tissue. Furthermore, alteration in the level of proteins such as Pik3r1 reflects compensatory responses to preserve cellular function under insulin deficiency conditions. These intricate molecular interactions emphasize the multidimensional nature of insulin secretion and diabetes pathophysiology, emphasizing that understanding genetic predispositions in combination with metabolic factors could improve therapeutic approaches towards treating diabetes, as documented by Ivanenko (2023).

5.2.1. Role of Glucose in Insulin Release

Release of insulin from the pancreatic beta cells is a finely regulated process, both crucial to glucose homeostasis and of central significance to the understanding of diabetes mellitus. Glucose itself plays the central role in this regulation and is the primary secretagogue for insulin. In hyperglycemia, following meals, for instance, glucose enters beta cells through the glucose transporter 2 (GLUT2). This uptake initiates a cascade of intracellular events, primarily leading to increased ATP levels and resultant closure of ATP-sensitive potassium channels. The resulting depolarization of the cell membrane initiates the opening of voltage-gated calcium channels, allowing the entry of calcium, which is essential for initiating insulin granule exocytosis. This mechanism recognizes the direct link between elevated levels of glucose and the release of insulin, demonstrating how dysregulation can lead to the defective release of insulin characteristic of type 2 diabetes mellitus. Insulin's physiological role is not restricted to the control of glucose but encompasses several metabolic actions, including lipid and protein metabolism. Insulin facilitates glucose uptake by peripheral tissues like muscle and adipose tissue, leading to decreased plasma glucose levels. It promotes glycogenesis within the liver, storing excess glucose as glycogen and inhibiting gluconeogenesis, the process of generating glucose from non-carbohydrate substrates. This intricate action of insulin demands its proper release in reaction to varying levels of glucose. In insulin-resistant or metabolically deranged patients, however, the beta cells get overwhelmed, predisposing them to beta-cell fatigue as well as reduced insulin response even when hyperglycemia is present. Understanding these interactions is critical for the management of metabolic disorders such as diabetes, especially since insulin sensitivity decreases with time. Moreover, the relationship between glucose metabolism and insulin secretion reveals the pathophysiology of diseases such as gestational diabetes mellitus (GDM). In pregnancy, hormonal changes predispose toward insulin resistance, increasing the requirement for insulin production to maintain normal glucose levels. In the event of an improper pancreatic response, this results in elevated levels of glucose in the blood and thus leads to GDM, which is defined by both maternal and fetal complications. The implications of GDM are dire and justify ascertaining glucoses role in insulin dynamics in pregnant women. Treatment of GDM is not merely of direct advantage for the health of the mother and child at present but also as a way of preventing the development of type 2 diabetes at a later date in both populations. It is therefore valuable to understand in detail how glucose stimulates insulin release, as this can inform the prevention and treatment of diabetes and related metabolic disorders (Figure 5.6).

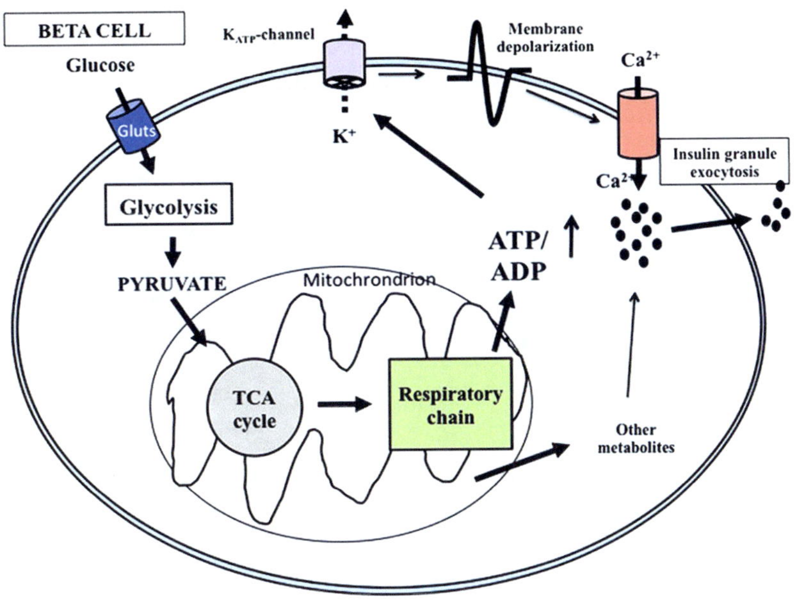

Figure 5.6. Key mechanisms of glucose-induced insulin secretion.

Source: https://www.researchgate.net/publication/317389671/figure/fig1/AS:11431281246776660@1716470538767/Key-mechanisms-of-glucose-induced-insulin-secretion-Glucose-enters-the-beta-cell-rapidly.tif.

5.2.2. Regulation of Insulin Secretion

Control of insulin secretion is a critical process in the maintenance of glucose homeostasis, critically important in diabetes mellitus management. Insulin is secreted by the pancreatic beta cells in response to rises in blood glucose levels, particularly after meals. The release of insulin is controlled by a complex series of signaling pathways involving glucose metabolism, ion channel function, and several hormonal signals. Specifically, the metabolism of glucose brings about an increase in ATP production, leading to the closing of ATP-sensitive potassium channels. This depolarization of the cell membrane brings about an influx of calcium, ultimately resulting in insulin granule exocytosis. These elaborate mechanisms ensure that insulin is released in the right manner in accordance with physiological needs, indicating the functionality of pancreatic beta cells in overall metabolic health. Furthermore, insulin release is strongly controlled by non-glucose factors. Hormonal messages, such as from incretins such as glucagon-like peptide-1 (GLP-1), are crucial for enhancing glucose-stimulated insulin release. It should be noted that GLP-1 is secreted from the intestines with the ingestion of nutrients and works to enhance the release of insulin from beta cells. In addition, elevated levels of circulating free fatty acids and certain amino acids are also able to evoke insulin secretion, illustrating the cross-talk between macronutrients and hormonal stimuli in glucose homeostasis regulation. In obesity and type 2 diabetes, this regulation may be disturbed, leading to inadequate insulin secretion and exacerbating hyperglycemia. These disturbances underlie the pathophysiology of metabolic diseases and underscore the value of a unified understanding of insulin signaling pathways. Moreover, dysfunction of adipose tissue has a significant impact on insulin release and metabolic health. As discussed in research, various forms of adipose tissue with varied functionality exist, particularly in obesity. In obesity, adipose tissue is pro-inflammatory and becomes highly resistant to insulin, which could interfere with the ability of the pancreas to release sufficient insulin in response to glucose.

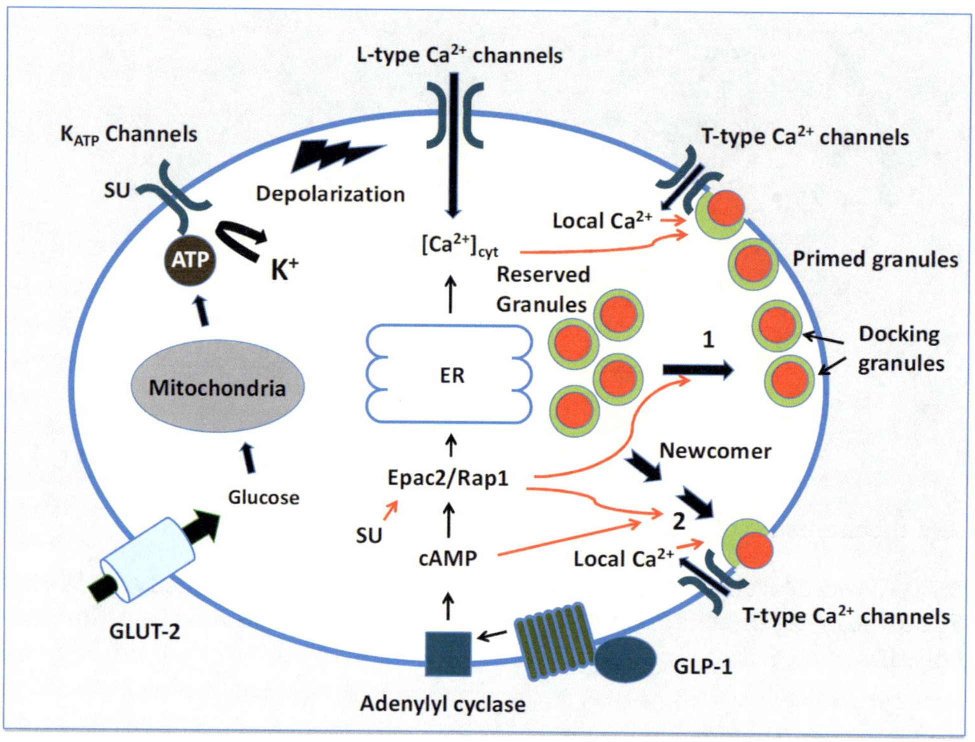

Figure 5.7. Regulation pathways of insulin secretion in a pancreatic β-cell.

Source: https://www.researchgate.net/profile/You-Lu-12/publication/329962001/figure/fig3/AS:708652054888448@1545967224667/Regulation-pathways-of-Insulin-secretion-in-a-pancreatic-b-cell.png.

This condition creates a vicious cycle, whereby augmented insulin resistance further exacerbates dysregulation of adipose tissue, leading to worsening of metabolic disturbance characteristic of type 2 diabetes mellitus. The association between insulin secretion and adipose tissue is not cause-and-effect but symbiotic, with both contributing essential functions within the overall environment of metabolic disease regulation. Understanding these interactions can unlock focused therapeutic interventions for the reestablishment of insulin sensitivity and glycemic control with a reduction of the adverse effects of excess body fat, particularly in diabetic individuals (Chait et al., 2020; Verdecchia et al., 2020) (Figure 5.7).

5.2.3. Impact of Other Hormones on Insulin Release

Insulin secretion by the pancreatic beta cell is under multifactorial control by other hormones alongside blood glucose. A specific group of hormones that affect insulin release are the incretin hormones, including GLP-1 and gastric inhibitory polypeptide (GIP). They are released from the gut after nutrient ingestion and play a key role in augmenting insulin release in a glucose-dependent manner. By enhancing the sensitivity of beta cells to glucose, incretins facilitate more balanced release of insulin, particularly with regard to diabetes mellitus. Dysregulation in the incretin pathway has been associated with insulin resistance, and therefore the pathogenesis of type 2 diabetes.

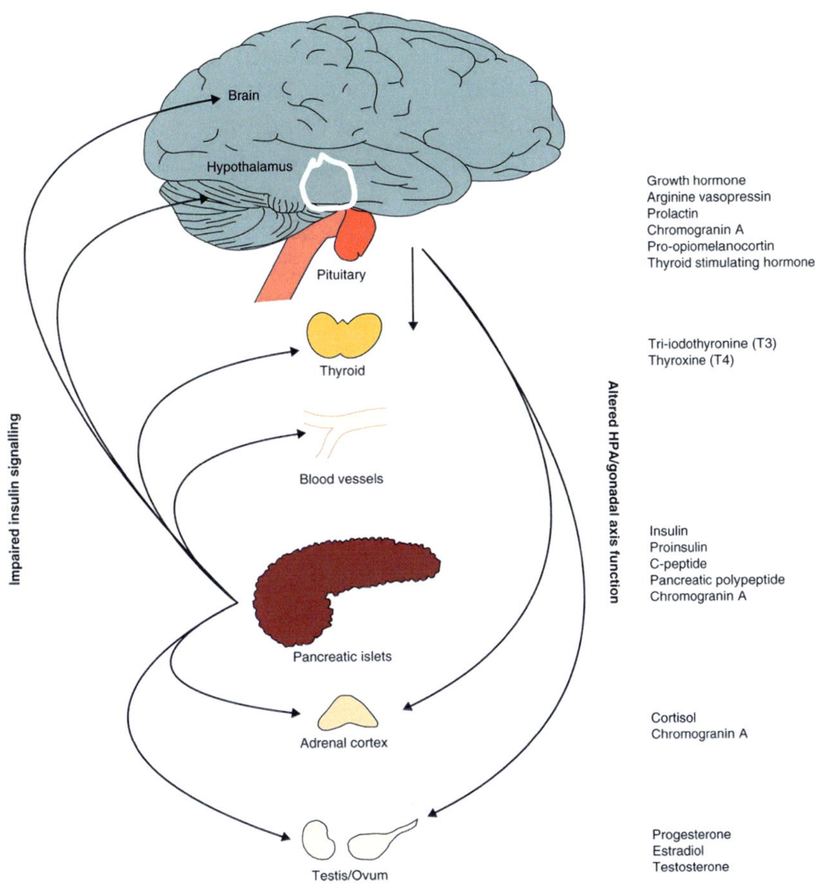

Figure 5.8. Potential effects of insulin resistance on the secretion of other hormones and bioactive molecules across the diffuse neuroendocrine system.

Source: https://www.researchgate.net/profile/Daniel-Martins-De-Souza-2/publication/236082991/figure/fig2/AS:216419468877828@1428609830345/Potential-effects-of-insulin-resistance-on-secretion-of-other-hormones-and-bioactive.png.

Therapeutic drugs that mimic or augment the effect of incretins have been developed, testifying to their important role in the management of diabetes-related metabolic disturbances. Apart from incretins, other endogenous hormones such as cortisol and epinephrine also play a role in influencing insulin release and could profoundly modulate glucose metabolism in stress. Cortisol is a glucocorticoid hormone released from the adrenal glands and could induce insulin resistance through modulating the receptor signal pathways and gluconeogenesis in the liver. Elevated cortisol levels, like those occurring in Cushing's syndrome, have the added insulin resistance lead to exacerbation of hyperglycemia and predispose to the creation of type 2 diabetes. Catecholamines, particularly epinephrine, are also known to inhibit insulin release in the state of acute stress responses, redirecting energy sources for the body's short-term demands. The complex interaction of these hormones highlights the importance of a general understanding of hormonal dynamics in the formulation of diabetes therapies aimed at both insulin release and peripheral insulin sensitivity. Adipose tissue is also involved in insulin secretion through the secretion of numerous adipokines that convey endocrine and paracrine signaling. As the body's largest endocrine organ, adipose tissue can develop into dysfunction during obesity, where an enhanced discharge of pro-inflammatory cytokines and low insulin signaling consequence. This disrupted environment not only impacts insulin discharge but also invokes a cascade of insulin resistance and systemic inflammation that plays a role in advancing type 2 diabetes mellitus. The specific role of adipokines such as leptin and adiponectin is highlighted; whereas leptin has the potential to increase insulin sensitivity, the role of adiponectin in regulating insulin action is more complex. Each interaction provides an opportunity for the creation of specifically designed interventions to increase adipose tissue function for optimal insulin secretion and restoration of metabolic homeostasis during diseases such as diabetes (Chait et al., 2020) (Figure 5.8).

Test Your Knowledge

1. How does glucose trigger insulin secretion from pancreatic beta cells?
2. Name two hormones that enhance insulin secretion and explain how.

5.3. Types of Diabetes Mellitus

Learning Outcome

1. Explain the causes and characteristics of type 1 diabetes;
2. Describe risk factors and symptoms associated with type 2 diabetes;
3. Understand gestational diabetes.

Diabetes mellitus has been mainly classified into two broad forms: Type 1 and Type 2 diabetes, each differing in pathophysiology, onset, and population prevalence. Type 1 diabetes mellitus (T1DM) is an autoimmune disorder where the immune system mistakenly attacks and destroys pancreatic beta cells that secrete insulin. This results in absolute insulin deficiency and the need for the patient to receive lifelong insulin therapy for proper blood glucose regulation. Typically diagnosed in children and young adults, T1DM is marked by acute onset of symptoms including polyuria, polydipsia, and weight loss. Its pathogenesis is multifactorial, involving an interplay of genetic predispositions and environmental triggers. Besides this, recent evidence hints at the potential role of viral infections in provoking autoimmune responses, which highlights the complexity of the disease. An understanding of these mechanisms is essential for the development of targeted interventions and prevention strategies in susceptible populations. By contrast, Type 2 diabetes mellitus (T2DM) is also associated with insulin resistance and relative impairment of insulin secretion. T2DM usually arises in adults but increasingly so in children and adolescents as a result of increased rates of obesity. The pathophysiological processes of T2DM are complex and include genetic susceptibility, lifestyle factors, and hormonal disturbances. Of specific interest is the Wnt signaling transcription factor Tcf7l2, known to be a critical genetic determinant for susceptibility to T2DM and to influence insulin secretion from beta cells. Experiments in tcf7l2 zebrafish mutant models show the genes impact on glucose regulation and islet formation, and what implications might be identified for therapeutic interventions. It should be noted that the complexity of T2DM since it causes 90–95% of diabetes within the world population, and effective management strategies are called for to prevent its associated complications. There also exists a third category known as gestational diabetes mellitus (GDM) which is found in pregnancy and presents unique challenges to maternal and fetal health. GDM generally results from hormonal changes that cause insulin resistance, combined with a failure to secrete enough insulin to counteract the resistance. GDM normally resolves post-pregnancy but makes the mother susceptible to the development of Type 2 diabetes later in life. It is a condition that requires screening, since if left unattended, it can have dangerous complications such as macrosomia and neonatal hypoglycemia. Management of GDM involves dietary modification, exercise, and in some cases, treatment with insulin. The increasing prevalence of obesity among pregnant women emphasizes the importance of extensive study and preventative measures to address this significant health problem. Differentiation between the diabetes mellitus forms is necessary to implement effective management and education intervention methods tailored to the specific needs of each patient group.

5.3.1. Type 1 Diabetes: Causes and Characteristics

Etiology of Type 1 diabetes is multifactorial but the majority is classified as an autoimmune disease that results in loss of insulin-secreting beta cells of the pancreas. The exact etiology is not yet clear, but it has been proposed on the basis of studies that susceptibility is largely under the control of genetic predisposition. Specific human leukocyte antigen (HLA) genes, particularly those involved in autoimmunity, are also largely found in the patients of this condition. Environmental factors, such as viral infections, have also been implicated, which has led to the hypothesis that infections may trigger the autoimmune process in genetically predisposed individuals. Additionally, nutritional deficiency, particularly during pivotal developmental periods, cannot be ruled out. All contribute towards the complexities of Type 1 diabetes and the need for ongoing research into its multifactorial etiologies and their interactions. The characteristics of Type 1 diabetes extend beyond its autoimmune etiology and include its presentation and course. Presentation is characteristically accompanied by symptoms of polydipsia, polyuria, and weight loss, which can occur very rapidly, and in some instances result in an episode of ketoacidosis. Unlike Type 2 diabetes, whose presentation is typically late in life, Type 1 diabetes typically presents in childhood or adolescence and thus is particularly frightening to families. The failure to make insulin necessitates a lifelong course of insulin therapy for glucose management, emphasizing the chronicity of the disease. Insidiously, patients also are at risk for long-term complications, including diabetic retinopathy, neuropathy, and cardiovascular disease, which result as a direct consequence of long-term hyperglycemia. These aspects demand a general management plan, including careful planning of blood glucose monitoring and lifestyle modification. Research into mechanisms for pancreatic endocrine cell differentiation informs Type 1 diabetes. Early in embryonic development, the process begins with the function of neurogenin 3 in the formation of pancreatic islets. As illustrated in research, neurogenin 3 expression is critical for the onset of endocrine cell differentiation and a mechanism for the development of insulin-secreting beta cells. The intricacies of such differentiation process are further governed by a set of transcription factors, suggesting the hierarchy that influences cell fate determination. Clarification of these simple biological processes contributes to the knowledge of Type 1 diabetes pathogenesis and potentially to the future direction of therapeutic intervention. By understanding how neurogenin 3 and other factors work together in this development cascade, researchers can build a plan for potential interventions that can salvage insulin secretion or preserve beta-cell function in at-risk individuals (Anderson et al., 2000; Chowdhury et al., 1994) (Figure 5.9).

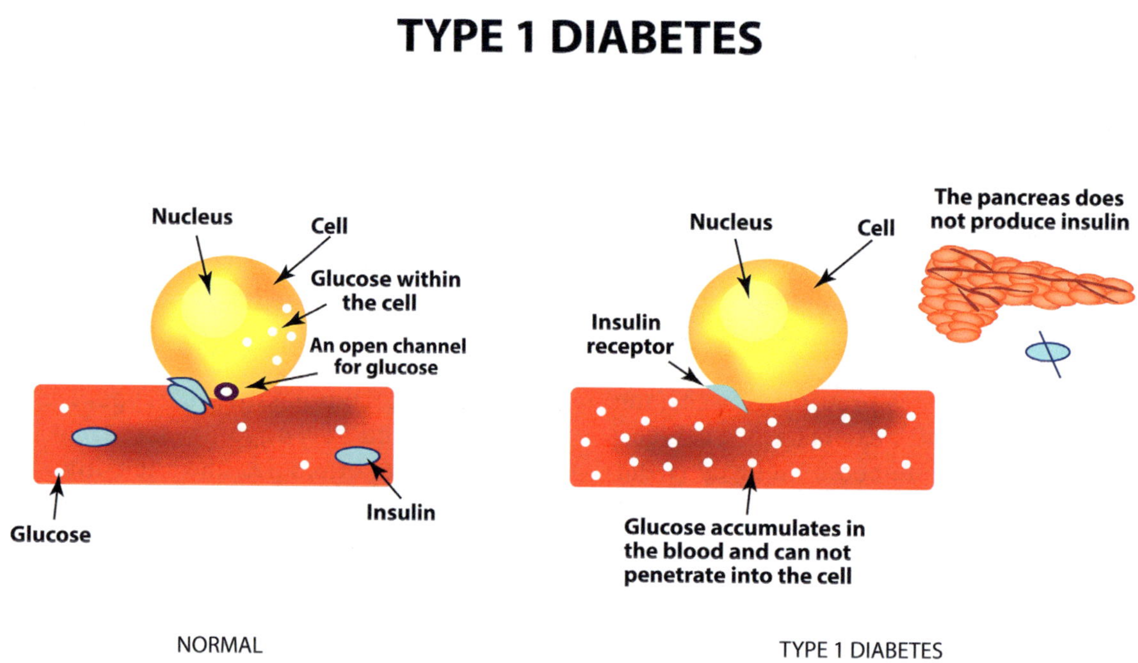

Figure 5.9. Illustration of type 1 diabetes.

Source: https://www.endocrineharmony.sg/wp-content/uploads/2024/10/type-1-diabetes-1024x700.jpeg.

5.3.2. Type 2 Diabetes: Risk Factors and Symptoms

The etiology of Type 2 diabetes mellitus is mainly dictated by the multifactorial interaction of risk factors upon lifestyle choices and hereditary predisposition. Obesity is one of the strongest risk factors for this disease, and more adipose tissue, particularly visceral fat, causes insulin resistance and impaired glucose metabolism. Sedentary lifestyle fuels this, as physical inactivity lowers the body's sensitivity to insulin. Other non-modifiable factors are age, ethnicity, and family history of diabetes, which contribute importantly to susceptibility. Therefore, knowledge of these risk factors is necessary for the identification of populations with increased risk and the application of prevention measures that might go a long way towards reducing the incidence of Type 2 diabetes. The presenting symptoms of Type 2 diabetes tend to develop insidiously and may be insidious in their onset, making it difficult to make an early diagnosis. The typical symptoms are increased thirst, increased urination, weakness, and blurred vision because of elevated blood glucose levels. Weight loss along with increased hunger also results in some patients as the body is unable to effectively utilize glucose for fuel. Skin problems such as dark spots or infection can also result, pointing to the systemic nature of the disease. These symptoms typically result from long-standing hyperglycemia and have the potential to significantly impact quality of life. Thus, their detection is important for the early treatment and management of the disease and ultimately improved patient outcomes as well as prevention of diabetes's long-term complications. The endocrine pancreas's relationship with Type 2 diabetes further shows the diseases' complexity. Compromised insulin release and synthesis are the characteristic of the pathogenesis of the condition, with gradual beta-cell dysfunction of the pancreas. This may be due to prolonged contact with raised levels of glucose, leading to a vicious cycle of worsening glycemic control. Furthermore, conditions such as pancreatic exocrine insufficiency (PEI) may be present, complicating the clinical picture further with compromised uptake of nutrients and overall metabolic status. In the management of Type 2 diabetes, these endocrine characteristics will need to be considered since they impact strongly on management plan. Manipulation of diet, e.g., consumption of fiber, can play an important role, but their efficacy can be contingent on particular pancreatic function and overall health (Arnelo et al., 2017; Badiali et al., 2019) (Figure 5.10).

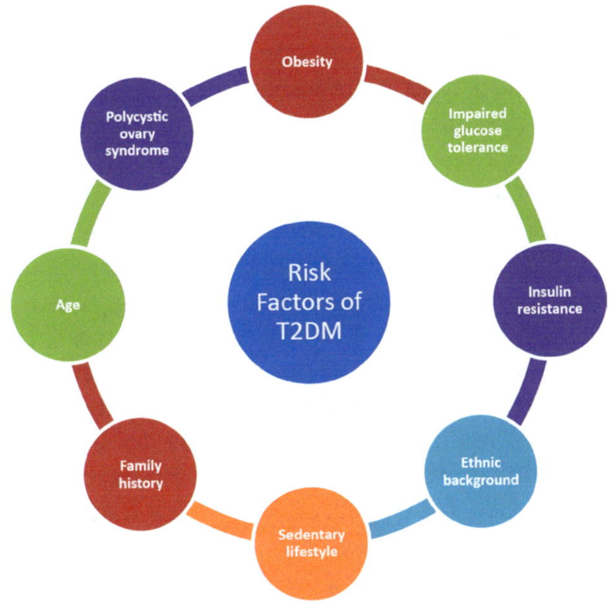
Obesity
Impaired glucose tolerance
Insulin resistance
Ethnic background
Sedentary lifestyle
Family history
Age
Polycystic ovary syndrome
Risk Factors of T2DM

Figure 5.10. Some of the main risk factors of type 2 diabetes mellitus.

Source: https://www.researchgate.net/publication/345718453/figure/fig1/AS:983871579492353@1611584672942/Some-of-the-main-risk-factors-of-type-2-diabetes-mellitus.png.

5.3.3. Gestational Diabetes: Implications for Mother and Child

Gestational diabetes mellitus (GDM) is a significant health problem since it happens during pregnancy, affecting both the maternal and fetal well-being. In GDM, females develop elevated blood glucose levels that typically revert to normal after childbirth but are associated with an increased risk of developing type 2 diabetes mellitus later in life. The pathogenic mechanisms are usually insulin resistance with added hormonal alterations during gestation. Maternal hyperglycemia has a direct effect on fetal growth, making the baby larger—a condition that is also known as macrosomia. Macrosomia fetal size is a cause of delivery complications like an elevated number of cesarean deliveries and potential birth traumas.

Aside from the direct pregnancy risks, GDM mothers are one to seven times more likely to develop type 2 diabetes, so their metabolic health must be followed up on in the postpartum period. The effects of gestational diabetes are not just on the mother's health but have significant implications for the neonate as well. Infants of GDM-affected mothers can experience a cascade of complications, from hypoglycemia, neonatal jaundice, and respiratory distress. In addition, premature exposure to high glucose levels can program the infant's metabolism, thereby making them vulnerable to obesity and adult-onset type 2 diabetes. Research has established that children who have had prior exposure to GDM exhibit alterations in their insulin secretion and sensitivity, potentially exposing them to future metabolic disorders. In a surprising turn of events, infants have been found to have a trend towards insulin resistance, which reflects the role of maternal prenatal pathology on their eventual health results. Thus, the interaction between GDM and metabolic outcomes in the offspring forms a core area of study in the broader picture of diabetes and the endocrine pancreas. To avoid the adverse effects of gestational diabetes, its early detection and treatment strategies are crucial. This would include general screening of GDM, preferably in the second trimester, and the implementation of lifestyle modifications that ensure optimal maternal weight gain, diet, and exercise.

Nutrition counseling is an important component of blood glucose control during pregnancy and can reduce the need for pharmacologic treatment. Postpartum care visits, including glucose derangements screening and prevention counseling for future diabetes, should also be prioritized by providers. Because GDM has implications for both mother and child, an interdisciplinary care system among obstetricians, endocrinologists, and pediatricians is required. Improved awareness and active practices of care can significantly improve the health outcomes of mothers and children, thus ameliorating the far-reaching impacts of diabetes on this vulnerable population (Figure 5.11).

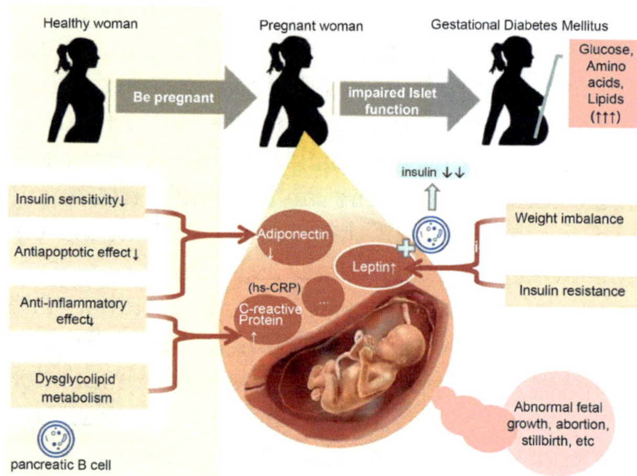

Figure 5.11. Mechanisms of gestational diabetes mellitus.

Source: https://www.researchgate.net/publication/375802292/figure/fig1/AS:11431281258253721@1720023044957/Mechanisms-of-gestational-diabetes-mellitus.jpg.

Test Your Knowledge

1. What is the primary cause of type 1 diabetes mellitus?
2. What are common risk factors for developing type 2 diabetes mellitus?
3. What is gestational diabetes and what risks does it pose?

5.4. Pathophysiology of Diabetes Mellitus

Learning Outcome

1. Understand the fundamentals of insulin resistance in type 2 diabetes;
2. Discuss about autoimmune destruction of beta cells in type 1 diabetes;
3. Understand long-term complications of uncontrolled diabetes.

Pathophysiology of diabetes mellitus is intrinsically linked with the malfunction of the endocrine pancreas, whose primary function is insulin release. Type 1 diabetes mellitus (T1DM) results due to autoimmune destruction of pancreatic beta cells with absolute insulin deficiency, thus producing hyperglycemia and elevated blood glucose levels. By comparison, type 2 diabetes mellitus (T2DM) is characterized by insulin resistance and relative insulin deficiency following the loss of pancreatic beta cells as a result of chronic hyperglycemia and lipotoxicity. Its later-stage effects are deranged glucose metabolism and defective lipid regulation, each with deep impacts on global metabolic homeostasis. Thus, understanding these mechanisms in relation to the endocrine pancreas is priceless in terms of shedding light on disease multifaceted nature. An investigation into such pathophysiological dynamics underlies the process of devising proper therapeutic interventions aimed at re-establishing normal metabolic processes in diabetic patients. Fatty pancreas disease (FPD) is a pivotal area of interest in diabetes research, particularly considering its role in type 2 diabetes and metabolic syndrome. It has been noted in studies that patients with newly diagnosed T2DM have much higher grades of hepatic steatosis along with much lower fecal elastase, indicating exocrine pancreatic insufficiency. The alterations suggest a deleterious effect of fatty infiltration of the pancreatic tissue on the duality of function of the organ that subsequently complicates clinical control of diabetes even more. The inverse association of fecal elastase levels with HbA1c underlines the intricate correlation between pancreatic function and glycemic control. Specifically, elevated HbA1c levels, which reflect chronic hyperglycemia, are inversely related to pancreatic function, implying metabolic disturbances more than a simple deficiency in insulin. Comprehensive metabolic studies employing assays of endocrine and exocrine functions are essential for the clarification of FPDs role in diabetes induction and therapy (Karaevren et al., 2025). Exocrine deficiency is a valuable but often underrated complication of diabetes mellitus, with clinical and quality-of-life consequences. The dual function of the pancreas is one in which if insulin release is impaired, the release of food enzymes can also be impaired and lead to malabsorption and associated gastrointestinal symptoms. Such a state makes it difficult to control diabetes since it can lead to weight loss and micronutrient deficiency. The high incidence of pancreatic exocrine deficiency among diabetic patients has been indicated by this recent finding, and clinicians should notice this aspect of pancreatic function. Moreover, the concurrent dysfunction of both exocrine and endocrine pancreatic functions can cause glycemic control and metabolic balance complexities and create a vicious cycle aggravating diabetic complications. The interplay between these pancreatic functions indicates the requirement for an integrative approach to the management of diabetes involving both hormonal control and nutrition support to achieve optimal patient outcomes (Valente et al., 2024).

5.4.1. Insulin Resistance in Type 2 Diabetes

Insulin resistance is a fundamental characteristic of Type 2 diabetes, with its most significant effect being upon the function of the endocrine pancreas. Resistance is produced once the cells of the body become less sensitive to insulin, a hormone secreted by the pancreas that enables the cells to take up glucose from the blood. With reduced sensitivity to insulin, the blood glucose level rises, and the pancreas secretes more insulin to compensate for the weakened cellular response. Over time, this compensatory mechanism can lead to pancreatic beta-cell dysfunction, which is a component of the progressive nature of Type 2 diabetes. The interaction between beta-cell dysfunction and insulin resistance creates a vicious cycle, ultimately worsening glucose dysregulation. Knowledge of these dynamics is critical in the design of effective interventions aimed at restoring insulin sensitivity and overall metabolic health among infected persons. The consequences of insulin resistance are not limited to glucose metabolism but extend to diverse physiological processes. For instance, obesity, which is a strong risk factor for Type 2 diabetes, is associated with insulin resistance. Increased adiposity and particularly visceral fat may secrete inflammatory cytokines and free fatty acids, which once more interfere with insulin signaling pathways. This dysregulation further places one at increased risk of acquiring other conditions of comorbidity such as cardiovascular disease and dyslipidemia. Additionally, the rise in childhood obesity has been directly responsible for the rapidly increasing rate at which Type 2 diabetes is being diagnosed among child populations, with insulin resistance occurring increasingly earlier and more aggressively. These lifestyle factors, such as diet and physical exercise, must be tackled in terms of controlling the incidence of obesity-related insulin resistance and resultant ailments (Kapke et al., 2015). Genetic factors, other than diet and obesity, also play an important role in the development of insulin resistance in Type 2 diabetes. Family history and some genetic markers have also been implicated in varying the sensitivity of individuals to insulin. Moreover, conditions such as tropical calcific pancreatitis put particular challenges to glucose homeostasis, as the fact that it is associated with fibrocalculous pancreatic diabetes, an insulin deficiency type of diabetes secondary to chronic diseases of the pancreas (Chowdhury et al., 1994). The convergence of genetic, environmental, and behavioral determinants highlights the multi-factorial nature of insulin resistance. As researchers continue to unscramble these interactions, the development of targeted treatments becomes increasingly critical. Recognition of the multifaceted nature of insulin resistance not only teaches prevention methods but also maximizes treatment options in individuals already suffering from type 2 diabetes (Figure 5.12).

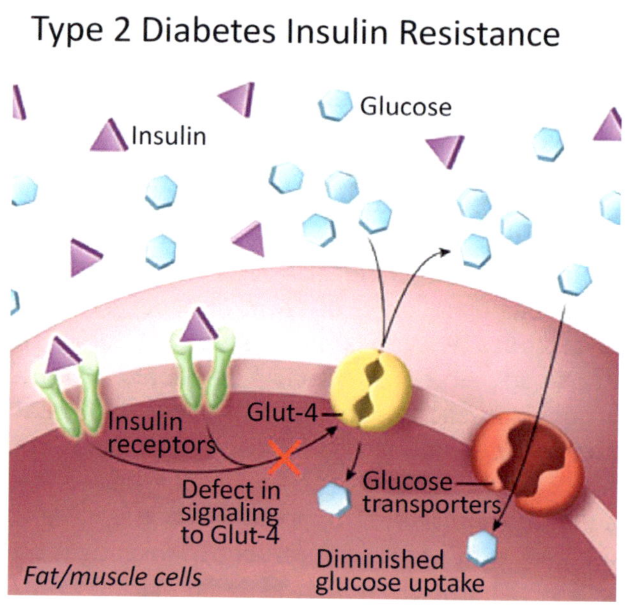

Figure 5.12. Insulin resistance is a fundamental characteristic of type 2 diabetes.

Source: https://diabetesteachingcenter.ucsf.edu/sites/g/files/tkssra6931/f/wysiwyg/insulin.jpg.

5.4.2. Autoimmune Destruction of Beta Cells in Type 1 Diabetes

The autoimmune destruction of pancreatic beta cells is a feature of Type 1 diabetes mellitus, an illness in which there is a deficiency of insulin production. In this illness, the immune system of the body mistakenly identifies beta cells as foreign and marks them for elimination. Such autoimmune attack has been suggested to result from a combination of predisposing genes and environmental insults such as viral infections or food antigens. As the disease advances, the loss of beta cell mass leads to a lack of insulin secretion, ultimately producing hyperglycemia. The intricacy of this autoimmune destruction highlights the need for continued research into the underlying mechanisms driving beta cell devastation, which can help the development of therapeutic approaches to stop or reverse the disease process. Recent studies have demonstrated that inflammatory signaling pathways play a key role in autoimmune destruction of beta cells. Of interest, studies have established that NF-κB signaling plays a role in mediating inflammatory responses associated with Type 1 diabetes. This established pathway of inflammation and immune response can lead to induction of pro-inflammatory cytokines that are detrimental to beta cell survival. In addition, cross-talk of NF-κB with other important signaling pathways may also complicate the immune attack on beta cells, causing dysfunction and further apoptosis. The understanding of such signaling dynamics is central to the creation of targeted therapy that could best protect beta cells from immune-mediated pathology, preserving insulin synthesis and improving clinical outcomes of Type 1 diabetes patients (Guo et al., 2024). With the autoimmune mechanism of Type 1 diabetes, therapy has increasingly turned to immune system modulation rather than the traditional control of blood glucose. New therapies are geared towards restorative therapies of immune tolerance and prevention of beta-cell destruction by a myriad of mechanisms, including monoclonal antibodies and immunotherapy. Combination therapies, too, that aim to target individual pathways involved in the autoimmune process may be more effective. Additional research in this area is important because advances in adjacent fields, e.g., the role of adipose tissue in the control of metabolism, can inform about the systemic interactions leading to beta cell loss. Thus, a full understanding of the endocrine function of the pancreas and the intricacy of immune dysregulation is needed to enhance treatment and potential remission of Type 1 diabetes (Dilworth et al., 2021) (Figure 5.13).

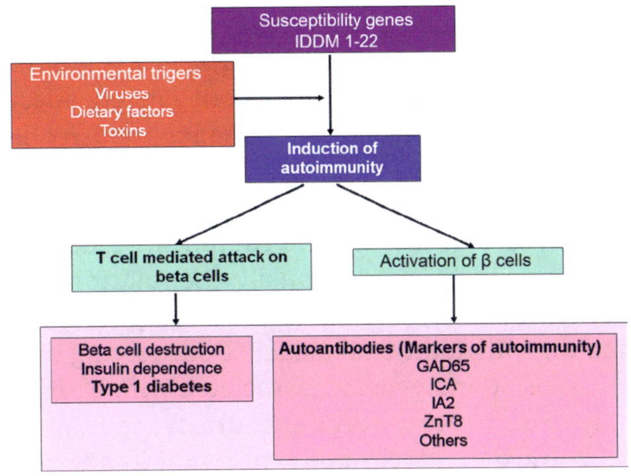

Figure 5.13. Simplified model of mechanism of autoimmunity and beta cell destruction in type 1 diabetes.

Source: https://www.researchgate.net/publication/267814388/figure/fig1/AS:1027976518975489@1622100109344/Fig-Simplified-model-of-mechanism-of-autoimmunity-and-beta-cell-destruction-in-type-1.png.

5.4.3. Long-Term Complications of Uncontrolled Diabetes

Long-term complications of uncontrolled diabetes are numerous and largely severe, significantly affecting several organ systems and overall health. Hyperglycemia, the hallmark of diabetes mellitus, is the pivotal feature in the pathogenesis of complications. As the sustained high blood glucose level goes on, it leads to endothelial dysfunction and promotes atherosclerosis, contributing to cardiovascular complications. Also, microvascular complications such as diabetic retinopathy, nephropathy, and neuropathy develop as a direct consequence of long-term exposure to high blood glucose levels. These result in significant morbidity in the form of blindness, renal failure, and amputations, thus making strict glycemic control essential to prevent these complications (Genta et al., 2015). Also, the prevalence of overlap between diabetes and obesity contributes to the complexity of the long-term complication picture. Obesity exacerbates insulin resistance, and glycemic control becomes impaired. Obesity is associated with a plethora of metabolic derangements that negatively affect many organ systems. For instance, obesity is often associated with chronic inflammation as well as dysregulation of lipids to produce cardiovascular disease and complicate diabetes care even further. Additionally, the relationship between obesity and diabetes can impact brain health, with additional evidence suggesting that metabolic derangements associated with obesity may accelerate neurodegenerative changes. This burden of co-morbidity highlights the importance of combined management strategies targeting both diabetes and obesity to maximize long-term health outcomes (Keller et al., 2019). Given these potential complications, timely intervention and active diabetes management are critical. Public health interventions must focus on the importance of regular screenings among the susceptible populations, along with dietary modifications such as a balanced diet and regular exercise. Furthermore, the healthcare providers must prioritize individualized treatment plans considering the risk factors of the patients and the related comorbid disorders. Innovative approaches to therapy such as novel antidiabetic agents can be employed for the optimization of blood glucose control. Multidisciplinary measures combining medical therapy with lifestyle interventions may also decrease substantially the development of long-term complications and enhance the quality of life in diabetic mellitus patients. Management of the multifaceted nature of diabetes is a matter of teamwork among patients, health practitioners, and society (Figure 5.14).

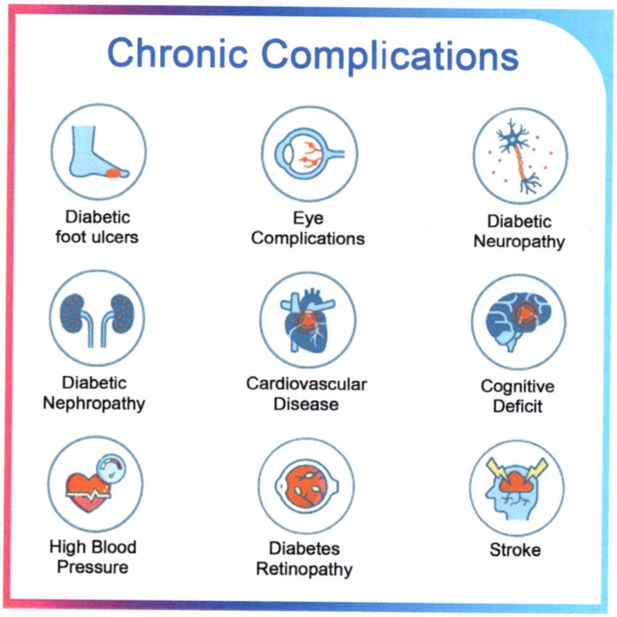

Figure 5.14. Chronic complications of uncontrolled diabetes.

Source: https://www.fitterfly.com/blog/wp-content/uploads/2022/10/internal-image-01_11zon.webp.

Test Your Knowledge

1. What is insulin resistance and how does it contribute to type 2 diabetes?
2. Name three microvascular complications of long-term uncontrolled diabetes.

5.5. Diagnosis of Diabetes Mellitus

Learning Outcome

1. Discuss about common diagnostic tests for diabetes mellitus;
2. Explain the criteria for diagnosing diabetes;
3. Understand the importance of early detection of diabetes mellitus.

Diabetes mellitus diagnosis remains a challenging process, encompassing diverse methodologies and factors to treat the variability of this endocrine illness. The diagnostic process is primarily constructed around the evaluation of blood glucose, traditionally measuring using criteria such as fasting plasma glucose, oral glucose tolerance tests, and the assessment of HbA1c. These are key because they provide information on short-term as well as long-term glucose metabolism control. In addition, more awareness of Type 3c diabetes mellitus (T3cDM) that occurs secondary to other pancreatic pathology, such as chronic pancreatitis, is also present. It further complicates the diagnostic picture, which indicates how the health of the pancreas has significant burden in glycemic control and needs an expanded method of diagnosis that considers the patients overall endocrine function (Diaconu et al., 2018). The integration of sophisticated technology in diabetes diagnosis is becoming ever more crucial as the medical fraternity struggles with the diseases chronic and intricate nature. Machine learning (ML) has been found to be a very promising tool in this context by identifying early-stage diabetes more accurately, which has previously been difficult owing to the frequently asymptomatic nature of the disease's progression. With the aid of sophisticated algorithms, ML also processes glucose data to recognize patterns that might not be sensed with traditional diagnostic methods. The approach not only facilitates early diagnosis but also facilitates personalized intervention programs based on individual glucose control profiles. The incorporation of synthetic data generated by biophysical models also further improves the analysis, with the potential to obtain high precision in identifying insulin resistance and improving clinical results (Jo et al., 2020). Further, education and patient awareness play a critical role in the diagnosis and management of diabetes mellitus. Patients present with nonspecific or symptoms associated with other conditions, which result in delayed diagnosis and increased risks of complications. Therefore, public health interventions to educate individuals on the risk factor awareness of diabetes, such as obesity, physical inactivity, and family history, are crucial. Parallel to these educational efforts, the medical professionals also need to pursue increasing access to the diagnostic tools and facilities. Effective diagnosis not only relies on clinical testing but also on fostering an open perception among patients regarding the necessity of taking their health into account and recognizing early manifestations of glycemic irregularities. Finally, a strategy that integrates technology, patient education, and good diagnostic practice will lead to improved outcomes in those at risk or with diabetes mellitus.

5.5.1. Common Diagnostic Tests (e.g., Fasting Glucose, HbA1c)

The clinical practice of diabetes diagnosis is heavily driven by the use of common diagnostic tests, and fasting glucose and HbA1c are cornerstones in this endeavor. Fasting glucose, which measures blood glucose following overnight fasting, provides essential insights into the body's baseline glycemic control. Values above 126 mg/dL are typically a sign of diabetes, whereas values from 100 to 125 mg/dL are indicative of prediabetes. This test is important in the sense that it offers a simple and cost-effective method for primary diabetes screening, in line with broader public health efforts at detecting at-risk populations. However, fasting glucose alone may be insufficient to detect the subtleties of diabetes and therefore necessitate such supporting tests as HbA1c in order to better evaluate glycemic control over time (Figure 5.15).

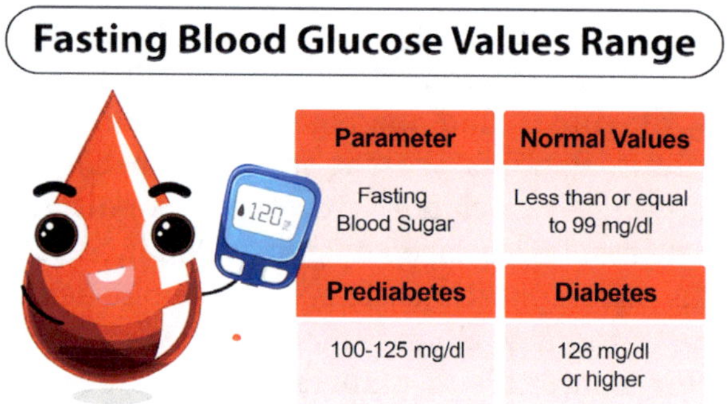

Figure 5.15. Understanding fasting blood glucose levels.

Source: https://img.freepik.com/free-vector/understanding-fasting-blood-glucose-levels_1308-178019.jpg.

HbA1c, or glycated hemoglobin, is an indicator of the two- to three-month average blood glucose level and is thus a primary diagnostic tool for long-term glycemia control. The test reflects the percentage of glycated hemoglobin, and levels at 6.5% or higher are used in a diagnosis of diabetes. Notably, HbA1c possesses over fasting glucose in that it is less influenced by the fluctuating day-to-day pattern of blood glucose due to food and stress. Furthermore, constant monitoring with the use of HbA1c allows clinicians to evaluate the effectiveness of current treatment programs and make necessary adjustments. It should be noted, however, to consider variation in HbA1c values due to hemolytic anemia or certain hemoglobinopathies that may skew results and make diagnosis more challenging, thus the need for clinician recognition and extensive patient assessment. Technological advancements over the years have also seen the incorporation of devices such as continuous glucose monitoring systems (CGMS) into mainstream diabetes management. These sensors offer immediate monitoring of blood glucose fluctuations, thus enhancing the understanding of the individual glycemic pattern. While research shows the possibility of the reduction of fasting blood glucose and glycemic excursions with CGMS, its usefulness in initial diagnosis is less than fasting glucose and HbA1c (Bonakdaran et al., 2013). Secondly, the concurrent use of these tests with CGMS can empower patients with information to help them make healthier lifestyle choices and thereby improve self-care management. Together, classic diagnostic procedures and emerging technologies constitute a multistep approach towards diabetes mellitus diagnosis and management as we progress to learn about this widespread endocrine illness, emphasizing the value of a comprehensive evaluation plan in practice (Abdul-Rasoul et al., 2016) (Figure 5.16).

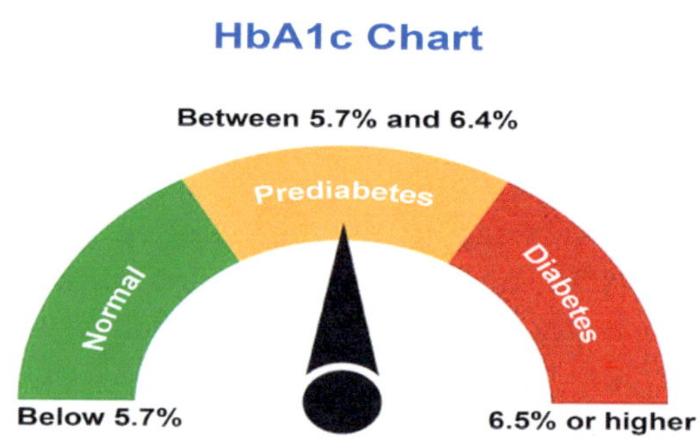

Figure 5.16. HbA1c chart.

Source: https://www.fitterfly.com/blog/wp-content/uploads/2024/01/HbA1c-Chart.webp.

5.5.2. Criteria for Diagnosing Diabetes

Diagnosis of diabetes involves the careful evaluation of a multitude of clinical criteria established by leading health organizations. Central to such evaluation is the measurement of blood glucose levels, which can be ascertained by various approaches. The American Diabetes Association (ADA) mandates that a fasting plasma glucose of at least 126 mg/dL confirms diabetes, and an oral glucose tolerance test (OGTT) with a blood glucose of at least 200 mg/dL two hours after it is another critical diagnostic marker. An HbA1c level of 6.5% or higher also establishes the diagnosis. Deserving of note are the occurrence of signs such as polyuria, polydipsia, and unexplained weight loss, which similarly result in testing, particularly in patients who have these classic findings, testifying to the importance of diligent clinical assessment in the diagnosis of diabetes. In the past decade, the experience with atypical manifestations of diabetes, including syndromic diabetes, has supplemented the classical diagnostic paradigm. Defined by clear-cut major and minor criteria, syndromic diabetes may indicate the simultaneous occurrence of diabetes with any abnormality of the organ systems other than the endocrine pancreas. For diagnosis to be established, a patient must display one major criterion—i.e., dysmorphic features, intellectual disability, or neurodevelopmental disorders—and a minor criterion from another organ system, or three minor criteria with no exclusion criteria if diagnosed under the age of 35. The exact knowledge allows more refined diagnosis and management, as with the findings of recent studies that show heterogeneity and variability of diabetes presentation within some populations (Stephen et al., 2025). Moreover, the novel onset of autoimmune Type 1 diabetes has been reported in patients following SARS-CoV-2 infection and offers a novel aspect to be taken into account in differential diagnosis. Such cases have established that diabetes is of multifactorial etiology, wherein autoimmune processes following infection lead to destruction of pancreatic beta cells that secrete insulin. In a significant case, a young adult in good health had developed markedly elevated blood glucose levels spontaneously shortly after recovery from COVID-19, along with the presence of coexistent autoantibodies, consistent with autoimmune diabetes (Taşkaldıran et al., 2023). This emerging understanding highlights the importance of considering recent viral illness as the precipitants of diabetes, thereby making healthcare professionals more vigilant when it comes to diabetes diagnosis and management in connection to existing conditions.

5.5.3. Importance of Early Detection

Early diagnosis of diabetes mellitus is significant to allow for proper management and prevention of disease-related complications. Diabetes mellitus may be an asymptomatic disease in most patients until there is severe damage to the pancreas and other organs. The endocrine pancreas plays a crucial role in glucose homeostasis, and any failure may lead to severe metabolic derangement. The importance of early diagnosis is not only to give early interventions but also to prevent long-term diabetes complications, such as cardiovascular disorders and metabolic syndrome (MetS). Because MetS is a cluster of predictive abnormalities for diabetes and cardiovascular disease, early identification of these individuals by screening can direct early therapeutic interventions to avoid the progression of these diseases (Fahed et al., 2022). By generating awareness and carrying out population-based screening programs, the healthcare systems can reduce the morbidity and mortality of diabetes significantly. The physiological effects of uncontrolled diabetes extend far beyond increased blood glucose levels and influence various organs and organ systems of the body. Chronic hyperglycemia can induce derangement of normal metabolic processes and complications in the form of neuropathy, nephropathy, and retinopathy. These challenges, as well as alterations in the composition and balance of the extracellular matrix (ECM) between matrix metalloproteinases (MMPs) and their inhibitors, could result in irreparable damage if not identified early (Griselda et al., 2020). Moreover, the disruption of ECM remodeling underlies the formation of diabetic degenerative conditions. Thus, early detection is crucial not only for immediate glucose control but also to preserve integrity and function of damaged tissues. Clinicians must emphasize routine monitoring and early interventions because early detection can guarantee more favorable clinical outcomes. Incorporating the highest-evidenced diagnostic methods can consolidate the early detection of diabetes to provide a better estimation of an individual's risk profile. Standard screening procedures including fasting blood glucose levels, hemoglobin A1c testing, and oral glucose tolerance tests are crucial for the identification of metabolic disturbances before they set in as overt diabetes. Furthermore, knowledge of associated risk factors such as obesity, genetic predisposition, and lack of physical exercise should prompt healthcare professionals to act with preventive measures and lifestyle change. Adoption of these strategies not only contributes to improved health of the individual but also reduces the public health burden of diabetes and its complications. Through early diagnosis, healthcare systems can develop an avenue for comprehensive prevention programs that improve quality of life as well as reduce healthcare costs associated with the management of end-stage disease.

Test Your Knowledge

1. What are the four main tests used to diagnose diabetes mellitus?
2. What is the diagnostic threshold for diabetes using fasting plasma glucose?
3. Why is early detection of diabetes important?

5.6. Management and Treatment Options

Learning Outcome

1. Explain the role of lifestyle modifications in the management and prevention of diabetes mellitus;
2. Discuss about pharmacological management of diabetes mellitus;
3. Discuss the importance of monitoring and self-management strategies for individuals living with diabetes mellitus.

Management and therapeutic treatment of diabetes mellitus, particularly that of the endocrine pancreas, has been an area of interest for physicians and scientists. Present treatment modalities are mostly founded upon insulin therapy in type 1 diabetes mellitus (T1DM), which is characterized by an absolute deficiency of insulin due to autoimmune destruction of pancreatic beta cells. In canine T1DM cases, the treatment usually includes twice-daily injections of insulin, along with daily checks on blood sugar levels. While the treatment works, it is problematic in terms of implementation and adherence and often leads to complications like hypoglycemia. Recent advances have opened the door for the creation of new therapeutic strategies, including regenerative medicine methods and designing artificial pancreas devices that will potentially make therapy more effective and reduce the economic burden on pet owners and their pets. These, as yet, experimental options provide an encouraging prospect for more effectively managing diabetes in veterinary medicine (Flavia et al., 2024). In clinical medicine, the term "diabetes" has expanded to encompass type 2 diabetes mellitus (T2DM), which is frequently linked with insulin resistance. It results from the interplay between genetic predisposition and environmental factors to become significant public health problems.

T2DM is commonly treated with lifestyle modification—diet and physical exercise—and drugs to increase insulin sensitivity and stimulate insulin release. More recent drugs, such as GLP-1 receptor agonists and SGLT-2 inhibitors, are acquired more prominence since they not only contribute to glycemic control but also yield cardiovascular and kidney benefits. Treatment of the mechanisms that cause insulin resistance is essential to the creation of more effective treatment strategies, as evidenced by ongoing research into the role of endocrine cell plasticity in the pancreas that could create therapeutic targets for reversing some of the symptoms of the disease (Sandra et al., 2024). The future of diabetes treatment seems to lean towards a twin focus on new pharmacotherapies and possibly curative therapies. Regenerative therapies, such as insulin-secreting beta cells derived from stem cell technology, have the potential to radically change the future of diabetes treatment. Clinical trials are already under way to examine the efficacy and safety of these therapies, representing a paradigm shift from symptom management to management of the causes of the disease itself. In addition, advancement in personalized medicine, driven by an increased understanding of genetic and environmental determinants for diabetes, can lead to tailored treatments that enhance patient outcomes. Ongoing studies, integrating outcomes from human and animal research, can promote understanding of the pathophysiology of diabetes and ultimately result in better treatment and control practices for the two groups (Flavia et al., 2024; Sandra et al., 2024).

5.6.1. Lifestyle Modifications (Diet and Exercise)

The role of lifestyle modification, specifically diet and physical exercise, cannot be overstressed in the prevention as well as treatment of diabetes mellitus, particularly with its endocrine pancreas function. Stabilization of blood glucose can be achieved through a diet of whole foods such as fruits, vegetables, whole grains, and lean proteins. Portion control and restriction of saturated fats and refined sugars are strategies that are in line with dietary recommendations for individuals at risk for the development of diabetes. Furthermore, apart from helping in glycemic control, these interventions reduce the resultant risks of metabolic syndrome, which is strongly connected to insulin resistance and chronic inflammation (Guo et al., 2022). By promoting a healthy diet regimen, long-term diabetic complications can be minimized, and overall metabolic health can be maximized. Exercise is also a key element of the lifestyle modification equation, both as a weight control agent and as an effective tool for increasing insulin sensitivity. Regular exercise, such as aerobic exercise, resistance training, or even walking can go a long way in regulating blood sugar levels. Exercise causes muscles to absorb more glucose and enhances the efficiency of the endocrine pancreas overall. Studies have shown that 150 minutes a week of moderate-intensity exercise can substantially lower the risk for Type 2 diabetes and promote cardiovascular health (Fahed et al., 2022). Furthermore, promoting an active lifestyle counters sedentary behavior embedded in modern life, which is a potent identified risk factor for the onset of metabolic disorders. Last but not least, both dietary adjustment and regular physical exercise combined can assist in facilitating meaningful modifications among individuals with diabetes mellitus. In addition to addressing the short-term requirements concerning glycemic management, these lifestyle modifications contribute to long-term improvements in health status through reduced incidence of comorbid conditions such as cardiovascular disease and obesity. The convergence of diet therapy and increased exercise is an interdisciplinary approach in the management of diabetes that makes the patient sensitive to managing their health. Therefore, medical professionals should place more emphasis on lifestyle modification counseling as a central aspect of diabetes control, citing its applicability in maximizing well-being and life expectancy (Fahed et al., 2022; Guo et al., 2022) (Figure 5.17).

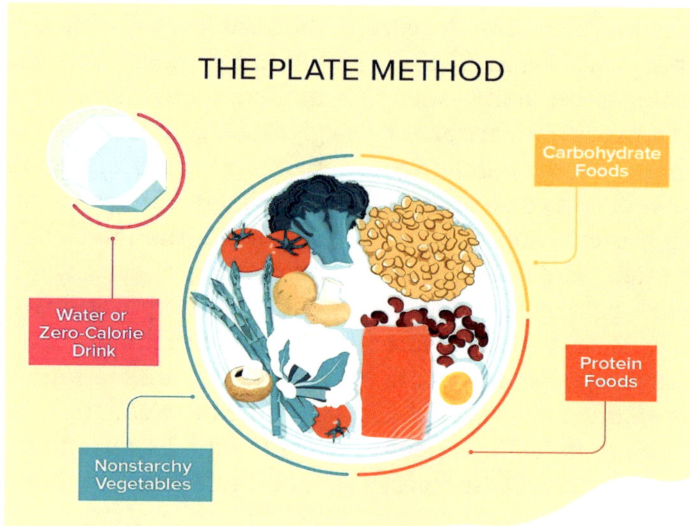

Figure 5.17. The plate method for management and prevention of diabetes mellitus.

Source: https://i0.wp.com/post.healthline.com/wp-content/uploads/2022/01/HL-1862499-The_Best_Diabetes_Friendly_Diets_to_Help_You_Lose_Weight-Infographic-The_Plate_Method-1296x1065-1.jpg?w=1155&h=2238.

5.6.2. Pharmacological Treatments (Insulin and Oral Medications)

Pharmacologic therapy of diabetes mellitus, particularly with insulin and oral therapy, has evolved significantly over the last few decades, reflecting the complex mathematical interrelations between glucose metabolism and the disease pathology. Insulin therapy remains a cornerstone treatment for type 1 diabetic patients and for the majority of type 2 diabetic patients, especially in late-stage disease. Insulin acts to increase the cellular transport of glucose, lowering blood glucose concentration and avoiding the threat of hyperglycemia. Insulins are available in various forms as rapid-acting, long-acting, and combination insulins to meet the individual need of every patient. Administration of insulin, however, can be problematic in terms of having the potential to induce hypoglycemia and in the need for frequent monitoring. Pharmacological effectiveness of insulin highlights its absolute necessity in the management of diabetes in spite of ongoing issues with compliance and lifestyle adjustments. In addition to insulin, various oral hypoglycemic agents have been introduced into clinical practice to regulate blood glucose levels in type 2 diabetic subjects. Examples of these drugs are sulfonylureas, biguanides, thiazolidinediones, and DPP-4 inhibitors, each with a different mode of action to increase insulin sensitivity, promote insulin release, or reduce glucose entry into the intestines. Metformin, for example, a commonly used biguanide, lowers glucose output from the liver and increases insulin sensitivity and thus is a first-line treatment for most diabetic patients. However, long-term use of oral drug is not constraint-free; they can cause gastrointestinal side effects or lead to weight gain, compromising patient compliance. As such, clinicians must move carefully through these facets while fine-tuning treatment based on patient profiles and maintaining glycemic control. Research into other drug therapies continues to assure better diabetes care by obliterating the imperfections of existing treatment. Priced analytically, natural products have become more popular, and their demand in diabetic management is increasing due to fewer side effects and greater affordability, as seen in existing research (Saha, 2024). Moreover, new treatment modalities such as injectable GLP-1 receptor agonists and SGLT-2 inhibitors have gained popularity as they not only lower blood glucose but also have cardiovascular advantages and aid in weight reduction, addressing multiple facets of diabetes mellitus and its complications. While efficacy and safety are always chief concerns in the development of such pharmacological agents, the ongoing need for effective treatments for diabetes underscores the need for ongoing research and investigation of synthetic and natural compounds to enhance the quality of life of patients afflicted with this disease (Marigliani et al., 2011) (Figure 5.18).

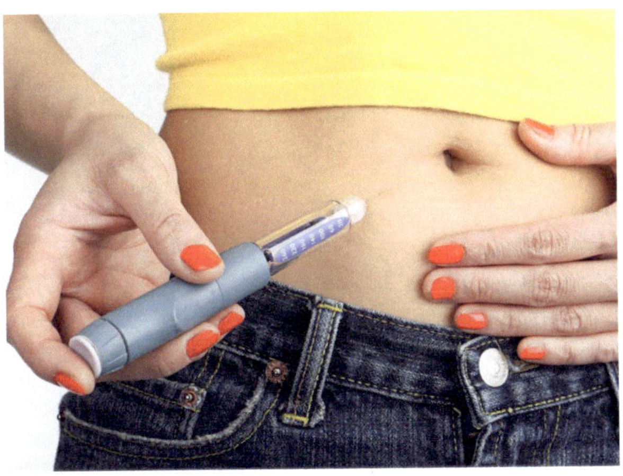

Figure 5.18. Insulin is a crucial medication for managing diabetes.

Source: https://www.knowdiabetes.org.uk/media/5727/shutterstock_234799480.jpg?anchor=center&mode=crop&width=800&height=600&rnd=133159229720000000.

5.6.3. Monitoring and Self-Management Strategies

Effective monitoring and self-management strategies are important for individuals with diabetes mellitus, particularly Type 1 diabetics. With continuous blood glucose monitoring, patients can be provided with real-time feedback regarding their glucose level, and therefore it is feasible for them to undergo appropriate interventions at the right time that can prevent acute complications such as hypoglycemia or hyperglycemia. Studies have proven that individuals with consistent monitoring practices are in a better position to manage their disease as they can readily adjust their insulin dosage or diet based on their readings. Advances in technology, including continuous glucose monitors (CGMs), have permitted much greater facilitation of tracking and managing blood glucose levels, blending into daily life without issue. But ongoing education regarding interpretation of such data continues to be crucial to empower patients and enhance their decision-making capacity regarding insulin injection and life change, eventually reducing the long-term health cost of diabetes (DiMeglio et al., 2018). Diabetes self-management extends from glucose monitoring to a range of lifestyle interventions that patients must adopt in order to manage the disease efficiently. Preparation of an equilibrated meal and adhering to a regular exercise regimen are fundamental self-management guidelines that can have a direct effect on glycemic control. Individualized meal plans such as carbohydrate counting enable patients to make proper food intake choices based on personal preferences and nutritional needs. Regular exercise also promotes weight management and enhanced insulin sensitivity, consequently enhancing metabolic status. Implementation of these strategies requires a systems-level understanding of the interaction among nutrition, physical activity, and control of diabetes. While studies persist in highlighting the importance of lifestyle modification in diabetes management, medical practitioners should prioritize these factors as the nucleus of their treatment protocols to facilitate an integrated approach to self-management (Adi et al., 2015). Technology has also greatly influenced diabetes self-management, offering innovative solutions to monitoring improvement and therapeutic adherence. The development of platforms like the Tidepool Platform has introduced an integrated and device-independent approach to diabetes management. The platform, based on the cloud, allows users to collect data from various glucose monitors and insulin pumps and see their patterns of glucose and treatment response in one easy interface. The technologies are particularly valuable, as they provide for breaking down silos of data that make diabetes management complex. In addition, these platforms enable the transparency required for successful diabetes education, which is necessary in creating a patient sense of agency. In the long term, through the utilization of technology in monitoring and self-management methods, diabetes patients can have more individualized attention and improved outcomes, making new platforms a requirement in the evolving environment of diabetes care (Adi et al., 2015).

Test Your Knowledge

1. What are two key lifestyle modifications recommended for managing diabetes?
2. Name two classes of oral medications commonly used to treat type 2 diabetes and their basic mechanisms.

SUMMARY

In conclusion, the intricate interaction between the endocrine pancreas and diabetes mellitus points to the outstanding importance of understanding these interactions in order to manage diseases properly. The role of the pancreas in glucose metabolism is of utmost importance, given its regulation of insulin and glucagon release in order to provide homeostasis. Disruption of these hormone pathways can lead to the onset and development of diabetes mellitus, both Type 1 and Type 2. When diabetes progresses, the complications can emerge and affect several organ systems and hence necessitate an interdisciplinary approach in treatment and management. Sophistication calls for constant research to understand the pathophysiological mechanisms involved in these diseases as acquisition of knowledge can be capable of driving new therapeutic schemes geared towards the optimized treatment of patients with diabetes (Ayaanuddin et al., 2025). The association between diabetes mellitus and other endocrine disorders, such as thyroid disorders, complicates clinical management further. Both conditions have intrinsic autoimmune mechanisms and genetic etiologies that complicate the worsening of symptoms and the intertwinement of treatment timelines. For instance, hypothyroid patients can present with impaired glucose tolerance, while diabetic patients can present with thyroids function impaired by the metabolic effects of insulins. This symbiotic relationship calls for an integrative approach where healthcare providers screen consistently for simultaneous endocrine diseases, with a perspective to administering comprehensive care. Integrated management may thus not only mitigate risks associated with each disease but maximize patient outcomes through endocrine condition management of the polyfactorial nature (Kumar et al., 2024). Future directions in diabetes mellitus management must involve individualized medicine with respect to the patient's unique endocrine profile. Enhanced technology, including electronic health devices and selective drug therapy with specific pharmacokinetic and pharmacodynamic effects, has the power to change clinical practice. Such technologies are capable of producing more precise diagnoses and treatment plans suited to the patient's unique metabolic demands. Furthermore, an emphasis on educating patients for lifestyle modification, such as exercise and diet, remains integral in the preventive model of diabetes management. With the establishment of an interdisciplinary relationship between patients and health professionals, we are able to maximize compliance with treatment plans and optimize the quality of life among diabetes mellitus patients. In short, the handling of diabetes' multifaceted character calls for collaborative convergence of research, practice, and patient care (Ayaanuddin et al., 2025).

The endocrine pancreas plays the role of regulating glucose homeostasis by releasing hormones such as insulin and glucagon. Diabetes mellitus is caused by derangement of the endocrine pancreas function, leading to abnormal glucose metabolism. The etiology of Type 1 diabetes is based on autoimmunity-mediated beta-cell destruction leading to insulin-secreting cells, while the etiology of Type 2 diabetes is caused by insulin resistance with consequent beta-cell failure. Both diseases demonstrate the role of the pancreatic endocrine system in maintaining normoglycemia and the noxious effects of its dysfunction. Additional studies are required to further clarify the pathophysiological mechanisms involved in these diseases and to create targeted treatment plans considering the endocrine pancreas dysfunction in their basis. The relationship between gut microbiome and metabolic disorders, like diabetes mellitus, has garnered significant attention in the past several years. Dysbiosis or imbalance of gut microbiota has not just been associated with gastrointestinal diseases but also pancreatic well-being (Solil et al., 2024). Specifically, chronic pancreatitis is linked with the gut microbiome composition, and it can be the cause of disease severity and impact the endocrine function of the pancreas. Pancreatic secretions, particularly enzymes like elastase, are reported to have a very important role in regulating intestinal microbiota and hence the metabolic activity. These linking highlights the necessity of a multidisciplinary approach to diabetes research, merging gastroenterology, endocrinology, and microbiology to better understand the determinants of health of the endocrine pancreas and its role in the development of diabetes. Linking birth weight and Type 2 diabetes risk provides crucial insight into metabolic disease early onset. Low birth weight (LBW) has always been associated with high risks of insulin resistance and subsequent diabetes, particularly in those who are born small for gestational age (Salmi et al., 2018). The relationship has been thought to be due to fetal programming, where adverse intrauterine conditions lead to alterations in pancreas development and function. It has been researched and documented that LBW has the propensity to cause both insulin resistance and insulin secretory dysfunction, a cumulative effect that predisposes the individuals to diabetes. Improved maternal health and antenatal care are therefore paramount in averting these risks, making it imperative to have a sustainable public health intervention that is geared towards optimizing birth outcomes to reduce the responsibility of chronic diseases like diabetes in adulthood.

KEY TERMS FROM THIS CHAPTER

- Autoimmune processes
- Blood glucose control
- Chronic pancreatitis
- Delta cells
- Diabetes pathology
- Diabetes treatment
- Dietary deficiency
- DPP-4 inhibitors
- Endocrine pancreas
- Beta cells
- Blood glucose regulation
- Cyanogenic compound
- Diabetes mellitus management
- Diabetes self-management
- Diabetic diagnostic criteria
- Disease-altering therapy
- Endocrine component
- GDM-affected mothers

CRITICAL THINKING QUESTIONS

1. **Which of the following pancreatic cells is primarily responsible for insulin secretion?**
   a. Alpha cells
   b. Beta cells
   c. Delta cells
   d. PP cells
2. **What is the primary trigger for insulin secretion by pancreatic beta cells?**
   a. Increase in glucagon
   b. Decrease in blood pressure
   c. Elevated blood glucose levels
   d. Increased oxygen demand
3. **Which of the following correctly describes Type 1 Diabetes Mellitus?**
   a. It is caused by insulin resistance.
   b. It usually presents in adulthood.
   c. It can be managed by oral hypoglycemic agents alone.
   d. It is an autoimmune destruction of beta cells.
4. **In Type 2 Diabetes Mellitus, which of the following pathophysiological mechanisms is most prominent?**
   a. Complete absence of insulin production
   b. Increased insulin receptor sensitivity
   c. Peripheral insulin resistance
   d. Autoimmune beta-cell destruction
5. **Which of the following is a diagnostic criterion for Diabetes Mellitus?**
   a. Fasting plasma glucose $<$ 100 mg/dL
   b. HbA1c $\geq$ 6.5%
   c. Random blood glucose $<$ 140 mg/dL
   d. 2-hour OGTT value $<$ 140 mg/dL

Short Answer Questions

1. Describe the structure and function of the endocrine pancreas.
2. Explain the mechanism by which glucose stimulates insulin secretion from beta cells.
3. Differentiate between Type 1 and Type 2 diabetes mellitus based on cause and onset.
4. What are the key pathophysiological differences between Type 1 and Type 2 diabetes?
5. List the common diagnostic tests for diabetes mellitus and the criteria for diagnosis.
6. Why is early diagnosis of diabetes important?
7. What are the main lifestyle and pharmacological strategies for managing diabetes?
8. How can self-management and education improve diabetes outcomes?

Answers to Critical Thinking Questions

1. (b); 2. (c); 3. (d); 4. (c); 5. (b)

REFERENCES

1. Abbott, D. H., Dumesic, D. A., Grogan, T., Nicol, L., et al. (2014). Abnormal infant islet morphology precedes insulin resistance in PCOS-like monkeys. https://core.ac.uk/download/323069697.pdf (accessed on 22nd July 2025).
2. Abdul-Rasoul, M., Agarwal, A., Ahlgren, U., Alejandro, R., American Diabetes Association, Anderson, D., Appleton, D., et al. (2016). What's in a name? Classification of diabetes mellitus in veterinary medicine and why it matters. https://core.ac.uk/download/76980783.pdf (accessed on 22nd July 2025).
3. Adi, S., Arbiter, B., Blum, M., Look, J., et al. (2015). A case study in open-source innovation: Developing the Tidepool Platform for interoperability in type 1 diabetes management. https://core.ac.uk/download/323073561.pdf (accessed on 22nd July 2025).
4. Anderson, D. J., Conners, J. R., German, M. S., Johnson, J. D., et al. (2000). Expression of neurogenin3 reveals an islet cell precursor population in the pancreas. https://core.ac.uk/download/4893026.pdf (accessed on 22nd July 2025).
5. Argenton, F., Ek, O. F. D., Facchinello, N., Grisan, E., et al. (2017). *Tcf7l2* plays pleiotropic roles in the control of glucose homeostasis, pancreas morphology, vascularization and regeneration. https://core.ac.uk/download/84923362.pdf (accessed on 22nd July 2025).
6. Arnelo, U., Haas, S. L., Löhr, J. M., Martin, C., et al. (2017). Pancreatic exocrine insufficiency after bariatric surgery. https://core.ac.uk/download/188827229.pdf (accessed on 22nd July 2025).
7. Ayaanuddin, S. K., Hizomi, A., Soju, S. M., Chagiashvili, A., Zehra, S. F., Bennetict, S. M., Sundaramoorthy, M., et al. (2025). Advancing management of pediatric celiac disease: Genetics, diagnosis, and health trajectories. *International Journal of Innovative Science and Research Technology*. https://www.semanticscholar.org/paper/47a473ea0aa0a536247f0a2bf90a79c254e07e4a (accessed on 22nd July 2025).
8. Badiali, D., Bruno, G., Ribichini, E., Rossi, M., et al. (2019). Role of fiber in nutritional management of pancreatic diseases. https://core.ac.uk/download/231748461.pdf (accessed on 22nd July 2025).
9. Balamurugan, A. N., Alexander, G. M., Allen, T. M., Amos, C. C., Barber, J. D., Barrou, Z. A., Bartlett, S. T., et al. (2002). *Pancreas and Islet Cell Transplantation*. https://core.ac.uk/download/12205582.pdf (accessed on 22nd July 2025).
10. Bonakdaran, S., Hezarkhani, S., Marjani, A., Rajabian, A., et al. (2013). Comparison of glycemic excursion in patients with new onset type 2 diabetes mellitus before and after treatment with repaglinide. https://core.ac.uk/download/52204666.pdf (accessed on 22nd July 2025).
11. Bykov, Y. V. (2023). Review article circadian disruption in pathophysiology of diabetes mellitus. *Fundamental and Clinical Medicine*. https://www.semanticscholar.org/paper/3a390fb457b4ac1301d69b4c62a906a08ce0d2ba (accessed on 22nd July 2025).
12. Cabral-Pacheco, G. A., Garza-Veloz, I., Castruita-De la Rosa, C., Ramirez-Acuña, J. M., Perez-Romero, B. A., Guerrero-Rodriguez, J. F., Martínez-Avila, N., et al. (2020). The roles of matrix metalloproteinases and their inhibitors in human diseases. *International Journal of Molecular Sciences, 21*, 9739–9739. https://doi.org/10.3390/ijms21249739 (accessed on 22nd July 2025).
13. Chait, A., & den Hartigh, L. J. (2020). Adipose tissue distribution, inflammation and its metabolic

consequences, including diabetes and cardiovascular disease. *Frontiers in Cardiovascular Medicine, 7*. https://doi.org/10.3389/fcvm.2020.00022 (accessed on 22nd July 2025).

14. Chowdhury, R., Harada, H., Matsumoto, S., Mizushima, N., et al. (1994). Tropical calcific pancreatitis: An overview. https://core.ac.uk/download/12529210.pdf (accessed on 22nd July 2025).

15. Cryan, J. F., O'Riordan, K. J., Cowan, C. S. M., Sandhu, K. V., Bastiaanssen, T. F. S., Boehme, M., Codagnone, M. G., et al. (2019). The microbiota-gut-brain axis. *Physiological Reviews, 99*, 1877–2013. https://doi.org/10.1152/physrev.00018.2018 (accessed on 22nd July 2025).

16. Da Silva Xavier, G. (2018). The cells of the islets of Langerhans. https://core.ac.uk/download/185508777.pdf (accessed on 22nd July 2025).

17. Diaconu, C. C., Diculescu, M., Ditu, G., Hainarosie, R., et al. (2018). Pancreatogenesis type 3C diabetes. https://core.ac.uk/download/216809675.pdf (accessed on 22nd July 2025).

18. Dilworth, L., Facey, A., & Omoruyi, F. O. (2021). Diabetes mellitus and its metabolic complications: The role of adipose tissues. *International Journal of Molecular Sciences, 22*, 7644–7644. https://doi.org/10.3390/ijms22147644 (accessed on 22nd July 2025).

19. DiMeglio, L. A., Evans-Molina, C., & Oram, R. A. (2018). Type 1 diabetes. https://core.ac.uk/download/228066211.pdf (accessed on 22nd July 2025).

20. Fahed, G., Aoun, L., Bou Zerdan, M., Allam, S., Bou Zerdan, M., Bouferraa, Y., & Assi, H. (2022). Metabolic syndrome: Updates on pathophysiology and management in 2021. *International Journal of Molecular Sciences, 23*, 786–786. https://doi.org/10.3390/ijms23020786 (accessed on 22nd July 2025).

21. Genta, S. B. F., Honore, S. M., & Sanchez, S. S. V. (2015). *Smallanthus sonchifolius* (Yacon) leaves: An emerging source of compounds for diabetes management. https://core.ac.uk/download/159286606.pdf (accessed on 22nd July 2025).

22. Grilo, L. F., Tocantins, C., Diniz, M. S., Gomes, R. M., Oliveira, P. J., Matafome, P., & Pereira, S. P. (2021). Metabolic disease programming: From mitochondria to epigenetics, glucocorticoid signaling and beyond. *European Journal of Clinical Investigation, 51*. https://doi.org/10.1111/eci.13625 (accessed on 22nd July 2025).

23. Guo, J., Huang, X., Dou, L., Yan, M., Shen, T., Tang, W., & Li, J. (2022). Aging and aging-related diseases: From molecular mechanisms to interventions and treatments. *Signal Transduction and Targeted Therapy, 7*. https://doi.org/10.1038/s41392-022-01251-0 (accessed on 22nd July 2025).

24. Guo, Q., Jin, Y., Chen, X., Ye, X., Shen, X., Lin, M., Zeng, C., et al. (2024). NF-κB in biology and targeted therapy: New insights and translational implications. *Signal Transduction and Targeted Therapy, 9*. https://doi.org/10.1038/s41392-024-01757-9 (accessed on 22nd July 2025).

25. Ivanenko, T. (2023). Determination of molecular mechanisms of development and course of experimental diabetes mellitus in Wistar rats. *Current Issues in Pharmacy and Medicine: Science and Practice*. https://www.semanticscholar.org/paper/f3f006fdab674f4223985cdb206914f881314f45 (accessed on 22nd July 2025).

26. Jo, J., Lee, W. S., & Song, T. (2020). Machine learning for the diagnosis of early-stage diabetes using temporal glucose profiles. https://arxiv.org/abs/2005.08701 (accessed on 22nd July 2025).

27. Kapke, D. R. (2015). Childhood type II diabetes: The risks and complications. https://core.ac.uk/download/58826199.pdf (accessed on 22nd July 2025).

28. Karaevren, T. T., Yorulmaz, R., Cerit, M., Şendur, H., Kalafat, B., Yaz Aydin, G., Gülbahar, Ö., et al. (2025). Fatty pancreas disease in newly diagnosed type 2 diabetes patients: A case–control study on relationships with glycemic control and exocrine function. *Diabetology & Metabolic Syndrome, 17.* https://www.semanticscholar.org/paper/fa6f33a4f782ead8f3b399f6ce93949014cfd30c (accessed on 22nd July 2025).

29. Keller, J. N., & Uranga, R. M. (2019). The complex interactions between obesity, metabolism and the brain. https://core.ac.uk/download/287882287.pdf (accessed on 22nd July 2025).

30. Kumar, U., Singh, J., & Singh, K. (2024). Epidemiological and clinical implications of coexisting thyroid dysfunction and diabetes mellitus. *International Journal of Clinical Biochemistry and Research.* https://www.semanticscholar.org/paper/7a2a7a8546bc662350517296cff3e4c1b8d27227 (accessed on 22nd July 2025).

31. Lokman, E. F., Kamaruddin, P. S. N. M., Muhammad, H., Zulkapli, A., Che Lem, S. Z. (2025). Investigating the effects of *Orthosiphon stamineus* on blood glucose regulation via pancreatic endocrine and exocrine functions in Type 3C diabetes mellitus Wistar Bonn/Kobori (WBN/Kob) pancreatitis rat model. *F1000Research.* https://www.semanticscholar.org/paper/9a3432ce6d9a9fd9c427dad4d920303551885e05 (accessed on 22nd July 2025).

32. March, C. A., Libman, I., Becker, D., & Levitsky, L. (2022). From antiquity to modern times: A history of diabetes mellitus and its treatments. *Hormone Research in Pediatrics, 95*, 593–607. https://www.semanticscholar.org/paper/937f5bb6fa1a2986be350c58ad450cd4781741ab (accessed on 22nd July 2025).

33. Marigliani, B., Aguiar-Yamaguchi, G. S., Ko, G. M., Miguel, G. P. S., Azevedo, J. L. C., Azevedo, J. L. M. C., Neves, K. F., et al. (2011). Organic consequences of ileal transposition in rats with diet-induced obesity. https://core.ac.uk/download/pdf/290138.pdf (accessed on 22nd July 2025).

34. Oliveira, F. C. M., Voorbij, A., Pereira, E. C., Alves e Almeida, L. M. M., Moraes, G. R., De Oliveira, J. T., Gouw, B. H. T., et al. (2024). Treatment of canine type 1 diabetes mellitus: The long road from twice daily insulin injection towards long-lasting cell-based therapy. *Organoids.* https://www.semanticscholar.org/paper/bfd856c3deb1f34a0a021f06739681a9deeec6e4 (accessed on 22nd July 2025).

35. Plows, J. F., Stanley, J. L., Baker, P. N., Reynolds, C. M., & Vickers, M. H. (2018). The pathophysiology of gestational diabetes mellitus. *International Journal of Molecular Sciences, 19*, 3342–3342. https://doi.org/10.3390/ijms19113342 (accessed on 22nd July 2025).

36. Rafaqat, S., Hafeez, R., Mairaj, R., Saleem, A., & Rafaqat, S. (2023). Pancreatic biomarkers: Role in diabetes mellitus. *Journal of Pancreatology, 6*, 169–177. https://www.semanticscholar.org/paper/278f544d93c5758062f3367005bb66d5ff35915b (accessed on 22nd July 2025).

37. Rinella, M. E., Neuschwander-Tetri, B. A., Siddiqui, M. S., Abdelmalek, M. F., Caldwell, S. H., Barb, D., Kleiner, D. E., et al. (2023). AASLD practice guidance on the clinical assessment and management of nonalcoholic fatty liver disease. *Hepatology, 77*, 1797–1835. https://doi.org/10.1097/hep.0000000000000323 (accessed on 22nd July 2025).

38. Saha, S. (2024). Novel antidiabetic therapeutics from some Indian medicinal plant kingdom. https://core.ac.uk/download/622439909.pdf (accessed on 22nd July 2025).

39. Salmi, I., & Hannawi, S. (2018). Birth weight and gestational age: Early life management strategy to population health for glucose disorders. *Volume (4)*. https://www.semanticscholar.org/paper/c63ee76e8c16219eb6316baffccee03c9ec8df0e (accessed on 22nd July 2025).

40. Schlünder, K., Cipriano, M., Zbinden, A., Fuchs, S., Mayr, T., Schenke-Layland, K., & Loskill, P. (2024). Micro physiological pancreas-on-chip platform with integrated sensors to model endocrine function and metabolism. *Lab on a Chip*. https://www.semanticscholar.org/paper/755919522be0ee0313fb738e916051f62261ceda (accessed on 22nd July 2025).

41. Solil, D., Dite, P., Přecechtělová, M., Uvírová, M., Dolina, J., & Martínek, A. (2024). Intestinal microbiome in patients with chronic pancreatitis. *Gastroenterologie a Hepatologie*. https://www.semanticscholar.org/paper/2ea12bd2796e4c9ca6a0a4d8c7dd5d585d3772ec (accessed on 22nd July 2025).

42. Stone, S. I., Urano, F., Yang, Y., Kirk, C., & Tosur, M. (2025). 75-OR: Novel syndromic forms of diabetes within the Rare and Atypical Diabetes Network (RADIANT). *Diabetes*. https://www.semanticscholar.org/paper/7070c898b563acee8562111c7816f42eaf7ce219 (accessed on 22nd July 2025).

43. Szlapinski, S. K., & Hill, D. J. (2024). *In vivo* models of gestational and type 2 diabetes mellitus characterized by endocrine pancreas cell impairment. *The Journal of Endocrinology*. https://www.semanticscholar.org/paper/2614cf9a725db9ed788eed794ce7dbc317d83e09 (accessed on 22nd July 2025).

44. Taşkaldıran, I., & Nar, A. (2023). A case of new-onset autoimmune type 1 diabetes mellitus following COVID-19 infection. *Endocrine, Metabolic & Immune Disorders Drug Targets*. https://www.semanticscholar.org/paper/d18fa2c294c741969e204a56d91adafc476c19d0 (accessed on 22nd July 2025).

45. Valente, R., Coppola, A., Scandavini, C., Halimi, A., Magnusson, A., Lauro, A., Sotirova, I., et al. (2024). Interactions between the exocrine and the endocrine pancreas. *Journal of Clinical Medicine, 13*. https://www.semanticscholar.org/paper/553f75ccae395169cae9c7e26bf129479ad4fe71 (accessed on 22nd July 2025).

46. Verdecchia, P., Cavallini, C., Spanevello, A., & Angeli, F. (2020). The pivotal link between ACE2 deficiency and SARS-CoV-2 infection. *European Journal of Internal Medicine, 76*, 14–20. https://doi.org/10.1016/j.ejim.2020.04.037 (accessed on 22nd July 2025).

47. Zhao, M., Xie, Y., Gao, W., Li, C., Ye, Q., & Li, Y. (2023). Diabetes mellitus promotes susceptibility to periodontitis—Novel insight into the molecular mechanisms. *Frontiers in Endocrinology, 14*. https://doi.org/10.3389/fendo.2023.1192625 (accessed on 22nd July 2025).

REPRODUCTIVE ENDOCRINOLOGY (MALE)

6

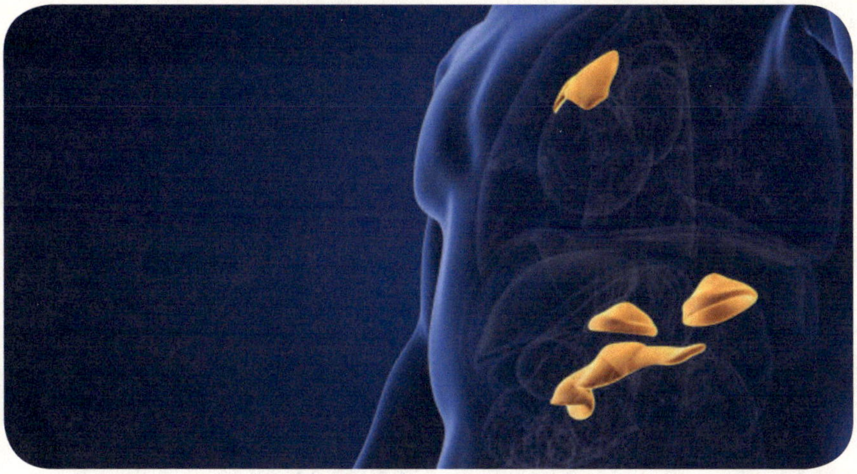

LEARNING OBJECTIVES

After studying this chapter, you will be able to:

1. Discuss the anatomy of the male reproductive system;
2. Understand the fundamentals of hormonal regulation of male reproduction;
3. Describe the process of spermatogenesis;
4. Explain the disorders of male reproductive endocrinology;
5. Focus on diagnostic approaches of male reproductive health issues;
6. Deal with range of treatment options available for addressing various male reproductive health disorders.

Introduction

Reproductive endocrinology, particularly in the male, is the intricate interaction of hormones that regulate much of male reproductive function. Knowing the hormonal blueprints that regulate functions such as spermatogenesis, secretion of testosterone, and physiological mechanisms of male fertility is essential. The male reproductive system is delicately sensitive to environmental factors, genetic determinants, and hormonal cues, hence making the subject of male reproductive health complicated. Factors like lifestyle, nutrition, and age also contribute to the intricacies of such interactions and therefore a thorough investigation is warranted. A good foundation in the field of reproductive endocrinology is important, particularly in the light of novel disorders like benign prostatic hyperplasia (BPH), which is increasingly being seen in young age groups due to hormonal disturbances and lifestyle patterns (Ye et al., 2023). Reproductive endocrinology knowledge is vital to the management of male-specific health issues such as aging-related reproductive impairment, endocrine disorders, and infertility. Recent research has identified that environmental exposures such as those to certain chemicals generally disrupt normal testicular development and function. Surprisingly, research has shown that prenatal chemical exposure to substances like bisphenol A and benzophenones could lead to reproductive hormone changes in later life, so exposures in early life are of special significance to male reproductive health (Holmboe et al., 2022). This cautionary awareness underlines the importance of incorporating environmental health issues into reproductive endocrinology study, presenting a challenge to increase sensitivity and allow for preemption by public health professionals and the public. The effects of reproductive endocrinology are felt beyond the individual organism, influencing broader societal trends. With growing recognition of men's reproductive health issues, it is necessary to examine preventative interventions and therapeutic mechanisms that offset hormonal imbalance and associated disorders. New data on the role of vitamin D in controlling reproductive mechanisms and its association with prostate health also demonstrate the significance of an interdisciplinary focus on men's reproductive health (Ye et al., 2023). All such integrative endeavors are important to set up holistic care plans, addressing the biological and environmental determinants of reproductive issues in concert, and formulating improved health results for men from all age brackets. As knowledge continues to evolve, collaborative research will play an essential role in providing valuable information on understanding the intricacies of male reproductive endocrinology and fostering overall male reproductive health.

Definition of Reproductive Endocrinology

Reproductive endocrinology is a core division of the broader field of endocrinology that deals exclusively with hormonal and cellular mechanisms governing reproductive systems. Reproductive endocrinology is the investigation of hormones, hormone pathways, and cell-to-cell relationships that govern reproduction. In research on male reproductive health, reproductive endocrinology examines key hormones such as testosterone, luteinizing hormone (LH), and follicle-stimulating hormone (FSH). These hormones not only play a critical role in regulating spermatogenesis but also perform significant roles in influencing libido, erectile function, and reproductive health in general. The fine balance of these hormones and their contribution to male fertility must be studied, especially in the wake of rising cases of infertility. The relevance of reproductive endocrinology is emphasized by research demonstrating the way in which external factors, such as obesity, can damage male reproductive health through hormonal derangements. Studies have shown that alterations in body mass index (BMI) can lead to significant declines in seminal parameters of significance, including sperm count and motility, and rises in reproductive hormone levels, all of which combine to make up male infertility (Yassin et al., 2025). Specifically, obese men have lower testosterone, LH, and FSH levels, which are all crucial to normal reproductive function. This correlation between metabolic health and reproductive endocrinology underscores the fact that optimal health is the key to ensuring hormonal homeostasis and, therefore, fertility. Furthermore, understanding about mitochondrial function enhances our knowledge regarding male reproductive endocrinology. Sperm motility and viability share intimate relationships with the function of mitochondria, whose functions are energy production and handling of reactive oxygen species. Mitochondrial dysfunction can lead to poorer quality sperm and ultimately the potential for fertility (Raad et al., 2024). The two-way interaction between mitochondrial integrity and endocrine control opens new avenues for investigating treatment strategies for male infertility. As work in this area continues to advance, it becomes ever more important to investigate these relationships so that effective interventions and better clinical outcomes may be developed for men with reproductive issues (Figure 6.1).

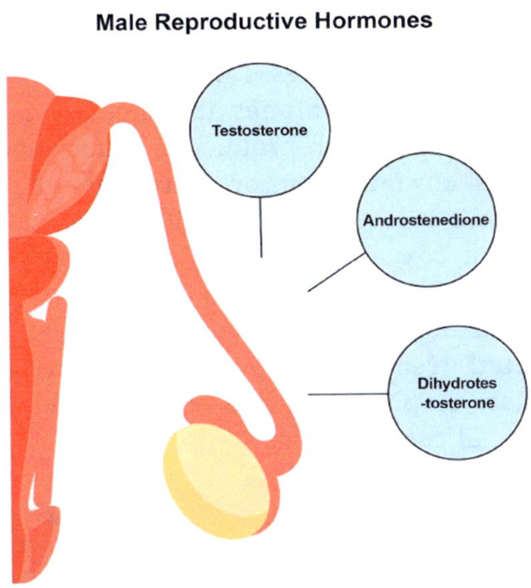

Figure 6.1. Male reproductive hormones.

Source: https://img.freepik.com/premium-vector/male-reproductive-hormones-human-endocrine-system-organ-producing_277904-18851.jpg.

Importance of Male Reproductive Health

The importance of male reproductive health is emphasized by its far-reaching influence on overall well-being, interpersonal relations, and public health. Men's reproductive capacity has a strong relationship with hormone function, particularly testosterone, which has the role of generating sperm, libido, and overall health. Decline in reproductive health can manifest in various ways, including hormonal imbalance, infertility, and sexual dysfunction, all of which will have a profound effect on an individual's quality of life. Moreover, maladies of male reproductive health, such as hypogonadism or infertility, may be an indicator of more comprehensive systemic conditions, such as cardiovascular or metabolic disease. Male reproductive health management is therefore not simply one of reproductive function but one that is an outgrowth of traditional paradigms of health and also of lifestyle determinants of health that may influence health outcomes over the lifespan. Environmental factors also significantly impact male reproductive health. Research has shown that exposure to low-dose ionizing radiation (LDIR) has profound impacts on the testicular immune microenvironment with numerous detrimental effects. LDIR exposure is associated with genotoxic stress and oxidative injury, ultimately leading to dysfunction in DNA repair mechanisms in reproductive cells. Deficiency of such a process weakens spermatogenesis and sperm quality deterioration. Given the critical role an intact immune microenvironment plays in maintaining normal reproductive function, such adverse effects heighten the urgency to investigate the mechanisms involved. Addressing outcomes of this study may have interventions able to mitigate such threats and ultimately bring about better male reproductive outcomes and usher an active reproductive endocrinology practice (Yin et al., 2025). Besides environmental hazards, infectious diseases also pose a tremendous threat to male reproductive health. For instance, brucellosis due to the Brucella bacteria can lead to severe reproductive disadvantage in infected males. This disease primarily impacts the reproductive tract, resulting in orchitis and diminished fertility. Moreover, the economic impact of brucellosis in animals demonstrates the broader impact of infectious diseases on male reproductive health aside from individual cases, as outbreaks can induce disruptions in herd fertility and significantly impact agricultural yields. In humans, transmission of brucellosis through contaminated animal products can lead to long-term health complications, which is a direct reflection of how animal health and public health interventions are interlinked.

Severe control interventions paired with public sensitization campaigns are needed in an effort to abrogate the occurrence and effects of such illnesses, thus guaranteeing male reproductive health on various fronts (N/A, 2024).

Overview of Hormonal Regulation in Males

Hormonal regulation in males is primarily coordinated through the interplay between the hypothalamus, pituitary gland, and gonads, giving rise to what is known as the hypothalamic-pituitary-gonadal (HPG) axis. It begins with the secretion of gonadotropin-releasing hormone (GnRH) by the hypothalamus, which stimulates the secretion of luteinizing hormone (LH) and follicle-stimulating hormone (FSH) by the anterior pituitary gland. LH acts on the Leydig cells in the testis to induce testosterone production, while FSH acts on Sertoli cells to support spermatogenesis. The intricate hormone feedback system ensures the optimal amount of testosterone, which is vital for secondary sexual trait development, libido, and overall male reproductive health. Furthermore, hormonal regulation in men extends far beyond the primary sex hormones; it is controlled by many proteins and factors that can affect fertility and reproductive capacity. Lipocalin 2 (LCN2), a protein that was initially described for its role in innate immunity, has been noted for its potential association with male reproductive well-being. Evidence suggests that the alterations in LCN2 expression are correlated with various reproductive disorders, which implies its regulatory role in male fertility. Curiously, LCN2 has also been seen to alter according to varying levels of hormone fluctuation, particularly testosterone. Elucidating the dynamics of LCN2 could help unveil the intricate hormonal interaction modulating male reproductive potential and potential biomarkers for reproduction. Apart from testosterone and LCN2, other hormones such as estradiol and inhibin also play important roles in male reproductive health. Estradiol, although a historically female biology term, is also present in males and has been used to describe various physiological processes, including libido and spermatogenesis. Inhibin, produced by Sertoli cells, inhibits FSH secretion by exerting negative feedback on the pituitary gland and thereby has a function in ensuring the fine tuning of the reproductive hormones. This multi-dimensional control of the hormones is reflective of the complexity of male reproductive endocrinology, such that any imbalance or interruption of these hormones creates disorders like infertility or impaired sexual health. As science develops further in this area of study, understanding these relationships will be important to developing targeted treatments for male reproductive disease, emphasizing the role of integrated hormonal control in male reproductive health.

6.1. Anatomy of the Male Reproductive System

Learning Outcome

1. Discuss the structure and function of the testes;
2. Explain the role of the epididymis and vas deferens;
3. Understand the importance of accessory glands (seminal vesicles, prostate).

The male system is a complex system of organs and tissues that permit the manufacturing and transportation of sperm as well as the secretion of male hormones. At the center of everything is the testes, which do spermatogenesis and testosterone production. Inside the testes, the seminiferous tubules are the primary sites for the manufacture of sperm. Supporting the work of these tubules are Sertoli cells that nurture young sperm cells and Leydig cells that secrete testosterone. The physiological processes of the testes have a close relationship to its anatomy;

any disruption in their organization can lead to severe hormonal imbalance and sterility. Thus, an understanding of this anatomy is essential in male reproductive endocrinology, especially for disorders that affect hormone levels and fertility. Once the sperm is formed inside the testes, the sperm are transported to the epididymis, where they mature and accumulate. The epididymis is a coiled organ that not only stores sperm but also enables them to develop motility and fertilizing capability. Sperm are ejaculated through the vas deferens into the seminal vesicles and prostate gland during ejaculation. These accessory glands play a vital role in producing seminal fluid that nourishes and protects sperm during its travel through the male genital tract. Secretions of these glands are mixed together to form semen, which plays a crucial role in reproduction. Disruption in any of this system's components leads to infertility and underscores the importance of intact anatomy to male reproductive success. Furthermore, an interaction between the male reproductive anatomy and the endocrine system plays a pivotal role in general reproductive health. Hormonal regulation is key since it governs processes such as spermatogenesis and male secondary sexual feature development. Disruptors, such as endocrine disruptors and environmental toxins, can interfere with this delicate balance. For example, it has been confirmed by research that the introduction of chemicals such as o,p´-DDT and EE2 can adversely affect the anatomy of male reproductive organs, resulting in disorders such as reduced semen production and dysfunctional hormone function (Hermansson et al., 2007). This highlights the intricate relationship between the anatomy and endocrinology of the male reproductive system and presents serious implications for environmental safety and reproductive well-being (Baskin et al., 2019). Hence, it is essential to have a deep sense of understanding how these two fields interact to solve the issues of male reproductive health today.

6.1.1. Structure and Function of the Testes

The testes are important glands of the male reproductive system, whose primary functions include spermatogenesis and secretion of hormones, particularly testosterone. Each of them is enveloped by a sheath known as the tunica albuginea that helps to retain its internal pressure required for spermatogenesis. The testes are also divided into numerous seminiferous tubules where spermatogenesis occurs. Within these tubules, germ cells undergo a series of development, ultimately differentiating into mature spermatozoa. The seminiferous tubules are covered by Leydig cells, which are tasked with testosterone synthesis, implying the double functional role of the testes in gamete production and endocrine regulation. The hormonal regulation of testes function is largely directed by the hypothalamic-pituitary-gonadal (HPG) axis. The hypothalamus releases gonadotropin-releasing hormone (GnRH), which, in turn, causes the anterior pituitary to release luteinizing hormone (LH) and follicle-stimulating hormone (FSH). LH, particularly, triggers Leydig cells to release testosterone, which, in turn, indirectly influences spermatogenesis as well as secondary sexual development. Concurrently, FSH is responsible for the stimulation of Sertoli cells, which provide nourishment and support for developing sperm cells. This intricate interaction emphasizes the dual function of the testes as an endocrine gland releasing hormones and an exocrine gland producing sperm, thereby maintaining both reproductive and endocrine function required for male fertility and well-being. Alterations in testes structure or function can lead to severe reproductive health issues. Hypogonadism, underproduction of testosterone, can significantly impair fertility as well as overall health. Also, the exposure to endocrine-disrupting chemicals (EDCs) contributes to impaired testicular function and hormone regulation disruption, which reflects the susceptibility of the testes to environmental insults. Such findings underscore the importance of maintaining healthy testicles and of establishing the potential adverse effects of various chemicals on reproductive endocrinology. As the research continues to explain the complexities of testicular function, it becomes increasingly clear that detailed knowledge of anatomical and physiological issues is critical for appropriate management of male reproductive health conditions (Michele et al., 2019; Teede et al., 2018) (Figure 6.2).

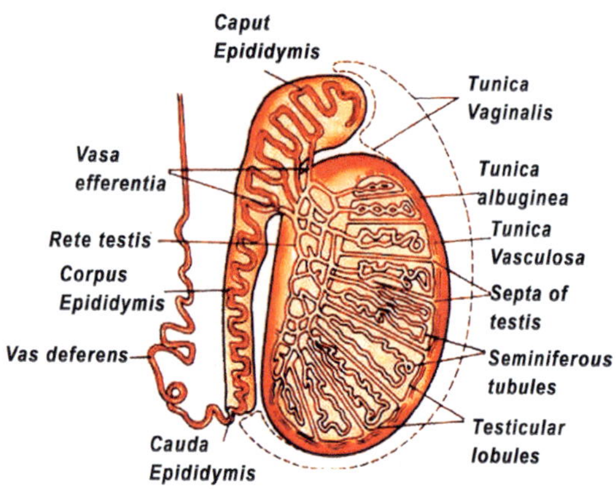

Figure 6.2. Structure of the testes.

Source: https://www.vedantu.com/question-sets/3ddc9bef-9907-420d-b8cb-027f7f56043b5994258399396555390.png.

6.1.2. Role of the Epididymis and Vas Deferens

Epididymis and vas deferens are critical structures of the male system, performing significant roles in sperm maturation and transport. The epididymis is a coiled, tubular structure behind the testes, where spermatozoa undergo multiple processes of maturation. During their journey through the epididymis, which could be weeks, sperm gain motility as well as the ability to fertilize an egg. This maturity is crucial, because immature sperm, upon release from the testes, lack the necessary abilities to facilitate successful fertilization. Moreover, the epididymis also secretes various substances that induce maturation of the sperm, e.g., glycoproteins and signaling molecules that regulate sperm functionality and viability in reproductive environments (N/A, 2024). Once matured, sperm are transported from the epididymis through the vas deferens to the ejaculatory duct. The vas deferens contains a muscular wall, which contracts to expel sperm during ejaculation. The duct is not just a passage but also a reservoir for sperm in which the release of sperm is controlled during sexual arousal. The vas deferens is integrated with hormonal signals that influence its contractions as well as overall function, thereby harmonizing properly with other parts of the male reproductive system like the prostate and seminal vesicles. In addition, the importance of the vas deferens is also attributed to its critical cellular composition that has been found to include specific proteins involved in normal sperm transport and protection, showing the need to research these body organs in reproductive endocrinology (Song et al., 2024). Since the epididymis and vas deferens play a critical role in male fertility health, their dysfunction is sure to lead to priceless fertility complications. Conditions such as epididymitis or vas deferens blockages can hinder sperm maturation and transport and thus lead to infertility. Furthermore, with recent research, the molecular regulation of these phenomena has been explored and the individual roles of signaling molecules such as hydrogen sulfide revealed in maintaining intact vas deferens and epididymal function. From these findings, selectively interrupting specific pathways has been suggested to offer therapeutic interventions for male reproductive illnesses. Finally, knowledge of the epididymis and vas deferens' functions is paramount in clinical practice and generally in reproductive health discourse, as both structures play vital roles in effective spermatogenesis and fertility (N/A, 2024; Song et al., 2024) (Figure 6.3).

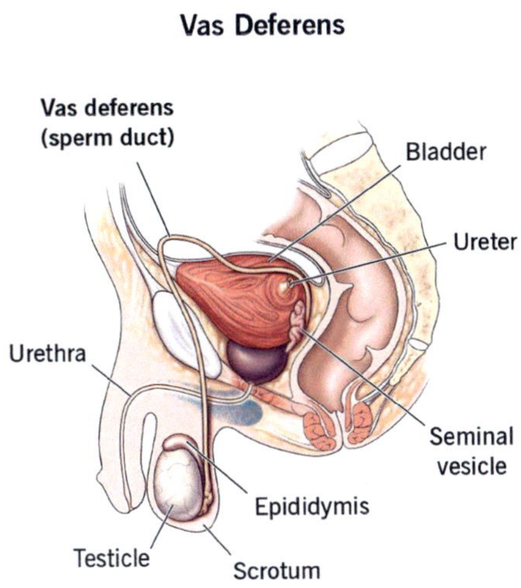

Figure 6.3. Vas deferens.

Source: https://my.clevelandclinic.org/-/scassets/images/org/health/articles/22763-vas-deferens.

6.1.3. Importance of Accessory Glands (Seminal Vesicles, Prostate)

The male reproductive system's accessory glands, including the seminal vesicles, prostate, and bulbourethral glands, carry out a vital role in reproduction. The glands add most of fluid that comprises semen and serves various purposes apart from merely carrying sperm. The seminal vesicles, for example, secrete fructose and other components that serve as energy sources for sperm motility. This form of energy plays a pivotal role in guiding sperms through the female reproductive system to the egg, thereby ensuring effective fertilization. The prostate secretions further assist in the addition of alkalinity to the semen, which is an essential component in counteracting the acidic content of the male urethra and the female vagina, enhancing sperm survivability and mobility during the reproduction process (Berger et al., 2024). Also, accessory glands not only produce seminal fluid but are also involved in the hormonal regulation as well as reproductive function. They are regulated by male sex hormones such as testosterone and estrogen in the process of their development and operation. Studies have demonstrated seminal vesicle and prostate expansion and function to be adaptive to reductions in estrogen signaling, underscoring the complexity of endocrine regulation of male reproduction (Berger et al., 2024). These glands' dysfunction is the cause of numerous diseases like benign prostatic hyperplasia and prostate cancer, prevalent among older men. To develop therapeutic strategies for preserving male reproductive functions and treating associated diseases, it is imperative that the mechanisms governing these glands are understood. Furthermore, the environmental components playing a role in modulating accessory gland health must be addressed. According to reports, treatment with certain toxicants, such as aluminum, adversely affects the morphology and functioning of these glands.

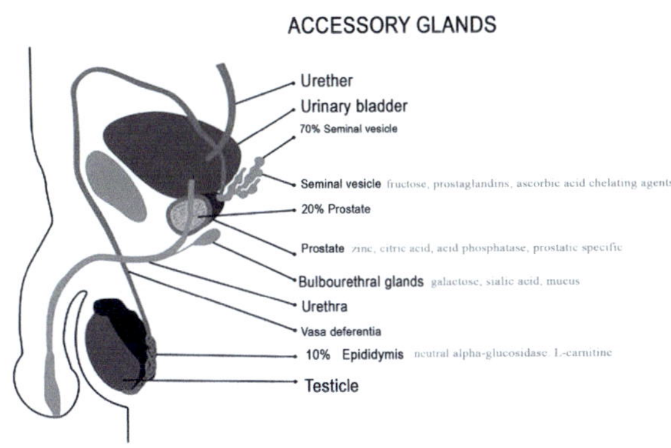

Figure 6.4. Male accessory glands and their main products of secretions.

Source: https://www.intechopen.com/chapters/60429.

For instance, aluminum can be implicated in interrupting hormone balance and altering the histoarchitecture of the prostate to disrupt reproductive capacity. The results pinpoint not only the necessity of discovering the biological roles of accessory glands but also stressors in the environment that might compromise their action. By controlling the intrinsic and extrinsic determinants of accessory glands, scientists and healthcare workers can more effectively work towards enhancing male reproductive wellness, improving outcomes, and consequently minimizing the impacts of many reproductive disorders (Figure 6.4).

Test Your Knowledge

1. What are the primary functions of the testes?
2. What role does the epididymis play in male reproduction?
3. What are the functions of the seminal vesicles?

6.2. Hormonal Regulation of Male Reproduction

Learning Outcome

1. Explain the role of testosterone in male physiology;
2. Understand the function of luteinizing hormone (LH);
3. Describe the role of follicle-stimulating hormone (FSH).

The endocrine regulation of male reproduction is a complex phenomenon involving a multitude of endocrine signals that coordinate the establishment and maintenance of male reproductive processes. Central to this system of regulation is the hypothalamic-pituitary-gonadal (HPG) axis, which is tasked with the regulation of production and secretion of key hormones such as gonadotropin-releasing hormone (GnRH), luteinizing hormone (LH), and follicle-stimulating hormone (FSH). The hypothalamus releases GnRH, which stimulates the anterior pituitary gland to release and secrete LH and FSH. The gonadotropins play a crucial role in initiating testosterone production in Leydig testicular cells and spermatogenesis in Sertoli cells. This intricate hormonal feedback loop aids in keeping testosterone levels strong within the physiological range, vital for male fertility and sexual health. In the past decades, environmental contaminants, particularly polystyrene nanoplastics, have been looked at with respect to their influence on hormonal regulation in male reproduction. Research indicates that exposure to these contaminants may disrupt endocrine processes, leading to male reproductive toxicity. Interference by these nanoplastics with hormone signal pathways is of concern regarding fertility and offspring quality in such affected males.

The reproductive system toxicological effects bring to the fore the importance of having a clean environment in guaranteeing improved male reproductive health. Hence, the understanding of hormonal reaction in male reproduction is not merely a matter of physiological interest but a matter of public health priority since new pollutants pose a threat to reproductive quality and duration (Marwa et al., 2024). Furthermore, novel data of the role of specific transcription factors in the integration of environmental inputs with hormonal controls required for male fertility are emerging. Work on Arabidopsis has demonstrated that basic helix-loop-helix (bHLH) transcription factors are essential for pollen development and fertility under varying light conditions. While plant systems have thus far received the most focus, these data suggest the potential for similar mechanisms to operate in vertebrates, including men. The bHLH protein family may be involved with elucidating how environmental stresses influence male reproductive hormone signaling, particularly in the context of environmental stressors. Research on these regulatory networks may inform mechanisms regarding how environmental influences impact male reproductive health and therefore to the broader topic of reproductive endocrinology and its translation into fertility in ecological as well as clinical contexts (Jordan et al., 2023).

6.2.1. Role of Testosterone in Male Physiology

Testosterone is a key component of male physiology, with its main role being the development and maintenance of male reproductive tissue and secondary sexual characteristics. Being a steroid hormone, it is produced mainly in the testes and is critical for spermatogenesis, the production of sperm cells. Elevated levels of testosterone are commonly associated with increased libido and sexual function, solidifying its worth in reproduction. Besides sexual development, testosterone has a general function in the wellbeing of men in relation to body muscle, bone mineral density, and fat distribution. Research has revealed that there exists a great relationship between luteinizing hormone (LH) levels and testosterone levels, which suggests that LH has a significant function in regulating the production of testosterone in other animals, e.g., mammals (Masram, 2025). Such intricate hormonal balance lies at the core of an understanding of male reproductive endocrinology and how it relates to fertility and wellness. The physiologic effects of testosterone extend far beyond mere reproductive processes but exert numerous systemic impacts that frame male wellness. Metabolic processes such as fat metabolism and insulin sensitivity are profoundly influenced by this hormone. In addition, testosterones' action in bone and muscle integrity cannot be overemphasized as it helps protein synthesis and maintenance of skeletal structure. Additionally, emerging studies indicate that testosterone has protective functions against a wide range of chronic illnesses such as cardiovascular disease by improving endothelial function and hemodynamics. Importantly, the interaction between testosterone and other controlling systems is complex as seen in the role of environmental factors in altering testosterone levels.

For example, contamination of the aryl hydrocarbon receptor (AhR) may result in hormonal dysregulation and dysfunctional spermatogenesis (Bustani et al., 2025). These observations highlight the need to pay attention to physiological as well as environmental components in male reproductive endocrinology research. The control of testosterone is mediated through a feedback mechanism of the hypothalamic-pituitary-gonadal (HPG) axis. Secretion of testosterone is controlled primarily by the pituitary gland releasing the gonadotropins, LH and FSH. This finely tuned control mechanism allows testosterone levels to remain exactly as demanded by the physiological requirements of the male body. Interruption of the axis can lead to hypogonadism or hypergonadism, both having profound influences on male fertility and well-being in general. Furthermore, the interaction of testosterone with other hormones, including estradiol, is critical to the optimal reproductive function. As continued research further explores the intricate roles of testosterone in male physiology, it will be knowledge regarding its interaction with other hormones as well as with the environment that will be crucial to unraveling male reproductive health and potentially fertility issues (Figure 6.5).

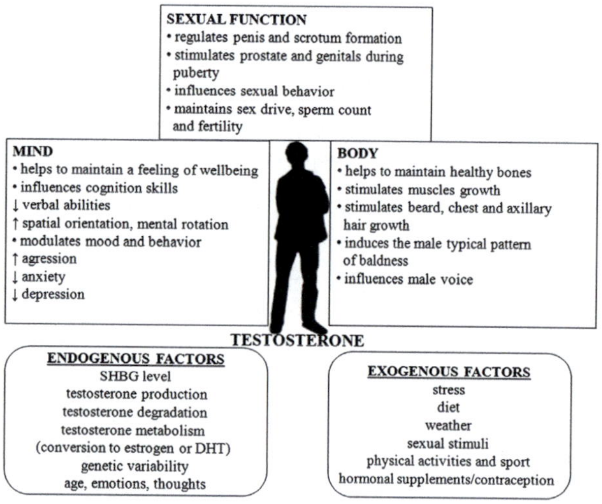

Figure 6.5. Schematic illustration of testosterone activity with factors modulating its levels and effects. (↑) Stimulation; (↓) attenuation. Androgen activity depends on testosterone levels, which are influenced by various factors. Testosterone affects body morphology and multiple physiological functions.

Source: https://www.researchgate.net/profile/Jaroslava-Durdiakova/publication/221740685/figure/fig3/AS:305557710884893@1449862043751/Schematic-illustration-of-testosterone-activity-with-factors-modulating-its-levels-and.png.

6.2.2. Function of Luteinizing Hormone (LH)

The function of luteinizing hormone (LH) in male reproductive endocrinology lies at the fore in testosterone production regulation and spermatogenesis. Secreted by the anterior pituitary, LH stimulates the Leydig cells in the testes to release testosterone, a critical hormone for male secondary sexual development and reproductive function. With inadequate LH levels, testosterone secretion may be impaired, leading to reduced fertility along with several symptoms of androgen deficiency. It has been observed that LH impacts not only gonadal function but also leads to extragonadal effects, and studies on this area of interest continue. The overall implication of LH in male reproductive wellness emphasizes its role in regulating disorders related to hormonal imbalance as well as infertility. In addition, its interaction with other hormones evinces its place in a tightly regulated hierarchy essential to male reproductive fitness. The stimulation of LH secretion is ordinarily provoked by gonadotropin-releasing hormone (GnRH) of the hypothalamus, illustrating a central nervous system-to-peripheral endocrine interface of key importance. This interaction is further regulated by feedback from testosterone and inhibins to maintain homeostasis of testosterone levels. Besides, LH is discovered to modulate many signaling pathways that indirectly affect spermatogenesis and thus make it an important regulator of male fertility. The subtle balance between these hormones discloses the complexity of male reproductive endocrinology that cannot be appreciated by straightforward comprehension of LH function. Modern studies plunge into the multifaceted functions of LH and suggest that its functions could be so much more than the long-held paradigms revolving around testicular activity. For example, evidence indicates that LH receptors in extragonadal tissues are capable of mediating important physiological reactions, but the significance of these interactions remains yet to be fully appreciated in their functional contexts. The role of LH must also be considered in relation to other hormones such as estradiol and neuroprogesterone, which interact with each other in the regulation of reproductive behaviors and functions across various species, including human beings. The expanding understanding of LH and its association with male reproductive well-being increasingly guides the management of infertility, underpinning the need for all-encompassing studies targeting the unravelling of hormone management in male reproductive endocrinology (Ahtiainen et al., 2007; Bentley et al., 2016) (Figure 6.6).

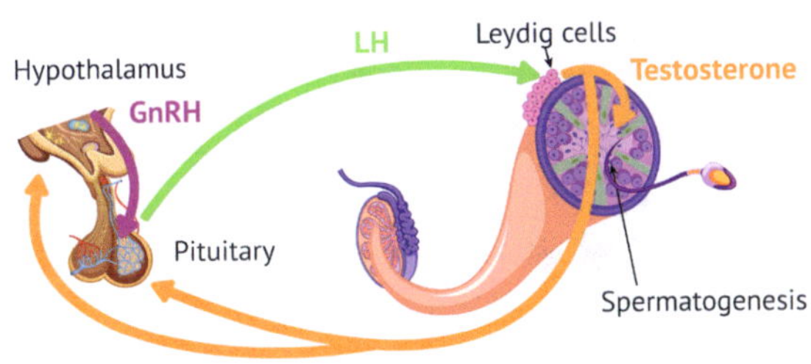

Figure 6.6. The function of luteinizing hormone (LH) in male reproductive endocrinology is pivotal for the regulation of testosterone production and spermatogenesis.

Source: https://www.invitra.com/en/wp-content/uploads/2014/05/hormone-regulation-spermatogenesis-lh-testosterone-1536x653.png.webp.

6.2.3. Role of Follicle-Stimulating Hormone (FSH)

Follicle-stimulating hormone (FSH) plays a critical function in the male's reproductive endocrinology that makes normal spermatogenesis possible. FSH is released by the anterior pituitary gland and acts primarily on Sertoli cells of the testis. Sertoli cells play crucial roles in nurturing and nourishing immature sperm cells. By activating Sertoli cells, FSH increases secretion and production of androgen-binding protein, which maintains high levels of testosterone within seminiferous tubules.

Testosterone is needed to promote the progression of spermatogenesis and finally produces viable sperm. Defects in the level of FSH through genetic disorders or hormonal imbalance may lead to the inappropriate formation of sperm and result in infertility. Understanding the mechanisms through which FSH functions offers evidence for the comprehension of potential treatments of male reproductive health diseases. Experimental studies through various animal models offers evidence on the function of FSH in regulating male reproductive function. For instance, research on Ames dwarf mice revealed that treatment with growth hormone and levothyroxine not only enhanced testicular weight and complete spermatogenesis but also resulted in increased FSH expression in the treated group. This is in direct contrast to control mice, who were low for FSH and failed to become sexually mature, indicating the significance of FSH for male fertility. Then, therapies that normalize FSH levels constitute a promising therapeutic solution to male infertility, an essential therapeutic area in endocrinology.

Finally, continuous monitoring of FSH levels can also play a role as a diagnostic criterion to evaluate reproductive health, and this suggests the primacy of the hormone in the male reproductive axis and endocrine balance in general (Azevedo et al., 2024). Furthermore, the interaction between FSH and other hormones, such as luteinizing hormone (LH) and testosterone, increases our understanding of male reproductive systems. For example, research also indicates that fluctuations in testosterone levels can influence the secretion of FSH, creating a closely regulated feedback mechanism that is required for fertility. Under diet or environmental exposures, studies have confirmed that chemicals such as zearalenone can interfere with normal hormone levels by reducing serum levels of FSH, testosterone, and other hormones required for spermatogenesis. The protective effect of dietary antioxidants, such as rutin, against interferences implies that restoring normal serum levels of the aforementioned hormones, such as FSH, is crucial to reproductive health. This insight is important in developing therapeutic approaches to improve male reproductive diseases (Sayed et al., 2024) (Figure 6.7).

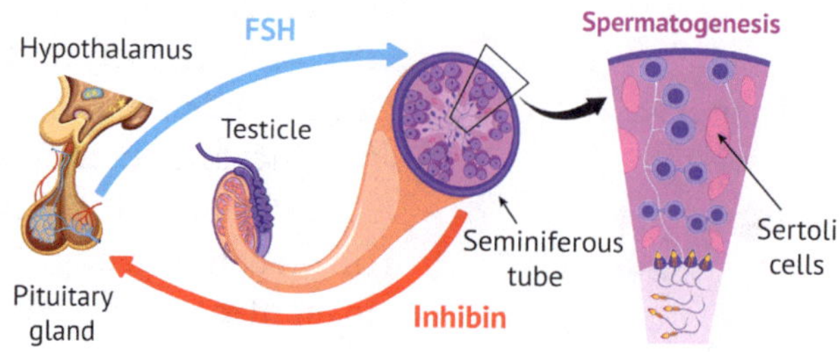

Figure 6.7. Regulation of spermatogenesis by FSH (follicle-stimulating hormone).

Source: https://www.invitra.com/en/wp-content/uploads/2014/05/espermatogenesis-fsh.png.webp.

Test Your Knowledge

1. What hormone is primarily responsible for the development of male secondary sexual characteristics?
2. What are three key physiological effects of testosterone in males?
3. What hormone from the hypothalamus regulates both LH and FSH release?

6.3. Spermatogenesis

Learning Outcome

1. Explain the stages of sperm development;
2. Describe factors influencing spermatogenesis;
3. Understand the role of Sertoli cells in sperm maturation.

Spermatogenesis is the complex biological process of the male reproductive system, namely in the seminiferous tubules of the testes. The process comprises proliferation and differentiation of spermatogonia into spermatozoa, comprising a series of major steps which encompass mitosis, meiosis, and spermiogenesis. Firstly, spermatogonia undergo mitotic divisions to yield primary spermatocytes. These early spermatocytes proceed to meiosis to produce secondary spermatocytes, which then have a second meiotic division to produce spermatids. Finally, spermatids undergo spermiogenesis, where they elongate into spermatozoa, maturing completely. The entire process of spermatogenesis takes around 64 to 72 days and is crucial for male fertility. Proper regulation of this intricate process is required for the formation of viable sperm, and this has implications for male reproductive health and fertility status in general. Spermatogenesis is largely controlled by hormones through an interaction between the hypothalamus, pituitary gland, and testes through a feedback loop that is significant in homeostasis. Hypothalamic gonadotropin-releasing hormone (GnRH) stimulates release of the anterior pituitary hormones luteinizing hormone (LH) and follicle-stimulating hormone (FSH), both of which are important for testicular function. LH acts on Leydig cells to stimulate the production of testosterone, which is important for male reproductive tissue development and maintenance, including the seminiferous tubules. Concurrently, FSH stimulates Sertoli cells to become more active, which provide necessary support, nutrition, and signaling to developing spermatocytes. Disruption of this endocrine axis might lead to dysfunctions in spermatogenesis. For instance, excessive exercise or endocrine-disrupting chemicals might have adverse effects on hormone levels and therefore compromise the production of sperm, as explained in revised reviews focusing on lifestyle determinants affecting male reproductive health (Adelowo et al., 2024). The impact of external sources on spermatogenesis, such as drug exposure and lifestyle, cannot be discounted in the context of male reproductive endocrinology. Certain pharmacologic drugs, particularly chemotherapeutic agents, have the proven effect of negatively affecting spermatogenesis through mechanisms such as oxidative stress and direct testicular damage. Examples of relevance are the cisplatin and cyclophosphamide disorders, which have been reported to lead to profound alterations in sperm quality and number through courses of therapy (Walker, 2024). Besides, lifestyle factors such as diet, exercise, and environmental exposures have been reported to significantly impact reproductive hormone levels and, consequently, spermatogenesis. Moderate exercise has been associated with improved sperm quality, but excessive physical stress could be detrimental to reproductive well-being (Adelowo et al., 2024). This understanding is thus relevant for developing interventions that can preserve male fertility in the presence of a multitude of drug and lifestyle-related challenges.

6.3.1. Stages of Sperm Development

The formation of sperm, or spermatogenesis, is a highly organized process that takes place in a sequence of well-defined stages in the seminiferous tubules of the testes. The biological process begins with the differentiation of spermatogonia, the stem cells at the basal layer of the tubule. When these cells undergo mitosis, they grow in number and then go on to meiosis, becoming mature primary spermatocytes. Internal cell changes involving a reduction of chromosome number are of significance since such spermatocytes move through meiotic divisions to form haploid spermatids. The smooth progression of the aforementioned phases is important for the formation of functional spermatozoa, which shall be capable of interacting with the oocyte for potential fertilization. Understanding these steps is crucial because any interruption can lead to infertility or sperm dysfunction, and thus it is absolutely necessary that a regulated process of sperm formation occurs. During the transformation from spermatogonia to mature spermatozoa, there occur structural and functional modifications that are crucial for fertility. Following meiosis, there occurs a sequence of morphological changes in round spermatids known as spermiogenesis. These are the transformations of condensation of nuclear material, acrosome development, and the elongation of the flagellum. These are the kinds of transformations that are required to make sperm establish the motility and fertilizing capacity. One should not underestimate the role of certain proteins and regulation factors in spermatogenesis; a case in point is the splicing factor heterogeneous nuclear ribonucleoprotein M (hnRNPM), which has been implicated as essential for sperm development. Research indicates that hnRNPM controls alternative splicing during spermatogenesis, a process crucial to guaranteeing proper development of functional sperm. Without such control factors, male infertility follows as exemplified in research illustrating the consequences of deficiency of the hnRNPM in reducing sperm counts and abnormalities (Lv et al., 2025). The broader applications of sperm genesis go beyond the immediate fertility outcomes, venturing into environmental and health implications influencing reproductive endocrinology. Exposure to environmental contaminants, such as per- and polyfluoroalkyl substances (PFASs), has proven to have adverse effects on sperm function and quality. They cause interference with endocrine mechanisms, leading to potential alterations in hormone levels that are pivotal for spermatogenesis. PFAS exposure has been discovered to impair sperm motility and viability, as indicated by research, further consolidating a fragile balance between toxins in the environment and reproductive health. Moreover, the epigenetic changes caused by PFASs, such as DNA methylation patterns in male germ cells, underscore the significance of environmental influences on the reproductive tract. Cumulatively, these factors stress the need for thorough examination of how genetic and environmental components regulate the stages of sperm development and their eventual influence on male fertility (DruAnne et al., 2025) (Figure 6.8).

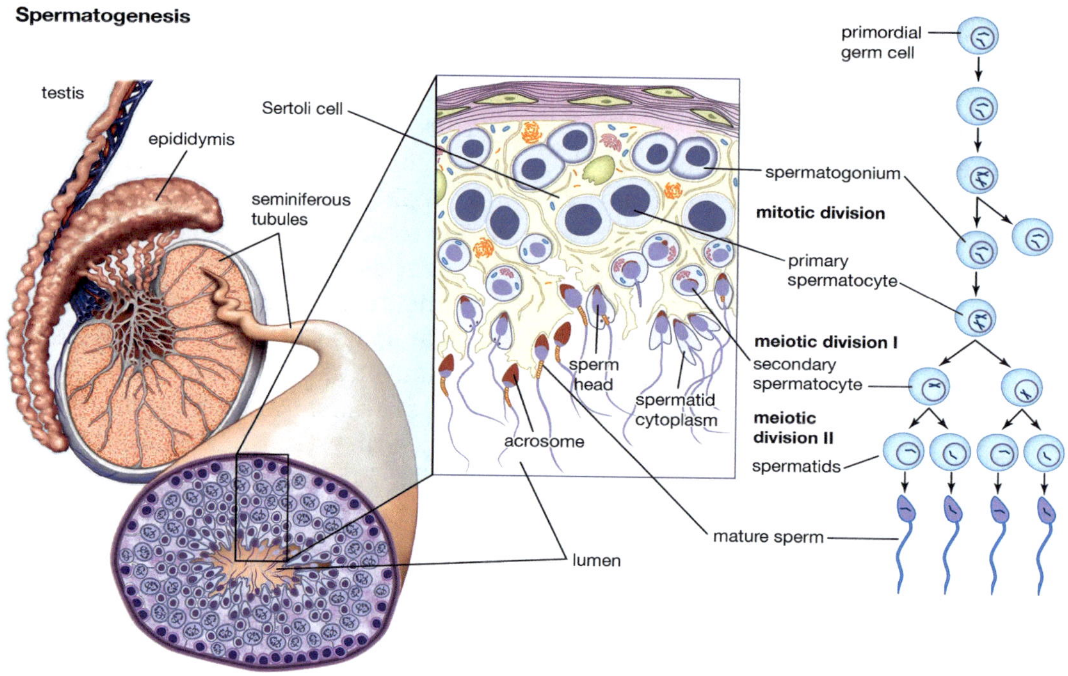

Figure 6.8. Spermatogenesis is the origin and development of the sperm cells within the male reproductive organs, the testes.

Source: https://cdn.britannica.com/49/135449-050-D1730B7E/spermatogenesis-human-anatomy.jpg.

6.3.2. Factors Influencing Spermatogenesis

Spermatogenesis, the complex biological process that produces sperm, is regulated by a thousand and one factors with a significant bearing on male reproductive health. The balance of hormones is of utmost significance; testosterone, secreted primarily by Leydig cells, has a critical contribution to make toward regulation of spermatogenesis through enabling the maturation of germ cells. Sertoli cells, which are in charge of nourishing and supporting maturing sperm, also rely on optimal metabolic conditions to perform their function optimally. For instance, metabolic diseases such as diabetes can skew the supply of energy needed for spermatogenesis because they disrupt glucose transport and lactate production in Sertoli cells. This relationship illustrates the intricacy of spermatogenic regulation, in which hormone and metabolic signals converge to be fertile and prevent sterility, complicated by other factors of environmental and lifestyle factors that can be additional stressors to the male reproductive system (Chen et al., 2025). Genetic factors also contribute to a significant factor in influencing spermatogenesis and male fertility. MicroRNAs (miRNAs) have been determined to directly participate in the regulation of gene expression at various stages of spermatogenesis. MicroRNAs are small non-coding RNA molecules that have the ability to modulate the function of Sertoli cells and germ cells, influencing sperm quality, quantity, and reproductive outcomes in general. Several miRNAs associated with faulty spermatogenesis have been revealed through research, demonstrating how the alteration in expression of miRNAs can result in fertilization and embryonic development failure. Hence, identifying miRNA profiles may not only serve to enhance the knowledge regarding male infertility but even prove beneficial as future biomarkers for diagnosing reproductive disorders. This intricate dance between genetic regulation, endocrine equilibrium, and metabolic health lies at the center of comprehending the numerous variables influencing spermatogenesis and masculinity (Shi et al., 2024). Exposures to toxins and endocrine-disrupting chemicals complicate the picture for spermatogenesis. These chemicals have the ability to interfere with normal endocrine communication, inducing hormone imbalance that negatively affects testicular function. For instance, it has been established that exposure to plasticizers, pesticides, and heavy metals reduces sperm motility and sperm production and consequently directly damages male fertility. Beyond the environmental factors, nutrition and physical exercise also play a significant role in spermatogenesis. Vitamin and trace element deficiencies necessary for reproduction result in defective sperm formation and quality. The multifactorial character of spermatogenesis highlights the importance of a comprehensive approach to male reproductive endocrinology in which interactions among genetic, hormonal, metabolic, and environmental factors have to be cautiously analyzed to manage effectively male infertility (Chen et al., 2025) (Figure 6.9).

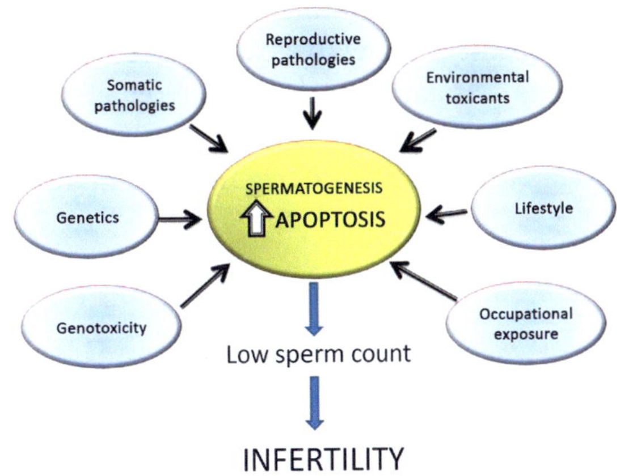

Figure 6.9. Factors affecting germ cell apoptosis in spermatogenesis.

Source: https://www.researchgate.net/profile/Ricardo-Moreno-21/publication/221818530/figure/fig1/AS:669128188784651@1536544000393/Factors-affecting-germ-cell-apoptosis-in-spermatogenesis.png.

6.3.3. Role of Sertoli Cells in Sperm Maturation

The Sertoli cells, or the nurse cells of the testes, play a pivotal role in the process of sperm maturation in the male reproductive system. The somatic cells within the seminiferous tubules provide the developing germ cells with the necessary structural and nutritional support. Sertoli cells play a vital role in the process of spermatogenesis, which transforms spermatogonia into mature spermatozoa through a sequential process. Aside from their support role, Sertoli cells play an active part in hormonal regulation of spermatogenesis through which they react to follicle-stimulating hormone (FSH) to release a series of factors important in the development of sperm. Their function is an expression of intricate cooperation between cell structure and hormonal control in ensuring male fertility and overall reproductive wholesomeness (Clavijo et al., 2018). Further, Sertoli cells help to create the blood-testis barrier, a specialized structure wherein a secure microenvironment can be developed in the germ cells. This barrier separates developing sperm from immune responses of the body, thereby preventing potential autoimmune reaction to sperm antigens. Apart from safeguarding germ cells, Sertoli cells also play a role in phagocytosis of cytoplasmic residue during spermatid maturation to enable clearance of cellular debris that would otherwise be detrimental to sperm motility and viability. This refined balance between structural support and immunological defense is critical for the optimal development of sperm. Any derangement in Sertoli cell function can lead to impaired spermatogenesis and reduced fertility, highlighting their significance in the broader context of endocrinology of male reproduction (Bellingham et al., 2016).

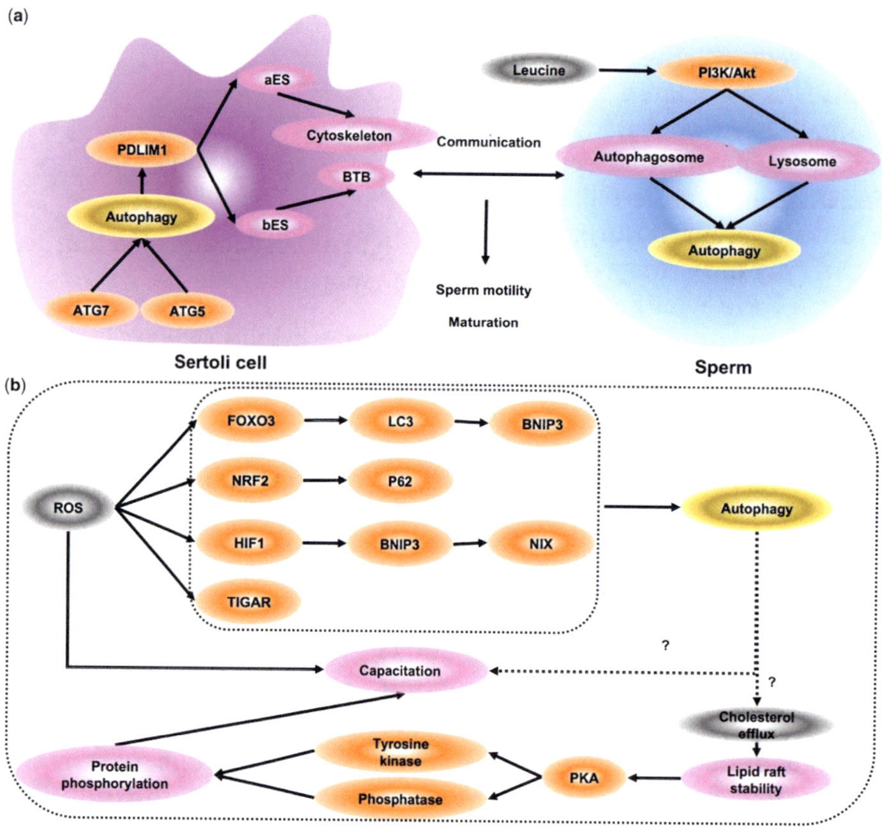

Figure 6.10. Role of autophagy in sperm maturation. (a) Sertoli cells. Cell-specific knockout of *Atg5* or *Atg7* results in spermatozoa with malformed heads and low motility. (b) Capacitation. ROS regulates autophagy through transcriptional and post-transcriptional pathways, including ROS–FOXO3–LC3/BNIP3–autophagy and ROS–NRF2–P62–autophagy.

Source: https://www.researchgate.net/publication/357459139/figure/fig2/AS:1131764248522756@1646845032966/Role-of-autophagy-in-sperm-maturation-a-Sertoli-cells-Cell-specific-knockout-of-Atg5.png.

The function of Sertoli cells is not merely physical support; they also release a family of signaling molecules that control the entire spermatogenic paradigm. For instance, inhibin and activin, both critical for feedback regulation of FSH levels and, in turn, spermatogenesis, are released from Sertoli cells. They release androgen-binding protein (ABP) that pins down testosterone in the seminiferous tubules to permit sperm maturation. This fine hormonal interplay demonstrates the central regulatory function of Sertoli cells in maintaining the delicate balance of hormone levels essential for fertility. Through the regulation of these processes, Sertoli cells not only facilitate sperm maturation but also ensure that the male reproductive system is sensitive to various internal and external cues, thus highlighting their significance in male fertility (Clavijo et al., 2018) (Figure 6.10).

Test Your Knowledge

1. What are the main stages of spermatogenesis?
2. Name three key factors that influence spermatogenesis.
3. What is the role of Sertoli cells in spermatogenesis?

6.4. Disorders of Male Reproductive Endocrinology

Learning Outcome

1. Define hypogonadism and its effects;
2. Understand disorders of sperm production;
3. Explain the impact of endocrine disruptors on male fertility.

The male endocrine system for reproduction is intricate, regulated by an exquisite balance of hormones governing a plethora of physiological processes. Systemic dysfunction can significantly influence male reproductive physiology and overall well-being. One frequent feature of these conditions is deficiency of testosterone, which can be due to primary or secondary hypogonadism. The causation may range from genetic conditions to chronic conditions and even drugs. Symptoms may include diminished libido, fatigue, and muscle wasting, with significant mental health and quality-of-life consequences. Diagnosis generally involves assessment of serum testosterone and extensive clinical assessment. Appropriate treatment choices can be hormone replacement therapy, lifestyle modification, and correction of underlying medical illness to restore hormonal balance and alleviation of symptoms. Hyperandrogenism is another important disorder in male reproductive endocrinology that may lead to varied reproductive and metabolic dysfunctions. Conditions like congenital adrenal hyperplasia (CAH), which is due to 21-hydroxylase deficiency, point to extensive hormonal assessment in the investigation of endocrine diseases. The condition leads to overproduction of adrenal androgens, resulting in virilization and infertility. These individuals typically require cautious follow-up and management steps, like glucocorticoid therapy, to rectify the hormonal imbalance and avoid complications. Male patients with CAH might also develop psychosocial problems due to the induced somatic changes, necessitating the need for multidisciplinary intervention including endocrinology, psychiatric management, and fertility counseling (Speiser et al., 2018). Such disorders such as Klinefelter syndrome also create severe problems in male reproductive endocrinology. Characterized by an extra X chromosome, this genetic anomaly typically results in hypogonadism and infertility. Physical defects such as gynecomastia, reduced testicular size, and intellectual disability may be present, making social integration and self-concept problematic. It has to be detected early and can be accomplished through the use of karyotyping and hormonal evaluations. Although no cure exists for Klinefelter syndrome, treatments such as testosterone replacement therapy and reproductive aid technology have been effective in increasing fertility and overall wellness. Thanks to increased awareness and knowledge regarding the influence of such disorders, medical providers are better placed to provide complete care specific to reduce issues involved while improving reproductive wellness and quality of life (Gausman et al., 2020).

6.4.1. Hypogonadism and Its Effects

Hypogonadism, which is characterized by inadequate release of testosterone, has significant effects on the reproductive health of men. Hypogonadism results from a variety of causes such as genetic disorders, illness, and lifestyle. Men with this disorder commonly manifest a range of symptoms, such as decreased libido, erectile dysfunction, and decreased muscle mass. Furthermore, hypogonadism results in infertility due to low levels of testosterone inhibiting the release of sperm. In reproductive endocrinology, knowing the underlying pathophysiology and treatment options of hypogonadism would serve to better enhance the patient's outcome. Not only does this hormonal imbalance improve one's fertility, but it also has a secondary function of improving overall physical and mental well-being. Hypogonadism is also increased by metabolic conditions, particularly among younger people. For instance, in a recent study highlighted that diabetes mellitus has strong association with hypogonadism and male erectile dysfunction and emphasized the importance of glycemic control in these patients. In a cohort of young adults with type 2 diabetes, hypogonadism was observed in more than 27% of patients, predominantly secondary hypogonadism (Raghuraman et al., 2024). Testosterone-metabolic health interaction is important and brings to the foreground the necessity of detailed assessments in the clinical setting, with the aim of not only controlling glucose levels but also endocrine balance.

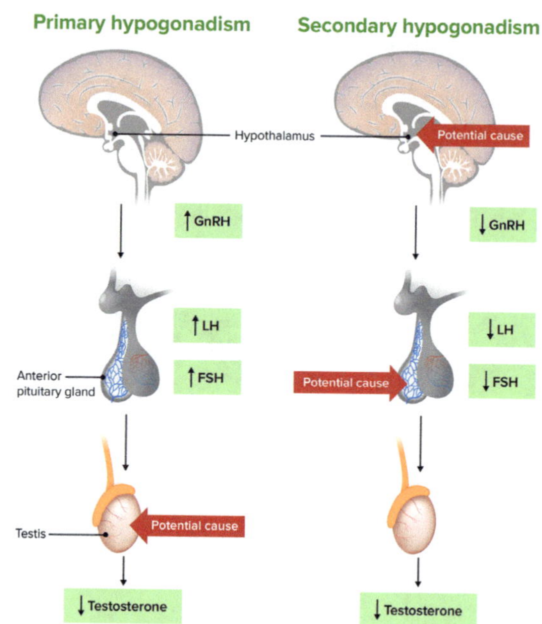

Figure 6.11. Pathogenesis of primary versus secondary hypogonadism.

Source: https://cdn.lecturio.com/assets/Pathogenesis-of-primary-vs-secondary-hypogonadism.jpg.

This multisystemic strategy may actually enhance the quality of life of individuals with diabetes as well as the effects of hypogonadism. Therapeutic control of hypogonadism, such as gonadotropin therapy, is also revealed to be irretrievably variable depending on the patient profile. A comparative trial of pulsatile gonadotropin-releasing hormone (GnRH) treatment and human chorionic gonadotropin and human menopausal gonadotropin (hCG/HMG) treatment revealed no difference in the rate of successful sperm production between the two treatment modalities. The pulsatile GnRH therapy was, however, associated with greater testicular volume and shorter treatment duration, which would be indicative of advantages in certain patients (Zheng et al., 2025). These findings lay the groundwork for a more sophisticated understanding of the management of hypogonadism and the virtue of individualized medicine. As research continues to evolve, the identification of effective therapeutic options will remain at the center of male reproductive medicine in reproductive endocrinology (Figure 6.11).

6.4.2. Disorders of Sperm Production (e.g., Azoospermia)

Sperm disorders of production are part and parcel in the diagnosis of male infertility, and azoospermia is one of the most significant conditions. Azoospermia is defined as the complete lack of sperm in the ejaculate that affects approximately 15% of men diagnosed with infertility. The condition can be classified into two broad categories: obstructive azoospermia (OA) and non-obstructive azoospermia (NOA). OA is caused by physical obstructions that hinder sperm from leaving the reproductive tract, whereas NOA is caused by intrinsic testicular failure or hormonal disturbances. Having an idea of the difference between the two is essential in planning effective treatment strategies. While the etiologies of azoospermia may never be forthrightly apparent, they are most often problems with the functioning of the reproductive apparatus, as compounded by chromosomal errors, that are likely to strongly hinder spermatogenesis and overall reproductive health in general (Sinwal et al., 2024). Klinefelter syndrome (KS), a chromosomal aberration characterized by the presence of an extra X chromosome, is a major cause of azoospermia and primary hypogonadism in men. Clinically, KS is defined by varied symptoms including delayed puberty, micropenis, and gynecomastia, along with biochemical markers such as low testosterone and elevated follicle-stimulating hormone (FSH) (Krueger et al., 2024). The extra X chromosome creates testicular fibrosis and impaired spermatogenesis due to dysfunctional testes.

This implies that KS men typically experience deep infertility problems. The heterogeneity of sperm production impairment underscores the need for adequate evaluations in order to provide early detection and adequate treatment interventions. Early diagnosis by karyotyping is critical since it informs fertility management and allows affected individuals to make informed decisions on the application of assisted reproductive technologies (Krueger et al., 2024). Refinement in reproductive technology has provided avenues for the treatment of sperm production disorders, particularly azoospermia. Techniques such as microdissection testicular sperm extraction (micro TESE) have revolutionized the technique of sperm recovery from the testes, especially for men diagnosed with NOA. The new microsurgical technique enhances the success of sperm recovery and, by extension, successful intracytoplasmic sperm injection (ICSI) for assisted reproduction. In addition, continuous research and investigation into hormonal therapies hold potential in maximizing spermatogenesis in men presenting with pre-existing hormonal deficiency. Despite the psychological and emotional trauma that accompany the diagnosis of azoospermia, optimism for effective treatment continues to increase, giving couples seeking children hope. Such developments are a testament to the interactive dynamic between male infertility treatment and reproductive endocrinology (Sinwal et al., 2024) (Figure 6.12).

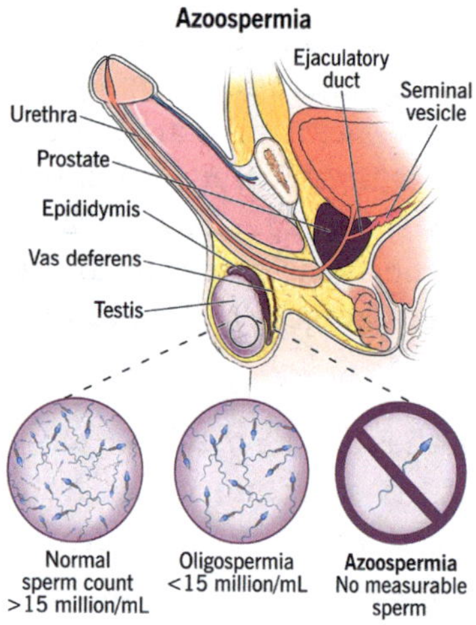

Figure 6.12. Azoospermia illustration.

Source: https://my.clevelandclinic.org/-/scassets/images/org/health/articles/15441-azoospermia.

6.4.3. Impact of Endocrine Disruptors on Male Fertility

The contribution of endocrine disruptors to male fertility is now a significant concern in the field of reproductive endocrinology, reflecting concerns about chemicals in the environment that undermine hormonal function. Such disruptors, from a variety of synthetic chemicals employed in plastics, pesticides, and industrial chemicals, have been linked with adverse reproductive outcomes. Over the decades, studies have revealed a disturbing trend that incorporates decline in male reproductive health, as exemplified by increasing rates of infertility and declining semen quality. The decline is hypothesized to be linked to chemicals that act as hormone mimics or blockers, yielding hormonal imbalances that interfere with spermatogenesis and overall reproductive function. It is important to appreciate the critical role those environmental elements, in their capacity as potential endocrine disruptors, take in determining male fertility and what this entails in terms of implications for public health programs in reducing exposure. Added to the complexity of the situation for male fertility is the contribution of oxidative stress, compounded by its occurrence as the result of exposure to endocrine disruptors. Experiments identify that a majority of these disruptors trigger excess ROS production, which overcome the cellular antioxidant defenses and lead to oxidative stress. As detailed below, oxidative stress is a significant contributor to male reproductive functions decline and affects sperm quality along with interfering in the delicate hormonal regulation by the hypothalamus-pituitary-gonadal (HPG) axis. The disruption is achieved through lowered testosterone levels, altering sperm mobility, and general fertility impairment. It is crucial to understand how environmental chemicals induce oxidative stress and consequent infertility, as control of these factors could offer promising ways for sustaining male reproductive health in a rapidly changing environment, bringing the findings closer to practical clinical applications. Cumulative effects of endocrine disruption and oxidative stress imply a multi-modal approach to addressing effectively male infertility. Studies, in recent findings, highlight the need to ensure total guidelines addressing prevention of exposure to toxic substances and creating awareness about their impacts. The discovery that endocrine disruptors are potent agents which can induce hormonal imbalance compels continued research into their mechanism of action on the male reproductive tract. With growing support for environmental health, pressure to reform policy to regulate the use of such chemicals grows, the implication being that action taken ahead of time may avoid the decrease in male fertility rates. This new awareness underscores the need for an interdisciplinary effort to bring together endocrinology, environmental science, and public health to counter the devious threat posed by endocrine disruptors to male reproductive health and fertility (Figure 6.13).

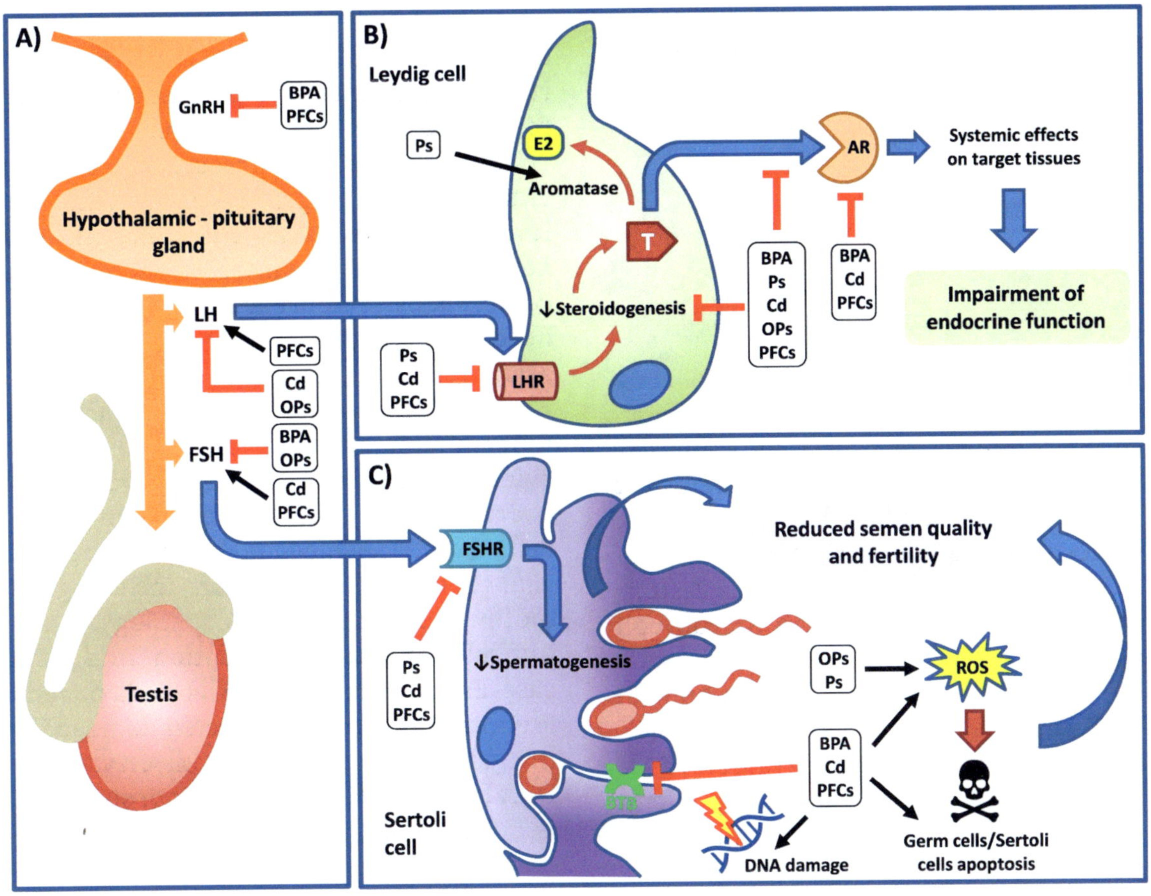

Figure 6.13. Schematic representation of endocrine disruptors' (EDs) effects on male fertility and the related mechanisms of toxicity. Results from both preclinical and clinical studies are summarized for each ED.

Source: https://www.researchgate.net/publication/330182728/figure/fig1/AS:963513870712877@1606731016976/Schematic-representation-of-endocrine-disruptors-EDs-effects-on-male-fertility-and-the.png.

Test Your Knowledge

1. What is hypogonadism in males, and what are its primary effects?
2. What is azoospermia, and what are its two main types?
3. How can endocrine disruptors affect male fertility?

6.5. Diagnostic Approaches

Learning Outcome

1. Describe hormonal assays and their significance;
2. Focus on semen analysis and interpretation;
3. Explain imaging techniques in reproductive endocrinology.

The etiological diagnosis of disorders of male reproductive health is a multiaxial process, because infertility can be caused by a number of anatomical, hormonal, and genetic factors. It starts with a proper medical history in which certain questions related to previous illnesses of health, habits of lifestyle, and the family history are inquired. This is followed by a thorough physical examination in which secondary sexual characters are assessed and any anatomical faults are recorded. Semen analysis is then performed to evaluate the parameters of sperm concentration, motility, and morphology. This step, which is typically reflective of oligozoospermia or asthenozoospermia, serves as the foundation of further investigations. Hormonal evaluation is also crucial, particularly in hypogonadism suspected on history, as it assists in determining the endocrine environment influencing spermatogenesis. Adherence to evidence-based guidelines enhances diagnosis quality and informs future treatment strategies, justifying the use of a systematic diagnostic strategy. Advances in the recent past have increased diagnostic methods to incorporate genetic assessment and radiologic assessment. Genetic assessment is recommended in cases of severe male infertility due to the fact that certain chromosomal abnormalities, such as Klinefelter syndrome or Y-chromosomal microdeletions, constitute significant reductions in fertility potential. In addition, imaging techniques such as ultrasound and magnetic resonance imaging (MRI) are employed to evaluate the presence of varicoceles or reproductive tract obstructive lesions. These diagnostic tools provide valuable information that informs appropriate interventions. Of significance, revised guidelines give paramount importance to the use of hormone therapies to treat some conditions, such as prescribing clomiphene citrate to treat oligozoospermia with reduced levels of testosterone, citing the inclusion of hormonal assessment in treatment regimens. This comprehensive approach is in response to the need to fuse traditional and advanced diagnostic approaches to improve male reproductive health. Bacteriospermia is also a significant determinant of male fertility, as growing evidence demonstrates its adverse effects on sperm quality and reproductive outcomes. Semen bacterial infection can produce significant changes in sperm parameters, including reduced motility and aberrant morphology, leading to difficulty in natural conception. In a particular case, Escherichia coli and Klebsiella pneumoniae identification led to suspected damaged sperm integrity, with evidence from elevated sperm DNA fragmentation. Treatment of such instances is normally by means of antibiotic therapy to eradicate the bacterial infection, supplemented with antioxidant supplements to alleviate oxidative stress-associated damage. Follow-up assessments have been promising, with dramatic improvement in sperm quality and successful assisted reproduction techniques thereafter. Though research points towards the correlation of bacteriospermia with male infertility, it is essential to incorporate elaborate microbiological evaluations as part of standard diagnostic plans to enhance the success of treatment.

6.5.1. Hormonal Assays and Their Significance

Hormonal assays play paramount significance in the clinical field of reproductive endocrinology, particularly in comprehending male reproductive physiology. The assays measure the level of various hormones such as testosterone, luteinizing hormone (LH), and follicle-stimulating hormone (FSH), which are of paramount significance in the control of spermatogenesis and male reproductive function. Clinician-measured quantitative levels of these hormones assist in the diagnosis of hypogonadism, infertility, and other endocrine disorders that affect reproductive functions. Hormonal imbalance can cause dramatic changes in bodily well-being and reproductive outcomes, and therefore the accuracy of these assays is essential to provide effective therapeutic interventions. Continuous monitoring by hormonal assays, thus, is a safe method to ascertain male reproductive health and guide therapeutic interventions. The role of hormonal assays is not merely diagnostic; they also inform the intricate feedback mechanisms involved in the control of the hypothalamic-pituitary-gonadal (HPG) axis. Hormones such as GnRH from the hypothalamus stimulate the pituitary gland to release LH and FSH, which in turn command the testes to release testosterone and facilitate spermatogenesis. Disruption of this axis is caused by a combination of factors, including genetic abnormality, environmental exposure, or lifestyle, and may result in impaired reproductive function. For instance, studies have shown that the control of such crucial factors as cFOS can directly control gonadotropin subunit expression in the pituitary and thus influence overall reproductive potential (Coss et al., 2015). Understanding these interactions through the use of hormonal assays allows for a complete evaluation of male reproductive endocrinology. Using hormonal assays can also be beneficial in tracking the effectiveness of therapeutic intervention to correct hormonal imbalance. For example, men on testosterone replacement therapy must be tested periodically with these assays to ensure testosterone levels are within a physiological range, thereby minimizing potential side effects and optimizing fertility outcomes. The actions of hormones in signaling cascades and cellular reactions—such as those controlled by c-Fos in gonadotropes—mirror the interlacing of functions within the reproductive endocrine system (Arnold et al., 2001). Hence, proper interpretation of hormonal assay results not only directs clinical practice but also forms the ground for enhancing our understanding about the biological basis of male reproductive health so that health professionals are able to tailor their therapeutic planning more appropriately (Figure 6.14).

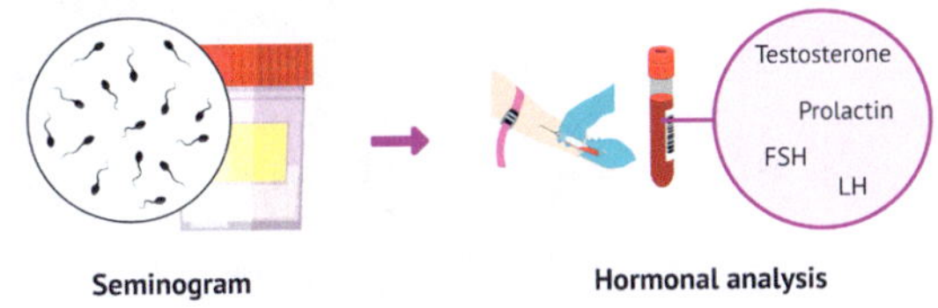

Figure 6.14. Male hormone analysis.

Source: https://www.invitra.com/en/wp-content/uploads/2022/08/male-hormone-analysis.png.

6.5.2. Semen Analysis and Interpretation

Semen analysis is a useful test tool in reproductive endocrinology that provides fundamental data concerning male fertility. It is an extensive assessment involving multiple parameters, including sperm concentration, motility, morphology, and total semen volume. Each of these makes individual contributions to reproductive function; for instance, an average concentration of over 15 million sperm per milliliter is normally adequate for fertilization. Abnormal results can suggest hidden pathology, be it hormonal disturbance or lifestyle factors, and necessitate more intensive investigation. Overall, semen analysis not only aids in the diagnosis of male infertility but also guides therapeutic interventions towards the revival of fertility and so is a valuable ally in reproductive care. The interpretation of semen analysis must rest upon an understanding of the male reproductive endocrinology, with special reference to the intricate balance of hormonal influences present. These hormones, including testosterone and follicle-stimulating hormone (FSH), regulate spermatogenesis and derangements can result in significant deviations of the semen properties. Quantification of these hormone levels alongside semen analysis allows clinicians to determine the cause of infertility. For example, a low level of testosterone can be linked with a reduction in sperm production, thereby informing practitioners of the necessity of hormonal treatments. Moreover, recognition of the link between endocrine function and quality of semen enhances the efficiency of treatment interventions to the enhancement of reproductive success, necessitating an integrated strategy in male fertility management (Clavijo et al., 2018).

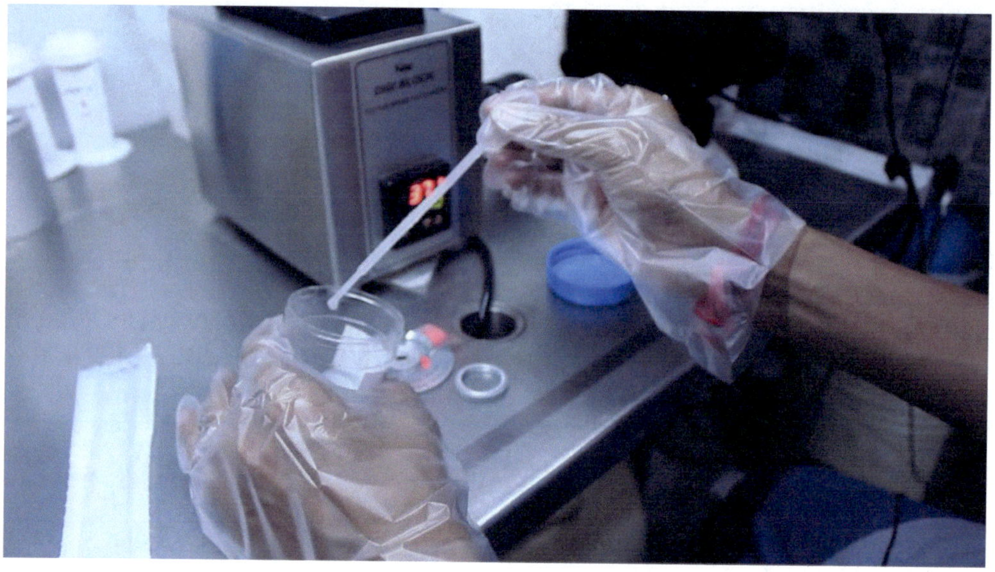

Figure 6.15. Semen analysis serves as a critical assessment tool in reproductive endocrinology.

Source: https://i.ytimg.com/vi/hMPTZrMiwF8/maxresdefault.jpg.

Besides biological factors, lifestyle choices have major impacts on semen quality and male fertility. Preliminary data indicate that lifestyle factors such as tobacco use, excessive alcohol use, and drug addiction are able to adversely affect sperm development and function. For instance, tobacco smoking has been linked to compromised sperm motility and abnormal morphology, whereas excessive alcohol intake can disrupt hormone regulation, leading to low fertility (Angelis et al., 2018). It is therefore crucial that, alongside traditional medical intervention, these lifestyle factors are also resolved in addressing male infertility issues. Promoting habit and behavior changes significantly enhances the chances of conception as a preventive intervention complementing therapeutic interventions. Hence, comprehensive understanding of biological and environmental determinants has to direct clinical practice in reproductive endocrinology with the objective of optimizing fertility outcomes for couples with fertility issues (Figure 6.15).

6.5.3. Imaging Techniques in Reproductive Endocrinology

Imaging modalities play a crucial role in the practice of reproductive endocrinology, particularly in the evaluation of the reproductive health of males. Modern imaging modalities, i.e., ultrasound, magnetic resonance imaging (MRI), and computed tomography (CT), have been of extreme usefulness in disclosing the anatomical and physiological details of male reproductive organs. For instance, ultrasound examination is utilized on a regular basis to assess the testes, scrotum, and surrounding structures in order that clinicians will be able to detect abnormalities like varicoceles, tumors, or hydroceles. MRI is increasingly utilized for its ability to provide high-resolution images of soft tissue so that lesions and infiltrative processes can be more clearly defined. This imaging modality application with modern techniques makes it possible to accurately diagnose and comprehensively understand many male reproductive illnesses, finally resulting in appropriate treatment regimes and therapy. In addition to structural assessment, imaging methods also furnish functional information on the male reproductive tract. For instance, Doppler ultrasound assesses blood flow in the testes, which can be relevant to the diagnosis of such conditions as testicular torsion or to the evaluation of the impact of varicoceles on spermatic cord blood flow. Scintigraphy and fluoroscopy have also developed applications in reproductive endocrinology so that clinicians are able to visualize dynamic processes such as sperm motility and distribution in the reproductive tract. Through the integration of these imaging modalities with endocrine studies, clinicians can achieve an extensive overview of reproductive function and dysfunction. Thus, the integration between imaging modalities and hormonal evaluation enhances the diagnostic accuracy and management of male reproductive endocrine disease. The uses of such imaging technologies are particularly relevant in the aspect of reproductive endocrinology personalized medicine. With additional research examining the correlation between imaging findings, hormonal status, and clinical outcome, a more tailored treatment approach may be achieved. For instance, by superimposing imaging data with knowledge from studies of transgender women (Defreyne et al., 2019), there is new understanding of how reproductive anatomy and function can be manipulated by hormonal interventions. In addition, findings from comparative studies in females, such as those highlighting alterations in reproductive organ morphology during the estrous cycle (Chatdarong et al., 2003), can inform imaging strategy in male reproductive health. With improving imaging technology, it will play an ever more vital role in advancing our understanding of male reproductive endocrinology and providing better patient outcomes.

Test Your Knowledge

1. What hormones are commonly measured in hormonal assays for evaluating male reproductive health, and why?
2. What are the key parameters assessed in a standard semen analysis?
3. Which imaging techniques are commonly used in the evaluation of male reproductive disorders?

6.6. Treatment Options

Learning Outcome

1. Explain how hormone replacement therapy (HRT) plays a pivotal role in addressing various reproductive endocrine disorders in males;
2. Discuss about assisted reproductive technologies (ART);
3. Deal with lifestyle modifications for improved reproductive health.

Within the discipline of reproductive endocrinology, understanding the range of possible treatments is critical while treating various disorders of male reproductive health. Infertility, hormonal imbalance, and sexual developmental disorders usually call for an all-encompassing approach that involves pharmacological treatment, surgery, and assisted reproduction methods. For instance, hormone replacement therapy is commonly administered to men who have testosterone deficiency to restore hormones and treat signs such as weakness and low libido. Additionally, medications such as clomiphene citrate can be useful in triggering the body's own testosterone synthesis in men with secondary hypogonadism. Decision-making is made individualized in nature with reference to patient-specific history, health status, and specific treatment goals while promoting open dialogue between patients and physicians. Surgery may be required for certain anatomical conditions responsible for causing male reproductive issues. Where physical abnormalities like varicocele, the condition where veins within the scrotum are dilated, are identified, surgical repair can yield dramatic gains in fertility. Hypospadias and cryptorchidism, also, which can disrupt normal genital function if unattended are managed operatively. Such surgery, performed by specialists as part of a team of experts, ensures the individualized treatment of each patient's own reproductive issues. Continuing evaluation of the effectiveness of such treatment is warranted, as patient and societal perceptions of reproductive health evolve. Integration of advances in surgical technique and postoperative care can make a significant difference in recovery and satisfaction rates for patients presenting with these challenging health concerns. Evolving treatment modalities also play an important role in resolution of the nuances of male reproductive health, particularly as related to transgender care. For transgender women, feminizing gender-affirming hormone therapy (GAHT) is a crucial component of treatment, comprising a range of hormone options with assumed physical and psychological advantages. Evidence indicates GAHT can significantly enhance quality of life and psychological functioning as well as produce physiological changes such as breast development. The associated risks, including cardiovascular disease and fertility issues, also need to be treated. As the body of evidence regarding the health care of transgender patients increases, ongoing studies are critical in order to determine long-term results of GAHT and to optimize treatment regimens according to patients' personal profiles to enhance the outcomes of health in the heterogeneous population (Defreyne et al., 2019).

6.6.1. Hormone Replacement Therapy

Hormone replacement therapy (HRT) is a central treatment for most reproductive endocrine diseases in men, particularly testosterone deficiency-related diseases. As a man ages, testosterone secretion declines naturally, leading to symptoms of which have a significant impact on the quality of life, including decreased libido, erectile dysfunction, and mood change. HRT brings the level of testosterone to within a normal physiological range, thereby alleviating these symptoms. Male reproductive and sexual medicine specialists must have an intimate knowledge of the male reproductive endocrinology physiology because this is the basis of hormone therapy. The effectiveness of

HRT depends on accurate diagnosis and strict observation of the hormone levels to ensure that treatment is tailored and specific to the patients' needs because unsuitable application can lead to unjustified side effects or exacerbate any existing conditions (Clavijo et al., 2018). Besides traditional testosterone therapy, the use of analogue hormones such as human chorionic gonadotropin (hCG) and low-dose aromatase inhibitors is becoming a significant area of male reproductive endocrinology. The aim of these alternatives is to stimulate endogenous testosterone production without causing much suppressive effect on the hypothalamic-pituitary-gonadal (HPG) axis. The incorporation of these adjunctive therapies into HRT regimens can prove particularly helpful for younger patients or those desiring to preserve fertility, as exogenous testosterone can lead to testicular atrophy and reduced sperm counts. Following that principle, sustaining therapeutic effect of HRT without compromising reproductive function necessitates a high degree of insight and strategic thinking by practitioners of the specialty of reproductive endocrinology (Clavijo et al., 2018). One of the determining factors for the efficacy of HRT in men is the ability of sex hormone-binding globulin (SHBG) to regulate hormone availability. SHBG is an estrogen- and androgen-binding protein with high affinity, effectively controlling the bioactivity of sex steroids. According to the free hormone hypothesis, the concentration of free, bioavailable hormones is critical to determine the outcome of HRT therapy. Research has shown that high levels of SHBG can enhance total levels of androgens but not the free testosterone concentration found in the body, potentially lowering the expected therapeutic effect on male reproductive organs. Therefore, both free and total hormone levels must be assessed to measure treatment efficacy and to make clinical judgments about HRT, as it shows the advanced nature of male reproductive endocrinology.

6.6.2. Assisted Reproductive Technologies (ART)

Assisted reproductive technologies (ART) have a critical role to play in the management of male infertility, particularly when traditional approaches are met with limited success. ART has transformed the discipline of reproductive endocrinology, allowing couples to conceive in spite of latent reproductive disorders in men. IVF and ICSI have become pillars of practice, particularly for men with reduced sperm count or motility defects. ART not only provides a means of conception but also allows for analysis and selection of potential sperm, which maximizes the chances of successful fertilization. Given that approximately 50% of infertile cases have a male component, the contribution of ART becomes replaceable no more in modern reproductive health management because it provides customized solutions to complex fertility problems (Konstantinidis et al., 2025). In particular, treatment of conditions such as retrograde ejaculation (RE) demonstrates the necessity and effectiveness of ART in reproductive endocrinology in men. Such a condition arises when sperm are unable to exit the body during ejaculation, often because of neurological or anatomical issues. ART interventions, especially sperm retrieval from urine after ejaculation, have been shown to be viable alternatives for couples experiencing the ramifications of RE. Advances in urine alkalization and sperm processing also allow for the use of recovered sperm in assisted reproduction. ART provides medical professionals with the means to successfully overcome the issues of male infertility, thereby finally granting afflicted patients their sought reproductive goals (Konstantinidis et al., 2025). With ongoing research further pursuing effective treatment options for unexplained infertility, the application of ART continues to become increasingly important. Studies indicate that up to 30% of couples struggle with infertility without an identifiable cause, complicating reproductive endocrinology assessments. In such scenarios, ART methods like IVF and IUI offer essential alternatives that can be adjusted based on patient demographics and previous outcomes. Notably, ART not only provides an avenue for conception but also fosters a deeper understanding of reproductive health and the nuances of male fertility. Modifying ART technologies to individual situations can render an enormous difference in rates of success and eliminate risks, underlining the ongoing revolution in reproductive medicine (Figure 6.16).

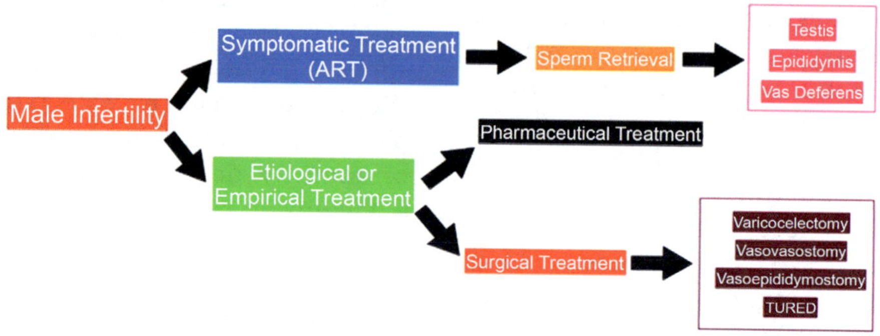

Figure 6.16. Symptomatic and etiological treatment of male infertility. [ART: Assisted reproductive technology; and TURED: transurethral resection of ejaculatory ducts].

Source: https://www.researchgate.net/profile/Aris-Kaltsas/publication/354534339/figure/fig1/AS:1075820407861250@1633506981870/Fig-1-Symptomatic-and-etiological-treatment-of-male-infertility-ART-Assisted.png.

6.6.3. Lifestyle Modifications for Improved Reproductive Health

Lifestyle interventions are an influential factor in enhancing reproductive health in men, particularly that of metabolic and endocrine health. The most crucial among the lifestyle interventions is the adoption of a healthy diet emphasizing whole foods and limiting processed foods and high-sugar foods. The nutritional content determines hormone levels, fertility, and overall reproductive function directly. Research recognizes the benefits of saturated fat-low, unsaturated fat-high diets that can improve overall metabolic health and insulin sensitivity. In essence, a rigorous diet intervention is capable of conquering all types of reproductive disorders because it regulates body weight and reduces the risk of disease caused by insulin resistance, thereby maintaining hormonal equilibrium. These changes form the foundation for the possibility of better fertility outcomes, so diet is a key element in male reproductive endocrinology and health discussions (Bernier et al., 2012). Another very important lifestyle change with significant consequences for male reproductive health is exercise. A consistent regimen has been associated with improved insulin sensitivity and cardiovascular health, both important factors in the maintenance of hormonal balance. Engagement in at least 150 minutes of moderate aerobic exercise weekly can be highly advantageous in improving metabolic function and testosterone levels, which are crucial for spermatogenesis and libido. Exercise is also beneficial in weight management, an important factor in the majority of endocrine disorders of the reproductive system. Because obesity negatively impacts fertility via its influence on hormone concentration and oxidative stress, incorporation of exercise into daily routines eliminates these health issues. Accordingly, a physically active lifestyle is not only healthy for general well-being but also essential for optimizing male reproductive potential, further supporting the connection between reproductive success and physical health (Ghazeeri et al., 2021). Proper stress management is also necessary to optimize reproductive well-being in men. Stress has the potential to induce elevated levels of cortisol, which has adverse effects on testosterone secretion and overall reproductive function. Mind-body treatments such as yoga, meditation, and mindfulness techniques have been shown to minimize stress, thus maintaining hormonal balance. Prioritizing mental health as a person prioritizes physical health allows men to design a favorable environment for the optimal reproductive outcome. The integration of stress management in a total lifestyle modification plan can significantly enhance chances of fertility. Therefore, learning about the heterogeneity of reproductive health and specifically addressing psychological and emotional issues alongside diet and exercise becomes essential in reproductive endocrinology's conversation (Bernier et al., 2012).

Test Your Knowledge

1. When is hormone replacement therapy (HRT) indicated in male reproductive disorders?
2. Name two assisted reproductive technologies (ART) used to help men with infertility.
3. What lifestyle modifications can improve male reproductive health?

SUMMARY

In summary, the identification of male reproductive endocrinology showcases the intricate relationship between hormonal regulation, environmental factors, and genetic backgrounds. Endocrine dysregulation may have dramatic effects on male reproductive physiology and, in turn, fertility and overall well-being. It is therefore crucial to determine how various factors control this hormonal environment in order to improve the design of targeted interventions. By examining endogenous and exogenous causes, including prenatal exposure to environmental disruptors, researchers can better explore the vulnerabilities that exist in male reproductive systems. This data is even more important in a time where there are rising incidences of reproductive disorders related to hormonal disturbances. Furthermore, the effect of prenatal programming on male reproductive health also highlights the necessity of gestational conditions. Evidence suggests that exposure to certain substances during pregnancy—such as certain environmental pollutants and hormone mimics—can trigger long-lasting changes in reproductive function and can influence not only the immediate offspring but also subsequent generations. These transgenerational effects raise questions instantly about the role of epigenetics in shaping the outcome of reproduction, supported by observations that suggest that actions on the GnRH neurosecretory system may be particularly significant during fetal life. Understanding these complex interactions is fundamental to public health planning for reducing reproductive endocrine disruption risks, and thus early action becomes an issue. Lastly, findings on endocrine disruptors, such as phytoestrogens, illustrate the pivotal position held by the environment in male reproductive endocrinology. For instance, studies on beta-sitosterol exposure and effect on gonadal cholesterol illustrate how these chemicals have a significant impact on reproductive hormone equilibrium. Elevated cholesterol in male subjects exposed to beta-sitosterol was accompanied by reduced testosterone production, indicating the intricate relationship between environmental chemicals and endocrine homeostasis. It thus becomes apparent that as reproductive endocrinology research progresses, there is a dire need for careful assessments of environmental effects. So, the future work would endeavor to describe the mechanistic connection between environmental exposures and endocrine responses, further expanding our understanding of male reproductive health in developing and developed worlds, as outlined by Bellingham et al. (2016) and Drolet et al. (2006).

Reproductive endocrinology in men encompasses a wide range of physiological and clinical conditions, with emphasis on the regulation by hormones of male reproductive health. Central to this discipline is the role of androgens, and particularly testosterone, which has a pivotal role in spermatogenesis and secondary sexual characteristics in men. Numerous hormonal disorders can follow from failure of the hypothalamic-pituitary-gonadal (HPG) axis, presenting as hypogonadism. The intricate interplay of these hormones is an actual indication of the need for a holistic approach to male reproductive endocrinology, especially considering the emerging problem of infertility and related disorders. With the incidence of such conditions continuing to grow, the need for proper diagnostic and treatment techniques becomes more imperative in both clinical and research settings, and recent research and interventions in the field are of growing urgency (Teede et al., 2023). A significant component of male reproductive endocrinology is the evaluation and treatment of erectile dysfunction and infertility, both of which are frequently due to the presence of underlying hormonal abnormalities. Evaluating them accurately entails measurement of serum levels of testosterone, luteinizing hormone (LH), and follicle-stimulating hormone (FSH) and aids in establishing the potential etiology of reproductive failure. Recent guidelines advise a uniform approach to diagnosis and treatment, highlighting the importance of patient history, clinical assessment, and laboratory findings. An awareness of the psychosocial factors affecting male reproductive health is equally important because these will have a lasting impact on treatment. Evidence-based, specialized management approaches according to individual patient-specific needs are followed by improved quality of life and fertility, supporting the importance of holistic treatment in male reproductive endocrinology (Teede et al., 2023). More evidence continues to unfold regarding the extensive implications of male reproductive endocrinology, particularly concerning metabolic status and lifestyle (Teede et al., 2023). There is mounting evidence to imply that such conditions as obesity and metabolic syndrome can have negative effects on male fertility and hormonal balance, pointing towards a two-way interaction between reproductive wellness and overall metabolic health. In addition, advancing treatments and technologies have extended the horizon for managing male reproductive diseases, including new frontiers such as hormone replacement therapies and assisted reproduction techniques. With the field expanding, the emphasis on multidisciplinary collaboration between specialists—like endocrinologists, urologists, and mental health experts—will be a decisive factor in developing inclusive care for men with reproductive problems. This collaborative effort will make it possible for both the physiological and psychosocial components of male reproductive health to be addressed (Teede et al., 2023).

KEY TERMS FROM THIS CHAPTER

Male fertility
Male infertility
Male reproductive endocrinology
Male reproductive tract
DNA methylation patterns
Dysfunctional testes
Environmental contaminants
Epididymitis
Fertility issues
Male germ cells
Male reproductive disease
Male reproductive system
Deficiency-related diseases
Doppler ultrasound
Ejaculation
Epididymal function
Estrogen signaling
Fluoroscopy

CRITICAL THINKING QUESTIONS

1. **Which structure in the male reproductive system is primarily responsible for the production of testosterone?**
   a. Epididymis
   b. Seminiferous tubules
   c. Leydig cells
   d. Sertoli cells
2. **Which hormone directly stimulates the Leydig cells to produce testosterone?**
   a. Follicle-stimulating hormone (FSH)
   b. Luteinizing hormone (LH)
   c. Gonadotropin-releasing hormone (GnRH)
   d. Prolactin
3. **Spermatogenesis occurs in which part of the male reproductive system?**
   a. Vas deferens
   b. Epididymis
   c. Prostate gland
   d. Seminiferous tubules
4. **Low levels of testosterone with high levels of LH and FSH in a male suggest:**
   a. Primary hypogonadism
   b. Secondary hypogonadism
   c. Normal gonadal function
   d. Hypergonadism
5. **What is the first-line hormonal diagnostic test for evaluating suspected hypogonadism in males?**
   a. Serum testosterone measurement
   b. Semen analysis
   c. Prostate-specific antigen (PSA) test
   d. Scrotal ultrasound

Short Answer Questions

1. What are the main components of the male reproductive system and their roles in reproduction?
2. How do the hypothalamic-pituitary-gonadal (HPG) axis and its hormones regulate male reproductive function?
3. What are the key stages of spermatogenesis, and which cells are involved in supporting and producing sperm?
4. What are the common endocrine-related disorders affecting male fertility, such as hypogonadism and androgen insensitivity syndrome?
5. What laboratory tests and imaging studies are typically used to evaluate male reproductive endocrine disorders?
6. How do testosterone, luteinizing hormone (LH), and follicle-stimulating hormone (FSH) levels help in diagnosing male reproductive endocrine disorders?
7. What are the primary treatment approaches for male hypogonadism, and when is hormone replacement therapy indicated?

Answers to Critical Thinking Questions

1. (c); 2. (b); 3. (d); 4. (a); 5. (a)

REFERENCES

1. Adelowo, O. E., Akindele, B. M., Adegbola, C. A., Oyedokun, P., Akhigbe, T. M., & Akhigbe, R. (2024). Unraveling the complexity of the impact of physical exercise on male reproductive functions: A review of both sides of a coin. *Frontiers in Physiology, 15*. https://www.semanticscholar.org/paper/33660bfb9750286b7cb745fc5f64f63b6cdf46b5 (accessed on 22nd July 2025).
2. Ahmed, S. F., & Markosyan, R. (2017). Sex assignment in conditions affecting sex development. https://core.ac.uk/download/150597685.pdf (accessed on 22nd July 2025).
3. Ahtiainen, P., Huhtaniemi, I., Pakarainen, T., & Poutanen, M. (2007). Extragonadal LH/hCG action–Not yet time to rewrite textbooks. https://core.ac.uk/download/159299787.pdf (accessed on 22nd July 2025).
4. Antonio, L., Blokland, M., Carmeliet, G., Claessens, F., et al. (2016). Sex hormone-binding globulin regulation of androgen bioactivity *in vivo*: Validation of the free hormone hypothesis. https://core.ac.uk/download/84044801.pdf (accessed on 22nd July 2025).
5. Arnold, B. S., Gross, T. S., McDonald, K., & Spulveda, M. S. (2001). Relations of environmental contaminants, algal toxins, and diet with the reproductive success of American alligators on Florida lakes. https://core.ac.uk/download/11016994.pdf (accessed on 22nd July 2025).
6. Baskin, L. S., Cao, M., Cunha, G. R., & Ricke, W. A. (2019). Reproductive tract biology: Of mice and men. https://core.ac.uk/download/323311356.pdf (accessed on 22nd July 2025).
7. Bellingham, M., Evans, N. P., & Robinson, J. E. (2016). Prenatal programming of neuroendocrine reproductive function. https://core.ac.uk/download/42371121.pdf (accessed on 22nd July 2025).
8. Bentley, G. E., Calandra, R. S., Micevych, P. E., & Paredes, R. (2016). Peripheral and central mechanisms involved in hormonal control of male and female reproduction. https://core.ac.uk/download/159295807.pdf (accessed on 22nd July 2025).
9. Berger, T., Guerrero, V., Boeldt, R., Legacki, E., Roberts, M., & Conley, A. (2024). Development of porcine accessory sex glands. *Animals: An Open Access Journal from MDPI, 14*. https://www.semanticscholar.org/paper/618f3e9300de9bc2dc4d9ec9aba9cfb478f4a8d4 (accessed on 22nd July 2025).
10. Bernier, D. (2012). Polycystic ovary syndrome: Pathogenesis, health consequences, and treatment of PCOS in relation to insulin resistance. https://core.ac.uk/download/72048051.pdf (accessed on 22nd July 2025).
11. Boczar, A., Dryja, P. M., Jarmołowicz, J., Stawicka, I., Orzołek, I., & Solisch, S. (2024). Comparison of the effectiveness of different assisted reproductive techniques (ART) in couples with unexplained infertility. *Journal of Education, Health and Sport*. https://www.semanticscholar.org/paper/157d4eddf1006c99c424fe27ff77de22ddeb31a1 (accessed on 22nd July 2025).
12. Bustani, G. S., Alghetaa, H., Mohammed, A., Nagarkatti, M., & Nagarkatti, P. (2025). The aryl hydrocarbon receptor: A new frontier in male reproductive system. *Reproductive Biology and Endocrinology: RB&E, 23*. https://www.semanticscholar.org/paper/a40cd2ef8aaf862d400785152210f0b9858de96f (accessed on 22nd July 2025).
13. Chatdarong, K. (2003). Reproductive physiology of the female cat. https://core.ac.uk/download/11694645.pdf (accessed on 22nd July 2025).

14. Chen, Z. F., Shen, Y. F., Gao, D., Lin, D. F., Ma, W. Z., & Chang, D. G. (2025). Metabolic pathways and male fertility: Exploring the role of Sertoli cells in energy homeostasis and spermatogenesis. *American Journal of Physiology. Endocrinology and Metabolism*. https://www.semanticscholar.org/paper/8f5d2d6e827067b6fb6c23a85b28f905d704871d (accessed on 22nd July 2025).

15. Clavijo, R., & Hsiao, W. (2018). Update on male reproductive endocrinology. https://core.ac.uk/download/323070097.pdf (accessed on 22nd July 2025).

16. Coss, D., Jonak, C. R., Kauffman, A. S., Xie, C., et al. (2015). Gonadotropin and kisspeptin gene expression, but not GnRH, are impaired in cFOS deficient mice. https://core.ac.uk/download/323311126.pdf (accessed on 22nd July 2025).

17. Darbandi, M., Darbandi, S., Agarwal, A., Sengupta, P., Durairajanayagam, D., Henkel, R., & Sadeghi, M. R. (2018). Reactive oxygen species and male reproductive hormones. *Reproductive Biology and Endocrinology, 16*. https://doi.org/10.1186/s12958-018-0406-2 (accessed on 22nd July 2025).

18. De Angelis, C. C., Di Dato, C., Gianfrilli, D., Isidori, A., et al. (2018). Smoke, alcohol and drug addiction and male fertility. https://core.ac.uk/download/153370850.pdf (accessed on 22nd July 2025).

19. Defreyne, J., Iwamoto, S. J., Motmans, J., Rothman, M., et al. (2019). Health considerations for transgender women and remaining unknowns: A narrative review. https://core.ac.uk/download/237010802.pdf (accessed on 22nd July 2025).

20. Drolet, M., MacLatchy, D. L., & Sharpe, R. L. (2006). Investigation of *de novo* cholesterol synthetic capacity in the gonads of goldfish (*Carassius auratus*) exposed to the phytosterol beta-sitosterol. https://core.ac.uk/download/143689350.pdf (accessed on 22nd July 2025).

21. Ebrahim, M. M., El-Dakdoky, M. H., El-shafiey, S. H., & Amer, A. S. (2024). Oral exposure to polystyrene nano plastics altered the hypothalamic–pituitary–testicular axis role in hormonal regulation, inducing reproductive toxicity in albino rats. *Birth Defects Research, 116*. https://www.semanticscholar.org/paper/13a55ac689e87080c77e09d1fb8ec09622f3f1b0 (accessed on 22nd July 2025).

22. Gausman, J., & Langer, A. (2020). Sex and gender disparities in the COVID-19 pandemic. *Journal of Women's Health, 29*, 465–466. https://doi.org/10.1089/jwh.2020.8472 (accessed on 22nd July 2025).

23. Ghazeeri, G., Hmedeh, C., et al. (2021). Nutritional management in polycystic ovary syndrome: Challenges and opportunities. https://core.ac.uk/download/161103740.pdf (accessed on 22nd July 2025).

24. Hermansson, A. (2007). Effects on the reproductive system in domestic fowl (*Gallus domesticus*) after embryonic exposure to estrogenic substances. https://core.ac.uk/download/11695140.pdf (accessed on 22nd July 2025).

25. Holmboe, S. A., Henriksen, L. S., Frederiksen, H., Andersson, A., Priskorn, L., Jørgensen, N., Juul, A., et al. (2022). Prenatal exposure to phenols and benzophenones in relation to markers of male reproductive function in adulthood. *Frontiers in Endocrinology, 13*. https://www.semanticscholar.org/paper/5c9afe8058ce96dcff3ae08e3b3eae739b05c839 (accessed on 22nd July 2025).

26. Konstantinidis, C., Zachariou, A., Evgeni, E., Çayan, S., Boeri, L., & Agarwal, A. (2025). Recent advances in the diagnosis and management of retrograde ejaculation: A narrative review. *Diagnostics, 15.* https://www.semanticscholar.org/paper/920b2a3a92eb95b3d8baaa3b977fb79fddb041a1 (accessed on 22nd July 2025).

27. Koreneva, Y. M., Bondarenko, V., Brechka, N., Smolienko, N., Belkina, I., Kustova, S., Boiko, M., et al. (2023). Fertility factors. D-hormone in prevention of reproducopathies caused by benign prostatic hyperplasia (literature review). *Problems of Endocrine Pathology.* https://www.semanticscholar.org/paper/e7acb87d0e69619b96b070cbe264959ce1bac3c0 (accessed on 22nd July 2025).

28. Križanac, M., Mass Sanchez, P. B., Weiskirchen, R., & Schröder, S. K. (2024). Overview of the expression patterns and roles of Lipocalin 2 in the reproductive system. *Frontiers in Endocrinology, 15.* https://www.semanticscholar.org/paper/1ae4fcb5c69050589ffd26fac66280209df6ad6d (accessed on 22nd July 2025).

29. Krueger, A., & Pelley, E. (2024). 6597 An unusual case of Klinefelter syndrome with both primary and superimposed secondary hypogonadism. *Journal of the Endocrine Society, 8.* https://www.semanticscholar.org/paper/aeb8e09e5fd2f5fbf54b934e5e8589bce6d4bfd3 (accessed on 22nd July 2025).

30. La Merrill, M. A., Vandenberg, L. N., Smith, M. T., Goodson, W. H., Browne, P., Patisaul, H. B., Guyton, K. Z., et al. (2019). Consensus on the key characteristics of endocrine-disrupting chemicals as a basis for hazard identification. *Nature Reviews Endocrinology, 16,* 45–57. https://doi.org/10.1038/s41574-019-0273-8 (accessed on 22nd July 2025).

31. Lakhe, G., Nair, N., Pareek, C., & Ugemuge, S. (2024). Bacteriospermia-related male infertility: A case report on diagnostic and therapeutic approaches. *Cureus, 16.* https://www.semanticscholar.org/paper/6118c4adbf8ecd5f84d2eb808d5a68d2ce39a6ea (accessed on 22nd July 2025).

32. Lv, P., Xu, W., Xin, S., Deng, Y., Yang, B., Xu, D., Bai, J., et al. (2025). HnRNPM modulates alternative splicing in germ cells by recruiting PTBP1. *Reproductive Biology and Endocrinology: RB&E, 23.* https://www.semanticscholar.org/paper/667e1ab4848c900741c668ad34e1691160e3fa4c (accessed on 22nd July 2025).

33. Masram, A. (2025). Study of reproductive physiology of male fruit bat *Rousettus leschenaulti* (Desmerest): A conservation effort of a crucial pollinator. *Uttar Pradesh Journal of Zoology.* https://www.semanticscholar.org/paper/2b0ed314d96d1a7b63db584c8d2a349c35c5042e (accessed on 22nd July 2025).

34. Maxwell, D. L., Petriello, M. C., Pilsner, P. M. J., Gaskins, A. J., & Minguez-Alarcon, L. (2025). PFAS exposure and male reproductive health: Implications for sperm epigenetics. *Seminars in Reproductive Medicine.* https://www.semanticscholar.org/paper/c1a8db64d44b1e24258ccc8307d7746b54b9e60c (accessed on 22nd July 2025).

35. Muselin, F., Dumitrescu, E., Doma, A., Degi, D., Dégi, J., Savici, J., Grigorescu, C., et al. (2024). Effect of *Sempervivum tectorum* extract on some biomarkers of reproductive function and levels of some trace elements in male rats exposed to aluminum. *Animals: An Open Access Journal from MDPI, 14.* https://www.semanticscholar.org/paper/7ba4a38f6ce8ac91c3d7e48034a328ae8662229a (accessed on 22nd July 2025).

36. Raghuraman, R., Bhuyan, A., Baro, A., & Saikia, U. (2024). Male sexual dysfunction and hypogonadism in young adults with type 2 diabetes mellitus: A cross-sectional study. *Journal*

of Human Reproductive Sciences, 17, 170–177. https://www.semanticscholar.org/paper/625cc3401d94485d2d915585ce60c47559e4e687 (accessed on 22nd July 2025).

37. Robson, J. K., Tidy, A. C., Thomas, S. G., & Wilson, Z. (2023). Environmental regulation of male fertility is mediated through *Arabidopsis* transcription factors bHLH89, 91, and 10. *Journal of Experimental Botany, 75*, 1934–1947. https://www.semanticscholar.org/paper/e556904882c242436f71c9180c452f42f6ff90ea (accessed on 22nd July 2025).

38. Sayed, H., Zhang, Q., Tang, Y., Wang, Y., Guo, Y., Zhang, J., Ji, C., et al. (2024). Alleviative effect of rutin on zearalenone-induced reproductive toxicity in male mice by preventing spermatogenic cell apoptosis and modulating gene expression in the hypothalamic–pituitary–gonadal axis. *Toxins, 16*. https://www.semanticscholar.org/paper/5f37dcec25f1ef1099a7f0dbdc593f477c8b7271 (accessed on 22nd July 2025).

39. Shi, Z., Yu, M., Guo, T., Sui, Y., Tian, Z., Ni, X., Chen, X., et al. (2024). MicroRNAs in spermatogenesis dysfunction and male infertility: Clinical phenotypes, mechanisms and potential diagnostic biomarkers. *Frontiers in Endocrinology, 15*. https://www.semanticscholar.org/paper/b41fc9de4ffedb0c3e43a183c3aeb196217af243 (accessed on 22nd July 2025).

40. Singh, H. (2025). The impact of sodium valproate on male reproductive health: A comprehensive review. *Communications on Applied Nonlinear Analysis*. https://www.semanticscholar.org/paper/fa6056c4d3f6d6720a83747e6642cee965826021 (accessed on 22nd July 2025).

41. Sinwal, A., Bhardwaj, M., & Nair, M. (2024). Azoospermia–An overview. *International Journal of Science and Healthcare Research*. https://www.semanticscholar.org/paper/e068140b518ec5791baa1b4f7045bb4d94d14c1b (accessed on 22nd July 2025).

42. Song, Y., Mao, C., Zhong, Q., Zhang, R., Jiang, D., & Sun, X. (2024). Role of hydrogen sulfide in the male reproductive system. *Frontiers in Endocrinology, 15*. https://www.semanticscholar.org/paper/e5a067bcc1d165ef2cb15823e873726905ca6def (accessed on 22nd July 2025).

43. Speiser, P., Arlt, W., Auchus, R. J., Baskin, L. S., Conway, G. S., Merke, D. P., Meyer-Bahlburg, H. F. L., et al. (2018). Congenital adrenal hyperplasia due to steroid 21-hydroxylase deficiency: An Endocrine Society* clinical practice guideline. *The Journal of Clinical Endocrinology & Metabolism, 103*, 4043–4088. https://doi.org/10.1210/jc.2018-01865 (accessed on 22nd July 2025).

44. Teede, H., Misso, M., Costello, M., Dokras, A., Laven, J. S. E., Moran, L., Piltonen, T., et al. (2018). Recommendations from the international evidence-based guideline for the assessment and management of polycystic ovary syndrome. *Clinical Endocrinology, 89*, 251–268. https://doi.org/10.1111/cen.13795 (accessed on 22nd July 2025).

45. Teede, H., Tay, C. T., Laven, J. J. E., Dokras, A., Moran, L., Piltonen, T., Costello, M., et al. (2023). Recommendations from the 2023 international evidence-based guideline for the assessment and management of polycystic ovary syndrome. *The Journal of Clinical Endocrinology & Metabolism, 108*, 2447–2469. https://doi.org/10.1210/clinem/dgad463 (accessed on 22nd July 2025).

46. Teede, H., Tay, C. T., Laven, J. S. E., Dokras, A., Moran, L., Piltonen, T., Costello, M., et al. (2023). Recommendations from the 2023 international evidence-based guideline for the assessment and management of polycystic ovary syndrome. *Fertility and Sterility, 120*, 767–793. https://doi.org/10.1016/j.fertnstert.2023.07.025 (accessed on 22nd July 2025).

47. Tsujimura, A., Iijima, M., Umemoto, Y., Kobayashi, H., Komiya, A., Shiraishi, K., Chiba, K., et al. (2025). Summary of the clinical practice guidelines for male infertility by the Japanese Urological Association with the support of the Japan Society for Reproductive Medicine. *International Journal of Urology: Official Journal of the Japanese Urological Association*. https://www.semanticscholar.org/paper/7af12992d588435adf39615a06a76cc9698fb282 (accessed on 22nd July 2025).

48. Vahedi Raad, M., Firouzabadi, A. M., Tofighi Niaki, M., Henkel, R., & Fesahat, F. (2024). The impact of mitochondrial impairments on sperm function and male fertility: A systematic review. *Reproductive Biology and Endocrinology: RB&E, 22*. https://www.semanticscholar.org/paper/546278f8570ad15aa962ed79b41e35a5e5045eb2 (accessed on 22nd July 2025).

49. Viscardi Azevedo, B., Marques, J. M., Trigueiro, N., Yariwake, V., Veras, M., Tamashiro, L. K., Cruz, R., et al. (2024). Fertility induction associated with improved peripheral reproductive parameters in male *Prop1df/df* mice subjected to GH and levothyroxine replacement. *Archives of Endocrinology and Metabolism, 68*. https://www.semanticscholar.org/paper/4b25f79bb602f0021320ce0962f4aeefbb1787b1 (accessed on 22nd July 2025).

50. Walker, T. (2024). Progress in the study of toxic effects of drugs on the male reproductive system. *Asia-Pacific Journal of Pharmacotherapy & Toxicology*. https://www.semanticscholar.org/paper/f18f1e18db9170f0ceec3370fd1c12e4eb536f27 (accessed on 22nd July 2025).

51. Yassin, M., Mwafy, S., & Laqqan, M. (2025). Association of obesity with reproductive hormones alterations, DNA fragmentation and protamine deficiency in human spermatozoa. *Middle East Fertility Society Journal*. https://www.semanticscholar.org/paper/a302c8f099427a865fc70b9a9f43629fd4c88729 (accessed on 22nd July 2025).

52. Yin, J., Ye, Y., Gao, Y., Xu, Q., Su, M., Sun, S., Xu, W., et al. (2025). Low-dose ionizing radiation and male reproductive immunity: Elucidating subtle modulations and long-term health implications. *International Journal of Molecular Sciences, 26*. https://www.semanticscholar.org/paper/686ffb6365502024ad4fe7c340a858a5c948e7b2 (accessed on 22nd July 2025).

53. Zheng, Y., Bai, H., Zhao, G. C., Tian, K., Yue, J., Li, D., Jiang, X., et al. (2025). Comparison of outcomes between pulsatile gonadotropin releasing hormone and combined gonadotropin therapy of spermatogenesis in patients with congenital hypogonadotropic hypogonadism. *Reproductive Biology and Endocrinology: RB&E, 23*. https://www.semanticscholar.org/paper/8957c21aa9cb7286b63cc77a593671b8940bba84 (accessed on 22nd July 2025).

REPRODUCTIVE ENDOCRINOLOGY (FEMALE)

7

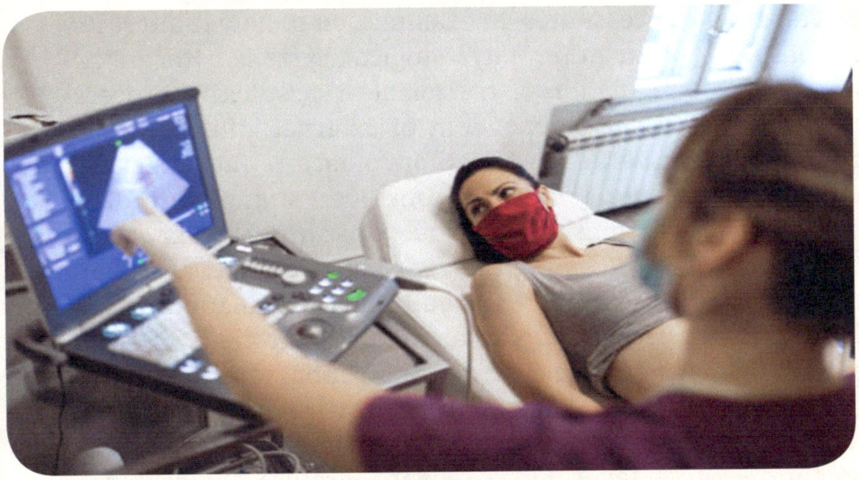

LEARNING OBJECTIVES

After studying this chapter, you will be able to:

1. Understand the anatomy of the female reproductive system;
2. Discuss about hormonal regulation of the menstrual cycle;
3. Describe common disorders in female reproductive endocrinology;
4. Explain diagnostic techniques in reproductive endocrinology;
5. Deal with treatment options for hormonal imbalances;
6. Focus on advances in reproductive technology.

Introduction

Reproductive endocrinology is a key specialty encompassing the hormonal interaction affecting female reproductive health and fertility. Throughout women's reproductive years, the complexity of hormonal regulation is more apparent. Several factors including age, body composition, and prior conditions greatly influence hormonal balance and consequently reproductive outcome. For instance, body adiposity excess is linked to a range of reproductive dysfunctions, highlighting the intricate relationship between obesity and menstrual characteristics. It has been established that not only adiposity parameters in general but even central adiposity correlate strongly with key reproductive hormones such as estrogen, progesterone, and prolactin, highlighting the necessity of the understanding of these dynamics for women's health (Ezeala et al., 2025). The theory of ovarian reserve is the foundation of reproductive endocrinology and defines the number and quality of a woman's remaining oocytes. It is a significant concept because its relationship with fertility potential is straight forward and becomes all the more relevant during the trend of delayed childbearing. Decreased ovarian reserve (DOR) is extremely difficult to treat, affecting the potential of conception and necessitating thorough assessment and treatment modalities. Each of these markers is used to assess ovarian reserve, with anti-Müllerian hormone levels and antral follicle count being most central to clinical evaluation. These markers offer clinicians important information regarding ovarian function, even if variability in results based on such factors as hormonal contraceptives and body composition make clinical life more difficult (Ufnal et al., 2025). Through integration of knowledge based in reproductive endocrinology, clinicians can gain a deeper understanding of the interrelatedness of hormonal health, ovarian reserve, and fertility problems. More recent interventions, such as lifestyle modifications and new therapies, offer the promise of optimizing reproductive results in women with compromised fertility potential. With continued unfolding of female reproductive health, future research will have to strive to refine assessment tools as well as to explore the broad range of determinants of ovarian function and hormonal regulation. To address these challenges in the field of reproductive endocrinology is to give women a complete experience addressing their own unique reproductive journeys.

Definition of Reproductive Endocrinology

The discipline of reproductive endocrinology is primarily devoted to the complex interaction between hormones and female reproductive physiology. It encompasses the study of various hormones like estrogens, progesterone, and gonadotropins that are crucial in regulating the menstrual cycle, ovulation, and pregnancy. This is an important discipline to understand not just normal reproductive physiology but also reproductive disorder pathophysiology. By the elucidation of hormonal interactions and their downstream effects, reproductive endocrinology illuminates such conditions as polycystic ovary syndrome (PCOS), endometriosis, and infertility. Furthermore, advances in reproductive endocrinology have far-reaching implications in reproductive health, informing therapies that enhance fertility and maximize control of hormonal imbalance, ultimately resolving women's health outcomes. Understanding the intricacies of reproductive endocrinology further necessitates an examination of how it interacts with other physiological systems. Hormonal regulation of the female reproductive process is not independent of external influence; it is governed by a plethora of factors, including age, heredity, and environmental stimuli. Circadian rhythms, for instance, are an important factor in regulating the reproductive cycle, including the estrus cycle and timing of ovulation. These biological cycles and their connections with the endocrine system are essential to reproductive success, aligning reproductive events with the most advantageous environmental conditions. As taken up in recent literature, the research highlights the importance of an integrated approach to reproductive health, examining how external body rhythms can affect hormonal pathways and consequently fertility and pregnancy outcomes (Boden et al., 2013). Besides, the field of reproductive endocrinology is constantly evolving on the basis of research development and new findings that expand our understanding of women's reproductive well-being. Out of this research emerged novel diagnostic technologies and treatments that have enabled clinicians to treat a variety of reproductive health ailments more effectively. For example, hormone-targeted therapies have undergone a significant evolution due to improved hormonal profiling and customized treatment strategies. The ongoing pursuit of knowledge in reproductive endocrinology not only assists in uncovering solutions to current reproductive health problems but also makes way for upcoming innovations that could enhance women's fertility and reproductive health in general. Thus, as an emerging domain of research, reproductive endocrinology will remain a crucial determinant in formulating women's healthcare policies (Arnold et al., 2001) (Figure 7.1).

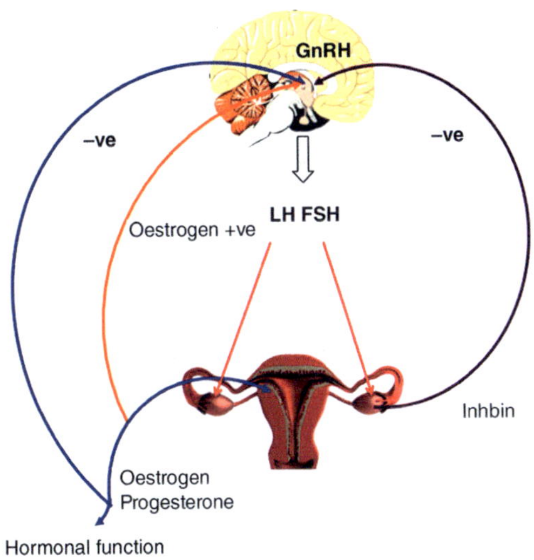

Figure 7.1. Female reproductive endocrinology. GnRH released from the hypothalamus stimulates the release of luteinizing hormone (LH) and follicle-stimulating hormone (FSH) from the anterior pituitary.

Source: https://i0.wp.com/basicmedicalkey.com/wp-content/uploads/2020/04/c03f002.gif?w=960.

Importance of Female Reproductive Health

The significance of women's reproductive health extends far beyond mere capability to bear and conceive children. It encompasses a complex array of biological, physiological, and psychological elements that are essential to women's overall health and well-being. Accurate understanding of reproductive endocrinology reinforces the fact that hormonal balance is the basis on which this health rests. Hormones like estrogen and progesterone, instrumental in managing the menstrual cycle and maintaining pregnancy, are also part of various bodily systems. Dysregulation of these hormones causes reproductive diseases, including polycystic ovary syndrome (PCOS) and endometriosis. These conditions not only affect fertility but also have far-reaching implications for metabolic health, implying that a woman's reproductive well-being is irrevocably tied to her overall physiological condition. Those endocrine imbalances, therefore, are capable of being treated with appropriate medical intervention, hence enhancing the quality of life of women, and therefore the significance of target healthcare strategies. In addition, awareness of the impact caused by endocrine disruption is significant in regard to environmental and lifestyle determinants for women's reproductive well-being. Endocrine-disrupting chemicals (EDCs) are likely to lead to less-than-optimally reproductive outcomes because evidence shows that such chemicals impersonate or interfere with hormone-related processes. Studies on the potential impacts of EDCs indicate a call for greater awareness and legislation to prevent exposure. To illustrate, whereas studies on vertebrates have indicated significant reproductive harm through exposure to EDCs, effects on invertebrates such as shore crabs have indicated patterns of endocrine disruption that are somewhat distinct from vertebrates (Brian et al., 2005). Thus, more research on the drugs is needed to develop effective public health policies that will protect women's reproductive health more generally. Finally, encouraging women's reproductive health should also be culturally responsive and focus on addressing access to health care services. Many women have economic constraints, ignorance, and stigma that block their accesses to essential reproductive health services. Offering universal coverage for healthcare, reproductive health education, and access to medical facilities like contraceptives and fertility therapy are fundamental. Coupled with this, fighting against system issues like gender imbalance in healthcare can empower women to make informed decisions on their reproductive rights. Initiatives promoting sexual education and open discussion about reproductive health at the community level can breed an educated populace, contributing to a healthier society in the long run. Hence, the worth of women's reproductive health transcends personal well-being to encompass broader public health, economic stability, as well as social justice in society (Figure 7.2).

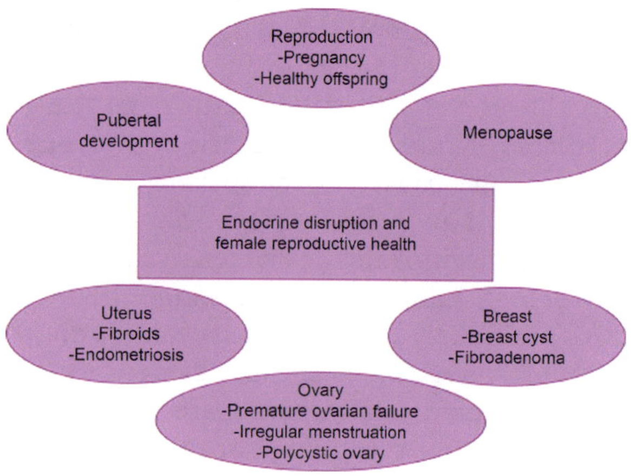

Figure 7.2. Endocrine disruption and female reproductive health.

Source: https://ars.els-cdn.com/content/image/3-s2.0-B9780128011393000089-f08-01-9780128011393.jpg.

Overview of Hormonal Regulation in Women

The endocrine regulation in females is a highly complex interaction of multiple endocrine glands with primary functions by the hypothalamus, pituitary gland, ovaries, and adrenal glands. The intricate mechanism enables precise regulation of reproductive processes, including the menstrual cycle, ovulation, and pregnancy. Gonadotropin-releasing hormone (GnRH), secreted by the hypothalamus, stimulates the release of follicle-stimulating hormone (FSH) and luteinizing hormone (LH) from the anterior pituitary. These hormones then influence the ovaries to cause growth of follicles and subsequent secretion of progesterone and estrogen. This regulatory hierarchy needs to be appreciated because dysregulation is often the cause of conditions such as polycystic ovary syndrome (PCOS) or ovarian insufficiency that can have a profound impact on women's reproductive health and general wellbeing, highlighting the importance of hormonal equilibrium in women's health. Furthermore, both progesterone and estrogen have key roles in the regulation of many aspects of physiology outside of reproduction. Estrogen is essential to secondary sexual development, bone mass, and cardiovascular regulation. Progesterone, meanwhile, is key to making the endometrium receptive to potential implantation and pregnancy maintenance. The fluctuation of these hormones through the menstrual cycle, then, not only signifies reproductive readiness but influences mood and mental function as well. The dynamic nature of these hormone fluctuations is to highlight the need for holistic treatment of menstrual irregularities and other hormonal imbalance, hence giving priority to the broader implications of reproductive endocrinology in the management of women. To this hormonal state is added the activity of other hormones, such as the androgens and adrenal gland hormones. While androgens are classically associated with male physiology, women produce them in lesser quantities, but those that are important to libido and overall energy. The adrenal glands contribute to this hormonal state through the secretion of hormones like cortisol, which is a role in stress. In addition, age, health status, and way of life could potentially have an effect on the hormonal balance of women. Understanding this holistic approach is integral, especially in the context of ongoing research into contraceptive methods, as discussed in prior research, Alsaadi et al. (2013) and established male reproductive endocrinology principles as a comparative model (Clavijo et al., 2018). Such data offers useful context to the field of reproductive endocrinology, shedding light on the unique hormonal complexities characteristic to women's health.

7.1. Anatomy of the Female Reproductive System

Learning Outcome

1. Understand structure and function of ovaries;
2. Explain the role of the fallopian tubes;
3. Discuss the importance of the uterus and endometrium.

The female reproductive system is a sophisticated collection of reproductive organs specialized for menstrual cycling, hormonal regulation, and reproduction. The central organ is the ovary, which produces the ova and secretes hormones such as estrogen and progesterone. Not only do they regulate the menstrual cycle but also play crucial roles in maintaining pregnancy and regulating secondary sexual characteristics. Fallopian tubes, extending from the ovary to the uterus, are the pathways for egg transport and site of fertilization. The uterus, characterized by its muscular walls, is the nurturing place for the developing embryo, readjusting itself each month for potential implantation. In the beauty of the anatomy of the female reproductive system, one enjoys the fine balance of the hormonal cues to facilitate successful reproduction and overall female health that is at the core of the overall theme in reproductive endocrinology. Holding the anatomical structures together is the histological composition that defines their functional qualities and traits. The ovaries are encapsulated by a germinal epithelium and contain primordial follicles that ripen during a woman's reproductive years. This process is tightly regulated by hormonal communication that originates in the anterior pituitary gland, including follicle-stimulating hormone (FSH) and luteinizing hormone (LH). The cyclical change of the ovaries is accompanied by endometrial lining changes in the uterus that are correspondingly responsive to the hormonal milieu determined by the ovulatory cycle. All phases of the menstrual cycle predispose the uterus to potential implantation and are also related to changes in vaginal discharge, uterine contractions, and other bodily functions. Normal anatomy, histology, and physiology of these organs all graphically illustrate the complexity of female reproductive endocrinology, how hormonal variation controls a multidimensional reproductive capacity (Justin et al., 2018). Significantly, understanding of embryological development in the female reproductive system enhances familiarity with potential reproductive disorders. The embryological development in the fetus of the female reproductive system occurs during a time when differentiation is influenced by genetic and environmental factors. For instance, changes of the hormonal environment during this time are able to cause congenital anomalies such as congenital adrenal hyperplasia, affect the equilibrium of sex steroids, and lead to failure of the reproductive system. The puberty age, which marks the onset of reproductive capacity, varies among individuals and is dependent on environmental influences such as diet and exposure to endocrine disruptors. Successful treatment of disorders of the reproductive endocrine is critical in the restoration of normal function and maximum health, as outlined in clinical practice guidelines (Speiser et al., 2018). Thus, the anatomical details of the female reproductive system not only provide a complete understanding of the functions but also are crucial in addressing the myriads of health issues that can arise.

7.1.1. Structure and Function of Ovaries

The structure of the ovary is central to ovarian function within the female reproductive system. Composed of a cortex and a medulla, the ovaries are filled with numerous developing follicles, each containing an oocyte, or immature egg. The ovarian follicles go through numerous stages, including primordial, primary, secondary, and tertiary, before ovulation, when a fully developed ovum is released. Such intricate architecture not only supports the maturation of oocytes but also contributes fundamentally to hormone release. Follicles release estrogen and progesterone that are vital in regulating the menstrual cycle and maintaining pregnancy. Cumulatively, the hierarchical organization of these ovarian structures lies at the heart of the reproductive endocrinology overall, affecting not just fertility but broader physiological ramifications in females throughout their reproductive life (Figure 7.3).

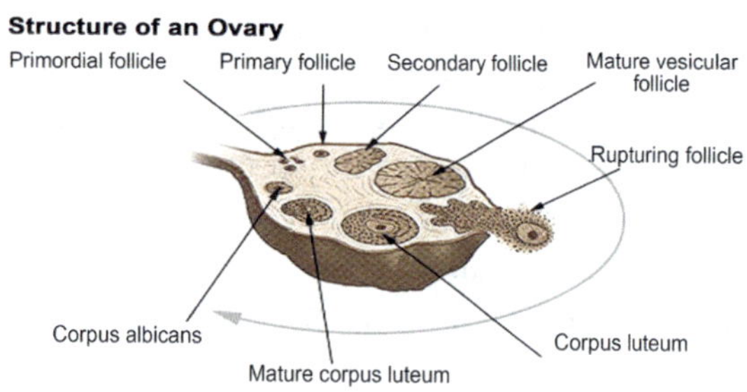

Figure 7.3. Structure of ovary.

Source: https://training.seer.cancer.gov/images/anatomy/reproductive/ovary.jpg.

The function of the ovaries is more than their role in producing oocytes; they are an important endocrine system that regulates a lot of women's health. Gonadotropins, primarily luteinizing hormone (LH) and follicle-stimulating hormone (FSH), secreted by the anterior pituitary gland stimulate ovarian function. This interaction of hormones is important to follicular maturation and ovulation. As mentioned in sturgeon research, the activities of FSH and LH in follicular growth and steroidogenesis are important, wherein their supplementation can significantly impact ovarian dynamics (Aizen et al., 2016). Moreover, ovarian endocrine function influences other physiological functions aside from reproduction, such as bone density and mood regulation, further linking ovarian function to overall health and well-being. Hence, the ovarian hormonal controls are of fundamental significance in the endocrinology of female reproduction. Local control within the ovaries also plays a significant role in the regulation of ovarian function. A case in point is the neuropeptide RFRP3, which is present both in the hypothalamus and in the ovaries, and has been observed to inhibit the secretion of gonadotropins and, by association, the growth of follicles and steroidogenesis. Experiments in domestic cats have indicated expression of RFRP3 and its receptors in the ovarian tissue, suggesting a function in maintenance of follicular integrity and survival (Bentley et al., 2019). The nuanced interaction betrays the complexity of ovarian function, integrating systemic hormonal signals and local mechanisms in the control of reproductive life. Understanding these interactions is essential, not just to reproductive health, but in formulating methods in wildlife conservation and population control, and therefore determining the bigger picture in ovarian function in species in general (Figure 7.4).

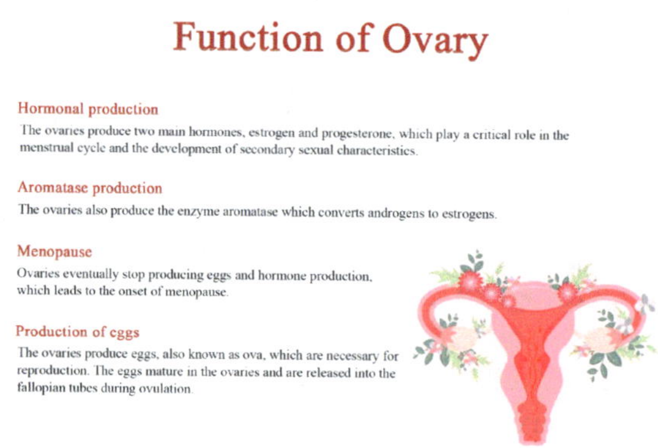

Figure 7.4. Functions of ovary.

Source: https://assets.lybrate.com/imgs/tic/enadp/functions-of-ovary.webp.

7.1.2. Role of the Fallopian Tubes

The fallopian tubes are the key structures in female reproductive endocrinology, and their primary role is the transport of oocytes and spermatozoa. The two structures have a strategic location to hold up the oocyte released from the ovary in the menstrual cycle, and their fimbriae play a crucial role in this context. After fertilization, which normally occurs in the ampulla of the fallopian tube, the zygote traverses the tube to the uterus for implantation. This is a required passage since any distortion or obstruction in the anatomy and physiology of the fallopian tubes will cause infertility or ectopic pregnancies, and their significant function in reproductive health becomes evident. Lastly, understanding the dynamics of fallopian tube function is used to highlight the interdependence of the reproductive endocrine system. Also, the impact of hormones on the fallopian tubes plays a crucial role in regulating their function. Estrogen and progesterone, in particular, control the motility of the ciliated epithelial cells of the tubes, which has implications for the transport processes that are part of both gamete interaction and embryo transit. The cyclical fluctuations of these hormones regulate not just the timing of ovulation but also prepare the uterine environment for potential implantation of an embryo. Any hormone irregularities, such as in cases of disorders like polycystic ovary syndrome, can result in dysfunctional fallopian tubes, thereby affecting fertility levels (N/A, 2022). Investigating these pathways of hormones illuminates more about the mechanisms of reproductive well-being and emphasizes the significance of endocrine balance within the female reproductive system. In addition, existing research has also investigated the possible influence of environmental factors on the normal functioning of the fallopian tubes, centering on exposure to nanoparticles and other chemicals. They have been studied to penetrate more than one biological barrier and get deposited within reproductive tissues, having a damaging effect on fertility by destroying the physical integrity of the fallopian tubes and disrupting hormonal communication (Wang et al., 2018). Exposure may lead to oxidative stress and inflammation, having a deleterious effect on the motility and reactivity of the tubes, thus impairing their basic functions. These findings suggest an urgent need for further investigation of the ways in which environmental toxins not only affect the reproductive health of individuals but also influence broader public reproductive endocrinology policies. The understanding of these interfaces will be essential for designing methods of minimizing risks to women's reproductive health (Figure 7.5).

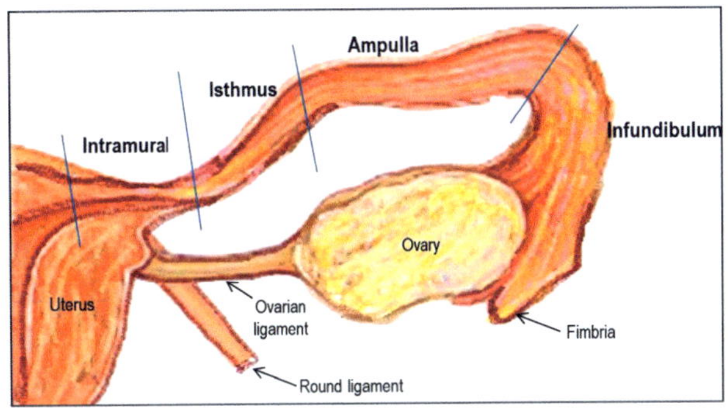

Figure 7.5. Drawing demonstrating the fallopian tube segments.

Source: https://www.researchgate.net/profile/Teresa-Cunha-3/publication/264763891/figure/fig1/AS:295831862300675@1447543220494/Drawing-demonstrating-the-fallopian-tube-segments.png.

7.1.3. Importance of the Uterus and Endometrium

The endometrium and uterus serve crucial roles in female reproductive biology, providing the structural and functional basis for conception and pregnancy to be successful. The endometrium, a mucous membrane overgrowth of the uterus, undergoes cyclic hormone-controlled alterations throughout the menstrual cycle. These hormonal alterations prepare the endometrium for potential implantation of an embryo and are thus critical to fertility. In addition, the endometrial tissue takes a key position in the physiology of pregnancy and menstruation, actively responding to both the presence of a fertilized ovum and to hormonal signals. Thus, disruptions in the endometrium can lead to very serious reproductive health problems, including infertility and conditions such as endometriosis. The current research on endometrial biology emphasizes its pivotal role within the field of reproductive endocrinology, confirming the immediate impact its health has on female reproductive success in general. Current research into the immunological function of the endometrium has revealed intriguing correlations between its cellular composition and reproductive outcome. Research indicates that B cells, a minor cell population of the human cycling endometrium, play pivotal functions in local immune processes during implantation. These immune competent cells are crucial to both maternal immune tolerance and defense against infection. Pathologies such as chronic endometritis have highlighted the importance of better understanding the immune mechanisms of the endometrium. Furthermore, B cells have a role beyond immunity and participate in the repair and regeneration of endometrium required for embryo implantation. And thus, the study of the immune microenvironment of the endometrium, the B cell lineage in particular, sheds more light on the issues and complexities of reproductive health and pregnancy maintenance (Kitaya, 2025). The evolution in regenerative medicine and tissue engineering has also put more stress on the significance of the uterine environment in reproductive endocrinology. Recent studies on decellularized uterus extracellular matrix (UEM) and its capacity to promote endometrial organoid growth highlight the intricate interplay between structure and function in tissue. UEM was reported to enhance epithelial regeneration as well as pregnancy rates in endometrial injury models, suggesting it as a therapy. Proteomic analysis highlights the functions of specific proteins, such as fibronectin and decorin, in supporting endometrial development and function, further illustrating the dynamic role of these extracellular matrix molecules in the reproductive process (Cha et al., 2024). This novel approach not only makes blastocyst implantation easy to understand but also lays the path open to advanced treatment of infertility and other reproductive diseases. Finally, uterus and endometrium are irreplaceable in reproductive endocrinology whose health and functioning significantly determine women's fertility and general reproductive success (Figure 7.6).

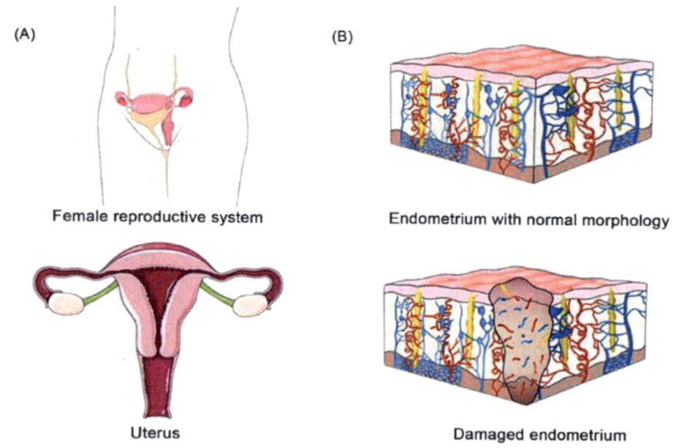

Figure 7.6. Diagram of the uterus and the structure of the endometrium. The endometrium includes veins, arteries, and many glands that, if damaged, can affect fertility-related functions. (A) Normal morphology of the uterus; (B) schematic diagram of the structural stratification and damage of the endometrium.

Source: https://www.researchgate.net/publication/368310661/figure/fig1/AS:11431281246062668@1716282865982/Diagram-of-the-uterus-and-the-structure-of-the-endometrium-The-endometrium-includes.png.

Test Your Knowledge

1. What are the key structural components of the ovaries?
2. How does the process of follicular development within the ovaries contribute to the menstrual cycle and ovulation?
3. What are the major layers of the uterus?

7.2. Hormonal Regulation of the Menstrual Cycle

Learning Outcome

1. Explain the phases of the menstrual cycle;
2. Understand the role of gonadotropin-releasing hormone (GnRH);
3. Describe the interaction between estrogen and progesterone.

Control of the menstrual cycle is a balanced interaction of several hormones that choreograph the physiological activity occurring within the female reproductive system. At the orchestra's center are the ovaries, pituitary gland, and hypothalamus, which work in harmony cyclically to enable successful ovulation and endometrial preparation for potential implantation. In the initial stage of the cycle, the hypothalamus releases gonadotropin-releasing hormone (GnRH), triggering the anterior pituitary to release follicle-stimulating hormone (FSH) and luteinizing hormone (LH). The gonadotropins induce ovarian follicles to mature and to release estrogen, primarily estradiol, to continue regulating the cycle by inhibiting the secretion of FSH but encouraging LH in a positive feedback system. This balance gives an indication of the importance of changes in hormones for reproductive integrity and fertility. During the course of the menstrual cycle, the role of progesterone is central, most notably the luteal phase. The ovulation, which is triggered by a surge in LH, results in the ruptured follicle being transformed into the corpus luteum that secretes the hormone progesterone. The hormone plays a vital role in preparing the endometrium for implantation of a fertilized egg by maintaining the uterine lining intact. In the absence of fertilization, the corpus luteum is destroyed, leading to a reduction in the levels of progesterone and estrogen, ultimately to the loss of the endometrial lining, which is called menstruation. These hormones are also controlled by metabolic and energy status, as is clear from research that indicates leptin and insulin as influential factors between reproductive and metabolic hormones and that reflects the close association between energy status and reproduction (Dynnik et al., 2025). Moreover, the contribution of mineral intakes towards hormonal regulation has also witnessed significant advancements. Minerals like selenium, magnesium, and zinc are essential in playing numerous reproductive roles such as hormone production and ensuring regular menstruation. Recent research highlights that poor mineral intake is likely to interfere with the balance of hormones, thereby resulting in reproductive disorders like polycystic ovary syndrome, among other reproductive disorders. By examining the effect of minerals on hormonal health, clinicians can potentially develop nutritional recommendations that can enhance the fertility of women, on a specific basis for different stages of the menstrual cycle. Such a precise study indicates that considering nutrition in the context of hormonal regulation can yield further information about optimizing reproductive health and thereby fill a critical need in current reproductive endocrinology literature (Kapper et al., 2024).

7.2.1. Phases of the Menstrual Cycle

The menstrual cycle represents an interactive dynamic balance between hormonal and physiological events occurring in the female reproductive tract and typically lasting approximately 28 days. The menstrual cycle has traditionally been divided into four phases: the menstrual phase, the follicular phase, the ovulatory phase, and the luteal phase. The menstrual phase is the shedding of the uterine lining, which occurs when endocrine support, primarily by progesterone, diminishes. Following menstruation, the follicular phase begins when the growth of ovarian follicles induced by follicle-stimulating hormone (FSH) occurs. Estradiol levels increase during this period as the dominant follicle develops, in preparation for potential ovulation. These phases are worth comprehending, as they can forecast a series of health outcomes, more specifically concerning reproductive endocrinology and the corresponding cognitive capacity, showing the definitive relationship between the fluctuation of the hormones and overall well-being throughout the cycle (Egli et al., 2017). Throughout continued development of the cycle, ovulation occurs approximately halfway through, where a spike in luteinizing hormone (LH) triggers the expulsion of a matured egg from the ovary. This ovulatory phase is significant when it comes to fertility due to the fact that the egg must be fertilized within a specific amount of time. Estrogen peaks in this phase and is responsible for physiological reactions such as cervical mucus production, promoting the movement of sperm. The luteal phase following ovulation is typically about 14 days long. During this phase, the corpus luteum forms, which secretes progesterone that is responsible for maintaining the uterine lining, in case of conception. Where there has been no fertilization, progesterone levels reduce, and the menstrual stage commences. The intricate regulation of the stages by hormones highlights their function not just in reproduction but also for potential impacts on women's health as the fluctuation in the levels of hormones will affect cognitive ability and mood (Anderson et al., 2017). The interaction between such phases often brings about enormous health outcomes, particularly in reproductive health, with regard to how external factors such as exercise and stress influence it. Overexercise and loss of energy, which is very common among sportswomen, has been shown to interfere with the hormonal equilibrium necessary for regular menstrual cycle. Conditions such as hypothalamic amenorrhea can be developed, highlighting the susceptibility of the hypothalamic-pituitary-gonadal (HPG) axis to the energy status of the person (Anderson et al., 2017). This disruption can lead not only to reproductive impairment but also affect bone status and psychological functioning, forming a part of the female athlete triad. Thus, understanding the phases of the menstrual cycle in the broader perspective of life determinants is key to developing plans for enhancing women's reproductive health and general health quality, representing the critical interdependence of reproductive endocrinology and physiological well-being (Egli et al., 2017) (Figure 7.7).

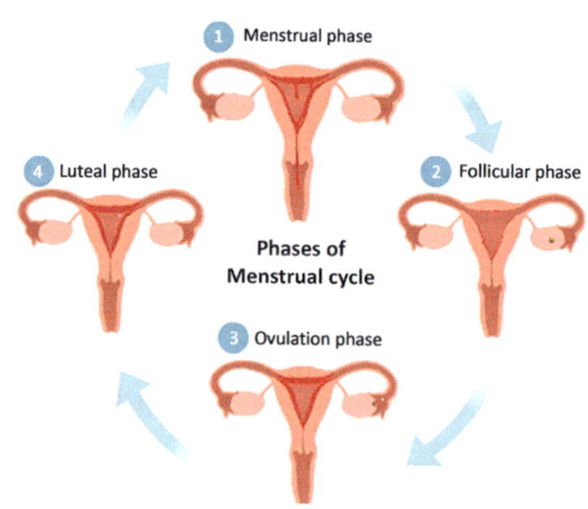

Figure 7.7. Menstrual phases.

Source: https://www.menstrupedia.com/assets/quickguide/physiology/pysiology-menstrual-phases.jpg.

7.2.2. Role of Gonadotropin-Releasing Hormone (GnRH)

Gonadotropin-Releasing Hormone (GnRH) is an initiator of the female reproductive endocrine cascade. It is secreted and released by the hypothalamus and functions as a crucial regulator of anterior pituitary release of gonadotropins, Follicle-Stimulating Hormone (FSH) and Luteinizing Hormone (LH). The gonadotropins play a crucial role in regulating ovarian functions including folliculogenesis and ovulation and thereby estrogen and progesterone synthesis directly. One of the characteristics of GnRH action is its pulsatile release, which is crucial to the balance and integrity of the reproductive system. An impairment in the pulsatile release of GnRH has been implicated in reproductive disease and highlights the role of GnRH as a gatekeeper for female reproductive health. This system of regulation enables both the endocrine and behavioral components of the reproductive cycle to be simultaneously coordinated so that reproduction can proceed successfully. The text with GnRH and other hormone signals also defines its importance in the female reproductive system. Recent research has unraveled the complex interplay between GnRH and neuroendocrine determinants, like kisspeptin, which controls GnRH neuron activity. For instance, estradiol produced during the menstrual cycle has a positive feedback effect on kisspeptin secretion, which subsequently stimulates GnRH release and leads to the LH surge necessary for ovulation. Furthermore, the roles of various molecular pathways of estrogen and progesterone in this control mechanism are under investigation. Signaling cascades coupled to GnRH have been found not only to influence reproductive capacity but also to play functions in other physiological responses, further demonstrating the multilateral effects of GnRH on female reproduction. These interactions affirm GnRHs pervasive role in reproductive endocrinology and its central importance to fertility. It is known that the broader use of GnRH also extends to agricultural and clinical settings. In cattle, for instance, alterations of GnRH dynamics exert a significant impact on reproductive performance as attested by evidence referencing decreased fertility in dairy cows with high yields. Long-term exposure to increased metabolic stress has been shown to be correlated with decreased estrous behaviors, which is inclined to suggest that GnRHs regulatory actions are highly determined by metabolic status. In addition, advances in the reproductive technologies, based on increased understanding of GnRH signal pathways, will introduce optimal schemes for breeding. This intersection of reproductive endocrinology and its application points to the necessity of continued investigation into GnRHs role, particularly in the context of emerging new reproductive issues in humans as well as farming. Knowledge gained through this ongoing research can pave the way for targeted therapies and interventions aimed at improving female reproductive health, validating the central position of GnRH in reproductive endocrinology (Bentley et al., 2016; Beerda et al., 2010) (Figure 7.8).

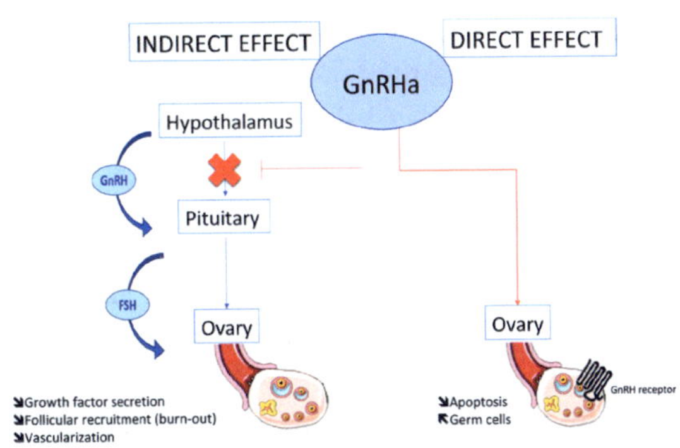

Figure 7.8. Gonadotropin-releasing hormone (GnRH) serves as an essential initiator of the reproductive endocrine cascade in female.

Source: https://patient9.com/wp-content/uploads/2023/02/Gonadotropin-Releasing-hormone.png.

7.2.3. Interaction of Estrogen and Progesterone

Estrogen and progesterone work together to play a key role in controlling female reproductive physiology. Both hormones are synthesized within the ovaries, where estrogen is synthesized primarily by maturing follicles and progesterone by the corpus luteum after ovulation. Estrogen is the key hormone in the proliferation and differentiation of the lining of the endometrium to prepare it for potential implantation of an embryo. Conversely, progesterone transforms proliferative endometrium into secretory after ovulation, to support implantation and early pregnancy. The subtle equilibrium between the hormones is indispensable for menstrual cycle function and fertility, with any variation leading to reproductive ailments such as amenorrhea or infertility. In addition, estrogen-progesterone interaction transcends simple hormonal equilibrium to complex molecular dynamics in ovary-target cells. Recent reports applying immunoprecipitation-mass spectrometry have identified a diverse set of proteins binding to progesterone receptors (PGR) in granulosa cells, particularly after luteinizing hormone (LH) surges that cause ovulation. The research identified coactivators that enhance PGR action as well as chaperone proteins whose removal might limit PGR activity. These isoform-specific interactions show how estrogen and progesterone build up a network of molecular signals amplifying the ovarian response to LH necessary for successful ovulation and the following luteal function, emphasizing the intricate interdependence of these hormones in reproductive endocrinology (Natalie et al., 2025). Environmental factors also have a significant impact on the hormonal balance of estrogen and progesterone that influences reproductive outcomes. One experiment that studied the effects of gasoline vapor exposure on the female Wistar rat found remarkable alterations in the levels of reproductive hormones, including reduced levels of estrogen and progesterone. This deficit was contrasted with honey intake, where not only was hormone balance regained but ovarian histology also improved. These findings illuminate the potential of exogenous forces in destabilizing the fine equilibrium between estrogen and progesterone towards malfunction in reproduction. It is important to understand such environmental effects so as to devise measures to counteract reproductive health hazards, emphasizing the need to conduct more research in how such interactions are regulated to enhance female reproductive health (Ridwanu et al., 2025) (Figure 7.9).

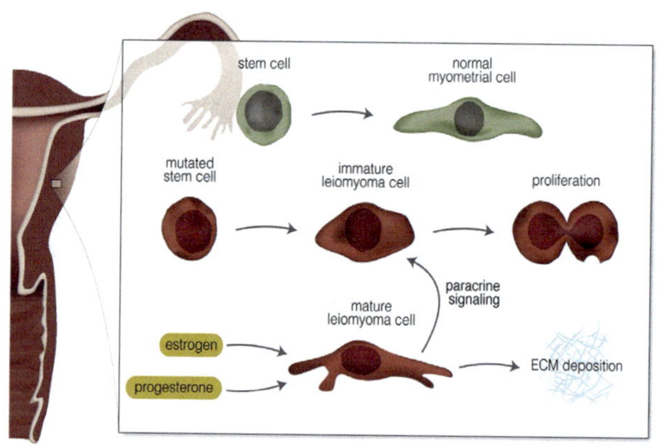

Figure 7.9. Diagrammatic representation of the roles of estrogen and progesterone in the pathogenesis of uterine fi broids.

Source: https://www.researchgate.net/profile/Enrrico-Bloise/publication/284797214/figure/fig1/AS:313993798406144@1451873363237/Diagrammatic-representation-of-the-roles-of-estrogen-and-progesterone-in-the-pathogenesis.png.

Test Your Knowledge

1. What are the four main phases of the menstrual cycle, and how are they hormonally regulated?
2. How does gonadotropin-releasing hormone (GnRH) from the hypothalamus control the secretion of FSH and LH during the menstrual cycle?

7.3. Common Disorders in Female Reproductive Endocrinology

Learning Outcome

1. Define polycystic ovary syndrome (PCOS);
2. Understand endometriosis;
3. Describe premenstrual dysphoric disorder (PMDD).

The interaction between body mass index (BMI) and various female reproductive diseases offers insight into significant topics of reproductive endocrinology. Of specific interest, it appears there is a strong genetic correlation between elevated BMI and other reproductive diseases, including endometrial cancer and gestational diabetes mellitus (GDM) (Shao et al., 2025). This correlation highlights the multi-dimensionality of the association between metabolic status and reproductive well-being, with the inference that the genetic factor may be underlying both illnesses. Pleiotropic loci shared pinpoint underlying biological mechanisms involved in RNA metabolism and pancreatic cell function, and therefore interventions aimed at BMI management are inferred to decrease the incidence or severity of these reproductive endocrine disorders. Prevention of female obesity would therefore not only improve overall health but offer a principal method for preventing risk factors for reproductive endocrine disorders, offering new targets for preventive therapy in women's health. Another prevalent disorder in female reproductive endocrinology is female hypogonadism (FH), which is characterized by the inadequate secretion of hormones due to multiple underlying factors. The condition is particularly prevalent in women who are of premenopausal age and could be caused due to premature ovarian insufficiency (POI) or hypothalamo-pituitary dysfunction (Jayasena et al., 2024). Treating FH is very challenging because guidelines do not adequately capture its numerous presentations, which lead to heterogeneity in practice. The present efforts at formulating integrated management plans highlight the necessity of a multidisciplinary approach involving specialists in endocrinology, gynecology, and reproductive health. This collaborative strategy will serve to benefit in the provision of an integrated model for the treatment of hypogonadism, potentially resulting in enhanced treatment outcomes in different patient contexts without compromising on individualized care coverage of both physiological and psychosocial dimensions. Apart from FH and its complications, other conditions such as polycystic ovary syndrome (PCOS) also portray a scenario of diversity in the case of female reproductive endocrine disorders. This intricate disorder is defined by hyperandrogenism, menstrual dysfunction, and polycystic ovaries and occurs in approximately 5–10% of reproductive-age women. The heightened prevalence of insulin resistance inherent in PCOS complicates its treatment, interconnecting metabolic and reproductive disturbances with abnormalities such as infertility and endometrial hyperplasia (Shao et al., 2025). As seen with ongoing discoveries about the endocrine and genetic pathways of PCOS, the development of treatments for this intricate disorder holds promise. Technological advancements in this field may not only alleviate symptoms but also overall reproductive health, and propose that a combined comprehension of female reproductive endocrinology can contribute to effective management and improve quality of life for those afflicted with these common disorders.

7.3.1. Polycystic Ovary Syndrome (PCOS)

Polycystic Ovary Syndrome (PCOS) is a complex endocrine disorder that affects a large percentage of women over the duration of their childbearing years. Characterized as being difficult to understand, PCOS is a triad of hyperandrogenism, ovulatory dysfunction, and the presence of polycystic ovaries. It is not merely a reproductive disorder, though, as it is also associated with chronic diseases such as type 2 diabetes and cardiovascular disease. Management for this disorder requires thorough knowledge of etiology and symptomatology to make proper diagnosis and management. The chronic nature of PCOS also complicates management, where a patient-focused strategy that combines lifestyle modification with pharmacotherapeutic measures is required to provide optimal results in affected individuals.

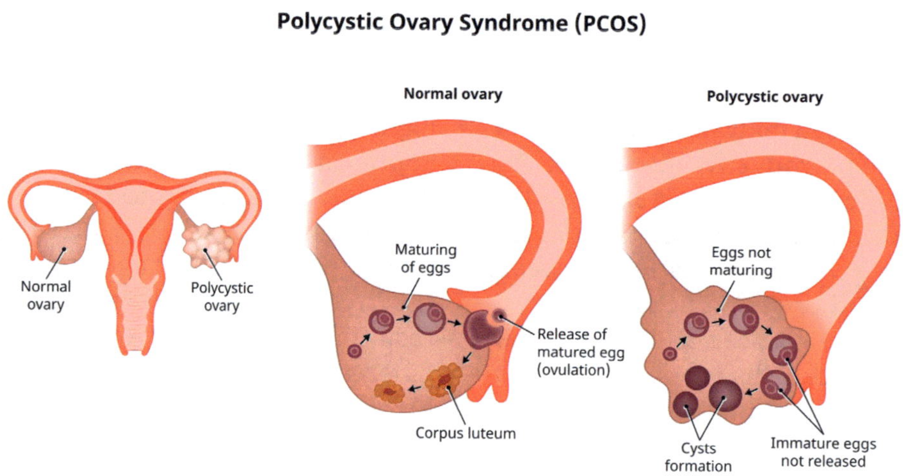

Figure 7.10. Diagram showing polycystic ovary syndrome (PCOS).

Source: https://cdn-assets-eu.frontify.com/s3/frontify-enterprise-files-eu/eyJwYXRoIjoiaWhoLWhlYWx0aGNhcmUtYmVyaGFkXC9maWxlXC96aEdCUm1VcXBCdHp4QUVZYnFiMi5qcGcifQ:ihh-healthcare-berhad:4Sd7u2CPOmdM7rtQYwsRuB6J_WcMj2S2sMcW_F3B9cE?format=webp.

There has been greater emphasis on cost-effective management of PCOS over the last few years, where therapeutic modalities are integrated with paradigms of chronic disease management. Vasudevan et al. (2025) discusses the need to capitalize on early diagnosis using primary care and establishing multidisciplinary clinics to provide comprehensive treatment. All these practices will attempt to make the treatment process less cumbersome without sacrificing on giving patients complete care that caters to their specific needs. Lifestyle changes like diet and routine physical exercise are usually recommended as first-line treatments because they can likely lower symptoms and improve overall health outcomes. In addition to these lifestyle changes, the use of pharmacologic treatments, such as generic drug therapy, is also central to the treatment of the complex presentations of PCOS in a cost-efficient and efficacious fashion. The changing diagnostic technologies also extend the range of management of PCOS, particularly through advances in machine learning approaches. As seen in Kumar et al. (2024), recent research has focused on non-invasive diagnostic systems that use clinical data to enhance the accuracy of PCOS classification. Through the application of various machine learning algorithms, researchers have significantly enhanced diagnostic sensitivity and specificity, thereby facilitating earlier detection of the syndrome. Hybridization of these models with optimization algorithms, such as Particle Swarm Optimization (PSO), has been surprisingly effective in making earlier and more accurate diagnosis possible. Not only are such developments better for the individual patient, but they can potentially revolutionize health care practitioners' approach to targeting PCOS, making more rational treatment decisions and improving quality of life for women with this exceedingly common endocrine disorder (Figure 7.10).

7.3.2. Endometriosis

Endometriosis is a significant health problem in women of reproductive age, often overlapping with infertility and chronic pelvic pain. Endometriosis is characterized by the growth of endometrial-like tissue outside the uterus, leading to a range of signs that can effectively jeopardize quality of life. It is a fascinating piece of information that between 6–10% women of reproductive age are affected, and of those with infertility, this percentage can rise to 25–35%. The pathophysiology of how endometriosis causes infertility is multifactorial and involves alteration of hormonal microenvironments, inflammatory responses, and disruption of ovarian dysfunction. Detailed understanding of these factors is necessary because effective management does not just involve the alleviation of symptoms but also addressing intrinsic reproductive problems. Treatment for endometriosis has evolved over the years in response to varying phases and presentations of the condition. From mild conservative hormone therapy to more invasive surgical options, particularly in the case of ovarian endometriomas (Salam et al., 2025), treatment options are highly diverse. Laparoscopic surgery, for instance, is a routine procedure used to remove endometriomas and adhesions and is a cornerstone for improving fertility in women who have severe symptoms. Current studies highlight the efficacy of combination treatment regimens, e.g., dienogest and atorvastatin, which have proven to be effective in ameliorating pain and reducing the size of endometrioma (Salam et al., 2025). Hence, tailoring treatment regimens according to patient profiles, including endometriosis severity and personal fertility goals, remains a crucial role of reproductive endocrinology. The intricate interaction of ovarian function and endometriosis further makes the reproductive scene more complex, emphasizing the true nature of holistic care intervention. Research has indicated that endometriosis not only impacts ovarian reserve but also decreases sensitivity to ovarian stimulation during ART treatment (Salam et al., 2025). This makes the achievement of successful pregnancy rates even more challenging and indicates the necessity for early detection and treatment. Doctors must adopt a comprehensive style of managing fertility that considers such aspects as hormonal examination and individual patient parameters, such as age and concomitant reproductive disease. With an expanding literature base, the improvement and development of treatment protocols to optimize reproductive outcomes among women battling the challenges posed by endometriosis are imperative (Figure 7.11).

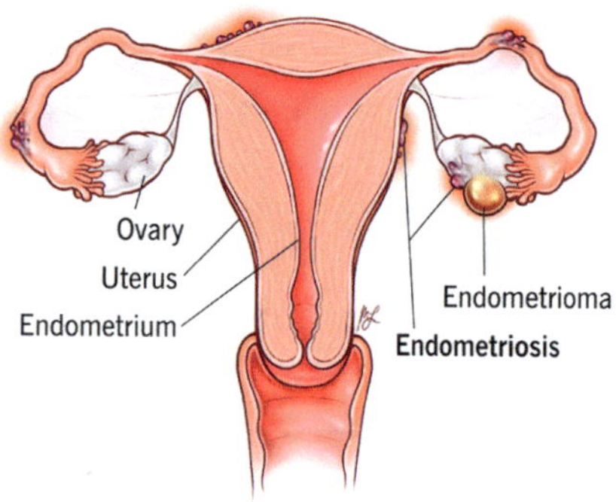

Figure 7.11. Illustration of endometriosis.

Source: https://my.clevelandclinic.org/-/scassets/images/org/health/articles/10857-endometriosis.

7.3.3. Premenstrual Dysphoric Disorder (PMDD)

Premenstrual Dysphoric Disorder (PMDD) is a disabling and hard-to-treat illness that occurs during the late luteal phase of the menstrual cycle, and is characterized by a pattern of emotional and somatic symptoms that significantly impair functioning. Affecting approximately 3–8% of menstruating women, PMDD represents more than the more common premenstrual syndrome (PMS), involving extreme disturbance of mood in the constellation of depression, anxiety, and irritability, along with physical complaints of fatigue and pain in the body. Diagnosis is often elusive since most doctors will likely fail to identify these symptoms because there are no certain biological markers. Improved insight into the impact of PMDD on quality of life is an imperative because the majority of individuals face challenges in their personal, academic, and professional life while coping with the distress of this disorder (Shahzad et al., 2025). New evidence has also indicated the broader impact of PMDD, and how it relates to other mental conditions, such as bipolar disorder and increased risks for suicidal thoughts. Women with PMDD typically report more depressive symptoms than the general population and are urgently in need of comprehensive mental health intervention. Socioeconomic status, a history of exposure to violence, and age have been noted as complicating factors for subjects with PMDD and underscore the need for multidisciplinary treatment modalities. Moreover, some studies suggest that PMDD may influence the chance of future perinatal depression, and therefore, treatment is required for not only the presenting symptoms but also long-term psychological consequences (Gupta et al., 2024). These multifaceted relationships justify the significance of PMDD in female reproductive endocrinology. PMDD treatment must be a multidisciplinary approach with respect to early diagnosis, increased awareness, and education regarding its influence on women's health. In the majority of the world, in nations like Pakistan, cultural taboo inhibits free exchange of information on menstruation and related disorders, and hence delays diagnosis and treatment. There is a need for immediate public awareness campaigns at all levels, particularly targeting men, to create a supportive environment for the targeted population. Initiatives targeted towards vulnerable groups in rural areas would enhance access to services, but the healthcare providers themselves must be adequately skilled to diagnose and manage PMDD effectively. In addition, more research on PMDDs prevalence and impact in various cultures will be necessary to further inform treatment approaches with the aim of improving the quality of life in so-affected individuals (Shahzad et al., 2025) (Figure 7.12).

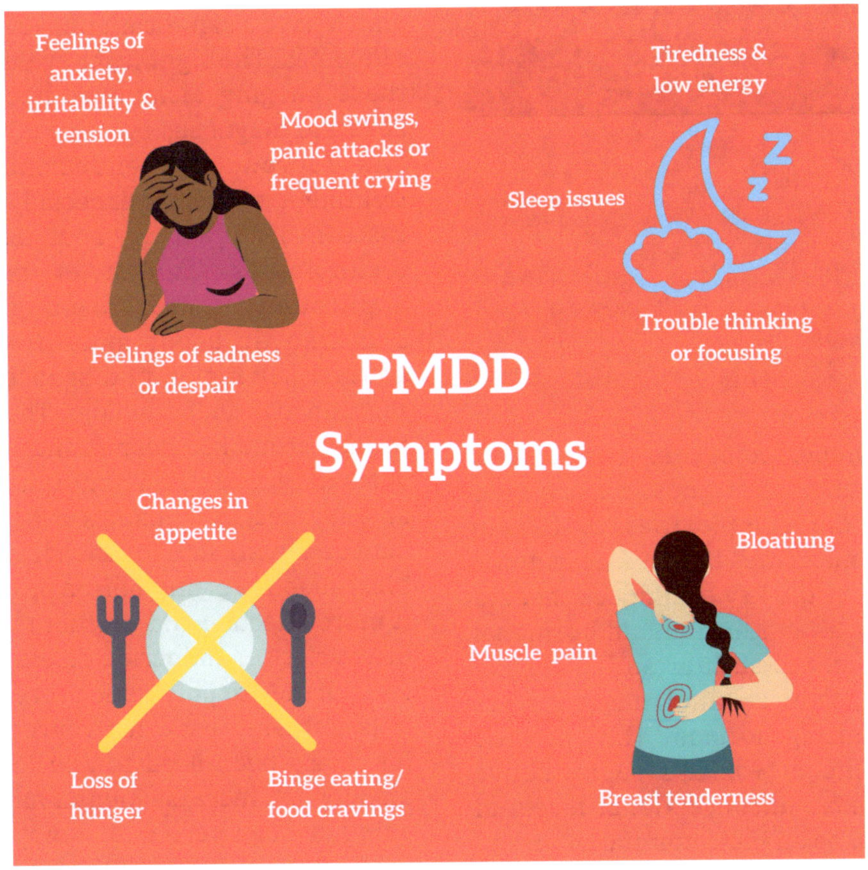

Figure 7.12. PMDD symptoms.

Source: https://www.hotteamama.com/cdn/shop/articles/PMDD_Symptoms_infographic.png?v=1712928867.

Test Your Knowledge

1. What are the key hormonal imbalances associated with Polycystic Ovary Syndrome (PCOS), and how do they affect ovulation and fertility?
2. How is Premenstrual Dysphoric Disorder (PMDD) different from premenstrual syndrome (PMS), and what are its primary psychological and physical symptoms?

7.4. Diagnostic Techniques in Reproductive Endocrinology

Learning Outcome

1. Discuss the assessment of hormonal blood tests for women facing fertility challenges;
2. Understand imaging techniques such as ultrasound and MRI in assessing female reproductive health;
3. Describe biopsy procedures.

Reproductive endocrinology is a discipline that employs a range of diagnostic techniques for unraveling the complexities of female infertility and endocrine diseases. Hormonal evaluation is one of the key techniques that aid in ascertaining ovarian function and hormonal balance. Key hormones such as anti-Müllerian hormone (AMH), follicle-stimulating hormone (FSH), and luteinizing hormone (LH) provide useful insight into a woman's reproductive status. For instance, unconventional levels of AMH and FSH can be an indicator of diminished ovarian reserve or primary ovarian insufficiency. These endocrine evaluations allow practitioners to create a specific treatment plan, such as controlled ovarian stimulation in patients with the mentioned conditions. The value of such testing is demonstrated in cases where tailored treatment protocols for *in vitro* fertilization (IVF) are designed to the hormonal profile, yielding higher success rates and assisting patients in improving certain reproductive disorders (Sanket et al., 2025). Apart from hormonal assessment, imaging techniques are part of reproductive endocrinology diagnostic protocols. Transvaginal ultrasound remains a first-line tool for imaging ovarian function, endometrial thickness, and any congenital defects that could impact fertility. Magnetic resonance imaging (MRI) is yet another sophisticated modality that further clarifies structural defects, including congenital uterine defects. For instance, MRI can illustrate defects like a unicornuate uterus, which have a significant impact on reproductive outcomes. The significant evaluation offered by these imaging techniques not only facilitates accurate diagnoses but also educates surgeons and reproductive endocrinologists during treatment planning, especially in complicated cases involving surgery or assisted reproductive technologies (Sanket et al., 2025). The application of micronized progesterone as a diagnostic agent and therapeutic tool is another key region of diagnostic techniques in reproductive endocrinology. This form of natural progesterone has been found to be effective in evaluating menstrual abnormality, for instance amenorrhea, as it enables withdrawal bleeding, hence enabling subsequent hormonal testing. The bioavailability of micronized progesterone makes it more effective and useful in the management of a variety of endocrine diseases from primary amenorrhea to polycystic ovary syndrome. Also, it is not only used for reproductive reasons, for it has been used to alleviate symptoms of anxiety and increase mental function in women going through peri- and menopause. The safety profile of micronized progesterone—specifically related to metabolic effects and cardiovascular risk—is desirable as an option for the treatment of reproductive-related conditions. With further research shedding light on its potential uses, micronized progesterone is set to open the door to new frontiers of diagnostic and therapeutic methods in reproductive endocrinology.

7.4.1. Hormonal Blood Tests

The analysis of hormonal blood work is a priority part of the reproductive endocrinology specialty, particularly among women of infertility. The hormonal blood tests assess major hormones such as estrogen, progesterone, and the other pituitary hormones to determine the hormonal climate affecting reproductive health. For instance, monitoring estradiol and progesterone levels can provide one with information regarding ovarian function, control of the menstrual cycle, and the prevalence of such conditions as polycystic ovary syndrome and endometriosis. The importance of such hormonal tests is emphasized by research evidence indicating significant correlations between hormone imbalance and female sexual dysfunction (FSD), which further aggravates reproductive outcomes. Specifically, patients with endometriosis had decreased estradiol levels compared to normal controls, implying how blood work for hormones can detect underlying issues that may prevent conception and successful pregnancy (Semeniuk et al., 2025). Furthermore, the diagnosis of hormonal profiles from blood work not only reflects reproductive health but also helps develop patient-specific treatment regimens. With the understanding of each patient's individual hormone levels, clinicians can design interventions that aim to restore hormonal balance and enhance fertility outcome. Profound changes in hormones during treatment were achieved in clinical trials in women with FSD and endometriosis, demonstrating the responsiveness of hormonal profiles to treatment. For example, with continued therapy, notable increases in estradiol were seen among women without endometriosis, but those who had endometriosis continued to present with hormone abnormalities following treatment. This implies that hormone blood tests are not only reserved for diagnosis purposes; they play a significant role in continuous monitoring and adjustment of treatment protocols in reproductive health care (Semeniuk et al., 2025). In addition to hormonal assessment, advances in reproductive endocrinology over the past few years have been characterized by endocrinological assessments based on the synthesis of hormonal measurement and observational methods. As an example, research on shark reproductive biology has utilized blood sampling to investigate the relation of estrogen to reproductive maturity, illustrating the taxonomic generality of hormonal insight. The knowledge gained through hormonal testing has extensive implications in the management of reproductive health in women, particularly when conception should happen and when hormonal imbalance that can affect the viability of pregnancy needs to be determined. Therefore, integrating hormonal blood testing into a general model of reproductive health not only assists with assessing immediate problems but also allows for preventive care to mitigate risks surrounding FSD and infertility (Figure 7.13).

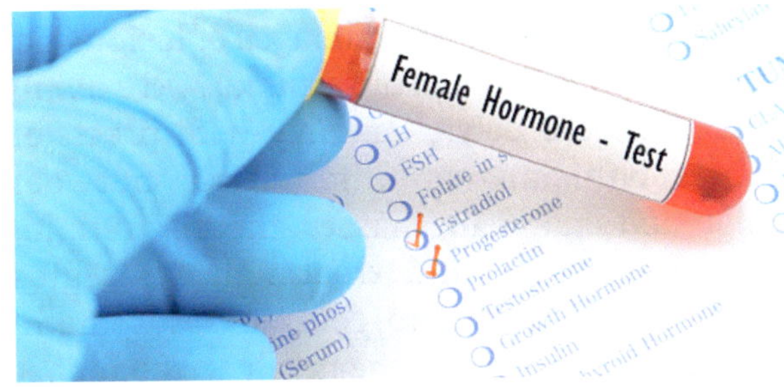

Figure 7.13. Hormonal blood tests play a crucial role in the field of reproductive endocrinology in females.

Source: https://diagnear.com/files/blog_images/1050x500/FEMALE_HORMONE__TEST_2.png.

7.4.2. Imaging Techniques (Ultrasound, MRI)

Imaging modalities such as MRI and ultrasound play a central role in reproductive endocrinology in the assessment of female reproductive health. Ultrasound, being non-invasive, is particularly renowned for its application in providing real-time imaging of the pelvic organs and fetal development. The technique is well-capable of monitoring conditions such as ovarian cysts, uterine fibroids, and reproductive abnormalities, which significantly impact fertility and overall hormonal function. For instance, research has noted the effectiveness of high-frequency ultrasound in tracking menstrual cycle structural changes to the advantage of practitioners making diagnoses for any type of menstrual abnormality. Moreover, ultrasounds application also overlaps with obstetrics, where it estimates gestational age and identifies potential congenital abnormalities, thus facilitating early medical intervention and enhancing maternal-fetal health outcomes (Brunetti et al., 2019). Magnetic resonance imaging (MRI) complements ultrasound in the landscape of reproductive imaging by offering superior soft tissue contrast. This imaging modality is particularly beneficial in evaluating complex gynecological conditions such as endometriosis, where it provides detailed images of lesions not typically visible through ultrasound. MRI's ability to visualize the pelvic anatomy with precision enables clinicians to differentiate between benign and malignant masses, thereby refining surgical planning and treatment strategies. The addition of MRI to routine assessments of female reproductive health has broadened the diagnostic capabilities of physicians to include information on anatomy and pathology that is critical to wise decision-making. These advances make reproductive health care simpler and make significant contributions to female endocrinological understanding (Defreyne et al., 2019). In addition, ultrasound and MRI are of significant importance in the latest technology of reproductive medicine, particularly assisted reproductive technologies. They are of tremendous use in the monitoring of ovarian response during *in vitro* fertilization (IVF) cycles, where ultrasound provides real-time measurements for follicular development. Monitoring is necessary in scheduling the optimal time for oocyte retrieval to enhance the chances of successful fertilization. MRI can also be utilized in assessing uterine anomalies that may significantly impact the rates of implantation success. The combination of these imaging techniques enhances the efficacy of interventions such that clinicians can tailor treatments according to individual patients' needs and conditions. With evolving field, ongoing research into female reproductive health applications of these imaging modalities will be essential to address unresolved issues (Brunetti et al., 2019; Defreyne et al., 2019) (Figure 7.14).

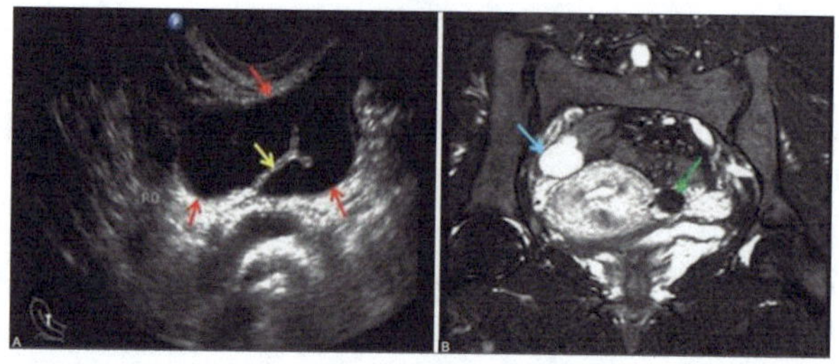

Figure 7.14. (A and B) Imaging studies of a 35-year-old woman with secondary infertility. The transvaginal ultrasound study (A) reveals a right-sided hydrosalpinx (red arrows) showing an incomplete septum within (yellow arrow). Pelvic MRI (B) of the same patient reveals a small fibroid at the left cornua of the uterus (green arrow) in addition to the dilated right fallopian tube (hydrosalpinx, blue arrow).

Source: https://www.researchgate.net/publication/340268880_Niche_role_of_MRI_in_the_evaluation_of_female_infertility.

7.4.3. Biopsy Procedures

Biopsy is included in the diagnosis and evaluation of most reproductive endocrinologic disorders in women, particularly in the diagnosis of abnormal uterine bleeding (AUB). The prevalence of AUB is significantly elevated in women who are perimenopausal and postmenopausal, and it is reported that 70% or more of women in both perimenopause and postmenopause may experience this symptom. Due to the diverse possible causes of AUB, from structural abnormalities to endocrine disturbances and malignancy, a thorough diagnostic approach is necessary. Among the methods employed, endometrial biopsy stands out because it allows direct sampling of the uterine lining. Schaeffer et al. (2020) concluded that Pipelle is a valuable method for sampling the endometrium due to the high sensitivity and specificity of the procedure, especially in comparison with traditional hysteroscopy. This advancement in biopsy techniques enables more accurate diagnosis of pathological conditions without raising the level of invasiveness, improving patient comfort and outcomes (Kashif et al., 2022). More scrutiny of biopsy procedures indicates them occupying a pivotal position in fertility testing, especially regarding assisted reproductive technologies such as *in vitro* fertilization (IVF). The use of preimplantation genetic testing for aneuploidy (PGT-A) following embryo biopsy is a radical shift in the practice of reproductive endocrinology. It has been established through studies that the use of euploid embryos—a euploid embryo containing the normal number of chromosomes—can successfully enhance pregnancy and reduce the incidence of miscarriage, particularly in women of older maternal age. Clinical outcomes further suggest that the psychological stress of having to wait after embryo transfer can also be alleviated through PGT-A. This procedure provides women with a sense of empowerment and control over their choice of IVF treatment, suggesting the varied benefits of emerging biopsy techniques, extending beyond physical health to encompass emotional (Forte et al., 2021). In general, biopsies are a routine part of reproductive endocrinology, facilitating accurate diagnosis and management of most clinical conditions of female reproductive health. The evolution in these technologies, more particularly the advent of less invasive techniques such as the Pipelle endometrial biopsy and embryo biopsy during IVF cycles, describes milestone advancements in patient care. As reproductive endocrinology continues to evolve, the emphasis on combining biophysics with counseling support becomes an urgent priority, allowing women to navigate their reproductive cycle with greater confidence and lower degrees of anxiety. Thus, ongoing research and technological advances in biopsy methods will go a long way in further enhancing the approaches used in the diagnosis and management of women's reproductive system diseases in the future (Forte et al., 2021; Kashif et al., 2022).

Test Your Knowledge

1. What key hormones are typically measured in blood tests to assess female reproductive endocrine function?
2. How is transvaginal ultrasound used to evaluate ovarian structure and uterine abnormalities?

7.5. Treatment Options for Hormonal Imbalances

Learning Outcome

1. Understand the role of hormone replacement therapy (HRT) in managing menopausal symptoms;
2. Discuss about lifestyle modifications and their impact;
3 Focus on surgical interventions in the management of various reproductive endocrine disorders in female.

Hormonal imbalances in females are proven to lead to a myriad of reproductive health issues, which significantly impact their lifestyle. The treatment methodologies for hormonal imbalances vary and can range from lifestyle adjustments to medication. Dietary changes and added exercises are one of the initial measures that need to be implemented to treat hormonal imbalances in a majority of situations. These natural interventions are proven to naturally put hormonal levels into check. For instance, a balanced diet rich in nutrients and omega-3 fatty acids and whole grains can improve the sensitivity of insulin, which plays a critical role in maintaining hormonal balance. Additionally, weight control through exercise has been known to regulate the levels of progesterone and estrogen, particularly in individuals with conditions such as PCOS. Lifestyle changes are therefore integral components of a comprehensive treatment regimen for maintaining hormonal balance. Pharmacological therapies provide another vital avenue for the management of hormonal imbalances, particularly when lifestyle changes are insufficient. Hormonal therapies, such as oral contraceptives, are typically prescribed to regulate menstrual cycles and alleviate symptoms of hormonal disorders. The medication can also level out by providing the body with equal hormone levels, thereby averting irregularities. In more severe cases, however, where there is significant endocrine malfunction, more refined treatments like hormone replacement therapy (HRT) come into play. This treatment is especially applicable in women going through menopause, when estrogen and progesterone levels drop drastically. Hormonal contraceptives and HRT have proven to be effective in alleviating symptoms and preventing long-term health effects of hormonal imbalance, underscoring the importance of informed medical advice in selecting appropriate treatments. Newer therapies like stem cell therapy have a promising future in managing hormonal imbalance. Current advances indicate that mesenchymal stem cells (MSCs) have gained attention because of their regenerative potential in treating reproductive diseases. MSCs can be harvested from various tissues like bone marrow and adipose tissue and are also revealed to show potential in restoring cellular function in hormonally related disorders. Studies indicate that MSCs could potentially contribute to the support of the endocrine system through hormone-secreting cell differentiation or immune response modulation, thereby addressing root causes of hormonal imbalance. This innovative treatment strategy is echoed in the growing trend towards personalized medicine and wholistic treatments in reproductive endocrinology, evidenced in ongoing clinical trials examining these options for optimizing therapeutic gain (Bryan et al., 2021; Duc et al., 2022).

7.5.1. Hormone Replacement Therapy (HRT)

The role of Hormone Replacement Therapy (HRT) in menopausal symptom management and women's reproductive endocrinology has been of much interest. The primary role of HRT is to manage symptoms such as hot flashes, night sweats, and mood swings that result from the decline in estrogen levels during menopause. Beyond symptom management, HRT is also a consideration when thinking about long-term health results for women who have reached menopause. Estrogen is also discovered to potentially offer neuroprotective benefits, maintaining cognitive function during the aging process. The effect of HRT on cognition, however, is controversial and complex. Findings show that while HRT can be related to improved cognitive functioning at certain times, age remains the most prominent predictor of change in cognitive ability over time, requiring close attention as to when and under what conditions HRT is to be delivered (Watermeyer et al., 2025). Further, some populations will experience different impacts from HRT, including those with genetic predispositions, e.g., BRCA1/2 mutations. Women undergoing risk-reducing salpingo-oophorectomy (RRSO) are left to deal with abrupt estrogen deficiency, worsening already menopausal symptoms and influencing cellular mechanisms that are in a healthy state. Utilization of HRT in such persons has been shown to be helpful, most significantly in enhancing urogenital symptoms and global health-related quality of life. Research indicates that HRT would directly decrease the intensity of urogenital pain and indirectly influence other symptoms of menopause, making it a holistic approach of treating symptoms (Ali et al., 2024).

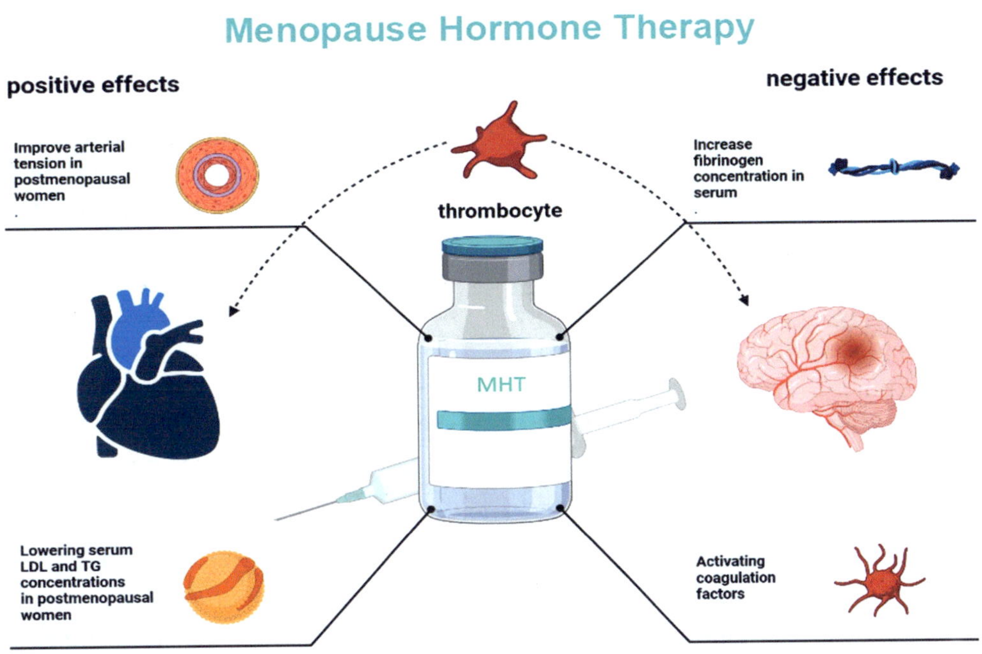

Figure 7.15. Menopause hormone therapy.

Source: https://media.springernature.com/lw685/springer-static/image/art%3A10.1186%2Fs12905-023-02788-0/MediaObjects/12905_2023_2788_Fig4_HTML.png.

However, HRT must be customized, as some cancer-inflicted women may exacerbate the symptoms, illustrating the requirement for personalized treatment regimens in reproductive endocrinology (Ali et al., 2024). The current debate of HRT sheds light on its benefits and limitations, and this is crucial in advancing female reproductive healthcare. It has become increasingly evident that HRT is not a generic solution; rather, its success is inextricably tied to numerous factors like genetics, age, and lifestyle choices. Widespread research, for instance, which examines the interaction of HRT use with cognition in later life, needs to guide evidence-based clinical guidelines. Further, exploring lifestyle factors, for instance, eating habits and physical activity levels, as well as HRT, allows opportunities to enhance therapeutic benefits in women. Future studies must overcome the hurdles associated with HRT, particularly formulation and duration of treatment, in a bid to enjoy its full potential for quality-of-life improvement in postmenopausal women (Watermeyer et al., 2025) (Figure 7.15).

7.5.2. Lifestyle Modifications and Their Impact

Lifestyle modification constitutes a critical aspect of reproductive health, particularly among reproductive-aged women who hope to improve their overall quality of life. The modifications can include various practices like dietary changes, increased physical activity, and stress management techniques. Research has confirmed that implementation of individualized lifestyle modifications has been capable of leading to impressive reproductive health outcomes. For instance, a study among teachers in Nigeria's Osun State confirmed a moderate positive relationship between reproductive health outcomes and health literacy, with an emphasis on the importance of awareness of one's health and the making of informed decisions. These decisions are related to the type of simple but useful changes like the augmentation of healthier food and routine physical exercise, which in combination have beneficial impacts on reproductive functioning and healthier menstrual cycles (Osu et al., 2025). The emphasis on complementary and alternative therapies (CATs) also indicates the direction of lifestyle changes impacting reproductive health. Dysmenorrheic female medical students, for instance, demonstrated a propensity to use CATs as well as standard pain management procedures. This trend indicates a general higher awareness of the need for holistic care methods that aim at long-term health over symptom control only. The study revealed that a major proportion of the respondents chose CATs, such as bed rest and heat application, in place of conventional painkillers, as they were worried about the safety and effectiveness of prolonged use of analgesics. The trend suggests an increased awareness among women of the potential beneficial impact of adding lifestyle modifications in their health care plan, hence increasing the management of reproductive health problems such as dysmenorrhea (Tahir et al., 2025). Finally, the integration of lifestyle modifications into reproductive care not only empowers women but also promotes a proactive way of life towards wellness. By fostering habits such as good diet, physical activity, and stress elimination, healthcare providers can have a significant influence on women's reproductive well-being. Policymakers and health educators are responsible for making these efforts easier by supporting accessible health information and resources. With empowerment through knowledge and skills to make decisions, women are able to take charge of their reproductive health, enhancing their quality of life and reproductive health. From the findings in the education field, there is a clear need to campaign for and implement lifestyle modification programs that favor women's reproductive health needs (Osu et al., 2025).

7.5.3. Surgical Interventions

Surgical intervention plays a central role in treating many reproductive endocrine disorders, such as PCOS, endometriosis, and female infertility. As an ultima ratio, surgical options become necessary in the treatment of recalcitrant patients with conservative management and for the restoration of fertility function and symptom relief. A good example is laparoscopy for repetitively carrying out endometrial extraction in endometriosis, which can dramatically improve pain and fecundity. In addition, ovarian drilling has also been employed as an intervention of minimal invasiveness to address anovulation among female PCOS patients and has led to improved ovulatory and menstrual regularity. The complexity of such conditions requires patient-specific surgical treatment, which places great importance on individually based interventions based on patient profiles and the extent of their reproductive endocrine pathologies, which were identified in findings of Lu et al. (2024). In addition, surgical implant integration has been a significant advancement in gynecologic surgical interventions. These implants, particularly polypropylene meshes, are employed to re-establish anatomical integrity for pelvic organ prolapse, which may be coincidental with reproductive endocrine disorders. By providing a supportive matrix, these meshes facilitate tissue ingrowth, thereby enhancing long-term success of surgical interventions. Research has established that successful placement of the implant helps to curb complications by reducing the development of scar tissue, hence ultimately providing improved operative prognoses. The new application ensures operative interventions targeted at correcting structural defects in conjunction with therapy of the underlying hormonal disorder at the root of female reproductive disorders, as emphasized in the discussion by Lytvak et al. (2024). Also, success in surgical treatment relies on an interdisciplinary program with expertise from surgery, reproductive endocrinology, and gynecology. Detailed understanding of the complex interactions between metabolic pathways and reproductive physiology brings prospects for improved management. Improved surgical outcomes are increasingly linked with pre- and postoperative metabolic evaluations, as evidence by recent studies employing Mendelian Randomization to investigate metabolite effects on reproductive endocrine disease. Accurate diagnoses can inform surgical management and permit individualized postoperative care strategies that promote recovery and endocrine homeostasis. As ongoing advances are made in the field of reproductive endocrinology, integrating advanced surgical techniques with principles of metabolism will be important to improving quality of life and fertility in women, imposing a need for ongoing research within the field.

Test Your Knowledge

1. In what clinical situations is hormone replacement therapy recommended for women?
2. How does HRT help manage symptoms of menopause, and what factors must be considered before initiating treatment?
3. What surgical options are available for treating endometriosis and uterine fibroids, and how do they impact hormonal balance and fertility?

7.6. Advances in Reproductive Technology

Learning Outcome

1. Explain the fundamentals of in vitro fertilization (IVF);
2. Discuss the role of genetic screening and counselling for female reproductive health;
3. Focus on emerging research in endocrinology.

The dynamic field of reproductive technology has seen dramatic advancements with the aim of addressing several problems in female reproductive endocrinology. Progress has been made immensely in Assisted Reproductive Technology (ART) as it enables couples that are infertile to reproduce, a condition that can bring severe emotional as well as physical suffering. All these advances in technology not only include the procedures like IVF and ICSI but also latest cryopreservation technology by which preservation of oocytes and embryos can be achieved. Therefore, women have more control over their reproductive options, especially the timing of childbearing. Furthermore, there are also current ethical concerns about ART that provoke controversy among religious and medical communities about its effect on community health, order, and human dignity as they pertain to reproductive rights in contemporary society (Gresham et al., 2020). Since the most important aspect of understanding reproductive technology's influence on women's endocrinology is the physiological basis of menstruation and fertility. Current research has provided insight into neuropeptide regulation of the reproductive hormones that have a key function in the onset of puberty and maintenance of reproductive well-being. For instance, binding of Substance P (SP) to NK1R has been reported to modulate gonadotropin secretion from the pituitary gland. It is pivotal in the regulation of the onset of puberty and fertility, so it is crucial for reproductive endocrinologists to comprehend these nuances. Research has confirmed that increases in SP signaling prior to puberty contribute to the coordination of hormone release, ultimately resulting in successful reproductive outcomes (Carroll et al., 2015). This information helps to further advance ART protocols and success of treatments administered to women with reproductive concerns. In addition, the overlap of advances in reproductive technology and understanding of female reproductive endocrinology also raises significant questions that involve issues of accessibility as well as ethics. While ART has opened new doors to family planning as well as the treatment of infertility, disparities in access to such technologies remain a live issue. Socioeconomic status, geographic location, and various healthcare policies have the ability to heavily impact a patients ability to benefit from such advances. Furthermore, there are constant ethical debates about the manipulation of reproductive processes like embryo selection and genetic screening, which need thoughtful examination of implications on society's norms and values. Addressing these inequalities not only demands public enhanced awareness and education regarding reproductive health but also intersectional analysis to guarantee that advancements in reproductive technology benefit all women equally (Gresham et al., 2020).

7.6.1. In Vitro Fertilization (IVF)

The introduction of *in vitro* fertilization (IVF) as a breakthrough technology in reproductive endocrinology is a milestone in the management of female infertility. IVF involves oocyte retrieval, lab fertilization, and embryo implantation within the uterus afterward. This targeted procedure allows doctors to overcome various reproductive barriers, from idiopathic infertility to diseases like polycystic ovary syndrome (PCOS). The International Evidence-based Guidelines on PCOS identify the imperative of person-centered care and treatment protocols, necessitating a multi-disciplinary endeavor that improves the

IVF experience for women with this condition. Compliance with these guidelines can lead to improved outcomes and patient satisfaction despite continued challenges of delayed diagnosis and gaps in care that continue to bedevil the treatment of PCOS and fertility issues (Teede et al., 2023). Hysteroscopy holds core relevance to the diagnosis and management of suspected uterine pathology that may impact IVF success. By the use of this imaging gold standard for the uterine cavity, healthcare providers can diagnose and correct illnesses such as fibroids, polyps, and adhesions before embarking on IVF. These intracavitary lesions can significantly impair implantation and ongoing pregnancy growth, and hence early diagnosis is crucial. Hysteroscopy can be employed to allow direct visualization and thereby enable specific intervention in this respect, ultimately contributing to improved reproductive outcomes. This procedure is consistent with the results discussed in new research studies, indicating that the correction of uterine pathology, in addition to the optimization of embryo culture environment, constitutes a more holistic strategy to improve fertility in IVF women (Parry et al., 2019). Furthermore, the development in reproductive endocrinology also underscores the need to achieve the hormonal and physiological substrate that influences IVF success rates. Both oocyte retrieval and embryo development demand appropriate hormonal equilibrium, with the therapies employed to stabilize hormone levels typically prior to IVF treatment. Varying treatment protocol according to individual patients hormonal profile can enhance endometrium synchronization, hence implantation opportunities. Future advances in reproductive endocrinology will similarly continue to emphasize individualized treatment with evidence-based therapy to lead women through IVF. As research continues, insights from fields such as endocrinology and reproductive surgery will also work to further techniques of IVF, resulting in better reproductive outcomes for women (Teede et al., 2023) (Figure 7.16).

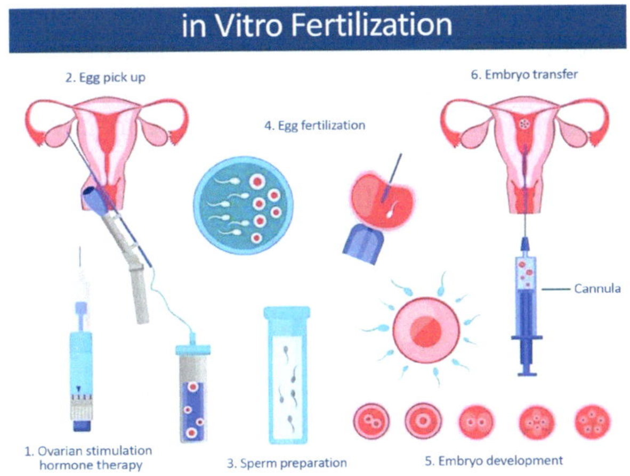

Figure 7.16. *In vitro* fertilization (IVF), as a transformative technology in reproductive endocrinology, signifies a pivotal advance in addressing female infertility.

Source: https://www.news-medical.net/image-handler/picture/IVF%20process%20infographic%20-%20ectorPot%20_thumb.jpg.

7.6.2. Genetic Screening and Counseling

Genetic counseling and screening form a critical part of reproductive endocrinology, particularly in assessing potential risk for genetic illness in pregnancy. The availability and sophistication of genetic testing technologies are widely accepted and contribute significantly to the knowledge of hereditary illnesses that affect the mother and the fetus. These screenings enable the identification of chromosomal defects and genetic illness, thus educating healthcare providers on the knowledge needed to counsel future parents on decision-making. Additionally, genetic counseling forms the core of reporting the implications of screening results, addressing the emotional impacts of genetic risk, and decision-making about reproductive options. This pro-active approach not only enhances maternal-fetal care but also underscores the importance of personalized medicine in obstetrics, where individual genetic histories can have a very real influence on outcomes. The use of genetic screening encourages a greater understanding of reproductive health concerns likely to be faced by women. The complexity of reproductive health necessitates genetic screening being regularly tailored to the risk factors of individual patients. Women who have previous histories of reproductive challenges, maternal age issues, or established family histories of genetic disorders are routinely given more priority for in-depth genetic testing and counseling. For instance, in the case of congenital cardiac anomalies, somatic maternal well-being and genetic predispositions that may elevate the risk in offspring toward such defects should be considered. Studies have shown that maternal conditions like cardiovascular and endocrine disease can have a deleterious effect on fetal outcomes, thus making intensive screening regimens essential. With both non-invasive prenatal testing (NIPT) and diagnostic invasive tests, if necessary, health care practitioners can efficiently examine the genetic health of the fetus and prepare families for any potential challenges in the future. These rigorous approaches are essential to promote the chances of healthy pregnancy and reduce the incidence of congenital malformations, as reflected in the result of a recent study that reported the prevalence of various congenital cardiac defects in screened populations (Helner et al., 2019). Moreover, the new landscapes of genetic screening technologies stimulate ethics with regard to access, interpretation, and implications of genetic information. With mounting application of genetic testing, disparities in access to such services become a pressing issue, raising questions about reproductive healthcare equity. In addition, the psychologic implications of genetic findings need to be managed delicately; family members may experience reproductive decision-making dilemmas in relation to test results, leading to severe emotional trauma. Effective genetic counseling is not merely a medium of information exchange, but a support mechanism to allow families to understand and accept their genetic susceptibility. As such, as part of reproductive endocrinology, the addition of genetic screening and counseling must also attend to not only medical accuracy, but to compassionate support systems that are able to alleviate the burdens imposed by the uncertainty of genetic disease. Ultimately, a multidisciplinary approach to genetic counseling can really make a difference in the reproductive options and quality of life for women and their families (Cheetham et al., 2019).

7.6.3. Emerging Research in Endocrinology

Recent studies in the area of endocrinology, i.e., women's reproductive health, have significantly enhanced our understanding of the complex interplay of hormones and their functions in a variety of health outcomes. Recent investigations have enlightened us regarding how differences in hormone levels may not only influence reproductive health but other health conditions like cardiovascular illness and metabolic disorders as well. For instance, the role of sex hormones such as progesterone and estrogen has become increasingly realized for their cardioprotective functions, suggesting that hormonal abnormalities can contribute to risks of heart disease in women. This intersection of reproductive hormone research and overall health is what underscores the necessity of comprehensive treatment modalities that consider the reproductive endocrinology of female patients alongside their general health needs, as emphasized in recent scholarship in the field. The significance of thyroid function as a factor in reproduction has also been emphasized, particularly with the aim of considering evaluation of thyrotoxicosis and its impact on female fertility and pregnancy outcome. Thyroid hormones are of critical significance for the control of metabolic processes and, when disrupted, may lead to severe reproductive ailments such as irregular menstruation and pregnancy-related issues. The existing guidelines released by the American Thyroid Association emphasize the necessity of proper evaluation and management of thyrotoxicosis for achievement of the best possible health status in women across all ages. These guidelines highlight that it is the role of clinicians to actively monitor and control thyroid function in women, thus enhancing our understanding of the subtleties of reproductive endocrinology as well as the interrelatedness of hormonal health at the systemic level (Douglas et al., 2016). Another significant area of continued research is the influence of external factors, such as environmental exposure and life habit, on women's reproductive endocrinology. Investigation is increasingly focusing on the effect of endocrine-disrupting chemicals (EDCs) that are present in many products on endocrine equilibrium as well as on reproductive well-being. Moreover, the COVID-19 pandemic has revealed unequal access to reproductive health care, as observed with challenges faced by pregnant women during the pandemic. Analysis of these stressors illuminates the strength of women's reproductive health systems and points to the need for policy safeguarding hormonal welfare under the influence of socio-economic stress. The more that research into these areas evolves, the more the findings can be utilized to inform more equitable health practices that take account of women's diverse reproductive requirements across groups (Gausman et al., 2020).

Test Your Knowledge

1. What are the key steps involved in the IVF process, and how is hormone regulation critical to its success?
2. In which reproductive endocrine disorders is IVF most commonly indicated, and what factors influence its success rates?
3. How does genetic counselling support patients undergoing fertility treatments, and what ethical considerations are involved?

SUMMARY

The intricate relationship between female fertility and reproductive endocrinology reflects the importance of understanding various pathological and physiological processes. What was noted in the case of visceral adipose tissue (VAT), for instance, is the ability of such obesity factors to significantly affect infertility outcomes. Particularly, the excessive levels of the Chinese Visceral Adiposity Index (CVAI) have been associated with extremely increased risk of female infertility, which highlights that metabolic health is an integral component of reproductive function. These publications reveal a need for attention and potential interventions with weight management as one of the fertility preservation strategies, which may be a sound measure for persons who have issues of infertility (Guo et al., 2024). Furthermore, the role of formal reproductive endocrinology consultations is key in fertility preservation, particularly among vulnerable populations such as children and adolescents with cancer. Research has confirmed that patients who are consulted are far more likely to select fertility preservation treatments, thereby safeguarding their reproductive capacity if they undergo gonadotoxic therapy. Perhaps most intriguingly, women are found to be more likely to both be consulted and take up fertility preservation, an imbalance by gender that merits further study. A systemic implementation of formal consultations can reinforce the debate on reproductive health, ultimately resulting in enhanced decision-making among these patients (Lindsay et al., 2024). Lastly, the implication arising from the interaction between obesity, reproductive health, and the application of endocrinology consultations is the necessity for systemic changes in managing reproductive health. This, in turn, demands greater investigation into the mechanisms of infertility and a re-evaluation of fertility preservation clinical practice. As females do have unique problems in the field of reproductive endocrinology, their specific needs must be understood in depth. By the elimination of the gap between research findings and clinical practice, medical practitioners are able to enhance the safety and the quality of care for infertile women, providing a friendly environment that ensures reproductive freedom and informed decision-making in any scenario (Guo et al., 2024; Lindsay et al., 2024).

In reproductive endocrinology, and more so in women, the interplay of hormones exerts a dramatic effect on physiological and behavioral processes. Women's hormonal changes, in major focus, have occurred during various stages of a woman's reproductive cycle, from menarche to menopause. The periodic pattern of estrogen and progesterone plays a significant role not only in fertility but in overall health implications as well. For instance, variations of such hormones have been correlated with diseases such as polycystic ovary syndrome (PCOS) and endometriosis, which both impact fertility and health in general. Through the understanding of the intricate balance of hormones and their impacts, researchers aim to solidify treatment therapy as well as improve health measures independently developed for women's reproductive well-being. As research progresses, it becomes increasingly necessary to consider gender-specific physiological response in medicine. Exercise and sports science, in particular, are beginning to realize that women may respond differently to training protocols due to hormonal influence. In doing so, calls have been made for robust research examining female physiology across those disciplines, as traditional models underestimate or overlook gender-specific responses. Moreover, integrating women-focused perspectives into education curricula will help future professionals treat women's unique health problems more effectively. Consequently, there is more activity aimed at revolutionizing research methods to embrace diverse life experiences and states of being in order to integrate more heterogeneous clinical observations in women's reproductive endocrinology and other areas of study (Hackney et al., 2024). Moreover, it is important to investigate the effect of supraphysiological levels of hormones, as during pregnancy or *in vitro* fertilization treatment, on a woman's physiology. Investigations into these special hormonal milieus provide insights worth expanding our current reproductive endocrinology knowledge. For instance, the changes of pregnancy not only optimize reproductive success but also provide the opportunity to explore the effects of increased hormone levels on various body systems. Such research can potentially account for unknown hormonal effects and their meanings to clinicians, ultimately providing a better understanding of female biology. Finally, advance in female reproductive endocrinology studies should be propelled by an integrative philosophy that embraces the complexity of hormonal regulation and innovation in research methods (Dhungana et al., 2025).

KEY TERMS FROM THIS CHAPTER

- Abnormal uterine bleeding (AUB)
- Assisted Reproductive Technology (ART)
- Chronic pelvic pain
- Clinical trials
- Endocrine-disrupting chemicals (EDCs)
- Environmental toxins
- Female sexual dysfunction (FSD)
- Genetic counseling
- GnRH signal pathways
- Anti-Müllerian hormone (AMH)
- Cardiovascular regulation
- Circadian rhythms
- Embryological development
- Endometriosis
- Estrogen
- Fertility problems
- Genetic disorders
- GnRHs regulatory actions

CRITICAL THINKING QUESTIONS

1. **Which of the following hormones is primarily responsible for ovulation?**
   a. Progesterone
   b. Luteinizing hormone (LH)
   c. Follicle-stimulating hormone (FSH)
   d. Estrogen
2. **Where are the Graafian follicles located?**
   a. Uterus
   b. Fallopian tubes
   c. Ovaries
   d. Cervix
3. **Polycystic Ovary Syndrome (PCOS) is often associated with which of the following features?**
   a. Hypothyroidism, amenorrhea, and hypoglycemia
   b. Hyperandrogenism, irregular menstruation, and insulin resistance
   c. Elevated prolactin, infertility, and galactorrhea
   d. Menorrhagia, endometriosis, and low estrogen
4. **Which diagnostic technique is most commonly used to monitor follicular development?**
   a. Pelvic X-ray
   b. Laparoscopy
   c. CT scan
   d. Transvaginal ultrasound
5. **What is the primary site of estrogen synthesis in premenopausal women?**
   a. Ovarian follicles
   b. Adrenal glands
   c. Pituitary gland
   d. Corpus luteum

Short Answer Questions

1. What are the main anatomical structures of the female reproductive system, and what are their specific functions in reproduction?
2. How do the levels of FSH, LH, estrogen, and progesterone fluctuate during the different phases of the menstrual cycle?
3. What is the role of negative and positive feedback loops in the regulation of gonadotropin-releasing hormone (GnRH) and subsequent hormone release?
4. What are the endocrine features of PCOS, and how do they affect ovulation and fertility?
5. How does endometriosis influence reproductive hormone balance and contribute to infertility or menstrual irregularities?
6. What hormonal blood tests are commonly used to assess female reproductive function, and what can abnormal values suggest?
7. How are ultrasound and endometrial biopsy used to diagnose reproductive endocrine conditions such as ovarian cysts or endometrial abnormalities?

Answers to Critical Thinking Questions

1. (b); 2. (c); 3. (b); 4. (d); 5. (a)

REFERENCES

1. Abubakar, R. Z., Bello, S. O., Chika, A., Umar, M., & Abubakar, M. (2025). Ameliorative effects of honey on petrol vapor-induced oxidative stress in the reproductive system of female Wistar rats. *Pharmacology and Toxicology of Natural Medicines* (ISSN: 2756-6838). https://www.semanticscholar.org/paper/d47fcc790263e7871680e3ab0a1c5754ef54efb5 (accessed on 22nd July 2025).

2. Aizen, J., Boehm, B., Degani, G., Golan, M., et al. (2016). Gonadotropins in the Russian sturgeon: Their role in steroid secretion and the effect of hormonal treatment on their secretion. https://core.ac.uk/download/323072349.pdf (accessed on 22nd July 2025).

3. Ali, A. M., Al-Dossary, S. A., Laranjeira, C., Amer, F., Hallit, S., Alkhamees, A. A., Aljubilah, A., et al. (2024). Effects of hormonal replacement therapy and mindfulness-based stress reduction on climacteric symptoms following risk-reducing salpingo-oophorectomy. *Healthcare, 12*. https://www.semanticscholar.org/paper/5ae16ee6a623f8204872c93ac5ec00531df79858 (accessed on 22nd July 2025).

4. Alsaadi, M., Ferro, V., Garside, D. A., Gebril, A., et al. (2013). An update on the potential for male contraception: Emerging options. https://core.ac.uk/download/9843862.pdf (accessed on 22nd July 2025).

5. Anderson, R. A., Gifford, R. M., Greeves, J., Reynolds, K., et al. (2017). Reproductive dysfunction and associated pathology in women undergoing military training. https://core.ac.uk/download/74208327.pdf (accessed on 22nd July 2025).

6. Arnold, B. S., Gross, T. S., McDonald, K., Spulveda, M., et al. (2001). Relations of environmental contaminants, algal toxins, and diet with the reproductive success of American alligators on Florida lakes. https://core.ac.uk/download/11016994.pdf (accessed on 22nd July 2025).

7. Beerda, B., Boer, H. M. T., Veerkamp, R. F., Woelders, H., et al. (2010). Estrous behavior in dairy cows: Identification of underlying mechanisms and gene functions. https://core.ac.uk/download/pdf/29246031.pdf (accessed on 22nd July 2025).

8. Bentley, G. E., Calandra, R. S., Micevych, P. E., Paredes, R., et al. (2016). Peripheral and central mechanisms involved in hormonal control of male and female reproduction. https://core.ac.uk/download/159295807.pdf (accessed on 22nd July 2025).

9. Bentley, G., Comizzoli, P., & Wilsterman, K. (2019). RFRP3 influences basal lamina degradation, cellular death, and progesterone secretion in cultured preantral ovarian follicles from the domestic cat. https://core.ac.uk/download/323081743.pdf (accessed on 22nd July 2025).

10. Boden, M., Kennaway, D., & Varcoe, T. (2013). Circadian regulation of reproduction: From gamete to offspring. https://core.ac.uk/download/19445268.pdf (accessed on 22nd July 2025).

11. Brian, J. V. (2005). Inter-population variability in the reproductive morphology of the shore crab (*Carcinus maenas*): Evidence of endocrine disruption in a marine crustacean? https://core.ac.uk/download/333887.pdf (accessed on 22nd July 2025).

12. Brunetti, A., Cocchia, N., Fatone, G., Greco, A., et al. (2019). Noninvasive ultrasound monitoring of embryonic and fetal development in *Chinchilla lanigera* to predict gestational age: Preliminary evaluation of this species as a novel animal model of human pregnancy. https://core.ac.uk/download/pdf/201590430.pdf (accessed on 22nd July 2025).

13. Carroll, R. S., Gill, J. C., Kaiser, U. B., Maguire, C. A., et al. (2015). Substance P regulates puberty onset and fertility in the female mouse. https://core.ac.uk/download/227069712.pdf (accessed on 22nd July 2025).
14. Cha, E., Choi, Y. S., Lee, M. J., Kim, M., Seo, S. J., Kwak, S. M., Park, S., et al. (2024). Uterus-mimetic extracellular microenvironment for engineering female reproductive system. *Advanced Functional Materials, 35*. https://www.semanticscholar.org/paper/5678a8a17305fefb355fae14ba02114a9281df38 (accessed on 22nd July 2025).
15. Cheetham, T., Fearon, K., Hanna, E., Herbrand, D., et al. (2019). The lived experience of Klinefelter syndrome: A narrative review of the literature. https://core.ac.uk/download/287585205.pdf (accessed on 22nd July 2025).
16. Clavijo, R., & Hsiao, W. (2018). Update on male reproductive endocrinology. https://core.ac.uk/download/323070097.pdf (accessed on 22nd July 2025).
17. Defreyne, J., Iwamoto, S. J., Motmans, J., Rothman, M., et al. (2019). Health considerations for transgender women and remaining unknowns: A narrative review. https://core.ac.uk/download/237010802.pdf (accessed on 22nd July 2025).
18. Dhungana, P., Wei, X., Kang, D. S., & Sim, C. (2025). A head-specific transcriptomic study reveals key regulatory pathways for winter diapause in the mosquito *Culex pipiens*. *Archives of Insect Biochemistry and Physiology, 118*(2), e70032. https://www.semanticscholar.org/paper/ff334719302df92148cbde267b4a8f1b611b4112 (accessed on 22nd July 2025).
19. Dynnik, V., Dynnik, O., & Bagatska, N. (2025). The relationships of the pituitary-gonadal regulation link of the menstrual cycle and hormones of energy metabolism in adolescents with abnormal uterine bleeding at different times of menstrual disorders debut. *Reproductive Health of Woman*. https://www.semanticscholar.org/paper/7e810d98a833b1da5f74a0a7e47f6a86bc6a531c (accessed on 22nd July 2025).
20. Egli, M., Geraedts, K., Hengartner, M. P., Ille, R., et al. (2017). Lack of associations between female hormone levels and visuospatial working memory, divided attention and cognitive bias across two consecutive menstrual cycles. https://core.ac.uk/download/141696144.pdf (accessed on 22nd July 2025).
21. Ezeala, O. S., Adienbo, O., & Amah-Tariah, F. S. (2025). Correlation of anthropometric indices with menstrual characteristics and female reproductive hormones. *Scholars Journal of Applied Medical Sciences*. https://www.semanticscholar.org/paper/a6400063689ac338cd46005ebc241a3e7e2ca7be (accessed on 22nd July 2025).
22. Foot, N. J., Dinh, D. T., Emery-Corbin, S. J., Yousef, J., Dagley, L. F., & Russell, D. L. (2025). Comparative analysis of the progesterone receptor interactome in the human ovarian granulosa cell line KGN and other female reproductive cells. *Proteomics*. https://www.semanticscholar.org/paper/bd9f1a4f413c376b5ca8bada636cc394c961ceca (accessed on 22nd July 2025).
23. Forte, M., Faustini, F., Venturella, R., Rania, E., Alviggi, E., Trabucco, E., Cimadomo, D., et al. (2021). P–500 Euploid embryo-transfer reduces advanced maternal age patients' anxiety in the waiting period before the pregnancy-test. *Human Reproduction*. https://www.semanticscholar.org/paper/35d5e8a241f6c7b58f6ba4a5a14259f9a77c401d (accessed on 22nd July 2025).
24. Gausman, J., & Langer, A. (2020). Sex and gender disparities in the COVID-19 pandemic. *Journal of Women's Health, 29*, 465–466. https://doi.org/10.1089/jwh.2020.8472 (accessed on 22nd July 2025).

25. Gresham, M. E. (2020). *Inconceivable: An Analysis of Assisted Reproductive Technology for The Church*. https://core.ac.uk/download/322850911.pdf (accessed on 22nd July 2025).

26. Guo, D., & Wang, R. (2024). Association between visceral adipose surrogates and infertility among reproductive-aged females: A cross-sectional study. *Frontiers in Endocrinology, 15*. https://www.semanticscholar.org/paper/7f3d63a496e871e392256546ed094739837fc94e (accessed on 22nd July 2025).

27. Gupta, K., & Patel, S. J. (2024). Prevalence and management of premenstrual dysphoric disorder (PMDD): Literature review. *Research Review International Journal of Multidisciplinary*. https://www.semanticscholar.org/paper/58a1a65d0b4145acbd073d51cca6ab13d5272bf0 (accessed on 22nd July 2025).

28. Hackney, A. C., & Elliott-Sale, K. (2024). Female physiology-endocrinology: Education is lacking and innovation is needed! *Women in Sport & Physical Activity Journal, 32*(1). https://www.semanticscholar.org/paper/13c5c06021607f82a07d37935940669911931fc5 (accessed on 22nd July 2025).

29. Hartup, L. A., Go, V. A., & Robinson, R. D. (2024). Standardized reproductive endocrinology and infertility consultation for pediatric and adolescent oncology patients. *Journal of Adolescent and Young Adult Oncology*. https://www.semanticscholar.org/paper/fc12f583f2c5700822b8beb4369d6c2c1a24973e (accessed on 22nd July 2025).

30. Helner, N. (N.), Makukh, H. (H.), Prokopchuk, N. (N.), Sharhorodska, R., et al. (2019). Medical genetic counseling of women with congenital heart diseases of fetus. https://core.ac.uk/download/301580705.pdf (accessed on 22nd July 2025).

31. Hoang, D. M., Pham, P. T., Bach, T. Q., Ngo, A. T., Nguyen, Q. T., Phan, T. T. K., Nguyễn, H. G., et al. (2022). Stem cell-based therapy for human diseases. *Signal Transduction and Targeted Therapy, 7*. https://doi.org/10.1038/s41392-022-01134-4 (accessed on 22nd July 2025).

32. Jayasena, C., Devine, K., Barber, K. A., Comninos, A., Conway, G. S., Crown, A., Davies, M. C., et al. (2024). Society for Endocrinology guideline for understanding, diagnosing and treating female hypogonadism. *Clinical Endocrinology, 101*, 409–442. https://www.semanticscholar.org/paper/0e17ecc5ce08aea029dbb5bd723eb350f89d4285 (accessed on 22nd July 2025).

33. Kapper, C., Oppelt, P., Ganhör, C., Gyunesh, A. A., Arbeithuber, B., Stelzl, P., & Rezk-Füreder, M. (2024). Minerals and the menstrual cycle: Impacts on ovulation and endometrial health. *Nutrients, 16*. https://www.semanticscholar.org/paper/df9758ce9b571b6b45d5198925708415d95101d6 (accessed on 22nd July 2025).

34. Kashif, S., Iftikhar, G., Jabbar, S., Khawar, N., Qureshi, M. N., & Choudhry, S. S. (2022). Comparison between Pipelle sampling and hysteroscopy guided biopsy in histologic evaluation of endometrium in tertiary care hospital in Pakistan. *Pakistan Journal of Medical and Health Sciences*. https://www.semanticscholar.org/paper/a1724ea4347016216cf23d51d1a3d0179cd38064 (accessed on 22nd July 2025).

35. Kitaya, K. (2025). B cell lineage in the human endometrium: Physiological and pathological implications. *Cells, 14*. https://www.semanticscholar.org/paper/18e2572a479e6119468f9656a639efdbdb0de731 (accessed on 22nd July 2025).

36. Kumar, A., Singh, J., & Khan, A. A. (2024). A comprehensive machine learning framework with particle swarm optimization for improved polycystic ovary syndrome (PCOS)

diagnosis. *Engineering Research Express, 6*. https://www.semanticscholar.org/paper/ff25383e1c212dcf3fe76b9b61e96327d821b64b (accessed on 22nd July 2025).

37. Lu, F., Wang, Z., Yang, Q., Yan, F., Xu, C., Wang, M., Xu, Z., et al. (2024). Investigating the metabolomic pathways in female reproductive endocrine disorders: A Mendelian randomization study. *Frontiers in Endocrinology, 15*. https://www.semanticscholar.org/paper/fbc98086105cf2aac9e5d00a53e16aad11d5c013 (accessed on 22nd July 2025).

38. Lytvak, O., Tsapenko, T., Vitovskyi, Y. M., Narytnyk, T., & Mashkina, O. M. (2024). Practice of using implants in gynecological surgical interventions (scientific literature review). *Клінічна та профілактична медицина*. https://www.semanticscholar.org/paper/d3ac216c34b9c217362541c923918e431f76c0a1 (accessed on 22nd July 2025).

39. Mahajan, S. S., More, A., Shrivastava, D., Anjankar, N., Mamankar, D., & Nawale, N. (2025). Navigating infertility in unicornuate uterus: Clinical management and success with assisted reproductive techniques. *Journal of Pharmacy and Bioallied Sciences*. https://www.semanticscholar.org/paper/5c2247c207cb59eacccb030f404eca58fd0c90d5 (accessed on 22nd July 2025).

40. Memi, E., Pavli, P., Maria, P., Vrachnis, N., & Mastorakos, G. (2024). Diagnostic and therapeutic use of oral micronized progesterone in endocrinology. *Reviews in Endocrine & Metabolic Disorders, 25*, 751–772. https://www.semanticscholar.org/paper/c892504d3dbcdad5ca71bc5cd0f3c7b184972f63 (accessed on 22nd July 2025).

41. Mourier, J., Planes, S., & Mills, S. C. (2024). Steroid hormones as a non-lethal assessment of the reproductive biology in male and female blacktip reef sharks. *Frontiers in Fish Science*. https://www.semanticscholar.org/paper/073fd596dc9839e5729eb1be3fe6c0bd5e9f10c9 (accessed on 22nd July 2025).

42. Osu, U. C., Adegbite, O. O., Olunubi, T. O., Ogunniyan, F. G., & Afolabi, P. I. (2025). Empowering female teachers through health literacy, reproductive health and lifestyle modifications in Osun State, Nigeria. *Journal of Arts, Humanities and Social Science*. https://www.semanticscholar.org/paper/fb9f2b726e6c68ccf3350a0fdd94b218b3903192 (accessed on 22nd July 2025).

43. Parry, J. P., & Isaacson, K. (2019). Hysteroscopy and why macroscopic uterine factors matter for fertility. *Fertility and Sterility, 112*, 203–210. https://doi.org/10.1016/j.fertnstert.2019.06.031 (accessed on 22nd July 2025).

44. Rahman, F., Sultana, N., Rahman, F., Paul, R., Salma, U., Yeasmin, F., & Jesmin, N. (2024). Outcome of endometriosis treatment in infertile patients in a tertiary level hospital. *Journal of Dhaka Medical College*. https://www.semanticscholar.org/paper/69a470a3576f63861327f3119fca71448a33fb70 (accessed on 22nd July 2025).

45. Ross, D. S., Burch, H. B., Cooper, D. S., Greenlee, M. C., Laurberg, P., Maia, A. L., Rivkees, S. A., et al. (2016). 2016 American Thyroid Association Guidelines for diagnosis and management of hyperthyroidism and other causes of thyrotoxicosis. *Thyroid, 26*, 1343–1421. https://doi.org/10.1089/thy.2016.0229 (accessed on 22nd July 2025).

46. Salam, S., Deeba, F., Banu, J., Ishrat, S., Saha, C., Sinha, S., Patel, P., et al. (2025). Statins: Is it new weaponry against endometriosis? *Advances in Human Biology*. https://www.semanticscholar.org/paper/2a12e99ee3e3f186d7e62a3de6e36b957a4104c6 (accessed on 22nd July 2025).

47. Schneider, B. J., Naidoo, J., Santomasso, B., Lacchetti, C., Adkins, S., Anadkat, M. J., Atkins, M. B., et al. (2021). Management of immune-related adverse events in patients treated with

immune checkpoint inhibitor therapy: ASCO guideline update. *Journal of Clinical Oncology, 39*, 4073–4126. https://doi.org/10.1200/jco.21.01440 (accessed on 22nd July 2025).

48. Semeniuk, L., Pankiv, V., Kozachuk, Y., & Kryzhanovska, O. (2025). Determining the relationship between hormonal background characteristics and signs of female sexual dysfunction in women with and without endometriosis in the prediction of gestational success. *International Journal of Endocrinology (Ukraine)*. https://www.semanticscholar.org/paper/d91ba3ff208287cbadad74b7e3fb6f82f5a43d36 (accessed on 22nd July 2025).

49. Shahzad, M., Saeed, M., Shahzad, F., & Hassan, A. (2025). Revealing the unspoken battle: Limited awareness of PMDD and its invisible consequences on women's well-being in Pakistan. *JPMA. The Journal of the Pakistan Medical Association, 75*(4), 687–688. https://www.semanticscholar.org/paper/99ffe42d2bab2fa2ddc76420f503aa222b5e9569 (accessed on 22nd July 2025).

50. Shao, H., Xu, C., Wang, H., Lu, N., Gu, H., Zhang, C., Li, L., et al. (2025). Dissecting the genetic determinants and biological associations between body mass index and female reproductive disorders based on genome-wide association study. *Reproductive Biology and Endocrinology: RB&E, 23*. https://www.semanticscholar.org/paper/cde91d0c80fc2a4c06640e0b40091f2876d0c120 (accessed on 22nd July 2025).

51. Speiser, P., Arlt, W., Auchus, R. J., Baskin, L. S., Conway, G. S., Merke, D. P., Meyer-Bahlburg, H. F. L., et al. (2018). Congenital adrenal hyperplasia due to steroid 21-hydroxylase deficiency: An Endocrine Society* clinical practice guideline. *The Journal of Clinical Endocrinology & Metabolism, 103*, 4043–4088. https://doi.org/10.1210/jc.2018-01865 (accessed on 22nd July 2025).

52. Tahir, A., Naseer, B., & Shafaq, F. (2025). Perception of university students about the use of painkillers, other remedies and lifestyle modifications for primary dysmenorrhea; a cross-sectional study at KEMU. *BMC Women's Health, 25*. https://www.semanticscholar.org/paper/e3fb359e6816a889209bcc23277f103bccdae09e (accessed on 22nd July 2025).

53. Teede, H., Tay, C. T., Laven, J. J. E., Dokras, A., Moran, L., Piltonen, T., Costello, M., et al. (2023). Recommendations from the 2023 international evidence-based guideline for the assessment and management of polycystic ovary syndrome. *The Journal of Clinical Endocrinology & Metabolism, 108*, 2447–2469. https://doi.org/10.1210/clinem/dgad463 (accessed on 22nd July 2025).

54. Ufnal, J., Wolff, A., Morawska, M., Lewandowska, D., Rosińska-Lewandoska, D., Szewczyk, M., Kożuchowska, K., et al. (2025). Ovarian reserve: A critical indicator of female reproductive health. *Journal of Education, Health and Sport*. https://www.semanticscholar.org/paper/d5b5b11903aaf10ed72d8a9324c4b8d1d541587d (accessed on 22nd July 2025).

55. Vasudevan, S., & Asokan, A. (2025). Cost analysis and cost-efficient of polycystic ovary syndrome (PCOS) management: A narrative review. *International Journal of Medical Sciences and Nursing Research*. https://www.semanticscholar.org/paper/563a324151d29bfbff55958ade1e36442513bba0 (accessed on 22nd July 2025).

56. Vidal, J. D., Wood, C. E., Colman, K., Whitney, K. M., & Creasy, D. M. (2018). *Reproductive System and Mammary Gland*. CRC Press eBooks. https://doi.org/10.1201/9780429504624-20 (accessed on 22nd July 2025).

57. Wang, R., Song, B., Wu, J., Zhang, Y., Chen, A., & Shao, L. (2018). Potential adverse effects

of nanoparticles on the reproductive system. *International Journal of Nanomedicine, 13*, 8487–8506. https://doi.org/10.2147/ijn.s170723 (accessed on 22nd July 2025).

58. Watermeyer, T., Gregory, S., Leetham, E., Udeh-Momoh, C. T., & Muniz-Terrera, G. (2025). Hormone replacement therapy, menopausal age and lifestyle variables are associated with better cognitive performance at follow-up but not cognition over time in older-adult women irrespective of APOE4 carrier status and co-morbidities. *Frontiers in Dementia, 3*. https://www.semanticscholar.org/paper/0876d8def3c5423ff878b2443cb88f1e30e8c509 (accessed on 22nd July 2025).

GROWTH AND PUBERTY

8

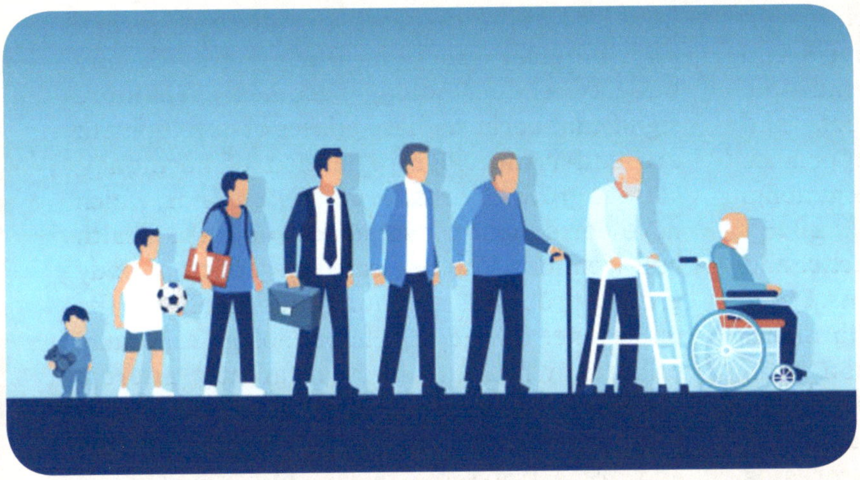

LEARNING OBJECTIVES

After studying this chapter, you will be able to:

1. Understand the endocrine system;
2. Describe growth hormone (GH);
3. Define the process of puberty;
4. Discuss about hormonal changes during puberty;
5. Explain disorders of growth and puberty;
6. Describe the role of nutrition and environment.

Introduction

It is essential in the field of endocrinology, a discipline that deals with the alterations in hormones that regulate such processes of growth and puberty. Puberty is a turning point, where extreme physiological changes transform a child into an adult. This stage is characterized by the activation of the hypothalamic-pituitary-gonadal (HPG) axis, which plays a critical role in growth and sexual development regulation. The study of these endocrine relationships allows researchers and clinicians to delineate not only typical patterns of development but also those deviations that are possible under the influence of either genetics or the environment. Through the utilization of evolutionary biology models, researchers are able to examine how an external factor, such as psychosocial stress, influences processes of maturation and, in the process, is able to inform the management of other developmental disorders and comment on healthy living approaches during puberty (Templeton et al., 2013). The complexity of puberty is also highlighted by the observation of various disorders that entail irregular patterns of growth, e.g., Turner syndrome (TS). Characterized by the absence or abnormalities of one of the X chromosomes, TS embodies the unparalleled influence of genetic influences on puberty and development. The symptoms of TS, including short stature and delayed puberty, illustrate the maximal influence of chromosomal abnormalities on pathways of development. Studies have systematically investigated the correlations between karyotype and TS clinical features and have given insight into the implications of early diagnosis and treatment. The prevalence of the multiple comorbidities such as cardiac defects and autoimmune diseases highlights the importance of longitudinal medical follow-up of TS patients throughout their lifetime (Abacı et al., 2015). The findings have important clinical practice and quality of care improvement implications. Other than genetic and chromosomal factors, hormonal signaling-environmental cue interaction is an important subject of research in the context of development as well as puberty. The ability of the body to adjust its developmental processes in response to energy supplies and social conditions is a type of advanced biological plasticity. Environmental factors, including nutrition and family psychosocial dynamics, may effectively modulate the hormonal regulation of growth. Further, studies have shown that such adaptations may be of evolutionary value so that optimal development may be promoted in light of contextual needs. Therefore, examining the endocrinological underpinning of puberty not only explains normal physiological processes but also addresses significant health issues related to alterations in growth patterns, thereby highlighting the necessity for multidisciplinary models in explaining these complex processes (Templeton et al., 2013).

Definition of Endocrinology

Endocrinology, as a medical specialty, is really all about the secretion of hormones and how those chemical messengers function in an effort to regulate many of the body's physiological functions. By gaining insight into the endocrine system, with glands such as the pituitary gland, thyroid gland, adrenal glands, and pancreas, endocrinologists are interested in understanding how hormones influence critical functions such as growth, metabolism, and reproductive processes. Therefore, the clinical practice of endocrinology is more than the study of hormones in isolation, encompassing the full range of knowledge of how endocrine diseases can disrupt normal physiological function. During growth and puberty, endocrinology becomes even more significant because these phases of development are under the close regulation of hormones, such as growth hormone and sex steroids, which have permanent consequences on one's health and wellness. The intricate interaction of body growth processes and hormones highlights the importance of studying endocrinology, especially puberty, when the body is greatly altered. Puberty is tightly regulated by the hypothalamic-pituitary-gonadal (HPG) axis, which controls and orchestrates the release of sex hormones like testosterone and estrogen, promoting physical change and sexual development. Notably, interruptions in this endocrine axis can trigger many growth illnesses, making it essential that endocrinologists monitor such conditions closely and bring them under control. As such experts apply their expertise, they not only aid in the physical development of teenagers but also guide their psychological and emotional existence, realizing that hormonal imbalance may affect quality of life. Clinically, endocrinologists apply emerging research and clinical guidelines to direct their management of common endocrine conditions, such as congenital adrenal hyperplasia and delayed puberty. For instance, updated clinical practice guidelines are focusing on patient-centered care that considers safety, quality of life, and effective treatment approaches (Speiser et al., 2018). Furthermore, the increasing understanding of the gut-brain axis and its dialogue with the endocrine system is indicative of dynamic interactions with growth and development (John et al., 2019). Overall, the interaction of endocrinology, growth, and puberty serves to underscore the significance of an integrated understanding of hormonal control as well as for the treatment of endocrine disorders in every phase of life.

Importance of Growth and Puberty

The significance of growth and puberty in endocrinology cannot be overstated, as they have a profound effect on the physical and hormonal status of an individual. Puberty is a critical transition from childhood to adulthood through a series of complex endocrine changes that regulate physical growth and sexual maturation. Puberty not only affects reproductive function but also has lasting effects on health. The intricate interdependence of the hormones, driven primarily by the hypothalamic-pituitary-gonadal (HPG) axis, supplies the foundation for adult physical and emotional wellness. Understanding the mechanisms behind development and puberty is essential for disease diagnosis, reducing treatment protocols, and aiding overall health at this formative stage of existence. New breakthroughs mention the role of individual biomarkers towards the assessment of development and pubertal growth and thus clinical understanding of these processes. For example, studies have identified serum phoenixin (PNX-14) as a potential marker for central precocious puberty (CPP) in girls. Its elevated levels correlate with other growth and development markers, including height and bone age, and therefore the value it can hold for diagnosis in clinical settings (Yang et al., 2025). Identification of such biomarkers enables physicians to monitor hormonal changes effectively and reverse any growth or pubertal development deviations. This targeted approach not only increases diagnostic accuracy but also enables interventions to achieve optimal health outcome among children and adolescents with growth-related problems. Assessment of growth and puberty must also be for variations in development across different groups, e.g., as presented by research focused on Danish boys with delayed puberty. These studies have led to the creation of puberty nomograms, a standardized instrument for pubertal onset and progression assessment (Lawaetz et al., 2015). Using these nomograms, healthcare providers will be able to separate normal variant development from actual pathologies, which will enable interventions to be made in a timely manner. Furthermore, the effects of interventions, such as oral testosterone undecanoate in boys with constitutional delay in growth and puberty, have been shown to improve both pubertal and growth outcomes. This two-way focus on clinical evaluation and targeted treatment underscores the importance of a broad understanding of growth and puberty within endocrinology, ultimately enhancing the health and well-being of adolescents (Figure 8.1).

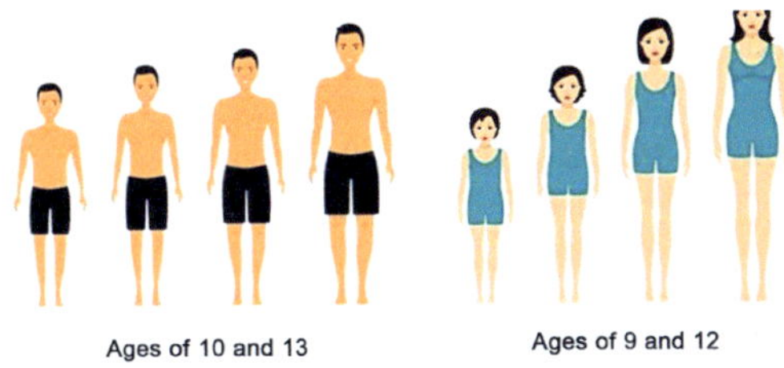

Figure 8.1. Understanding your body during puberty.

Source: https://media.licdn.com/dms/image/v2/D5612AQEuBaMlQxhr3w/article-cover_image-shrink_600_2000/article-cover_image-shrink_600_2000/0/1716444777095?e=2147483647&v=beta&t=OIMzT6rso5Ykg0HrDj4PbypjvqS7eM3wQn4E91eyYHE.

Overview of Hormonal Influences

Hormonal regulation plays a fundamental part in the complex process of growth and puberty that act as biological signals in directing development at these decisive phases of life. During the start of puberty, changes in hormone secretions, particularly by the hypothalamus, pituitary, and gonads, trigger a series of physiological events. Gonadotropin-releasing hormone (GnRH) is released from the hypothalamus to stimulate the pituitary gland to secrete luteinizing hormone (LH) and follicle-stimulating hormone (FSH). These hormones, in turn, stimulate the gonads to secrete sex steroids like estrogen and testosterone, which are required for secondary sexual characteristics. The intricate interplay of hormones not only causes growth stimulation of the reproductive system but also influences growth rate, creating the pubertal growth spurt characteristic of adolescents. The role of sex steroids during puberty goes beyond sexual growth to encompass their effect on patterns of growth and adult height. In males, for instance, testosterone has been shown to stimulate increased activity at the plates of growth, leading to accelerated growth. But in trans adolescents undergoing hormone therapy, the effect of sex steroids on growth is very different. A study among transgender teens revealed that trans girls exhibited a notable acceleration in growth during estradiol treatment, while trans boys had variable outcomes in the advancement of height. Specifically, half of the trans boys did not register expected increases in height prior to treatment, underscoring the necessity of dealing with hormonal impacts on growth trajectories in gender identity (Norup et al., 2024). This demonstrates the way in which hormonal effects need to be considered within the context of overall patterns of individual growth. Besides the sex steroids, other hormones also have vital functions during growth and puberty, namely growth hormone and insulin-like growth factors (IGFs). Growth hormone, produced by the anterior pituitary, is essential in the promotion of linear growth and the control of metabolism. Following increase of IGF-1, predominantly produced following stimulation by growth hormone, facilitates the growth of chondrocytes in growth plates, thereby increasing skeletal maturation. Astonishingly, more recent investigations have established a multidimensional association between rebound adiposity and the role of hormones in triggering puberty. For example, studies indicate that the age of adiposity rebound can vary surprisingly across children, particularly those born with birth weights less than gestational age, affecting not just their growth patterns but also pubertal onset (Kim et al., 2024). Such varied endocrine interactions indicate the necessity of an integrated perception of endocrine processes to affect growth and developmental health.

8.1. The Endocrine System

Learning Outcome

1. Explain major glands involved in growth;
2. Describe hormones regulating growth;
3. Focus on feedback mechanisms in hormone regulation.

The endocrine system plays a crucial role in sustaining development and growth during puberty, supported primarily by a complex interaction of hormones. The cornerstone to the process is the hypothalamic-pituitary-gonadal (HPG) axis that synchronizes the release of gonadotropins that stimulate sexual development. Sex hormones such as luteinizing hormone (LH) and follicle-stimulating hormone (FSH) play a vital role in this phase, which cause the development of sex organs and growth of secondary sexual features. Furthermore, steroid hormones, testosterone and estrogen, also play a major influence on the growth of the body and psychosocial development during puberty. These hormones not only facilitate reproductive growth but also influence bone density, muscle mass, and fat deposition. Overall, an understanding of the hormonal variation and the resulting effects can shed light on the ways in which the endocrine system drives the transforming phase of puberty. Prenatal impact on the endocrine system has significant consequences for pubertal growth and development. Recent evidence points to the intrauterine environment as a critical determinant of the neuroendocrine mechanisms that regulate reproductive function. Maternal diet, exposure to exogenous hormones, and environmental stressors may induce epigenetic modifications that can affect the offspring and even subsequent generations. For example, prenatal exposure to androgens may lead to abnormal development of the reproductive system, highlighting the fetal life sensitivity of the GnRH neurosecretory system. Prepubertally acting hormones may induce long-lasting changes that determine the onset of puberty as well as reproductive health thereafter, indicating the intricate interconnection between early hormonal milieus and terminal developmental outcomes (Bellingham et al., 2016). An understanding of these interactions lays a foundation for an understanding of growth and reproductive health disorders. Also, the action of steroid hormones extends into other physiological processes beyond reproduction, which illustrates the complexity of the endocrine system. As an example, estrogens and androgens play not only a key role in sexual differentiation but also in metabolic programming and in the risk for the development of diseases such as polycystic ovary syndrome (PCOS). It is an indication of the importance of hormonal regulation at puberty since dysregulation can lead to serious long-term illness. The neuroprotective action of progesterone in neurodegenerative diseases and the mechanism by which estrogens induce prolactin secretion are among the other facets of this complex interaction (Deniselle et al., 2016). As it is increasingly understood that the endocrine system has a deep effect on growth and adolescence, it is also increasingly important to consider how hormonal interactions impact not just health in the individual but overall public health as well.

8.1.1. Major Glands Involved in Growth

The endocrine system oversees growth and development through a web of glands that secrete hormones. Among the main glands that do this are the pituitary gland, thyroid gland, adrenal glands, and gonads. The pituitary gland, also referred to as the "master gland," secretes growth hormone (GH) that stimulates growth in various tissues, regulating general height as well as organ growth. It functions with thyroid hormones, which are pivotal in metabolism and have roles in child and adolescent growth. The adrenal glands also produce cortisol and adrenal androgens, which have roles in growth by changing metabolic processes and enabling the body's response to stress and ultimately affecting growth and development indirectly. In addition to the pituitary and adrenal glands, that of the thyroid gland is also of very crucial importance in regulating growth. The two principal hormones of the thyroid, thyroxine (T4) and triiodothyronine (T3), are the cornerstone of metabolic regulation, which is significant in the process of normal growth and development. Their deficiency will most probably lead to growth disorders, such as cretinism in infancy, resulting from arrested mental and physical growth. In addition, thyroid gland activity can significantly influence the onset of puberty as thyroid function plays a significant role in the synthesis of growth-stimulating hormones. With growth peaking during puberty, any change in thyroid function has a direct effect on the pattern of growth and final adult stature. The gonads, including the testes in men and ovaries in women, are also involved in the growth process through the production of sex hormones like testosterone and estrogen. These hormones not only allow secondary sexual characteristics to grow but also control the activity of the growth plate within the bones. Testosterone, for instance, builds muscle mass and promotes linear growth in puberty, while estrogen plays a pivotal role in the final closure of the growth plates, marking the completion of growth. The interplay among these hormones emphasizes the nature of endocrine control in growth and puberty. The endocrine climate during these stages of development is greatly influenced by a number of factors including genetics, nutrition, and overall health, demonstrating the intricate interactions between the major glands that govern growth and the resultant effect of these glands on human growth (Khare et al., 2025; Saroufim et al., 2022) (Figure 8.2).

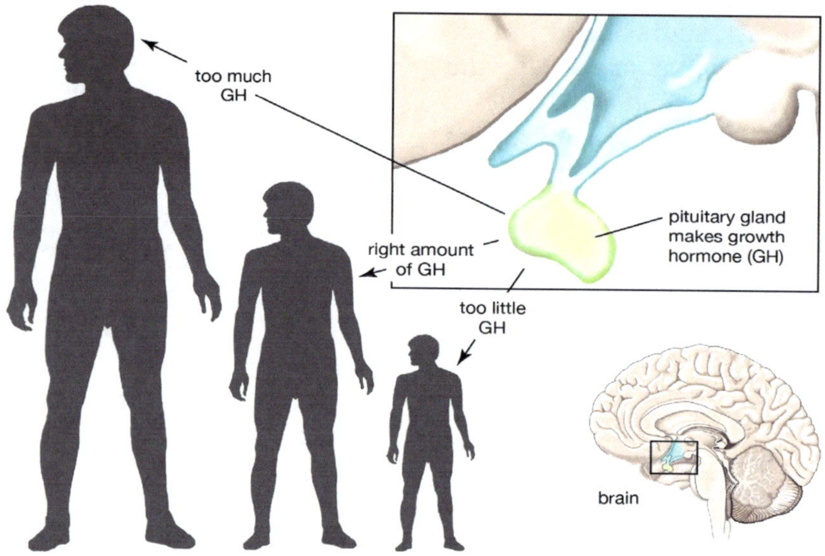

Figure 8.2. Growth hormone is secreted by the anterior lobe of the pituitary gland and is vital for normal physical growth in children.

Source: https://cdn.britannica.com/13/93313-050-6D750D77/Growth-hormone-pituitary-gland-anterior-lobe-growth.jpg.

8.1.2. Hormones Regulating Growth

The regulation of growth during adolescence is regulated by a multifaceted interplay of hormones, which have the central role of coordinating developmental activities. These critical hormones, such as growth hormone (GH), insulin-like growth factors (IGFs), and sex steroids (testosterone and estrogen), synergistically preside over the patterns of growth of individuals during this critical phase. Growth hormone released from the pituitary gland stimulates the release of IGFs from the liver, which leads to the proliferation of chondrocytes in growth plates that results in the elongation of bones that is essential during puberty when growth spurts are highest. Moreover, sex steroids do not only enhance the growth stimulation effect of GH and IGFs but also initiate epiphyseal closure, thereby marking the closure of longitudinal bone growth. Thus, hormonal regulation of growth is a subtle process to prepare individuals for adulthood along with reflecting overall endocrine functions in puberty. Thyroid hormones, excluding GH and IGFs, also play a significant role in regulating growth in puberty. Thyroid-derived hormones are crucial to normal development and maturation. They control metabolic processes influencing body composition and energy absorption and thus provide the basis for the adolescent growth spurt. Thyroid hormones interact synergistically with sex steroids to potentiate their anabolic effects on muscle and bone growth. Further, abnormalities in the production of thyroid hormones can lead to growth disorders such as delayed puberty or short stature. The interplay among thyroid hormone, GH, and sex steroids highlights the complexity of the hormonal interactions that not only dictate the timing of growth spurts but also the final height of an individual. Understanding these pathways is important in growth-related disorders that originate from imbalance of hormones during this important phase of growth. Recent research has also disclosed the role of the microbiota-gut-brain axis in altering hormonal responses and control of growth. The gut microbiome affects a range of metabolic processes and neuroendocrine signaling mechanisms that are important for growth. Microbial metabolites such as short-chain fatty acids are able to alter the secretion of hormones such as GH and insulin, and consequently influence growth dynamics. Secondly, stressors during periods of critical development have been found to alter composition of microbiota, which in turn may lead to hormonal dysregulation and affect growth patterns. These observations place importance on an understanding of the broader physiological context in which hormones operate, and also on the contribution of the microbiome to growth regulation. As we learn more about these interactions, therapeutic interventions that target the microbiota may be potential treatments for growth issues, synching endocrinology and microbiome research in new and promising fashions (Figure 8.3).

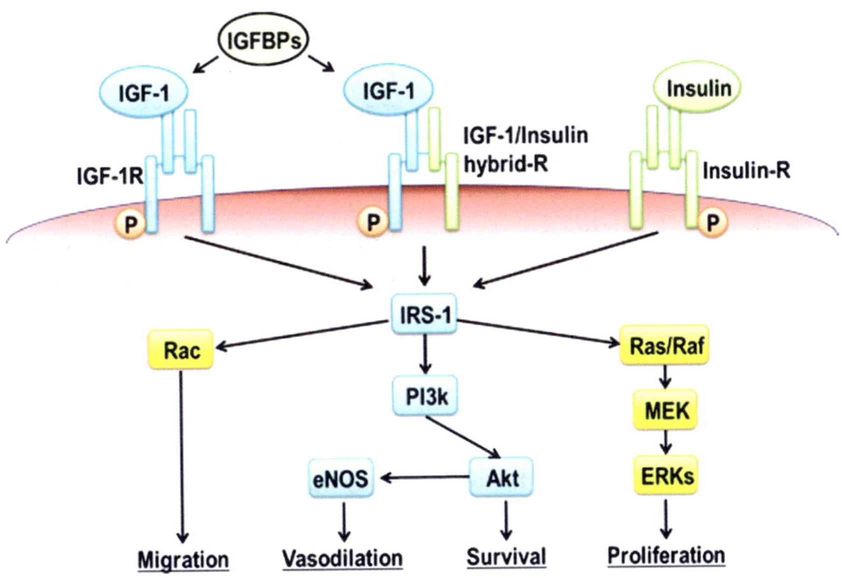

Figure 8.3. Insulin-like growth factor (IGF)-1 signal transduction. IGF-1 binds to IGF-1R and the IGF-1/insulin hybrid receptor, whereas insulin binds only to the insulin receptor (insulin-R) and triggers several signaling pathways.

Source: https://www.researchgate.net/profile/Patrice-Delafontaine/publication/223973394/figure/fig1/AS:304762013667333@1449672334912/Insulin-like-growth-factor-IGF-1-signal-transduction-IGF-1-binds-to-IGF-1R-and.png.

8.1.3. Feedback Mechanisms in Hormone Regulation

The intricate negative feedback mechanisms that control hormone regulation play a vital role in growth and puberty, particularly with regard to reproductive function. The hypothalamic-pituitary-gonadal (HPG) axis is at the heart of this system and serves as an exemplary model of negative feedback. The release of luteinizing hormone (LH) and follicle-stimulating hormone (FSH) from the pituitary gland is stimulated by gonadotropin-releasing hormone (GnRH) of the hypothalamus, which in turn stimulates the secretion of hormones in the gonads. Notably, the elevated levels of sex steroids like testosterone and estrogen stimulate the pituitary gland and the hypothalamus to inhibit the release of GnRH, FSH, and LH, hence ensuring hormone balance. Through this negative feedback mechanism, hormone fluctuation is maintained within a physiological range, a process which is important for the normal progression of puberty (Bellingham et al., 2016). Understanding these feedback mechanisms not only illuminates normal reproductive health but also shows potential mechanisms for the therapeutic treatment of reproductive pathology. Beyond the HPG axis, emerging studies show the contribution of various neuroendocrine factors that complicate hormone regulation throughout puberty. For instance, kisspeptin, a vital neuropeptide, appears to act as a gatekeeper for initiating the onset of puberty by modulating the release of GnRH (Bentley et al., 2016). This is evidence of the sensitivity of the neuroendocrine system to both internal and external cues, which can reprogram endocrine responses throughout an individual's lifetime. Stress, diet, and environmental exposures are among those factors that have been shown to influence kisspeptin signaling, thereby influencing the plasticity and functionality of the GnRH neurosecretory systems. The process behind such plasticity remains not so well understood yet but is pivotal as one thinks of how reproductive health is influenced over generations. The above discovery underscores the importance of further exploration on the interaction of hormonal feedback mechanisms with lifestyle and environmental factors. Research has also shown the significant role of epigenetic changes to the development of neuroendocrine pathways for the regulation of hormones. As seen in prenatal programming, the exposure to various external elements during pregnancy can have long-lasting effects on reproductive processes in offspring (Bellingham et al., 2016). For instance, the impacts of disturbed maternal diet or exposure to endocrine-disrupting chemicals can reprogramming the neuroendocrine axes regulating growth and reproduction with potential transgenerational consequences. Moreover, age-related hormonal changes complicate the feedback control more, particularly in women in whom kisspeptin regulatory effects on ovarian function decline with age (Bentley et al., 2016). It is an understanding of the complex processes of these feedback systems that underlies the planning of interventions that will optimize reproductive health during puberty and later, particularly in the face of increasing environmental stresses.

Test Your Knowledge

1. Which endocrine glands play a primary role in regulating human growth, and what hormones do they produce?
2. What is the role of growth hormone (GH) in the body?

8.2. Growth Hormone (GH)

Learning Outcome

1. Explain the role of GH in childhood growth;
2. Deal with regulation of GH secretion;
3. Discuss the effects of GH deficiency and excess.

The role of Growth Hormone (GH) in growth and development processes, particularly in adolescence, cannot be overstressed. GH, secreted from the anterior pituitary gland, is known to trigger linear growth, influence protein, fat, and carbohydrate metabolism, and general physiological development. GH release is pulsatile and sensitive to a wide range of stimuli such as sleep, exercise, and certain nutrient consumption, which reflects its adaptive role in addressing the body's needs during growth spurts. Of particular interest is GH's synergy with insulin-like growth factors (IGFs), by which the majority of its growth-stimulating action in peripheral tissues takes place and which generates a highly evolved endocrine environment that is accountable for development under normative conditions during times of critical growth, including in adolescence where rapid physiological growth occurs (Caroline et al., 2020). During puberty, the levels of GH secretion dramatically alter, secondary to the maturation of the hypothalamic-pituitary-gonadal axis.

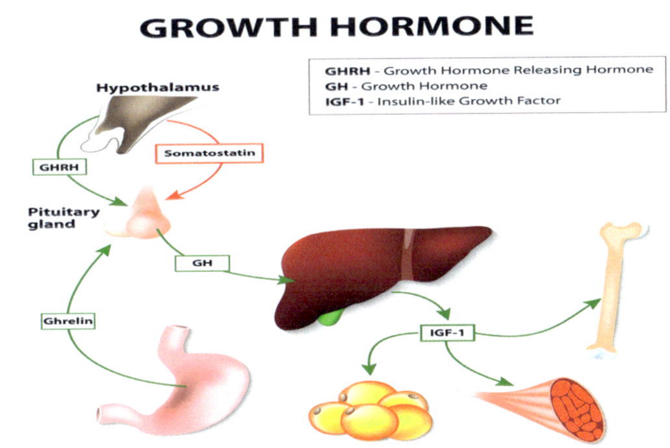

Figure 8.4. Growth hormone (GH).

Source: https://www.netmeds.com/images/cms/wysiwyg/blog/2021/08/1628665553_Hormone_big_450.jpg.

The pulsed secretion of GH also tends to mirror elevated circulating levels of the sex steroids that increase sensitivity and responsiveness of target tissues to GH. Such a correlation delineates the mechanism by which GH orchestrates a complex interaction of hormonal signals needed for optimal growth and development and activates not only linear growth but also ontogenesis of skeletal muscle and fat tissue. Furthermore, GH's influence on metabolic processes, including its role in maintaining body composition and augmenting lean mass accretion, is most prominent among adolescents, a time when increased physical activity and energy needs are typical among growing persons (John et al., 2019). Furthermore, heterogeneity of GH secretion and response is intended to further highlight its critical role in establishing growth patterns and outcomes. GH level variation may be brought about by environmental, lifestyle, and genetic factors, which play an important role in individuals growth patterns. This calls for the consideration of individualized hormonal effects in the study of growth and development in puberty. Most importantly, disruptions in GH signaling account for conditions such as growth hormone deficiency or excess, which can greatly impact normal development. Thus, recognizing the numerous functions of GH during adolescence is essential to prevent and treat growth disorders as well as optimize health benefits during this period of development (Caroline et al., 2020) (Figure 8.4).

8.2.1. Role of GH in Childhood Growth

The role of growth hormone (GH) in childhood development is one of the fundamental doctrines of endocrinology that emphasizes the importance of hormonal control in childhood years. GH released from the anterior pituitary gland has a crucial role to play in promotion of growth and proliferation of cells with deep impacts on longitudinal bone growth, increase in lean body mass, and overall physical growth in children. It works via insulin-like growth factor 1 (IGF-1), which in turn causes growth in various tissues. If the GH levels are in proportion, children undergo normal growth; however, when GH is above or below normal, it leads to serious developmental issues. In deficiency of GH, children may manifest with growth arrest, whereas overdose of GH may result in conditions such as gigantism, which is a definite indication of the fine balance required for normal growth and development in childhood. Furthermore, GH plays a key role in the intricate interaction between environmental stress and genetic factors during childhood growth. Experimental findings have established that the genetic component is largely involved in variance in GH levels and growth patterns. For instance, heritability of testosterone levels has been found to be approximately 50% in children and reflects a large genetic component to the control of hormones, as seen also with GH (Archer et al., 2005). In addition to genes, environmental forces, i.e., diet and chemical exposure, also play a role in influencing release and function of GH. This interaction affects the overall growth pattern and therefore the onset of puberty. Tackling the role of GH in this regard is particularly important because it illuminates how both intrinsic factors and extrinsic conditions interact to determine outcomes of growth.

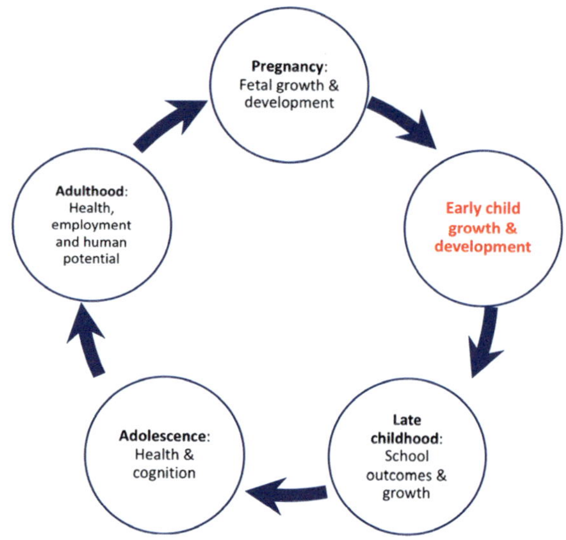

Figure 8.5. The cycle of child growth and development.

Source: https://www.researchgate.net/publication/337298800/figure/fig1/AS:962679653019649@1606532123733/The-cycle-of-child-growth-and-development.png.

Further, comprehending GHs role also includes an appreciation of the negative consequences that disruptions in the environment can have for children's growth and development. Exposure to toxic substances like endocrine-disrupting chemicals may damage not just GH signal pathways but also more general growth and developmental processes. Exposure is known to result in various health issues, for example, learning disabilities and behavioral disorders, which emerge through phases of basic growth and development (Hitchcock et al., 2011). Thus, avoiding such environmental dangers is central in the maintenance of childhood health. By knowing the double effect of the GH and the environment, pediatric health programs can be designed to optimize the growth and development of children so that passage through puberty and on into adulthood will be healthier (Figure 8.5).

8.2.2. Regulation of GH Secretion

The regulation process for the secretion of growth hormone (GH) is multifaceted and involves various hormonal stimuli, feedback, and physiological inputs. GH synthesis and release are primarily carried out by the anterior pituitary gland and are regulated by the effects of growth hormone-releasing hormone (GHRH) and somatostatin. GHRH release from the hypothalamus triggers GH release, and somatostatin inhibits it. The interaction between these two hormones guarantees the synchronization of GH secretion with the body's growth needs, particularly during phases like puberty. Notably, the pulsatile nature of GH secretion suggests that the concentration changes throughout the day and is specifically influenced by sleep, stress, and food intake, thereby further ensuring the influence of the environment on the regulation of growth. Along with these hormonal regulations, external factors considerably affect GH secretion. For instance, greater physical exercise and dieting, particularly among children, will trigger the release of GH, thus promoting linear growth. Moreover, sleep also plays a crucial role; most of the GH release occurs during deep phases of sleep. The physiological processes that cause these responses are interconnected, and factors such as age, sex, and metabolic rate affect general regulation of GH. In addition, this understanding of GH secretion is not exclusive to humans, as similar regulatory mechanisms exist in other species, wherein the evolutionary significance of GH during growth and development becomes evident. Further investigation into these dynamics is required to the management of growth disorders and to optimal health during the growth stages of life. More recent studies indicate that variability in stress response between individuals may impact GH secretion and therefore growth outcome. For instance, the association of behavioral characteristics with GH regulation indicates complicated interaction between psychological processes and endocrinological reaction. For fish, certain behavioral characteristics associated with growth rates and stress tolerance provide evidence of how variability in GH regulation may express itself among species (Gesto et al., 2016).

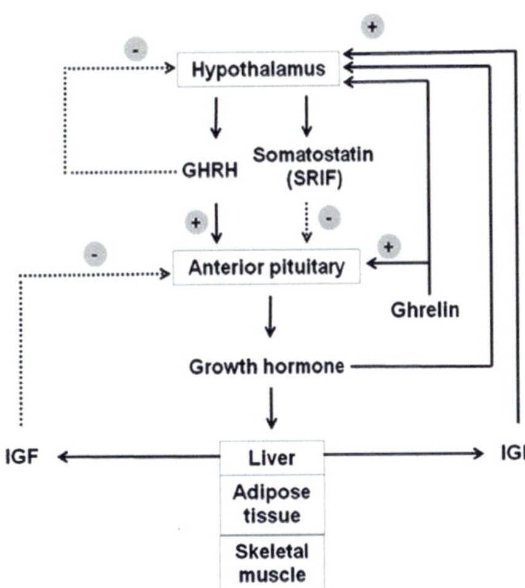

Figure 8.6. Regulation of growth hormone secretion.

Source: https://www.researchgate.net/profile/Valeria-Chaves/publication/235690936/figure/fig1/AS:341482977415191@1458427294844/Regulation-of-growth-hormone-secretion-GHRH-growth-hormone-releasing-hormone-IGF.png.

In humans, endocrine disorders such as hyperprolactinemia disrupt normal GH release patterns, which can cause growth and sexual development issues (Aversa et al., 2016). The endocrine pathologies need to be identified and addressed as they play essential roles in patterns of growth during significant periods of development. Understanding these regulatory mechanisms eventually leads to the formation of interventions in growth disease conditions and optimizing health outcomes during adolescence (Figure 8.6).

8.2.3. Effects of GH Deficiency and Excess

Growth hormone (GH) deficiency has profound physiological and developmental implications which resonate throughout an individual's pattern of growth. Children with GH deficiency commonly have suppression of growth, height far below normal expectation for age and gender. GH deficiency has more than just a statural implication; it has wide-ranging effects on metabolic function, including increased body fat, loss of muscle mass, and dyslipidemia. Besides, such a condition can also be further compounded by psychosocial consequences in the form of decreased self-esteem and social challenges resulting from physical inadequacy feelings. Successful management of GH deficiency requires early diagnosis and treatment, most often in the form of recombinant human GH treatment to restore normal growth rates and promote healthy results. In this case, understanding of the different consequences of GH deficiency becomes important for practitioners who are interested in catering to affected children through their growing years. Conversely, when too much GH exists, there are problems and complications that also manifest in the form of acromegaly in adults or gigantism in children depending on when the endocrine imbalance develops. While acromegaly includes bone and tissue growth beyond the normal threshold that produces unusual physical characteristics such as oversized arms and hands and facial structures, the metabolic effect is equally impressive. Adenoma patients who secrete excess GH are generally insulin resistant, which increases the possibility of type 2 diabetes and cardiovascular incidents. The differences in body composition, such as higher visceral fat and lower lean mass, have been implied by scientific evidence to produce severe long-term health consequences. Thus, management of GH excess also often involves a multidisciplinary team, with endocrinologists and surgical experts, to minimize associated morbidity and enhance quality of life in affected individuals. The interplay between GH physiology and metabolism underscores the pivotal role of this hormone in growth and puberty. Familiarity with the rudimentary mechanisms by which GH synthesis and release are regulated can offer insights as to why deficiency and excess both have such far-reaching manifestations.

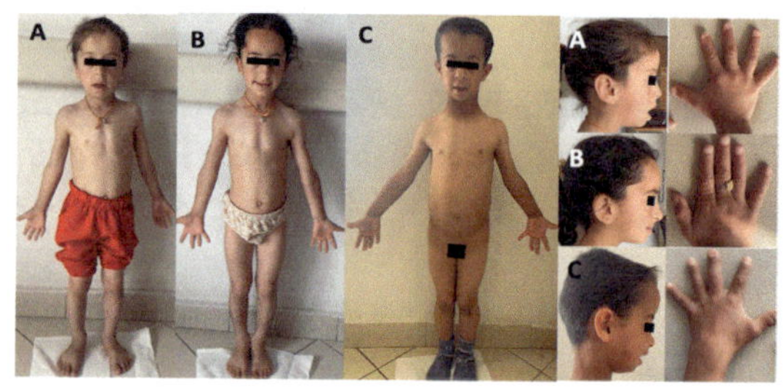

Figure 8.7. (A) Phenotypic features of the first case. Frontal bossing, maxillary hypoplasia, obtuse mandibular angle, disproportionate short stature, and brachydactyly can be noted. (B) Phenotypic features of the second case. Notice the prominent forehead, obtuse mandibular angle, and disproportionate short stature. (C) Phenotypic features of the third case. Frontal bossing, maxillary hypoplasia, obtuse mandibular angle, disproportionate short stature, and brachydactyly are evident.

Source: https://assets.cureus.com/uploads/figure/file/723831/lightbox_e3ffb7f03d3211eebf3891be6350f550-Ekran-Resmi-2023-08-17-22.08.16.png.

Determinants of GH concentration include rhythmicity of secretion, sensitivity to insulin, and interaction with other hormonal mechanisms, highlighting the complexity of endocrine control. Increasingly, researchers have begun to explore the interaction between GH and the gut-brain axis, acknowledging that hormones act in concert in the body. Interestingly, new evidence suggests that the gut microbiota composition may regulate GH secretion and, consequently, growth and metabolic homeostasis, particularly during sensitive developmental windows. More research here may shed vital light on targeted treatment for GH-linked metabolic and endocrinological disorders (John et al., 2019; Speiser et al., 2018) (Figure 8.7).

Test Your Knowledge

1. What is the role of growth hormone (GH) in childhood development?
2. Which hormones and factors regulate the secretion of GH from the anterior pituitary?
3. What are the common causes and clinical signs of growth hormone deficiency in children and adults?

8.3. Puberty: An Overview

Learning Outcome

1. Explain the definition and stages of puberty;
2. Discuss about timing and variations in puberty onset;
3. Understand psychological and physical changes during puberty.

Puberty is an important transition phase in human development, during which there occurs a sequence of physiological, emotional, and psychological changes. Puberty, as per the biological aspect, is initiated by activation of the hypothalamic-pituitary-gonadal (HPG) axis and subsequent release of sex hormones such as testosterone and estrogen. These hormones have been implicated in the development of secondary sex characteristics like female breast enlargement and increased muscle mass in males. The onset of puberty typically occurs around the ages of 9–14, with differences accounted for by genetic, dietary, and environmental factors. Recognition of these hormonal changes is crucial in determining how they influence not only body growth but also mental health, as adolescents navigate the process of establishing themselves and their connection to others. Nutritional status at puberty is critical because it can have significant impact on the timing and development of sexual maturation. Nutrition is relevant in meeting the energy needs of growth and hormone production during this period. For instance, proper nutrition rich in the required nutrients may enhance optimal growth patterns, while malnutrition may lead to delay of sexual maturation and an increased risk for negative long-term health consequences. Interestingly, the gut microbiota has emerged as a critical mediator in this context. The interaction between nutrition and the microbiota can make a difference in hormone activities and metabolic processes that are critical during puberty. Research suggests that an altered microbiota, with its function influenced by diet and environmental stresses, might be involved in the etiology of diseases in adulthood, thus closing the gap between early life exposures and later health (John et al., 2019). Moreover, the role of environmental exposures in the onset of puberty again highlights the need for a holistic understanding of this phase in endocrinology. There is new evidence that suggests exposure to endocrine-disrupting chemicals and environmental chemicals during windows of critical development can lead to changed hormonal signaling, ultimately affecting growth and reproductive health. These exposures, along with stress and diet, may predispose an individual to various health conditions ranging from obesity to reproductive disease (Jerrold et al., 2015). By understanding the determinants of puberty in complex terms, researchers are able to understand better how early life affects adult health. It is not only essential for the development of preventive strategies but also for constructing an integrated model of understanding endocrine health across the life course, where the biological and environmental determinants are equally salient.

8.3.1. Definition and Stages of Puberty

Puberty is the name that describes a highly significant period of human development characterized by a cascade of hormonal, physical, and psychological transformations. It typically marks the close of childhood and the start of adolescence and is initiated by endocrine stimulation, which is the turn on of the hypothalamic-pituitary-gonadal axis. With turn on, there occurs increased secretion of gonadotropin-releasing hormone (GnRH), leading to the secretion of luteinizing hormone (LH) and follicle-stimulating hormone (FSH). These hormones play extremely significant roles in sexual development, which leads to the occurrence of primary and secondary sex characteristics. Puberty occurs typically between 9 and 14 years for girls and 10 to 15 years for boys, but there can be a lot of variation based on heredity, environmental factors, and overall health condition of the body. Knowledge of the definition and process of puberty is vital in order to value its significance for adolescent development and growth. Puberty takes place in well-defined stages marked by unmistakable physical and biological changes, typically separated by the Tanner stages.

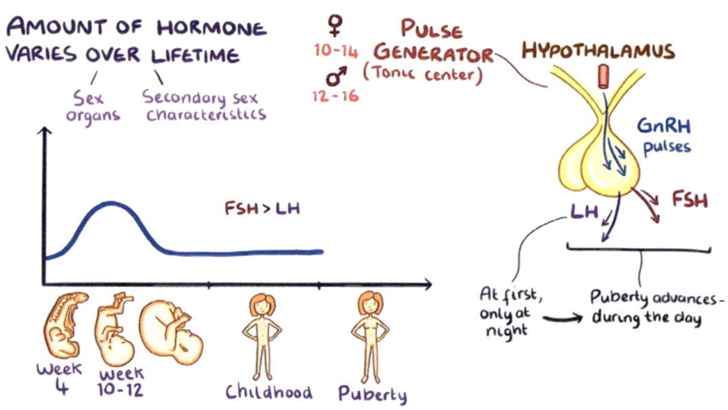

Figure 8.8. Puberty and tanner staging.

Source: https://d16qt3wv6xm098.cloudfront.net/QvyrvK9WR5GkIWYyk8noQU81SJalB3uD/_.jpg.

These assess breast and pubic hair maturation in females, and genital and pubic hair maturation in males. From Tanner stage 1, which is the prepubertal stage, to Tanner stage 5, which represents full sexual maturity, clinicians and researchers follow these progressions to determine normal growth patterns. Of special interest is the onset of menstruation (menarche), which is the culmination of female pubertal development, usually occurring in Tanner stages 3 to 4. In males, the progression of testicular development is an important indicator of the onset of puberty. This staged process not only allows for monitoring of individual growth but also permits detection of growth disorders, like delayed or precocious puberty, requiring clinical intervention. The endocrine component of puberty extends beyond its physical consequences, with significant impact on metabolic and psychological considerations. Pubertal changes in hormones influence growth hormone release patterns, which are important for optimal height gain and general physical development. For instance, studies indicate that small for gestational age (SGA) children may exhibit variability in the timing of onset of puberty based on growth hormone treatment, which further underscores the importance of interventions in aligning these schedules. Furthermore, factors such as adherence to GH treatment may play a pivotal function in maximizing growth potential at this critical period. Understanding the complex ballet of pubertal hormones, along with treatment adherence ramifications and response variability, is essential for accurate endocrinologists and practitioners to attain better patient outcomes (Boonstra et al., 2003; Carlo et al., 2017) (Figure 8.8).

8.3.2. Timing and Variations in Puberty Onset

Timings and variability of timing of onset of puberty are significant predictors of physical and reproductive health through life. Puberty is marked by a cascade of complex endocrine processes with the onset being the hypothalamic release of gonadotropin-releasing hormone (GnRH) that initiates the release of luteinizing hormone (LH) and follicle-stimulating hormone (FSH) from the pituitary gland. Small differences in the timing of these hormonal changes can have great impacts on sexual development and reproductive function. Recent work has suggested that late puberty is linked with adverse reproductive consequences in men, such as diminished semen quality and hormone changes. For instance, research has revealed that late-pubertal boys experienced reduced sperm counts and disturbed serum hormone profiles, emphasizing the importance of typical pubertal timing to male reproductive health (Jensen et al., 2016). Furthermore, genetic factors can also play an important role in the variation observed in the onset of puberty, particularly in females. There are some genotypes for FSH that have been discovered to influence reproductive hormone levels and ovarian development. In a study of healthy peripubertal girls, there were genetic variants that correlated with higher levels of FSH and estradiol, which play key roles in normal ovarian function and follicle maturation. These interactions between genes imply that an individual's genetic makeup may be predisposed to early or late puberty, subsequently influencing their overall reproductive health and functionality. Significantly, the interaction of genes with hormonal pathways highlights the complexity of puberty development and the necessity for further exploration into unravelling these interactions (Busch et al., 2016). The impact of changes in the onset of puberty reaches far beyond transient physiological alterations and may involve long-term determinants of health. Early or delayed development may be associated with growth patterns, psychosocial development, and risk of diseases like obesity and metabolic syndrome. In addition, delayed onset of puberty is not merely an indicator of current reproductive status but also a potential marker for future fertility issues. Because reproductive capacity is part of individual and population health, information regarding onset-of-puberty-associated factors will be crucial. Continuing studies in this area, and particularly in health correlates and genetic determinants, have the potential to guide intervention design that can maximize pubertal timing and result in healthier reproductive outcomes (Busch et al., 2016; Jensen et al., 2016) (Figure 8.9).

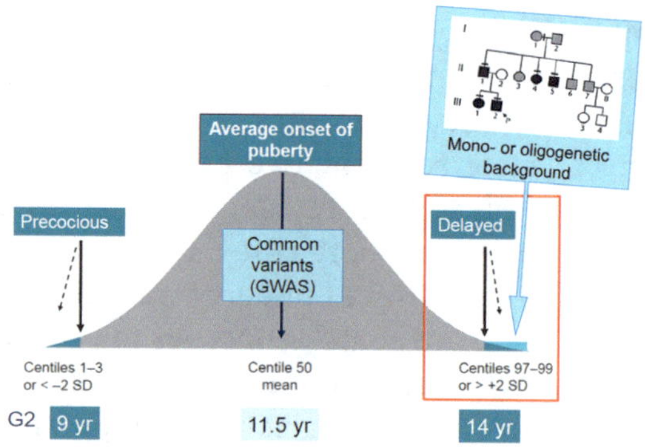

Figure 8.9. The genetics of pubertal timing.

Source: https://www.researchgate.net/profile/Sasha-Howard/publication/319887219/figure/fig1/AS:565626861490176@1511867360810/The-genetics-of-pubertal-timing-In-the-general-population-there-is-a-near-normal.png.

8.3.3. Psychological and Physical Changes During Puberty

The onset of puberty is a phase of highly critical psychological and physical transformations. The transformation is mostly brought about by hormonal alterations that lead to the development of secondary sexual characteristics and rebuilding of emotional and intellectual structures. They exhibit sudden spurts in growth, development of breasts among girls, and increased muscle and body hair for boys. Besides that, puberty is marked by altering body composition that impacts self-concept and mental health. These alterations can lead to body consciousness and unstable self-esteem due to the tendency of adolescents to compare themselves with others. Thus, the psychological landscape during puberty is irrevocably interconnected with the bodily transformations occurring, and hence understanding the connection between these elements is central to adolescent development and endocrinology. At such changes, adolescents' mental state also reflects the complexity of achieving social identities and intimate relationships. Adolescence typically begins around the time there is increased sensitivity to peer pressure and social life, which may in turn influence mental health significantly. Here, the desire to belong and be accepted socially during development may increase some towards anxiety or high-risk behavior. Further, heightened emotional instability, commonly linked with adolescence, is linked with increasing hormone levels, which contribute to mood swings and increased sensitivity to social derogation. Learning then why shifting hormones impact emotional regulation and social behavior is integral to learning fully about the psychological problems of this age, illustrating precisely how intertwined shifting hormones and psychological change are during puberty. Research emphasizes the salience of developmental environments, in this instance within an evolutionary context, to account for adaptations occurring during puberty. The theory argues that variations in timing of puberty and accompanying behavior can be influenced by the environment, as well as by psychosocial stressors. For instance, adolescents exposed to family stress could acquire life-history acceleration strategies that include early maturation and pursuing reproductive opportunities, which can shape social behaviors like aggression and risk-taking. This evolutionary perspective explains why some adolescents could exhibit abnormal psychological responses during puberty. Furthermore, research in studies of attractiveness judgments reveals that judgments of mate value change with physical development, and this implies that as growing up progresses, youngsters' preferences are largely in step with adaptive social cues for reproductive and social success (DeBruine et al., 2009; Templeton et al., 2013). Finally, being aware of these psychological and physical attributes gives us significant insights into the growing-up process, prioritizing the intervention of endocrinology in influencing the general maturing process (Figure 8.10).

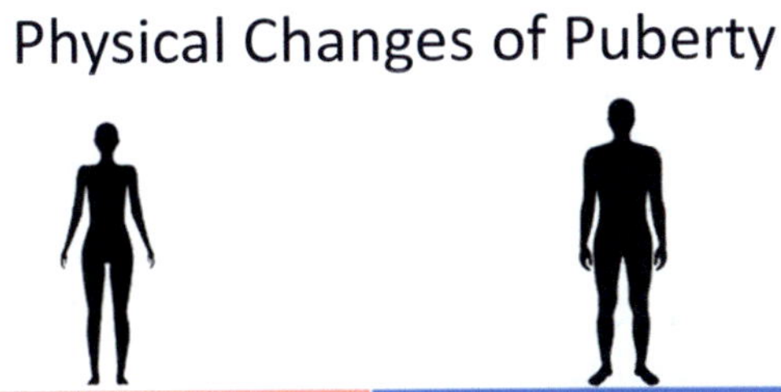

Females	Males
Breast Development	Testicular enlargement
Pubic hair, body odor, axillary hair	Pubic hair, body odor, axillary hair
Acne	Acne
Increased growth up to 8cm/year	Increased growth up to 10cm/year
Menstrual periods	Penis growth and Erections
Increased adiposity	Increased muscle mass, decreased adiposity
Increased ligamentous laxity	Sperm production/ejaculation
Risk for anemia with periods	Increased Hematocrit

Figure 8.10. Physical changes of puberty.

Source: https://ars.els-cdn.com/content/image/3-s2.0-B9780323999922000165-f03-03-9780323999922.jpg.

Test Your Knowledge

1. What is puberty, and what biological processes mark its onset?
2. What factors influence the timing of puberty onset, and what are the common variations such as precocious or delayed puberty?
3. How does puberty affect psychological and emotional development, and what challenges are commonly observed during this period?

8.4. Hormonal Changes During Puberty

Learning Outcome

1. Explain the role of sex hormones (estrogen and testosterone) during puberty;
2. Understand the impact of adrenal hormones in growth and puberty;
3. Discuss the interaction between growth hormone and sex hormones.

Puberty is an important period of transition marked by rapid hormonal changes that orchestrate development and maturation of sex characteristics. It is initiated when the hypothalamus secretes gonadotropin-releasing hormone (GnRH), which activates the anterior pituitary to secrete luteinizing hormone (LH) and follicle-stimulating hormone (FSH). These hormones, in turn, stimulate the gonads to increase production of the sex steroids estrogen and testosterone. The interaction of these hormones not only begins physical changes, such as breast growth and growth spurts, but also affects emotional and mental function. The significance of these hormonal changes is greater than mere superficial physical changes; they lay the groundwork for reproductive health and overall metabolic functioning in adulthood. Thus, understanding orchestration of these hormonal alterations is key to appreciation of their prime position within immediate developmental changes and long-term health effects. With progressing puberty, the growth hormone (GH) surge is of particular significance. GH, released from the anterior pituitary, is essential for stimulation of growth in numerous tissues, including muscle and bone, thus facilitating secondary sexual characteristics and increase of body mass. Besides its linear growth effect, GH also affects carbohydrate metabolism and is implicated in lipolysis, and hence composition of the body is altered. Such hormonal equilibrium is particularly important in individuals with certain inborn errors of metabolism (IEMs), whose unique metabolic patterns can further be disrupted by the pubertal hormonal shift. The research shows that high GH levels are capable of aggravating the metabolic derangements typically seen in such individuals, and this necessitates expert medical interventions at this juncture of crucial growth. Overcoming such adversity from an endocrinological point of view comes a long way in curing such adolescents who are experiencing both puberty and metabolic dysfunction (Lundqvist et al., 2025). Further, hormonal impact on puberty is also observed on the voice apparatus, illustrating the intricate interdependency between endocrine function and bodily development. Laryngeal and vocal cord structural development is highly influenced by hormones such as testosterone and estrogen. For instance, for males, when testosterone levels rise, the voice deepens due to the elongation and thickening of the vocal cords. Conversely, estrogen in women is the cause of voice changes which can add range and quality of tone. Surprisingly, voice changes have not only been linked with the sex hormones but thyroid hormones also play a significant role in voice in life stages like puberty. These disparities also attest to the sophisticated interaction between voice health and endocrinology, which warrants comprehensive evaluations considering hormonal influences on voice during this initial period (Kumar et al., 2016).

8.4.1. Role of Sex Hormones (Estrogen and Testosterone)

The role of the sex hormones, testosterone and estrogen is key to the development and growth experienced during puberty. Estrogen, which is produced primarily in the ovaries, controls some of the physiological processes experienced by women like the enlargement of the secondary sexual characteristics like breast growth and widening of the hips. These are signals of the onset of menstruation and the initiation of the child into adult life. Conversely, testosterone, secreted in the testes, triggers similar processes of development in males, stimulating muscle growth, voice change, and hair growth on the face and body. The interaction between these hormones not only allows for physical development but also influences psychological aspects, such as increased libido and mood changes. Coordination and timing of estrogen and testosterone are crucial to affording a normal and straightforward puberty. Apart from this, disturbances in the levels or activity of these sex hormones can have significant consequences on one's health. For instance, hypogonadism, where the body is unable to produce sufficient amounts of testosterone or estrogen, is responsible for delayed puberty and associated psychological consequences. Low levels of testosterone in men will delay the development of the secondary sexual characteristics of males and lead to infertility, while low levels of estrogen in females will result in irregular menstruation and blockage of normal breast development. Early diagnosis and therapy cannot be overemphasized in these individuals because hormone replacement therapy has the ability to produce the necessary change of physiology, allowing them to transition into adult life successfully. Treatment of such hormonal deficiencies underlines the primary role that estrogen and testosterone play in the health and well-being of adolescents. In addition, knowledge of sex hormones transfers into a variety of specific medical diseases, such as congenital adrenal hyperplasia (CAH) and congenital hypogonadotropic hypogonadism (CHH). CAH, which is the result of deficiencies in steroid hormone production, can lead to over-exposure to androgens, affecting physical development in both men and women. This highlights the necessity of clinicians exercising precaution with hormone therapy, particularly in complicated disorders involving normal hormone development. CHH is also challenging to reproductive health on account of the disrupted activity of gonadotropin-releasing hormone, such that puberty development is kept in abeyance and leads to sterility if not checked. These observations justify the essential role that estrogen and testosterone, together with their regulatory mechanisms, play in the multi-staged process of growth and development during puberty, preconditioning a person for life-long health (Boehm et al., 2015; Speiser et al., 2018).

8.4.2. Impact of Adrenal Hormones

Adrenal hormones' role in growth and puberty is fundamental, as they play the major role in the initiation and direction of developmental milestones. Adrenal glands manufacture a large number of steroids like cortisol, aldosterone, and adrenal androgens whose combination is responsible for sexual development and metabolic regulation. Puberty is triggered by the increase in secretion of adrenal androgens, namely dehydroepiandrosterone (DHEA) and its sulfate derivative (DHEAS). These hormones mainly induce secondary sexual features, such as pubic hair growth and modification in body composition. The delicate harmony sustained by these hormones is important; aberrations or malfunction in adrenal hormone secretion can cause conditions like congenital adrenal hyperplasia, which have a significant influence on growth patterns and sexual development. Thus, the influence of adrenal hormones on growth and puberty is important to comprehend in the context of endocrine mechanisms and how they impact health overall. In endocrinology, though, this interaction among adrenal hormones and growth is further complicated by external factors, such as stress and diet. The hypothalamic-pituitary-adrenal (HPA) axis is a fundamental mechanism in regulating the secretion of adrenal hormones, particularly cortisol, which affects metabolic processes and immune responses. Stressors, both environmental and physiological, are capable of precipitating premature release of cortisol at the expense of growth and pubertal development. To illustrate, elevated cortisol levels are capable of inhibiting the growth hormone axis, thus impairing linear growth in children. Furthermore, nutrition exerts a significant effect on adrenal function; nutritional insufficiencies in vital nutrients can disrupt hormone production and regulation, affecting growth and development. This complex interaction serves to underscore the importance of a regulated adrenal response to bodily demands and stress, with effects on physical as well as psychological aspects of growth in puberty. More recent research on the gut-brain axis also provides a clearer understanding of adrenal hormone roles in growth and puberty and underscores previously downplayed relationships between endocrine regulation. The gut microbiota cross-talks with the HPA axis, which modifies the adrenal hormone production by dietary and environmental factors. Modulation of the composition of the microbiota can influence metabolic health, which in turn has secondary effects on adrenal function, creating a feedback loop that regulates growth and development. Disequilibrium in the gut microbiome, for instance, has been linked to disease states such as obesity and anxiety, which have secondary effects on adrenal hormone secretion. With the intricate influences on growth and puberty, including interactions between adrenal hormone regulation and gut health, increased understanding of these processes is necessary. Understanding these interactions can give novel preventive and therapeutic strategies to cure disorders of maturation and growth, hence improving pediatric endocrinology clinical outcome (John et al., 2019; Speiser et al., 2018).

8.4.3. Interaction Between Growth Hormone and Sex Hormones

GH interaction with sex hormones is a significant component of physiological changes that occur during puberty. GH, the major hormone produced by the anterior pituitary, is accountable for stimulating growth and metabolic processes in a linear fashion. Notably, its release is not constant but pulsatile and subject to the influence of several factors, which include sex hormones, estrogens, and androgens. With the onset of puberty, the increased sex hormone levels induce GH secretion, and this secretion amplifies the growth-promoting activity of IGF-1. Complementarity for accelerating growth rates observed during adolescence is the cause of such acceleration. This places the endocrinological dynamics within the context of the process of pubertal development. In males, GH synergy with testosterone is particularly crucial for spermatogenesis and overall reproductive health. Testosterone, secreted by Leydig cells in the testes, has direct effects on the functioning of Sertoli cells, which support sperm development. Testosterone's action is complemented by GH, not only regulating the overall direction of growth but also making the testes more sensitive to gonadotropic hormones like luteinizing hormone (LH) and follicle-stimulating hormone (FSH). Notably, the action of hormones ensures that while GH promotes somatic growth, sex hormones promote the growth and functionality of the reproductive system to intertwine growth and reproductive health in males during puberty (Abel et al., 2009). In women, though, the interaction of GH and estrogens and progesterone is pivotal for growth and reproduction. Estrogen profoundly influences GH secretion, which indirectly controls the growth of the ovarian follicles—a process critical to ovulation and fertility. Paracrine effects in the ovaries, enhanced by GH, enable further growth through stimulation of local growth factors. This interaction suggests the central role of GH in not only physical growth but also in the acquisition of female reproductive function. Also, the regulation of the hypothalamic-pituitary-gonadal (HPG) axis at puberty emphasizes the central role of hormonal interaction, with estrogen moderating GH responsiveness and serving to mediate the overall transition to reproductive maturity (Bentley et al., 2016) (Figure 8.11).

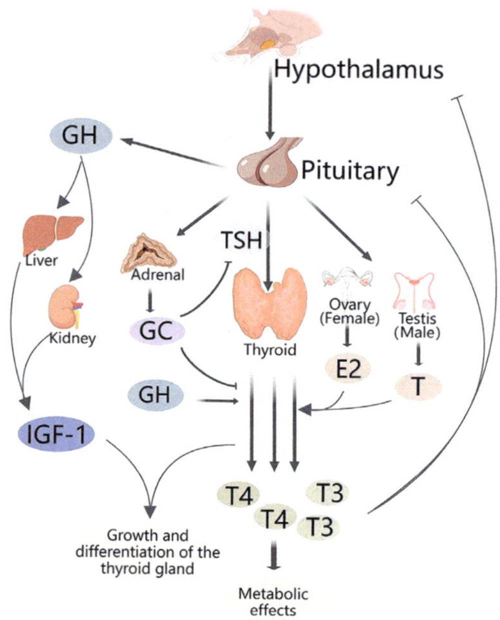

Figure 8.11. Hormones and hormone systems both directly and indirectly regulate thyroid growth and thyroid hormone secretion. The HPT axis regulates thyroid proliferation and production of THs. The GH/IGF-1 axis and sex steroids indirectly promote the secretion of THs and thyroid growth. The HPA axis inhibits the secretion of THs and TSH.

Source: https://www.researchgate.net/publication/382537996/figure/fig1/AS:11431281266544402@1722834234057/Hormones-and-hormone-systems-both-directly-and-indirectly-regulate-thyroid-growth-and.tif.

Test Your Knowledge

1. How do estrogen and testosterone contribute to the development of secondary sexual characteristics during puberty?
2. What is the role of adrenal androgens in the process of puberty, especially in adrenarche?
3. In what ways do growth hormone and sex steroids interact to influence the growth spurt observed during puberty?

8.5. Disorders of Growth and Puberty

Learning Outcome

1. Describe growth disorders;
2. Understand delayed or precocious puberty;
3. Discuss about psychological implications of growth disorders.

The interaction of the genetic, hormonal, and environmental factors is of very great importance in disorders of growth as well as puberty and hence merits a complete understanding in the field of endocrinology. These kinds of disorders like constitutional delay of growth and puberty (CDGP) and Turner syndrome create very difficult situations to measure normal growth patterns. CDGP refers to delay of growth, which is transient, with individuals affected by it eventually reaching up to peers in height during adolescence. On the other hand, Turner syndrome commonly leads to reduced growth potential and premature ovarian failure, and hence requires early treatment to maximize outcomes. Treatment of these disorders most often requires growth hormone therapies, which have been proven to enhance growth velocities and final heights of adults in case of judicious use. Physicians should be adept at differentiating these disorders from more severe underlying pathologies so that timely and appropriate care can be initiated. In addition to regular therapies, the use of anabolic agents such as oxandrolone has been useful in treating growth disorders, particularly in children. This synthetic anabolic steroid is known to promote growth and preserve lean body mass, particularly in patients with CDGP and after severe burn injuries. A systematic analysis of several studies demonstrates that oxandrolone increases growth velocity considerably with augmentation of final adult stature when administered in combination with treatments involving growth hormone. The clinicians need to weigh the benefit against potential side effects, such as virilization and premature skeletal maturation that occur at greater doses. Effective monitoring and selection of patients are key components of the treatment protocols with oxandrolone to ensure its administration safety and individualization, which maximizes its therapeutic action (Soliman et al., 2025). Artificial Intelligence (AI) is revolutionizing growth disorder and pubertal condition management with enhanced diagnostic accuracy and personalized treatment strategies. In child endocrinology, AI technology is being deployed to streamline diagnoses for conditions such as precocious puberty and growth disorders. AI is able to predict patient outcomes accurately using data analysis, allowing clinicians to tailor interventions based on a child's specific growth patterns and hormonal values. AI also allows risk factors to be detected for conditions such as childhood obesity, which is strongly linked with growth and developmental trajectories. With the advancement of such technologies, issues regarding algorithmic bias and data privacy need to be catered to, particularly in a pediatric environment where safeguarding sensitive information is paramount. Ultimately, the incorporation of AI in this domain promises improved outcomes while underscoring the irreplaceable value of the clinician-patient relationship in the management of growth and pubescence disorders (Dimitri et al., 2024).

8.5.1. Growth Disorders (e.g., Dwarfism, Gigantism)

The subtlety of growth disorders such as dwarfism and gigantism points to the delicate balance of endocrine regulation necessary for human development. Dwarfism, or primarily short stature, results from various genetic and hormonal abnormalities.

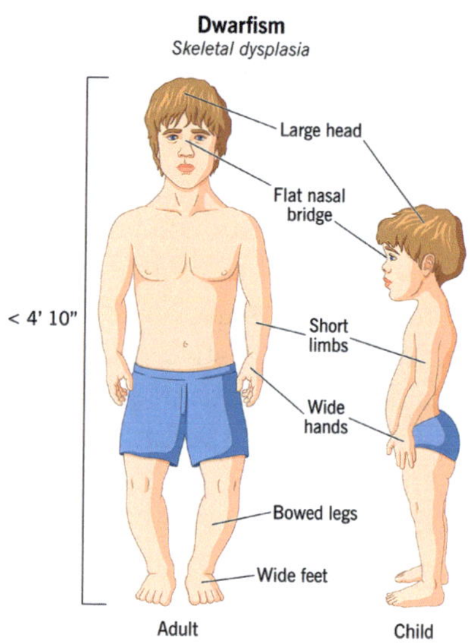

Figure 8.12. Illustration of dwarfism.

Source: https://my.clevelandclinic.org/-/scassets/images/org/health/articles/17862-dwarfism.

The best-known form is achondroplasia, resulting from a mutation in the FGFR3 gene, which regulates bone growth. On the other hand, gigantism is due to excessive growth hormone (GH) production in childhood caused by a benign growth on the pituitary gland. Pathophysiologic processes of these conditions illustrate the central role of hormones and growth factors in determining body size and skeletal development. Understanding these conditions not only provides us with clues to the health of a person but also highlights the larger implications of hormonal balance in the endocrine system on metabolic and physiological functions throughout life. The advances in endocrinology have better equipped us with knowledge about growth disorders, particularly through the work carried out on the growth hormone signaling pathway (Figure 8.12).

Growth Hormone Receptor (GHR) signaling pathway disturbance has been implicated in the pathogenesis and progression of disease conditions such as acromegaly, typically occurring in adult life following chronic excess of GH. Ger et al. (2020) reveals how alterations in GHR signaling can lead to many different chronic conditions, thus revealing that the effects of growth disorders extend beyond the disparity in size; they can predict underlying ailments such as metabolic disease and increased susceptibility to certain cancers. Such observations drive the need for early diagnosis and management of hormonal disturbances, validating the importance of hormonal assessment in clinical practice for mitigating the long-term implications of growth disorders on patients' health. Further, the treatment of growth disorders has slowly transitioned from utilizing naturally occurring growth hormone to developing biosynthetic alternatives. Initially, hGH was derived from cadaveric pituitaries, which raised safety issues, especially after the emergence of cases of Creutzfeldt-Jakob disease in treated children. Correction of this led to FDA approval of biosynthetic hGH, which significantly enhanced its availability and use. Alan et al. (2022) reminds us that the passage from the identification of GH differences to the clinic application of pure substances is a milestone for endocrinology. It resonates with both the progress of medicine and the need for ethical needs in treatment protocols of growth disorders. With more availability of biosynthetic substitutes, ongoing research regarding the efficacy of these therapies will be important in optimizing treatment for those with growth abnormalities (Figure 8.13).

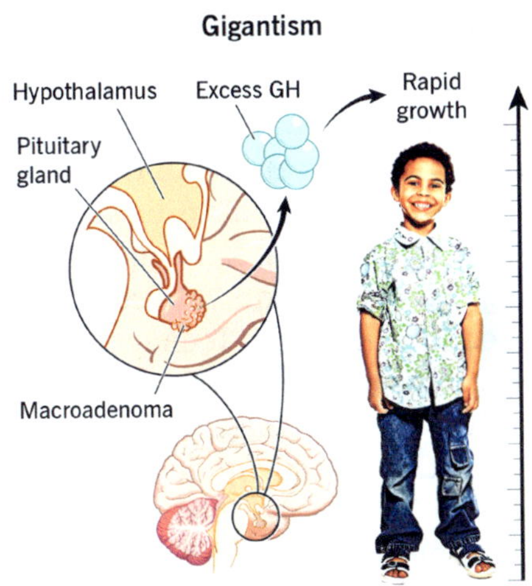

Figure 8.13. Gigantism.

Source: https://my.clevelandclinic.org/-/scassets/images/org/health/articles/22954-gigantism.

8.5.2. Delayed or Precocious Puberty

The status of delayed and precocious puberty, significant parts of endocrine development, is now a highlighted area due to increasing numbers of children developing abnormalities in developmental patterns. Delayed puberty refers to the inability to develop secondary sexual traits by the age of 14 years in males and 13 years in females, while precocious puberty encompasses the development of these traits before 9 years of age in males and 8 years in females. These conditions not only consist of physical problems, but they can also cause severe impacts on psychological health, social integration, and overall quality of life. It is important to learn about the below biological mechanisms that regulate the process of puberty because they are linked with a child's path of development and later on to health consequences, therefore it is an important field of inquiry in the field of endocrinology. Underlying reasons behind precocious or delayed puberty extend beyond genetic factors to encompass a variety of environmental influences. Population studies indicate a trend for earlier development, which is thought to be caused by improved socio-economic status, diet, and healthcare. The data also suggest, however, that exposure to endocrine-disrupting chemicals (EDCs) is likely to stimulate earlier pubertal development. For instance, phthalates and polychlorinated biphenyls have been found to be associated with alterations in hormone regulation resulting in premature puberty in some children. This association lends support to the concept that the mechanisms for regulating puberty are susceptible to genetic and environmental modification, and this indicates the potential advantage of multi-disciplinary research that integrates perspectives between endocrinology, epidemiology, and environmental science. The interaction between growth patterns and the timing of puberty is particularly tight in small-for-gestational-age (SGA) children. It has been found in research that such children are exposed to an early puberty onset, especially with sudden catch-up growth soon after birth. This may result in an aberrant sequence of development hindering the interpretation of normal pubertal development. Importantly, the disturbed perinatal environment, which is typically caused by exposure to EDCs, can disturb endocrine homeostasis as well as receptor sensitivity, and in so doing, can ultimately affect hypothalamic-pituitary-gonadal axis development. Hence, the influence of such interruptions can be extended to the puberty of the subject, which means that more research is needed to map out the causal pathways that connect environmental factors, growth patterns, and the timing of puberty in exposed children so as to pave the way for a more robust clinical response and prevention in the future (Adair et al., 2008; Templeton et al., 2013) (Figure 8.14).

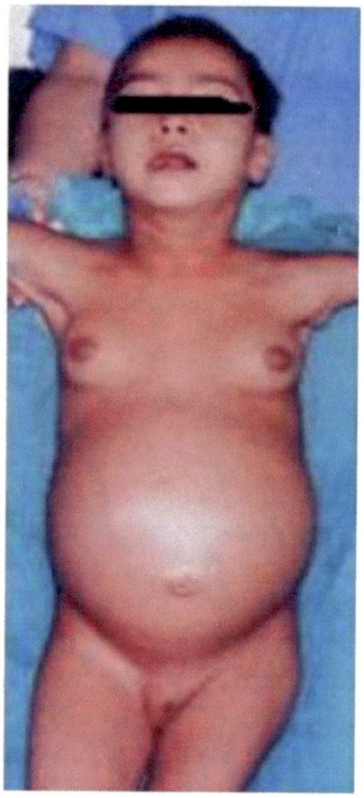

Figure 8.14. Four-year-old child showing signs of precocious puberty (developed breasts, hypertrophied labia majora, presence of pubic hair) and a large mass extending up to the xiphisternum.

Source: https://www.researchgate.net/profile/Shalini-Rajaram/publication/231614148/figure/fig1/AS:300394916925457@1448631137820/years-old-child-with-JGCT-showing-precocious-puberty-developed-breasts-hypertrophied.png.

8.5.3. Psychological Implications of Growth Disorders

The psychologic effect of disorders of growth is a multifaceted area of concern in the practice of endocrinology, particularly for the critical phases of growth and puberty. Children with growth disorders most often experience difficulties with self-image and self-esteem due to the significant difference from their peers in size. Discrepancies can feed the feelings of inadequacy and social self-consciousness, and therefore psychosocial disease is likely. There is a proven link between retarded growth and high anxiety and depression levels among the affected. Given that the adolescent years often enhance concerns regarding body image and social acceptability, suffering growth disorder patients can face double the trouble in the form of special psychological care and attention they require. To boot, growth disorders have further-reaching consequences than mere immediate psychological effects and reflect on long-term mental health outcomes. Teenagers who suffer from these disorders have emotionally complex lives, split between anger at their physical disability and their desire to be incorporated into society. This inner conflict can hamper intellectual and emotional growth, laying the groundwork for the creation of long-term psychiatric illness in adulthood. Families and caregivers must be vigilant, knowing that it is important to intervene early in treating not only the physical manifestations of growth disorders but also their psychological effects. Interventions that promote resilience, coping, and social skills have been shown to significantly contribute to enhancing the well-being of affected individuals. Research into the microbiota-gut-brain axis has begun to underscore the manner in which biological processes may further complicate this relationship, proposing that an integrated treatment plan is required in addressing the full spectrum of symptoms presented by these individuals (John et al., 2019). In the background of recent advances in clinical understanding and recommendations, as exemplified by revised guidelines for management of diseases like congenital adrenal hyperplasia, the requirement for personalized psychological support is evident. The association of endocrinological treatment with psychological counseling can enable a holistic approach to the management of growth disorders. For instance, efforts to treat the physiological component of alterations to body physiology with steroid treatment alongside providing mental health support can empower individuals. Not only do they better learn to be more mindful of their body maintenance, but also, they can better learn to be more aware of who they are and be good with themselves during their growth disorders (Speiser et al., 2018). With improvements in technology through research, practitioners need to start considering psychological methods in line with endocrinological treatment, making the environment more therapeutic for individuals living with growth disorders and the ensuing psychological impacts.

Test Your Knowledge

1. What are the primary causes and characteristics of dwarfism and gigantism, and how do they differ in terms of growth hormone involvement?
2. What are common causes of delayed puberty in adolescents, and how is it diagnosed clinically?

8.6. The Role of Nutrition and Environment

Learning Outcome

1. Understand nutritional factors affecting growth;
2 Describe environmental influences on puberty timing;
3. Focus on socioeconomic factors and their impact on growth.

Within the intricate balance of nutritional and endocrine regulation, environmental influences increasingly assume a central position, especially during the absolutely crucial phases of growth and puberty. At these periods, while adolescents are going through profound hormonal transformations, dietary habits have a direct impact on the trajectory of this process. Research highlights that nutrition deficiency, or in other words, the intake of very high energy-dense foods, can lead to obesity, which has been established as a key risk factor for most endocrinological disorders, including diseases that affect patterns of growth and metabolic status. Obesity in childhood and adolescence is usually followed by adiposity rebound, which initiates a cycle of weight-related complications, for instance, Type 2 Diabetes Mellitus and hypertension (Alvina et al., 2021). A well-balanced diet that includes all the nutrients necessary for growth is not just advisable; it is necessary in order to ensure maximum growth and control the influence of puberty over a person. Moreover, the surroundings in which children grow also play an important role in shaping their food habits and, in turn, their well-being. Psychological and social signals—e.g., peer and cultural influences—accountable for shaping the food relationships of adolescents. In some cases, the desire to conform to the norm can lead people to develop unhealthy eating habits, which come in the form of disorders like anorexia or binge-eating. The environment also encompasses access to healthy food; neighborhood access to healthy foods and socioeconomic conditions can limit healthy eating, which leads to reliance on convenience foods that promote obesity (Alvina et al., 2021). A supportive lifestyle with attention to nutrition and mental well-being is essential in order to counteract the detrimental effects of societal pressures and bad dieting habits during this pivotal developing phase. Moreover, a new area of research also establishes the connection between nutrition, gut microbiota, and hormonal regulation. The gut-brain axis, which focuses on the relationship between the gut microbiota and neural activity, is influenced by nutrient consumption during developmentally sensitive times. A number of mechanisms can influence microbiota structure—from the diet to environmental stressors—on neurodevelopment and general health. The right balance and diversity of the microbiome guarantees the healthful regulation of metabolic functions and immunity, while dysbiosis can exacerbate obesity and psychological illness that adversely affects growth and puberty. With increasing knowledge about the role of the microbiomes, including incorporating the promotion of balanced diets for gut health, will be essential for maximizing growth and endocrine function in teenagers (Figure 8.15).

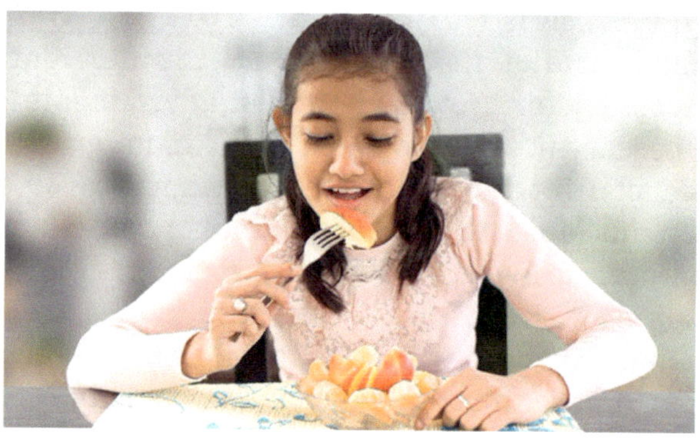

Figure 8.15. Nutrition plays a vital role in puberty, impacting both the timing and progression of this developmental stage.

Source: https://www.asknestle.in/sites/default/files/2023-06/Why%20good%20nutrition%20is%20important%20during%20puberty%20%28640x380%29px.jpg.

8.6.1. Nutritional Factors Affecting Growth

The interaction between nutrition factors and growth during puberty is intricate and very important. The basic nutrients, such as proteins, vitamins, and minerals, are essential in the physiological changes that occur during this state of growth. Adequate protein intake is particularly important since it aids in muscle growth and tissue repair, which are required since adolescents undergo rapid changes in the body. Moreover, vitamins such as D and minerals such as calcium are necessary for bone development; they help to reach the maximum bone mass, which is important for future skeletal health. Deficiency in these nutrients can discourage growth and may result in long-term health complications. Having a good balance of diet during puberty lays the foundation for healthy growth patterns and can buffer some of the risk associated with metabolic disorders later in life, various studies suggest. Recent research highlights the significance of macro and micro-nutrient balance and how these factors can modify the age of onset and tempo of puberty. For instance, a diet rich in animal protein accelerates menarche timing, possibly because it influences body weight as well as overall hormonal regulation. This conclusion points to the intricate relationship between diet and hormonal processes that regulate growth and sexual development. In contrast, deficiencies in nutrients have been linked to delayed puberty, illustrative of the delicate balance between nutrition and endocrine function. Environmental factors such as socio-economic status also contribute towards such effects, as they have a tendency to pre-determine diet patterns and availability. A study of such interactions can provide valuable information regarding how nutritional interventions could enable healthier growth patterns among adolescents, as several studies suggest. An understanding of the implications of dietary choice can result in improved health consequences for adolescents. More emphasis on educating parents and adolescents about nutrition is critical to promoting awareness of food consumption that enables healthy growth and development. Interventions specifically designed to enhance intake of key nutrients can combat the obesity challenge alongside halting stunted growth among disadvantaged populations.

Furthermore, research discoveries revealing the correlation between nutrient consumption and markers of development underscore the need for individualized nutritional advice. By integrating findings of research, such as those that examine the impact on body composition and bone mineral density, medical professionals are able to design effective interventions to guide adolescents through their growth spurt and beyond. Public health interventions that promote nutritional competence can thus be a powerful intervention in fostering integrated growth in a pivotal period of life, according to research evidence in this field.

8.6.2. Environmental Influences on Puberty Timing

Pubertal timing is a multifactorial process governed by an interaction of environmental and genetic determinants. During the progress from childhood to adolescence, psychological and physiological maturation can be greatly affected by a variety of environmental cues. Nutritional status is implicated to have a significant role where adequate food availability can induce precocious onset of puberty. In poor environments, delayed physical maturation may be an adaptive process optimizing survival and reproductive fitness. This phenomenon accounts for the concept of adaptive plasticity, where developmental trajectories are optimized on the basis of environmental limitation, reflecting directly on responses to fitness. Working in evolutionary developmental biology, the notion of puberty as an adaptive stage highlights that finding out how environmental factors, such as energy availability and social environment, affect this critical period of expansion and transformation in an individual's life and thereby contribute to the broader significance for development and health in the long term is essential (Templeton et al., 2013). Socioeconomic status (SES) also becomes an important environmental predictor of when puberty is attained. Research has shown that adolescent girls raised in lower-SES settings usually initiate menarche earlier than adolescent girls of more advantaged origin. Such difference tends to be attributed to varying stressors, of which is psychosocial stress from the family, capable of triggering adaptive reproductive processes. The correspondence between socioenvironmental circumstances and the biological process suggests that the rearing circumstances of an individual could play a substantial role in hormonal regulation and schedules of development. Moreover, the theory of evolutionary socialization would suggest that such rapid maturation could serve as an adaptive strategy for dealing with challenging environments, hence encouraging a short life history strategy. This interaction underscores the imperative call for an interdisciplinary endeavor, the integration of endocrinology and social sciences, toward a thorough understanding of contextual realities on human development and endocrine processes during adolescence (Templeton et al., 2013). Research on the genetic basis of the timing of puberty adds additional nuance to the environmental impact environment. Genetic predisposition has been shown to account for a significant majority of the variability in within-individual differences in menarcheal age, with studies estimating heritability at over 70%. New evidence, however, highlights gene-environment interaction as key, with environmental factors capable of having significant effects on the expression of genetically determined characteristics associated with the timing of puberty. For instance, certain genotypes are likely to cause later menarche, while environmental determinants such as too much stress or poor dietary intake can augment or modify these genetic determinations. This intricate interaction illustrates that despite the genetic models giving the basis for developmental trajectories, the environment within an individual has an ultimate deciding role in shaping these biological processes. These remarks underscore the complexity of puberty as not merely a biological phenomenon but rather a convergence of life history and environmental acclimatization, necessitating more exploration in endocrinology.

8.6.3. Socioeconomic Factors and Their Impact on Growth

The relationship between socioeconomic determinants and growth during adolescence is profound, such that the determinants can have a significant influence on the outcomes of development. Research highlights how environmental factors combined with socioeconomic status have the ability to influence patterns of growth. The availability of nutrition, for instance, is found to be associated with economic status, where poor households may provide inadequate food options to their children. Specifically, excessive intake of animal protein has been associated with earlier menarche, which suggests that nutrition is a key factor in development at this critical growth phase. Moreover, family structure, for instance, stressors associated with single parenthood, can adversely affect the emotional and physical health of the child, promoting or slowing down growth patterns. Therefore, socioeconomic determinants are of major significance to establish growth and puberty, confirming the necessity of the holistic approach to the research on these processes in endocrinology (Dvornyk et al., 2014). Additionally, psychological well-being can be significantly influenced by socioeconomic status, impacting children's development and growth during puberty. Studies find a correlation between deteriorating socioeconomic conditions and increased rates of psychiatric disorders in risk populations. For instance, kids with conditions like classical congenital adrenal hyperplasia (CAH) have high prevalence rates of attention-deficit hyperactivity disorder (ADHD) and anxiety disorders, further aggravated by socioeconomic issues. These issues not only impact emotional maturity but can also take place physically and, as a result, possibly alter normal growth patterns. The effects of stress and limited access to mental health services are measures of the worth of psychological care for youngsters who are experiencing puberty, particularly in those with poor socioeconomic statuses. Hence, a comprehension of the socioeconomic setting in which these kids grow is essential in enhancing healthier development settings (Ernst et al., 2010). Moreover, the relationship between socioeconomic components and development extends up to the policy implications of public health. Corrections to dietary deficiencies and mental health interventions for low-income children can enhance better outcomes in growth during puberty. Healthcare policies for increasing access to quality medical care, education material, and community support programs can reduce the detrimental effects of socioeconomic disadvantages. An investment in health education programs that involve balanced nutrition and mental well-being is an investment that can strengthen developmental pathways in at-risk adolescents. The positive association between socioeconomic status and growth indicates that advances in economic and social status may lead to positive alterations not just in the timing of puberty but also in long-term health outcomes. Proper attention to these factors is needed for public health interventions that will enable equitable growth and development (Dvornyk et al., 2014; Ernst et al., 2010).

Test Your Knowledge

1. How do specific nutrients influence normal growth and development in children?
2. How can environmentally factors like exposure to endocrine-disrupting chemicals affect the onset and progression of puberty?

SUMMARY

The complex interplay of the hormonal changes at puberty has a tremendous influence on growth patterns in teenagers. The action of the hormones such as growth hormone and sex steroids has the most significant role to play in the regulation of skeletal growth and the initiation of growth spurts. Disorder in hormonal regulation thus leads to disorders of growth, and pediatric endocrinologists must therefore understand these processes. For instance, treatment with oxandrolone has been reported to stimulate growth in the case of certain conditions like constitutional delay of growth and puberty (CDGP) and Turner syndrome, suggesting the applicability of personalized therapeutic intervention in the treatment of growth disorders. Nevertheless, clinicians must weigh very carefully the benefits of such interventions against side effects because there have been reports of premature skeletal maturation and changes in metabolism that are a cause for concern in this population (Soliman et al., 2025). Furthermore, understanding post-menarche growth in women adds another level to the practice of endocrinology. Evidence shows that while there may be some increase after menarche, it typically declines in comparison with menarcheal height and age. The findings reveal that girls who have later menarche and greater height can have limited post-menarche growth, emphasizing the necessity of individualized assessments in pediatric practice (Farahi et al., 2024). This highlights one of the principal concerns for clinicians who must counsel families about growth expectations at and after puberty. This information is critical for monitoring patterns of growth and counseling interventions, particularly in cases where premature or delayed menarche would impact overall patterns of growth. Lastly, the advances in our understanding of puberty and growth via endocrinological research offer promises as well as pitfalls. Subsequent research should aim to characterize the long-term metabolic consequences of such therapies as oxandrolone and explore further determinants of post-menarche growth in diverse populations. Such research will not only guide clinical practice, but also enhance standards of care for adolescents with growth disorders. Through integrating evidence-based practices into clinical settings and through ongoing research, the practice of pediatric endocrinology can further evolve, as adolescents are provided with the optimal care during developmentally critical growth periods in their life.

Pubertal and growth development is a critical phase of human growth heavily dependent on endocrine signaling. Interaction of hormones, particularly growth hormone and sex steroids, enables the physical features characteristic of adolescence to emerge. During this stage, an individual experiences a fast growth and development of secondary sexual features, synthesis of complex interactions between hormones initiated by the hypothalamic-pituitary-gonadal axis. Knowing about the mechanisms is crucial, as variations can lead to situations such as precocious puberty or growth diseases. In addition, the psychosocial climate in which this development occurs is also significant. Adolescent development involves not just physical change but emotional and social adjustment, which often creates challenges that must be treated with care by health professionals. As the incidence of childhood obesity increases, its impact on endocrine function becomes a problem that must be tackled. The increased body weight can disrupt normal hormonal equilibrium and exacerbate growth and puberty issues. Leptin and resistance to insulin are especially associated with altered timing of puberty and growth patterns, which highlights the need for a totalistic approach to reverse these conditions of ill health. Interestingly, with obesity emerging as a new condition among adolescents, so do the accompanying risks of comorbid disease such as Type 2 Diabetes Mellitus and dyslipidemia. In addition to putting physical health at risk, the conditions can also yield psychological complications such as negative body image and eating disorders. This relationship highlights the emergent need for comprehensive approaches that incorporate dietary and lifestyle change and counseling. Furthermore, the role of the gut–brain axis in the endocrine system opens up new possibilities for explaining puberty and growth control. The new studies point to the importance of the microbiota in controlling hormone pathways and metabolic processes. Imbalance of gut microbiota may exacerbate obesity, which, according to above, can lead to altered patterns of growth. Furthermore, the interaction between microbial metabolites and the endocrine system provides a novel perspective on how early life determinants such as diet and antibiotics shape long-term health outcomes. With increasing evidence being presented of a link between microbiota structure and disease conditions like obesity and neurodevelopmental disorders, additional study is necessary to identify microbial-based interventions that could promote health during puberty and potentially prevent some of the risks of hormonal imbalance (Alvina et al., 2021; John et al., 2019).

KEY TERMS FROM THIS CHAPTER

- Adolescent growth
- Autoimmune diseases
- Central precocious puberty (CPP)
- Congenital adrenal hyperplasia (CAH)
- Developmental health
- Emotional instability
- Endocrine control
- Endocrine-disrupting chemicals (EDCs)
- Environmental modification
- Anabolic effects
- Biosynthetic alternatives
- Clinical practice guidelines
- Cretinism
- Developmental patterns
- Endocrine climate
- Endocrine-disrupting chemicals
- Environmental forces
- Estradiol treatment

CRITICAL THINKING QUESTIONS

1. **Which hormone is responsible for the development of secondary sexual characteristics in males during puberty?**
   a. Estrogen
   b. Progesterone
   c. Testosterone
   d. Cortisol
2. **What triggers the onset of puberty in both males and females?**
   a. Increase in melatonin
   b. Activation of the hypothalamic-pituitary-gonadal axis
   c. Decrease in insulin levels
   d. Increased calcium absorption
3. **Which of the following is a possible result of growth hormone deficiency in children?**
   a. Acromegaly
   b. Precocious puberty
   c. Gigantism
   d. Dwarfism
4. **What environmental factor can delay the onset of puberty?**
   a. Exposure to sunlight
   b. Malnutrition
   c. Urban living
   d. Moderate exercise
5. **How does nutrition influence growth and puberty?**
   a. Only affects height, not hormones
   b. Has no significant impact on puberty
   c. Adequate nutrition supports normal hormonal function and growth
   d. Overnutrition always leads to early puberty

Short Answer Questions

1. Which endocrine glands are involved in regulating human growth and development, and what hormones do they secrete?
2. What is the role of growth hormone (GH) in childhood growth, and how does it interact with IGF-1 to promote tissue development?
3. What are the typical stages of puberty in males and females, and what physical changes occur during each stage?
4. How do estrogen and testosterone drive the development of secondary sexual characteristics during puberty?
5. How do growth hormone and sex hormones interact during puberty to produce the adolescent growth spurt?
6. What are the causes, signs, and treatment options for common disorders such as delayed puberty, precocious puberty, dwarfism, and gigantism?
7. How does nutrition—particularly protein, iron, and caloric intake—affect growth and pubertal development?

Answers to Critical Thinking Questions

1. (c); 2. (b); 3. (d); 4. (b); 5. (d)

REFERENCES

1. Abacı, A., Abalı, S., Adal, E., et al. (2015). Turner syndrome and associated problems in Turkish children: A multicenter study. https://core.ac.uk/download/227057395.pdf (accessed on 22nd July 2025).
2. Abel, M. H., Baker, P. J., Huhtaniemi, I., et al. (2009). Role of androgen and gonadotrophins in the development and function of the Sertoli cells and Leydig cells: Data from mutant and genetically modified mice. https://core.ac.uk/download/91350.pdf (accessed on 22nd July 2025).
3. Acerini, C. L., Lehwalder, D., Wac, K., & Bang, P. (2017). Optimizing patient management and adherence for children receiving growth hormone. https://core.ac.uk/download/146491367.pdf (accessed on 22nd July 2025).
4. Adair, L., Berg-Kelly, H., Blanck, H. M., Colon, I., DeCastro, F., Den Hond, E., et al. (2008). Endocrine disruptors and abnormalities of pubertal development. https://core.ac.uk/download/55877440.pdf (accessed on 22nd July 2025).
5. Ahmed, S. F., Chirita-Emandi, A., Corrigan, D., Devenny, A., et al. (2017). A retrospective analysis of longitudinal changes in bone mineral content in cystic fibrosis. https://core.ac.uk/download/96883054.pdf (accessed on 22nd July 2025).
6. Archer, J., Boomsma, D. I., Marshall, W. A., Bartels, M., Meikle, A. W., Rogol, A. D., et al. (2005). Heritability of testosterone levels in 12-year-old twins and its relation to pubertal development. https://core.ac.uk/download/2355.pdf (accessed on 22nd July 2025).
7. Aversa, A., Burnett, A. L., Corona, G., Isidori, A., et al. (2016). Endocrinologic control of men's sexual desire and arousal/erection. https://core.ac.uk/download/54532167.pdf (accessed on 22nd July 2025).
8. Bellingham, M., Evans, N. P., & Robinson, J. E. (2016). Prenatal programming of neuroendocrine reproductive function. https://core.ac.uk/download/42371121.pdf (accessed on 22nd July 2025).
9. Bentley, G. E., Calandra, R. S., Micevych, P. E., Paredes, R., et al. (2016). Peripheral and central mechanisms involved in hormonal control of male and female reproduction. https://core.ac.uk/download/159295807.pdf (accessed on 22nd July 2025).
10. Boehm, U., Bouloux, P. M., Dattani, M., de Roux, N., Dodé, C., Dunkel, L., Dwyer, A., et al. (2015). European consensus statement on congenital hypogonadotropic hypogonadism—Pathogenesis, diagnosis and treatment. *Nature Reviews Endocrinology, 11*, 547–564. https://doi.org/10.1038/nrendo.2015.112 (accessed on 22nd July 2025).
11. Boonstra, V. H. (Venje), Hokken-Koelega, A. C. S. (Anita), Mulder, P. G. H. (Paul), et al. (2003). Puberty in growth hormone-treated children born small for gestational age (SGA). https://core.ac.uk/download/19186358.pdf (accessed on 22nd July 2025).
12. Busch, A., Hagen, C., Almstrup, K., Main, K., & Juul, A. (2016). Genetic variations altering FSH action affect circulating hormone levels as well as follicle growth in healthy peripubertal girls. *Human Reproduction, 31*(4), 897–904. https://www.semanticscholar.org/paper/0af2e8d9b37a72c263a014644ad38e790750209a (accessed on 22nd July 2025).
13. Cryan, J. F., O'Riordan, K. J., Cowan, C. S. M., Sandhu, K. V., Bastiaanssen, T. F. S., Boehme, M., Codagnone, M. G., et al. (2019). The microbiota-gut-brain axis. *Physiological Reviews, 99*, 1877–2013. https://doi.org/10.1152/physrev.00018.2018 (accessed on 22nd July 2025).

14. DeBruine, L., Jones, B., Little, A., et al. (2009). Face and voice attractiveness judgments change during adolescence. https://core.ac.uk/download/9341126.pdf (accessed on 22nd July 2025).

15. Dimitri, P., & Savage, M. O. (2024). Artificial intelligence in pediatric endocrinology: Conflict or cooperation. *Journal of Pediatric Endocrinology and Metabolism, 37*, 209–221. https://www.semanticscholar.org/paper/935d8798e5ac4f2210cdf75e116e7b12ac1b597b (accessed on 22nd July 2025).

16. Dvornyk, V., & Yermachenko, A. (2014). Nongenetic determinants of age at menarche: A systematic review. https://core.ac.uk/download/38049488.pdf (accessed on 22nd July 2025).

17. Ernst, M., Green-Golan, L., Leschek, E., et al. (2010). Psychiatric characterization of children with genetic causes of hyperandrogenism. https://core.ac.uk/download/55802070.pdf (accessed on 22nd July 2025).

18. Farahi, H., Talebian, N., Falah Tafti, M., Akbarzadeh, N., & Razavi, Z. (2024). Evaluation of average post-menarche height growth and associated factors: A cross-sectional study. *Iranian Journal of Pediatrics*. https://www.semanticscholar.org/paper/6c666becb37f09da48e28f788fe320f860f7f2b4 (accessed on 22nd July 2025).

19. Gesto, M., & Jokumsen, A. (2016). Stress-resilience differences related to emergence time in *rainbow trout*. https://core.ac.uk/download/77086291.pdf (accessed on 22nd July 2025).

20. Gonzalez Deniselle, M. C., Lara, H. E., Recabarren, S. E., et al. (2016). Developmental and functional effects of steroid hormones on the neuroendocrine axis and spinal cord. https://core.ac.uk/download/159294623.pdf (accessed on 22nd July 2025).

21. Heindel, J. J., & Vandenberg, L. N. (2015). Developmental origins of health and disease. *Current Opinion in Pediatrics, 27*, 248–253. https://doi.org/10.1097/mop.0000000000000191 (accessed on 22nd July 2025).

22. Hitchcock, E., & Madsen, T. (2011). *Growing Up Toxic: Chemical Exposures and Increases in Developmental Disease*. https://core.ac.uk/download/71358334.pdf (accessed on 22nd July 2025).

23. Jensen, T., Finne, K. F., Skakkebæk, N., Andersson, A., Olesen, I. A., Joensen, U. N., Bang, A., et al. (2016). Self-reported onset of puberty and subsequent semen quality and reproductive hormones in healthy young men. *Human Reproduction, 31*(8), 1886–1894. https://www.semanticscholar.org/paper/d13ce99ff59cea3dd303845c2611e2ef2ba89896 (accessed on 22nd July 2025).

24. Kansra, A. R., Lakkunarajah, S., & Jay, M. S. (2021). Childhood and adolescent obesity: A review. *Frontiers in Pediatrics, 8*. https://doi.org/10.3389/fped.2020.581461 (accessed on 22nd July 2025).

25. Khare, J., Pendharkar, P. S., Kalra, S., & Jindal, S. (2025). Endocrinology and supernatural beliefs: A review. *Indian Journal of Endocrinology and Metabolism, 29*, 39–42. https://www.semanticscholar.org/paper/54ac7328523febca80ad1e22d1168e6ff737ba69 (accessed on 22nd July 2025).

26. Kim, J. H., Kim, S. J., Chung, I. H., & Lim, J. (2024). Adiposity rebound timing in small for gestational age children treated with growth hormone: Results from LG Growth Study data. *Journal of Korean Medical Science, 40*. https://www.semanticscholar.org/paper/17708478af9affe02053d1dafeaa59bae343291e (accessed on 22nd July 2025).

27. Kumar, K. H., Garg, A., Ajai Chandra, N. S., Singh, S. P., & Datta, R. (2016). Voice and endocrinology. *Indian Journal of Endocrinology and Metabolism, 20*, 590–594. https://www.semanticscholar.org/paper/0e3a66e759fba6693bdd2345ea8dc20ca2ba0924 (accessed on 22nd July 2025).

28. Lawaetz, J. G., Hagen, C., Mieritz, M., Blomberg Jensen, M., Petersen, J., & Juul, A. (2015). Evaluation of 451 Danish boys with delayed puberty: Diagnostic use of a new puberty nomogram and effects of oral testosterone therapy. *The Journal of Clinical Endocrinology and Metabolism, 100*(4), 1376–1385. https://www.semanticscholar.org/paper/d2841f08b5a03ecc5f7dad08be6c7b737d50a8cb (accessed on 22nd July 2025).

29. Lundqvist, T., Stenlid, R., & Halldin, M. (2025). Hormonal crossroads in inborn errors of the metabolism: Impact of puberty and dietary interventions on metabolic health. *Metabolites, 15*. https://www.semanticscholar.org/paper/960c7b5d410e4310debe582177d9c0cf478a0fcd (accessed on 22nd July 2025).

30. Müller, C., Caspers, B. A., Gadau, J., & Kaiser, S. (2020). The power of info chemicals in mediating individualized niches. *Trends in Ecology & Evolution, 35*, 981–989. https://doi.org/10.1016/j.tree.2020.07.001 (accessed on 22nd July 2025).

31. Must, A., Pickles, A., Towne, B., Sisk, C. L., Pillemer, D. B., Boomsma, D. I., et al. (2007). The familial clustering of age at menarche in extended twin families. https://core.ac.uk/download/pdf/11476781.pdf (accessed on 22nd July 2025).

32. Norup, P., Haahr, M., Christiansen, P., Aksglaede, L., Cleemann, L., Johannsen, T., Juul, A., et al. (2024). Growth and adult height attainment in Danish transgender adolescents treated with GnRH analog and sex hormones. *The Journal of Clinical Endocrinology and Metabolism, 109*, 2764–2773. https://www.semanticscholar.org/paper/5eaa43fe7484ef478e34a258f8193ab95fbae53d (accessed on 22nd July 2025).

33. Rogol, A. D., & Reiter, E. O. (2022). Growth and growth hormone through the ages: Art and science. *Hormone Research in Pediatrics, 95*, 515–528. https://doi.org/10.1159/000526440 (accessed on 22nd July 2025).

34. Saroufim, R., & Fuqua, J. (2022). The variability of growth and puberty in growth hormone-treated children born small for gestational age. *The Journal of Clinical Endocrinology and Metabolism, 107*, e4263–e4264. https://www.semanticscholar.org/paper/ec4de8c65899fa21c5a9bd97ef7a570b9236a452 (accessed on 22nd July 2025).

35. Soliman, A., Alyafei, F., Alaaraj, N., Hamed, N., Ahmed, S., AlHumaidi, N., Khalil, A., et al. (2025). Oxandrolone therapy in pediatric growth disorders: A comprehensive review of benefits, risks, and clinical implications. *World Journal of Advanced Research and Reviews*. https://www.semanticscholar.org/paper/b17128f69aa8bc41d7472e42a514fd0091ec9ee6 (accessed on 22nd July 2025).

36. Speiser, P., Arlt, W., Auchus, R. J., Baskin, L. S., Conway, G. S., Merke, D. P., Meyer-Bahlburg, H. F. L., et al. (2018). Congenital adrenal hyperplasia due to steroid 21-hydroxylase deficiency: An Endocrine Society* clinical practice guideline. *The Journal of Clinical Endocrinology & Metabolism, 103*, 4043–4088. https://doi.org/10.1210/jc.2018-01865 (accessed on 22nd July 2025).

37. Strous, G. J., Da Silva Almeida, A., Putters, J., Schantl, J., Sędek, M., Slotman, J. A., Nespital, T., et al. (2020). Growth hormone receptor regulation in cancer and chronic diseases. *Frontiers in Endocrinology, 11*. https://doi.org/10.3389/fendo.2020.597573 (accessed on 22nd July 2025).

38. Templeton, A., Arquitt, A. B., Migliano, A. B., Pesonen, A. K., Parent, A. S., Bogin, B., Campbell, B., et al. (2013). Evo-devo of human adolescence: Beyond disease models of early puberty. https://core.ac.uk/download/18528095.pdf (accessed on 22nd July 2025).

39. Yang, Y., Sun, J., Yang, S., Li, S., Zhang, J., Zhu, F., Pan, X., et al. (2025). Serum phoenixin levels and their diagnostic significance in girls with precocious puberty. *Journal of the Endocrine Society, 9*. https://www.semanticscholar.org/paper/fe0431789b4ddfb3fa8a05ea2e3b859325c7e57e (accessed on 22nd July 2025).

OBESITY AND METABOLIC SYNDROME

9

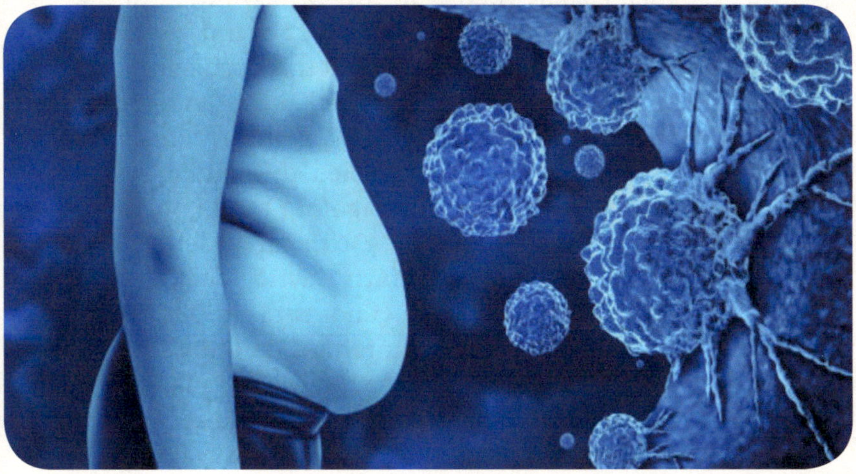

LEARNING OBJECTIVES

After studying this chapter, you will be able to:

1. Understand the pathophysiology of obesity;
2. Explain definition and criteria of metabolic syndrome;
3. Discuss the role of endocrine disruptors on obesity and metabolic syndrome;
4. Deal with relationship between obesity and insulin resistance;
5. Focus on interaction between psychological factors and obesity;
6. Describe effective treatment and management strategies for obesity and metabolic syndrome.

Introduction

Increasing prevalence of obesity and metabolic syndrome is a significant public health problem, attracting interest from a variety of different disciplines, one of which is endocrinology. Obesity, which involves the excess fat accumulation, is the primary cause of the development of metabolic syndrome. Metabolic syndrome is a cluster of risk factors that significantly increase the risk of cardiovascular disease, type 2 diabetes, and other disabling illnesses. It is essential to understand the complex relationship between metabolic syndrome and obesity in an effort to create effective prevention and intervention strategies. During the last decade, researchers have been trying to define biological as well as environmental determinants of these entities, with emphasis on genetic susceptibility and lifestyle. Accordingly, the role of endocrinology is pivotal to the resolutions of such interdependent issues of health and decisions regarding particular therapeutic regimens for the management and control of their impacts on populations involved. Recent studies have investigated novel predictive indicators for assessing the metabolic syndrome in patients with severe obesity. In fact, inflammation indexes derived from complete blood count, such as the Monocyte-to-HDL-C ratio (MHR), have been found to be useful for identifying patients at heightened risk of developing the metabolic syndrome. Metabolic syndrome patients had the significantly increased levels of these indexes compared to their controls without any such syndrome, indicating the potential of CBC-derive inflammation indexes as clinical diagnostic indices. Not only do the results attest to the utility of serological examinations for the diagnosis of metabolic disorder, but also to the inherent inflammatory process in obesity and metabolic syndrome. Such research is of paramount importance in defining the pathophysiological mechanisms that link obesity with metabolic syndrome and thereby enable clinicians to recognize people at high risk and implement early intervention aimed at these emerging health conditions (Marra et al., 2024). In addition, the implications of the association extend beyond traditional diagnostics; they provide a threshold for emerging therapies given the multifaceted nature of metabolic syndrome. The cause-and-effect relationship between type 2 diabetes, body mass index (BMI), and hypertension with lower limb ulcers demonstrates the multifactorial consequences of metabolic syndrome (Wang et al., 2024). They recognize both the system-wide effects of obesity and the necessity to fully understand the way in which metabolic syndrome leads to severe complications. Endocrinology science in the future will need to emphasize more these connections, encourage development of holistic management techniques that address obesity, metabolic syndrome, and their associated comorbidities. With an integrated strategy, like that utilized here, health care providers can more effectively combat the tide of disease related to obesity and enhance outcomes in clinical settings that are diverse.

Definition of Obesity

The classical definition of obesity is a surplus of body fat that poses severe health risks. The World Health Organization (WHO) defines obesity in Body Mass Index (BMI) terms, classifying anyone with a BMI of 30 or more as obese. Such a definition, while prevalent for its simplicity to apply and utilize, is restrictive in covering the full spectrum of health problems posed by obesity. Notably, obesity may take several forms, such as sarcopenic obesity, which refers to the presence of excess fat and loss of muscle mass. New research points out that this particular form of obesity has been identified as a risk factor for metabolic syndrome, or a grouping of conditions that consists of hypertension, dyslipidemia, and insulin resistance, highlighting the importance of clearly definition in clinical practice and epidemiology to identify with obesity the complexities involved (Choi et al., 2009). Apart from BMI, waist circumference and the ratio of waist to hip are gaining popularity as markers of obesity, and the focus is on body fat distribution. These are important because they may elucidate the relationship between visceral adiposity and metabolic comorbidity, including type 2 diabetes and cardiovascular disease. Its prevalence is particularly marked in older populations, where sarcopenic obesity may lead to lower muscle mass and physical function, which can again exacerbate existing health issues. Evidence for the prevalence of sarcopenia and its link with metabolic syndrome, particularly among older people, has been shown through research, and more comprehensive definitions that also consider muscle integrity and not just fat accumulation have been requested. Therefore, defining obesity in a multi-dimensional fashion will improve its management and perception of its health consequences (Choi et al., 2009). The impact of precise definition of obesity extends into the practice of clinical medicine and public health policy. A clear perception of the definition of obesity allows health practitioners to apply effective prevention and management strategies of disorders of obesity. For instance, reported associations between vitamin D status and metabolic syndrome illustrate the multifactorial nature of the etiology of obesity. Evidence indicates that metabolic syndrome can be prevalent in certain populations, such as postmenopausal women, necessitating differential preventive interventions. Therefore, examining various definitions and assessments of obesity not only adds to the debate in the field of endocrinology but also underscores the importance of utilizing the broader spectrum of obesity and resulting health disorders. The use of inclusive definitions will allow public health policy to better target interventions on halting the disease of obesity and its associated metabolic disorders (Figure 9.1).

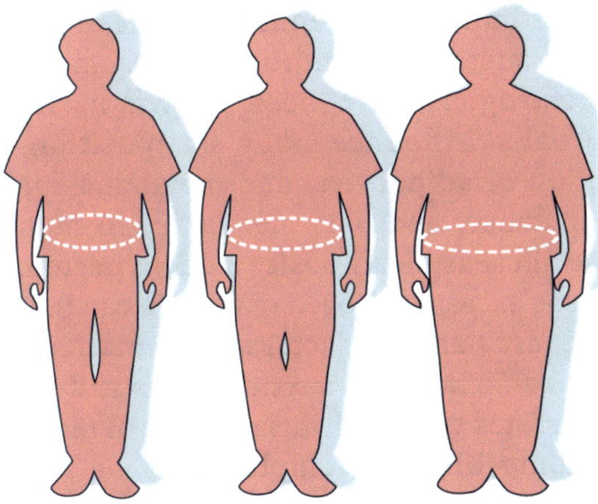

Figure 9.1. Illustration of obesity and waist circumference.

Source: https://upload.wikimedia.org/wikipedia/commons/thumb/0/08/Obesity-waist_circumference.svg/800px-Obesity-waist_circumference.svg.png.

Overview of Metabolic Syndrome

Metabolic syndrome represents a group of interrelated risk factors that dramatically enhance the risk of occurrence of cardiovascular disease, type 2 diabetes, and metabolic disorders. The most important components of this syndrome are abdominal obesity, hypertension, dyslipidemia, and insulin resistance. Pathophysiology of this syndrome is multi-factorial and in the majority of cases involves intricate interactions between genetic, environmental, and lifestyle determinants. Notable in particular is the pathogenic role of obesity, as excess fat tissue, particularly visceral fat, modulates lipid metabolism and alters insulin sensitivity. Current evidence indicates that hepatic impairment caused by chronic hypercorticosteronemia, as evident in conditions like metabolic syndrome, leads to inflammation and insulin resistance, with the implication of the profound impact of these metabolic derangements on liver function and overall metabolic health (Castro et al., 2016). Besides, lifestyle factors such as diet and exercise are responsible for the development and maintenance of metabolic syndrome. The rise in obesity rates across the world is directly related to dietary habits centered on processed food high in sugars and unhealthy fats. Concurrently, physical inactivity supports the deterioration of insulin resistance and other metabolic derangements. Additionally, contemporary work schedules, including shift work, have been investigated for their negative impacts on metabolic well-being. Circadian disruption and altered eating habits among shift workers not only compromise the quality of sleep but also have significant effects on gut microbiota and inflammatory processes, further contributing to the susceptibilities of metabolic syndrome (Lane et al., 2020). Understanding of these factors and how they interplay is essential for effective intervention strategies aiming to diminish the impact of metabolic syndrome. Management of metabolic syndrome effectively is a blend of managing lifestyle change and, if necessary, drug therapy. Weight loss by caloric restriction and increased exercise has been shown to increase insulin sensitivity, reduce visceral fat, and improve concomitant states like hypertension and dyslipidemia. Furthermore, healthcare professionals might need to turn to pharmacotherapy in patients who cannot achieve adequate control by means of lifestyle modifications only. The new awareness of the metabolic pathways affected by obesity and insulin resistance can lead to target therapies—highlighting the need for ongoing research in endocrinology. With metabolic syndrome a public health concern, preventive and therapeutic strategies will capitalize on the integration of endocrinological science into clinical practice and health policy.

Importance of Studying Obesity in Endocrinology

The significance of the study of obesity as an area of endocrinology cannot be overstated, given its close link to metabolic syndrome and its pervasive role in public health. Obesity is a disorder with multiple causations, whose multifaceted influence by genetic, environmental, and lifestyle factors ultimately results in a disturbance of hormonal balance and metabolism. Endocrinologists are curious about the contribution of adipose tissue, formerly conceived as a mere passive fat storage reservoir, to dynamic endocrine signaling and effecting metabolic processes. Given that obesity is typically associated with diseases such as diabetes and cardiovascular disease, the study of its effect on hormone regulation, particularly insulin and leptin, provides useful insights into therapeutic interventions that could temper resultant health risks. Consequently, increased understanding of obesity will inform treatment paradigms that augment endocrine function and metabolic health. Furthermore, the interrelatedness of obesity and endocrine dysregulation emphasizes the necessity for targeted research in this area. Turner syndrome illustrates the complexity of genetic defects in hormone regulation that can be exacerbated by obesity. In a large pediatric population, the prevalence of comorbidities such as insulin resistance and dyslipidemia suggests the possibility of obesity to amplify endocrine dysfunction, with elevated cardiovascular risk and other metabolic abnormalities. Recognition of such associations is crucial in developing interventions to not only alleviate obesity but also considering the subtle interaction between obesity and more widespread endocrine disease. As individuals with Turner syndrome possess heterogeneous karyotypes, knowledge of how these syndromes interact is essential for creating individualized treatment regimens. Lastly, examining the role played by sex hormones in endocrine modifications in obesity is critical towards building our understanding of gender-specific metabolic syndrome risks. Androgens and estrogens have been shown in studies to greatly influence body composition, the function of adipocytes, and metabolic control. For instance, androgen deficiency in men can cause increased adiposity and hypertension, whereas excess androgen in women can increase cardiovascular risk factors. This bidirectional relationship between sex hormones and obesity consolidates the multicausal nature of metabolic syndrome and the employment of tailored interventions. Furthermore, inflammation response pathways through hormones like NF-kB and obesity itself indicate the manner in which endocrine alterations are brought about by excess fat tissue. Continued research in this field will reveal the underlying mechanisms of such interactions, creating scope for new prevention and management strategies founded on individual hormonal profiles.

9.1. The Pathophysiology of Obesity

Learning Outcome

1. Define hormonal regulation of appetite
2. Describe the role of adipose tissue in metabolism
3. Explain the genetic factors influencing obesity

The pathophysiology of obesity is multi-factorial with a complex interaction of environmental, hormonal, and metabolic factors. Central to this is the role of adipose tissue, not just as an energy storage reservoir but also as an active endocrine organ. As obesity starts to develop, the adipocytes expand and become more numerous by hypertrophy and hyperplasia, leading to the release of pro-inflammatory cytokines and other bioactive molecules. This impaired function of adipose tissue underlies a chronic inflammatory state favoring insulin resistance, and hallmark of metabolic syndrome. The enzyme 11β-Hydroxysteroid dehydrogenase type 1 (11β-HSD1) is also key in this regard as gene overexpression in adipose tissue has been linked with augmented cortisol production and aggravation of metabolic derangements. This sequence of metabolic derangements establishes the need to understand clear pathological processes underpinning obesity and its systemic consequences (Aubert et al., 2003). Of equal importance in pathophysiologic association is the one between obesity and obstructive sleep apnea (OSA), which was identified as prevalent in obese patients. OSA can explain a large portion of metabolic abnormalities often associated with obesity, creating a two-way relationship that renders clinical treatment difficult. Mechanistically, sleep loss due to OSA-induced hypoxia disrupts usual metabolic pathways and possibly can impede glycemic control. Resistive insulin occurs in patients with OSA and dysregulation of hormones such as leptin, a vital energy balance hormone, also promotes weight gain. Recent studies stress that the impact of OSA is not merely weight gain but incorporates a factor of metabolic dysfunction that impacts cardiovascular health and morbidity rates overall. It is crucial to comprehend this multifaceted relationship to develop overall treatment strategies targeted at reversing the progression of metabolic syndrome in affected patients (Arble et al., 2018).

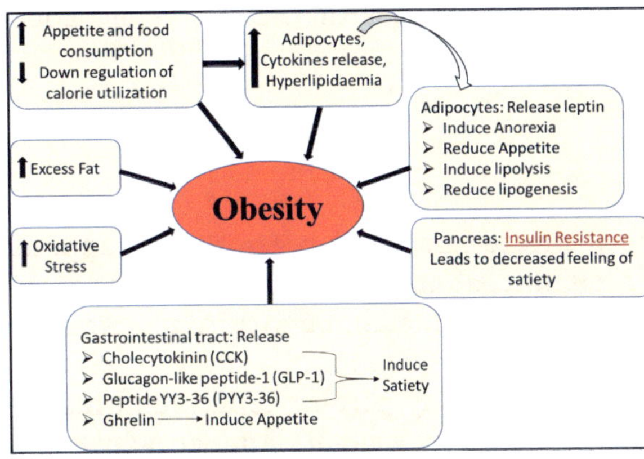

Figure 9.2. The diagrammatic representation of basic pathogenesis of obesity.

Source: https://www.researchgate.net/profile/Kiran-Patil-9/publication/329208017/figure/fig2/AS:699710989934595@1543835508912/The-diagrammatic-representation-of-basic-pathogenesis-of-obesity.png.

To maintain a big-picture perspective of the pathophysiology of obesity, its colossal physiological effect needs to be addressed. Among them, augmented systemic inflammation and activation of the renin-angiotensin system (RAS) are major mechanisms causing hypertension present in the metabolic syndrome of obesity. The findings on the overexpression of 11β-HSD1 demonstrate the manner in which this local glucocorticoid reactivation can lead to dyslipidemia, elevated blood pressure, and other cardiovascular problems. Further, the interconnectedness between these physiological adaptations and metabolic consequences of health compels attention to the multifactorial component of obesity. With its progression, there is considerable amplification of risk for the development of chronic conditions such as type 2 diabetes and cardiovascular disease, and there is a critical need to develop targeted therapeutic interventions. With the pathophysiology of obesity increasingly understood, it encourages the application of multidisciplinary approaches to effective management and complication prevention of its health (Aubert et al., 2003) (Figure 9.2).

9.1.1. Hormonal Regulation of Appetite

The intricate hormonal regulation of appetite is a significant mediator of the pathogenesis of obesity and metabolic syndrome. Appetite is regulated predominantly by a variety of hormones, namely ghrelin, leptin, and insulin, which collectively regulate hunger signals and energy balance. Ghrelin, released from the stomach, stimulates appetite and promotes fat storage and hence is an essential player in the short-term energy balance. On the other hand, leptin, produced by adipose tissue, relays the body's energy status to the hypothalamus, inhibiting hunger when fat stores are adequate. Insulin, produced by the pancreas, not only controls glucose homeostasis but also affects satiety, as high levels of insulin indicate that the body has adequate energy reserves. Dysregulation of these hormones causes hyperconsumption of energy and obesity and magnification of the metabolic derangements causing metabolic syndrome (Lin et al., 2021). Dysregulation of these appetite hormones in obesity produces incessant hunger and impaired satiety signaling. Circulating levels of ghrelin and resistance to leptin are typically increased in obese individuals, deranging the fine balance between energy intake and expenditure. This resistance is manifested as blunted response to leptins appetite-suppressing effects, leading to a paradox where individuals with increased fat stores feel hungry. In addition, insulin resistance also introduces an added layer of complexity to appetite regulation via carbohydrate consumption as it leads to ill-regulated insulin responses that fail to adequately convey satiety. The combined effect of these hormonal imbalances produces a cycle of hyperphagia and weight gain, which attests to the importance of exploring the mechanisms of hormones in an effort to develop effective treatment for obesity and metabolic syndrome (Chait et al., 2020).

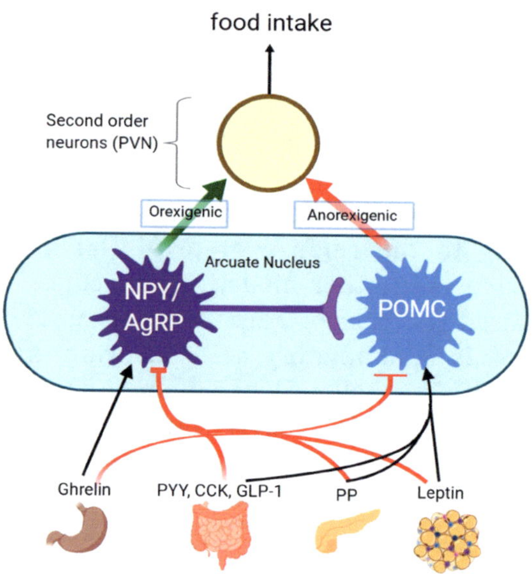

Figure 9.3. Signaling pathways involved in appetite regulation. This schematic diagram shows the effect of hormones on neuronal appetite signaling in the brain.

Source: https://www.researchgate.net/publication/348932892/figure/fig2/AS:11431281211454901@1702399059308/Signalling-pathways-involved-in-appetite-regulation-This-schematic-diagram-shows-the.tif.

Exploring the hormonal interactions involved in appetite regulation also directs towards potential treatment approaches to the prevention of obesity and its consequences. Pharmacologic agents targeting appetite-regulating hormones, such as leptin antagonists or ghrelin mimetics, have shown promise in the clinical setting. Moreover, lifestyle modification of diet and exercise has been shown to enhance hormonal sensitivity and normalize pathways of appetite regulation. For instance, a protein-rich diet could lead to lowered ghrelin levels and satiety, while regular exercise can enhance insulin sensitivity. These strategies not only aim to normalize levels of hunger and satiety hormones but also aim to trigger long-lasting changes in eating behavior and regulation of body weight. Thus, unlocking the hormonal regulation of appetite is key to managing the obesity epidemic and developing effective public health interventions that ameliorate the metabolic syndrome (Lin et al., 2021) (Figure 9.3).

9.1.2. Role of Adipose Tissue in Metabolism

The metabolic role of adipose tissue extends beyond the role of energy storage; it is an active endocrine organ with a key role in the regulation of systemic energy homeostasis. Adipose tissue has been found to secrete a variety of hormones and cytokines, all of which are referred to as adipokines, some of which include leptin, adiponectin, and resistin. These biomolecules have a central role in mediating insulin sensitivity, appetite, and inflammation. With obesity, there is an increase in certain adipokines, particularly leptin, which could lead to insulin resistance, a feature of metabolic syndrome. Such dysfunction creates a multi-way interaction between adipose tissue and other metabolic systems that disrupts overall endocrine function and exposes organisms to metabolic syndrome complications. Understanding these interactions is also key to the development of therapeutic interventions aimed at adipose tissue pathways to reverse the effect of obesity and related metabolic derangements. The effect of glucocorticoids on adipose tissue also identifies the fat storage-metabolism complexity. These steroid hormones involved in stress responses modulate the function of adipocytes through glucocorticoid receptors (GR). Surprisingly, inappropriately increased glucocorticoids may enhance an increase in fat mass, especially during visceral depots, and is of special concern in patients with metabolic syndrome. Studies have shown that the local activation of cortisol to cortisone by adipose tissue, catalyzed by 11b-hydroxysteroid dehydrogenase type 1 (11b-HSD1), may exacerbate adipocyte differentiation and function. By modulating the function of this enzyme, it is to be hoped that glucocorticoid action can be modulated within adipose tissue and metabolic dysregulation related thereto corrected. Collectively, these studies of glucocorticoid signaling highlight the adipose tissue as a critical controller of metabolic homeostasis, leading to a need for further investigation of target-directed therapeutic interventions (Harris et al., 2018). Adipocyte differentiation is another subject of significance of the metabolic function of adipose tissue. When exposed to glucocorticoids, human preadipocytes are seen to increase their differentiation, which is regulated by the activity of 11b-HSD1. This change not only enhances the deposition of lipids in adipocytes but also stimulates the expression of key adipogenic markers to improve the function of adipose tissue. Furthermore, after selective 11b-HSD1 inhibitor treatment, one can distinguish easily between adipocyte differentiation and function, which suggests a robust causal connection between glucocorticoid activity and adipose tissue metabolism. Therefore, an understanding of how adipose tissue interacts with hormonal signaling pathways may yield novel targets for therapeutic intervention in obesity and metabolic syndrome. With further studies in this field, a better understanding of adipose tissue functions can create new avenues to combat these health problems, ultimately resulting in improved metabolic health outcomes (Bujalska et al., 2008) (Figure 9.4).

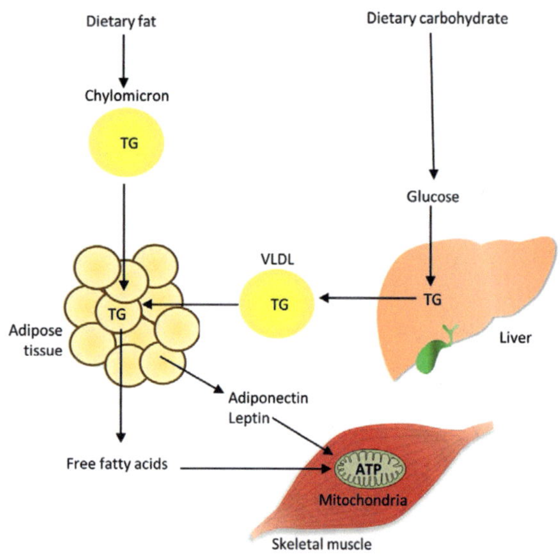

Figure 9.4. Metabolic and endocrine functions of adipose tissue. [TG: Triglycerides; and VLDL: very-low-density lipoproteins].

Source: https://www.researchgate.net/profile/Ivan-Torre-Villalvazo/publication/380392080/figure/fig1/AS:11431281243933984@1715777485042/Metabolic-and-endocrine-functions-of-adipose-tissue-TG-triglycerides-VLDL.ppm.

9.1.3. Genetic Factors Influencing Obesity

The intricate interaction between obesity and genetics highlights the significant role genetic factors play in determining one's susceptibility to weight gain and linked metabolic disease. Multiple genetic variants that influence adiposity and fat distribution have recently been implicated, and understanding how particular alleles cause individuals to be at risk of obesity. For instance, a study examining the cannabinoid receptor-1 (CNR1) locus has shown that some single nucleotide polymorphisms, such as A3813G and G1422A, have been shown to be linked with increased total fat depots and android fat distribution in some populations, indicating that genetic susceptibility is an important factor in shaping body composition and health risk factors for obesity (Milewicz et al., 2009). Understanding these genetic markers is essential to the development of specific interventions treating obesity, particularly in those with a genetic predisposition. In locating genetic factors, medical practitioners will be in a better position to customize the treatment programs for obesity according to the personal needs of each patient. In addition to the specific body weight effects of genes, the overall effects of genetic susceptibility contribute a level of complexity to obesity as a multidimensional disorder. Some people with specific genetic profiles may be impacted by variations in metabolic processes such as insulin sensitivity and lipid metabolism to make it harder to manage weight. For example, many chromosomal conditions such as Turner syndrome have been identified as being associated with risks of dyslipidemia as well as insulin resistance (Abacı et al., 2015). These conditions serve to underscore the need to understand the genetic origins of obesity in the context of a more comprehensive metabolic syndrome model. By knowing how genetic variables interact with environmental variables, such as exercise and diet, endocrinologists are better able to screen individual risk factors and formulate overall strategies for diminishing obesity, treating thus both the symptoms and etiology of the disease. Ultimately, using genetic data in obesity research and treatment is to enhance prevention and therapy. With future development of genomic medicine, there is promising potential for pharmacogenetic approaches to treating individual genetic differences leading to obesity. For instance, understanding the impact of CNR1 variants could lead to personalized pharmacological intervention targeted towards the modulation of endocannabinoid signaling as an intervention against obesity. Consequently, this genetic insight not only guides treatment but also can result in early identification of high-risk populations, prompting pre-excess weight lifestyle modification. Continued research on the obesity genetic profile remains a critical priority for endocrinology that will further bridge basic science and clinical application, ultimately resulting in healthier populations through informed healthcare interventions (Figure 9.5).

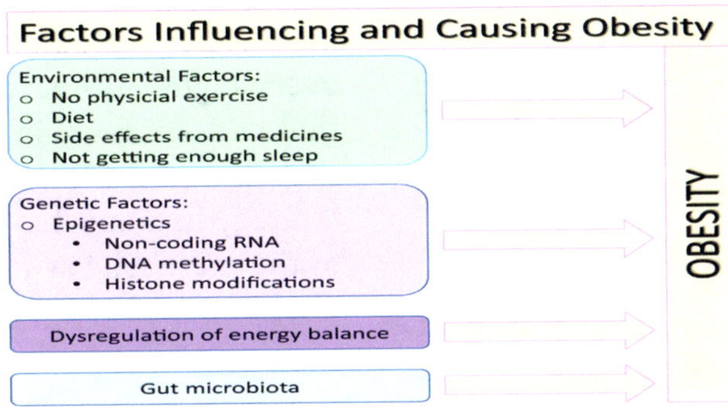

Figure 9.5. Genetics and obesity highlight the significant role that inherited traits play in influencing an individual's propensity to gain weight.

Source: https://www.researchgate.net/publication/343948848/figure/fig2/AS:929734158450695@1598677305969/Factors-influencing-and-causing-obesity-Obesity-can-be-caused-by-several-different.png.

Test Your Knowledge

1. What roles do hormones like leptin, ghrelin, and insulin play in regulating appetite and energy balance?
2. In what ways does adipose tissue function as an endocrine organ?
3. How do genetic predispositions interact with environmental factors such as diet and physical activity to influence obesity risk?

9.2. Metabolic Syndrome: Definition and Criteria

Learning Outcome

1. Identify the components of metabolic syndrome
2. Describe the diagnostic criteria according to the american heart association
3. Explain the prevalence rates in different populations

The metabolic syndrome is a cluster of metabolic risk factors that significantly increase one's risk of developing cardiovascular diseases and type 2 diabetes. Definitions may vary, but it is typically described as being linked with the occurrence of abdominal obesity, dyslipidemia, hypertension, and elevated fasting plasma glucose levels. These criteria emphasize the interconnectedness of these conditions, demonstrating how excess adiposity can culminate in metabolic dysfunction. In the endocrinology context, the significance of metabolic syndrome is underscored due to its common co-occurrence with obesity. The interaction between hormonal imbalance and visceral fat accumulation results in a pathological condition that significantly raises the risk of serious health outcomes, and thus precise conceptualization of definition and criteria constituting this syndrome is crucial. Identification of metabolic syndrome requires careful assessment based on some clinical guidelines established by various health organizations such as the American Heart Association and the National Heart, Lung, and

Blood Institute. Prominent among these measures is the measurement of waist circumference, followed by the evaluation of triglyceride levels, HDL cholesterol levels, blood pressure, and fasting glucose levels. All these markers translate underlying metabolic processes, such as insulin resistance and disturbed lipid metabolism. Thus, three or more of these risk factors are required for a diagnosis of metabolic syndrome. The criterion allows clinicians to stratify the risk of their patients and implement focused interventions that potentially prevent the onset of these complex metabolic disorders that are linked to obesity. Metabolic syndrome is particularly relevant in populations that are suffering from obesity because it represents a complex interaction between body composition and metabolic health.

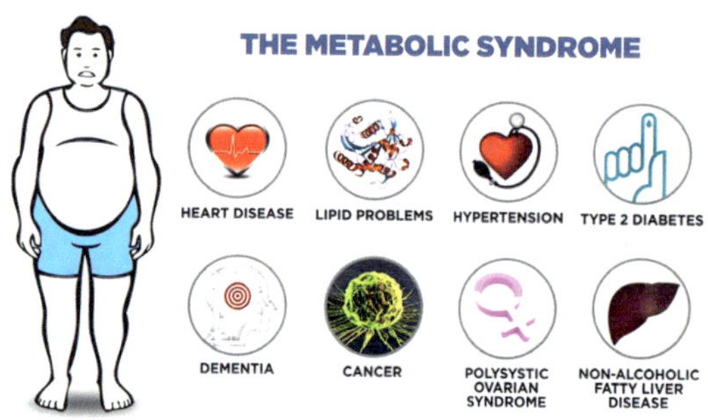

Figure 9.6. Illustration of metabolic syndrome.

Source: https://www.beltrebariatricsfl.com/wp-content/uploads/2023/04/symptoms-metabolic-syndrome-obesity-high-blood-pressure-glucose-intolerance-high-cholesterol-Orlando.jpg.

For instance, research has documented differential prevalence of metabolic syndrome by obesity phenotype. Specifically, research has described how the obese state of sarcopenic obesity, characterized by its coexistence of excess fat with reduced muscle mass, can be closely associated with elevated metabolic risk. Research has indicated that individuals with sarcopenic obesity are far more likely to develop metabolic syndrome, with adverse long-term health consequences. This information also underscores the necessity of comprehensive metabolic evaluations in patients who are overweight, ultimately guiding interventions that address fat gain and muscle preservation, thereby providing a more comprehensive strategy in managing obesity within the setting of the metabolic syndrome (Bonin et al., 2013; Choi et al., 2009) (Figure 9.6).

9.2.1. Components of Metabolic Syndrome

The components of metabolic syndrome (MetS) consist of a cluster of related risk factors, which significantly raise the likelihood of cardiovascular disease, type 2 diabetes, and other severe health conditions. Central obesity, in which there is abnormal fat deposition in the abdominal area, is one significant indicator. It is not merely cosmetic; this visceral fat actually generates insulin resistance and deregulation of metabolic pathways. All of the other essential factors are elevated blood pressure, elevated triglycerides, low high-density lipoprotein cholesterol (HDL-C), and impaired fasting glucose. All of these interact with each other to create a complex metabolic dysfunction with a resulting multiplier effect in the risk of chronic disease. Identification and diagnosis of these components matter in the establishment of effective interventions to lower the adverse health implications of obesity and MetS, giving rise to the need for total screening and early identification measures. In recent studies, the role of iodine status in the context of the components of metabolic syndrome has been a significant area of interest. Specifically, research has indicated that urinary iodine concentration (UIC) variations relate to the prevalence of MetS in adult populations in the U.S. Those with higher UIC indicated higher risk factors, such as high triglyceride levels and central obesity compared to those with normal iodine concentration. Interestingly, evidence suggests a nonlinear relationship wherein low UIC has been linked to lower risks of such metabolic disorders, an indication of the complex interplay of dietary nutrients and metabolic health. Thus, the interaction between iodine status and MetS components broadens understanding on nutritional determinants of obesity and suggests that dietary interventions may be a component of prevention and management strategies (Shen et al., 2023). MetS conceptualizations vary in a non-standard fashion, especially in youths. Currently used criteria to diagnose MetS in youths rely on the existence of abdominal adiposity as well as other parameters such as increased triglyceride, low HDL-C, high blood pressure, or low glucose levels. The present cut-offs do not change and do not take into account age and sex differences and result in misclassification of risk in the pediatric population. New guidelines propose the use of age- and sex-specific percentile cut-offs for abdominal obesity and elevated blood pressure to define, placing stress on the importance of individually tailored measures in pediatric assessment. The absence of specified international criteria results in problems with estimation of MetS prevalence between regions. Thus, more rational sets of criteria for MetS detection in youth are required for effective global health surveillance and intervention programs (Xin'nan et al., 2022) (Figure 9.7).

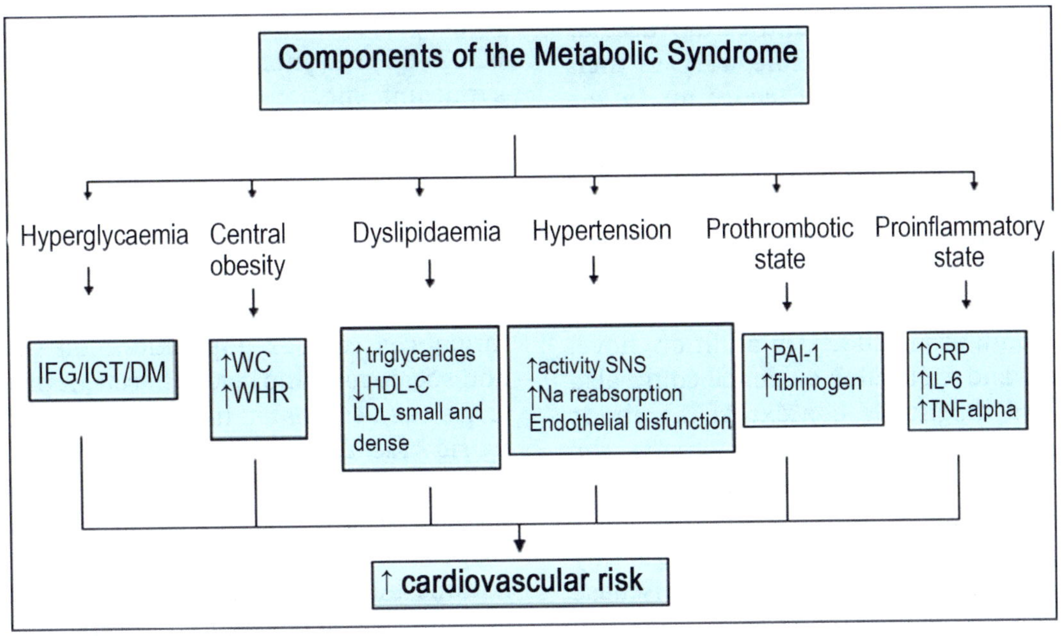

Figure 9.7. Metabolic syndrome components.

Source: https://lllnutrition.com/mod_lll/TOPIC24/Old_Version/images241/image001.jpg.

9.2.2. Diagnostic Criteria According to the American Heart Association

The American Heart Association (AHA) diagnostic criteria for metabolic syndrome are important in establishing obesity and cardiovascular disease interfaces. The syndrome is a set of risk factors that encompass increased waist circumference, elevated triglycerides, decreased high-density lipoprotein (HDL) cholesterol, hypertension, and hyperglycemia. A correct diagnosis involves the presence of at least three of these factors. The AHA places emphasis on these criteria because they assist in the identification of patients who are at greater risk of developing cardiovascular disease and type 2 diabetes, both of which are common conditions associated with obesity. Thus, not only do these diagnostic criteria serve as a clinician tool but also as a public health intervention model to assist in the reduction of obesity-related disease in the population. In addition to direct implications on diagnosis, the AHA criteria also provide a basis for individualizing treatment approaches. Awareness of the unique risk factors allows the clinicians to create tailored treatment choices to address the specific metabolic derangements in each patient. For instance, some of the metabolic syndrome phenotypes, as given by research on such diseases as polycystic ovary syndrome (PCOS), give an insight into how varying combinations of features can influence insulin resistance and cardiovascular risk. PCOS women, for example, vary in their rates of insulin resistance according to the phenotypic classification given in the diagnostic criteria. This latent understanding underscores the importance of applying AHA criteria for evaluating and treating metabolic syndrome effectively so that screening and intervention may be prioritized based on individual patient profiles (Bonin et al., 2013). In addition, novel biomarkers and molecular evidence could also enhance the diagnostic context of metabolic syndrome. Recent studies have shown the potential role of microRNAs, i.e., miRNA-93 and miRNA-223, as diagnostic indicators for conditions like PCOS and subsequently metabolic syndrome. Elevated levels of these microRNAs in PCOS women suggest that they can serve as markers of hidden metabolic abnormality regardless of normal parameters like insulin resistance. The integration of these high-level diagnostic tools with the AHAs set standards would make our detection system more accurate. Integrating these and other diagnostic tools could lead to plans for earlier intervention, finally reducing the burden of obesity complications on the healthcare system along with for those at risk (Atkin et al., 2015) (Figure 9.8).

Component	Clinical Cutoff Values
Waist Circumference	≥102 cm in men ≥88 cm in women
Triglycerides	≥150 mg/dL
HDL Cholesterol	<40 mg/dL in men <50 mg/dL in women
Blood Pressure (BP)	≥130 mmHg Systolic BP or ≥85 mmHg Diastolic BP
Fasting Glucose	≥100 mg/dL
Diagnosis	Any 3 of the 5 features above

Figure 9.8. Diagnostic criteria for metabolic syndrome.

Source: https://www.researchgate.net/profile/Daniel-Benyshek/publication/257881066/figure/tbl1/AS:669347202748434@1536596217763/Diagnostic-criteria-for-metabolic-syndrome.png.

9.2.3. Prevalence Rates in Different Populations

The global epidemic of obesity and metabolic syndrome is a primary public health concern that influences various populations on geographic and socioeconomic levels. In recent projections, it has been estimated that over 1.5 billion adults worldwide are overweight, of which at least 500 million are clinically obese with body mass indexes greater than 25 kg/m^2 and 30 kg/m^2, respectively. This is not specific to Western nations but also to emerging economies with speeding up urbanization and lifestyle change driving the obesity pandemic. The World Health Organization has indeed characterized obesity as an epidemic globally, identifying its importance as an under-played element of public health agendas. These statistics point out that the health consequences of obesity are extensive, with effects beyond mere weight gain that encompass severe ailments such as diabetes, cardiovascular diseases, and metabolic syndrome, which are increasingly on the rise in all population groups (Kyrou et al., 2010). Children and teenagers constitute a very vulnerable population, with obesity escalating at an alarming rate that can adversely affect their long-term health trajectory. In the United States, approximately 17% of children and adolescents belong to the obesity category, a percentage that indicates a trend towards increasing severity. Of those, severe obesity, which is defined as at or above 120% of the 95th percentile for BMI-for-age or a BMI of 35 kg/m^2 or more, is increasing rapidly, currently affecting nearly 6% of kids and teens. This subgroup is linked to increased risks for comorbidities, including coronary heart disease and type 2 diabetes, which have been proven to establish itself in a dose-dependent manner with regard to the severity of obesity. In this regard, therefore, the imperative for effective intervention tools becomes the primary concern, given the fact that traditional treatment strategies have low success rates in tackling this severe level of obesity (Ameer et al., 2018). The differences in obesity rates across various groups point to the complexity of this public health issue, which depends on ethnicity, socioeconomic status, and environment. The most susceptible are low-income groups with limited availability of nutritious food and green outdoor spaces, demonstrating a cause-and-effect relationship between structural inequalities and heightened obesity risk. Furthermore, cultural attitudes to health and body image can influence food behavior and lifestyle choices, driving the plague of obesity in specific populations. Holistic strategies addressing these social determinants are crucial in preventing obesity and related health conditions, including metabolic syndrome. Individualized interventions considering the unique attributes of various populations are essential to develop effective public health policies that will reduce obesity levels and improve overall health outcomes (Kyrou et al., 2010).

Test Your Knowledge

1. What is metabolic syndrome, and why is it considered a cluster of interrelated risk factors?
2. What are the five main components of metabolic syndrome commonly assessed in diagnosis?

9.3. The Role of Endocrine Disruptors

Learning Outcome

1. Understand the endocrine disruptors
2. Identify the sources of endocrine disruptors
3. Define impact on obesity and metabolic syndrome

The impact of endocrine disruptors on metabolic syndrome and obesity is an emerging research area in endocrinology. Endocrine disruptors, some of which are numerous environmental chemicals, have the potential to interfere with hormone signaling and regulation. Such interference can significantly alter metabolic processes and result in weight gain as well as the development of metabolic syndrome. Recent evidence suggests that certain chemicals can trigger adipogenesis, thereby increasing fat cell development and influencing energy balance. With the increasing prevalence of obesity worldwide, it becomes necessary to learn about the mechanisms through which such endocrine disruptors exert their effects so that effective means to combat concomitant health ailments can be developed. The obesogen hypothesis postulates that such compounds enhance susceptibility to obesity in individuals and highlight the necessity of examining environmental determinants of health in conjunction with genetic and life-style determinants (Blumberg et al., 2020). In addition, recent multidisciplinary professional workshops have highlighted the importance of exploring a broader class of compounds known as metabolic disruptors, which includes but is not limited to obesogens. This change in terminology is reflective of the nuance of these environmental exposures and their metabolic consequences since these disruptors possess several routes through which they can manifest their impacts, such as hormonal pathways critical to appetite and energy homeostasis. There is evidence for a staggering linkage between exposure to these disruptors and the onset of obesity and related metabolic conditions, drawn from epidemiological research as well as from animal model studies. By bringing together these observations, the scientific community aspires to gain a unifying theory of the contribution of environmental influences on the obesity epidemic and thus expand our paradigm for reactions to public health interventions and policy (Janesick et al., 2015). Finally, critical evaluation of existing literature demonstrates that there are several gaps in current understanding of endocrine disruptors and their role in contributing to obesity. Because the etiology of metabolic syndrome is multifactorial, research methods must be developed through multidisciplinary efforts that investigate these chemicals long-term health effects and how they compromise with genetic predispositions and lifestyles. There is a need for ongoing research to investigate more specifically the pathways through which metabolic disruptors impair metabolic processes and endocrine balances. Close these gaps would not only make our knowledge of the etiology of obesity more robust, but it would also allow healthcare providers and policymakers to make informed decisions towards minimizing exposure to toxic environmental chemicals. Overall, this comprehensive approach is necessary for responding to the increase in obesity and obesity-related complications in the broader endocrinology context (Blumberg et al., 2020; Janesick et al., 2015).

9.3.1. Definition of Endocrine Disruptors

Endocrine disruptors is a class of chemicals that can interfere with an organism's hormone system to cause adverse health effects. Such chemicals can either simulate naturally occurring hormones in an organism, disrupt the procedure of hormone production, or interfere with how an organism responds to hormones.

It is particularly worrying as it can aid in the metabolism of metabolic disease and the epidemic of obesity. With growing research in the area, it now becomes more apparent that exposure to such disruptors, most commonly from an environmental source, can affect body weight regulation through complex mechanisms like altering appetite control and fat accumulation. Unraveling the definition and scope of endocrine disruptors becomes pivotal to understanding their role in the growing prevalence of obesity and metabolic syndrome, illnesses involving complex physiological processes fueled by hormonal derangement. Novel evidence indicates that endocrine disruptors can also act as obesogens, which are chemicals that cause obesity by interfering with metabolic pathways. The obesogen hypothesis assumes that such chemicals increase an individual's predisposition to weight gain, potentially aiding fat accumulation by interfering with hormone function and altering energy balance. This perspective moves focus away from classic risk factors of diet and exercise to a broader viewpoint that encompasses environmental influences. Emerging data in animal model studies and human epidemiological information agree with claims that the occurrence of endocrine disruptors is long-term in its effect on metabolic well-being, maybe being responsible for some of the trend towards record levels of obesity observed globally. The sophistication of these interactions points to the need for additional research, namely in the domain of explaining how various environmental chemicals interact with endocrine pathways responsible for body weight regulation. Existing workshops and expert panels have spurred an expansion of the definition of obesogens to encompass metabolic disruptors, which embrace a more expansive group of environmental chemicals participating in obesity and metabolic syndrome. According to consideration in a seminal workshop in Parma, Italy, there is a pressing need for comprehension of the role of such disruptors in modulating health impact, specifically obesity and metabolic disease. The findings point to significant relationships between chemical exposure and physiological response predisposing to disease metabolic outcomes. When researchers attempt to close research gaps, there is no question that awareness of endocrine disruptors will be an important factor in the generation of effective prevention and intervention approaches against obesity. By synthesizing knowledge across disciplines, researchers attempt to put into words a comprehensive understanding of how exposure to the environment can affect metabolic health and thus cure the growing public health concern of obesity and metabolic syndrome (Blumberg et al., 2020; Janesick et al., 2015) (Figure 9.9).

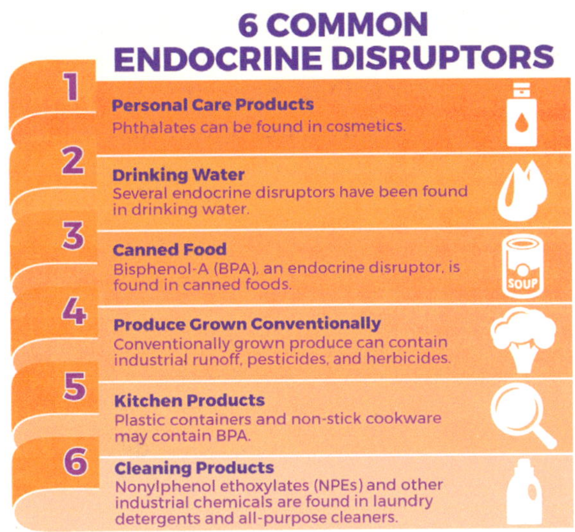
6 COMMON
ENDOCRINE DISRUPTORS
1
Personal Care Products
Phthalates can be found in cosmetics.
2
Drinking Water
Several endocrine disruptors have been found in drinking water.
3
Canned Food
Bisphenol-A (BPA), an endocrine disruptor, is found in canned foods.
SOUP
4
Produce Grown Conventionally
Conventionally grown produce can contain industrial runoff, pesticides, and herbicides.
5
Kitchen Products
Plastic containers and non-stick cookware may contain BPA.
6
Cleaning Products
Nonylphenol ethoxylates (NPEs) and other industrial chemicals are found in laundry detergents and all-purpose cleaners.

Figure 9.9. Infographic of six common endocrine disruptors.

Source: https://www.drlamcoaching.com/images/infographic-6-common-endocrine-disruptors.jpg.

9.3.2. Sources of Endocrine Disruptors

The widespread presence of endocrine disruptors in modern society presents serious challenges to public health, especially when it comes to obesity and metabolic syndrome. The chemical substances, present in a wide variety of everyday products ranging from plastics and detergents to pesticides, cause disruptions in normal hormonal functions in the human body. For instance, bisphenol A (BPA) and phthalates have been widely used in the production of food and drink packaging, resulting in widespread environmental contamination and unintended human exposure. Studies have linked the presence of these pollutants with the disruption of metabolism, suggesting that they may be crucial in inducing the rising epidemic of obesity through the regulation of appetite and fat deposition. The prevalence of such disruptors renders their sources important to assess to value their role in the etiology of metabolic diseases like obesity and to strategize preventive measures in advance (Younes et al., 2024). Additionally, the food environment itself is teeming with endocrine disruptors that originate not only industrially but also agriculturally. The widespread application of synthetic pesticides and fertilizers in agriculture has led to nutritional vectors of endocrine disruption, which contribute to the food chain chemicals that may have harmful effects on human health. Several studies offer evidence that exposure to these chemicals results in metabolic impairment and is associated with disease conditions such as insulin resistance and obesity. Of special interest is the evidence showing that such disruptors can act as obesogens, chemically inducing an increase in fat storage and altering energy balance. The crossroads between diet and environmental exposures illustrate the intricacy of tackling obesity in the modern era, as consumers are often unaware of the endocrine-disrupting nature of their food source (Carrel et al., 2009). Finally, the effects of endocrine disruption extend beyond immediate physical health issues, resonating within economic and social circles. Solutions to rising obesity and metabolic syndrome rates need a comprehensive approach in terms of public policy, education, and regulation of industry. As evidence continues to show the connection between endocrine disruptors and adverse effects, effective interventions must be given due consideration in order to properly mitigate their impact. For instance, legislation that reduces the application of particularly hazardous chemicals in consumer products and agriculture can be a public health intervention to limit exposure. Collective action, including promoting organic farming and sensitizing consumers about possible disruptors, is required to address such pressing health concerns. Without a comprehensive strategy to regulate and limit endocrine disruptor sources, the obesity and metabolic syndrome vicious cycle will persist (Younes et al., 2024) (Figure 9.10).

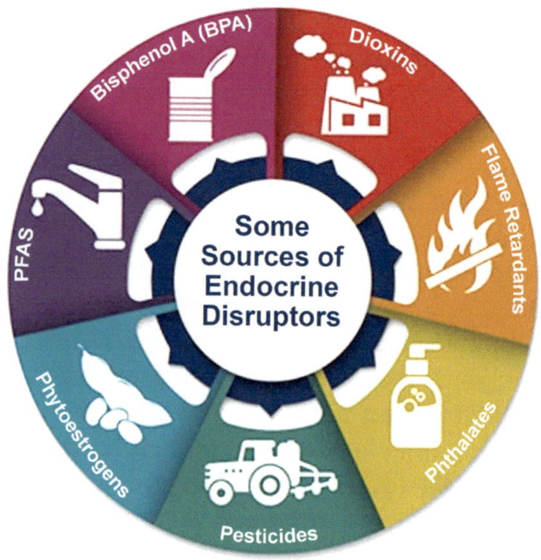
Some Sources of Endocrine Disruptors
Bisphenol A (BPA)
Dioxins
Flame Retardants
Phthalates
Pesticides
Phytoestrogens
PFAS

Figure 9.10. Endocrine disruptor sources.

Source: https://www.niehs.nih.gov/sites/default/files/health/assets/images/endocrine_disruptor_sources.jpg.

9.3.3. Impact on Obesity and Metabolic Syndrome

The progressively high incidence of obesity is strongly related to the rising prevalence of the metabolic syndrome, a cluster of conditions that very much predispose to cardiovascular disease and diabetes. Underlying the situation is a multifaceted interaction of genetic, behavioral, and environmental determinants that contribute to excessive body fat deposition. Specifically, dietary quality, as measured by the Healthy Eating Index (HEI, 2015), has been shown to be a central component in avoiding metabolic syndrome risk. Data substantiates that individuals on higher dietary quality have reduced risk of developing metabolic syndrome, with an odds ratio of 0.80 in participants who were at the 75th percentile of HEI (2015) scores (Li et al., 2024). Thus, the enhancement in diet can be an effective public health measure in the prevention of obesity and associated metabolic derangement. The function of obesity is not limited to heightened weight gain; it encompasses a number of biochemical alterations that are the very foundation of metabolic syndrome. Body mass index (BMI) has been found to be linked with greater systemic inflammation, an element central to metabolic derangement pathogenesis. For instance, logistic regression analysis revealed obesity as a main risk factor for acute radiation-induced skin toxicity and indicated broader implications of adiposity to health outcomes (Joseph et al., 2024). In addition, inflammatory status not only aggravates metabolic syndrome but also renders treatment approaches to diseases like breast cancer problematic because well-managed control is based on patient-specific information. Recognition of the multi-action of obesity on metabolic processes underscores the importance of comprehensive interventions addressing weight management and systemic inflammation concurrently. Tipping the balance of obesity-linked metabolic syndrome necessitates a multi-component approach involving lifestyle change, pharmacologic treatment, and community involvement. Interventions that promote dietary improvements, as highlighted by the associations validated using HEI (2015), play a pivotal role in guaranteeing healthier metabolic and weight profiles. Furthermore, the identification of the potential mediating functions of systemic immune-inflammation and uric acid level provides key insight into the ways in which increased dietary improvement is related to enhanced metabolic health (Li et al., 2024). These activities need to be accompanied by healthcare strategies that encompass adequate treatment protocols for the obese patient, thereby creating an environment that is conducive to effective practice along with enhanced quality of life. As obesity complications become better understood, prevention and intervention become more vital in addressing the multifaceted problems of obesity and metabolic syndrome in endocrinology.

Test Your Knowledge

1. How do endocrine disruptors alter hormonal signaling pathways involved in metabolism and energy balance?
2. In what ways have endocrine disruptors been implicated in the development of obesity?
3. How might long-term exposure to endocrine disruptors contribute to components of metabolic syndrome?

9.4. The Relationship Between Obesity and Insulin Resistance

Learning Outcome

1. Understand the mechanisms of insulin resistance
2. Identify the consequences of insulin resistance on health
3. Describe the role of weight loss in improving insulin sensitivity

The co-relationship between insulin resistance and obesity is of extreme significance in the pathogenesis of metabolic syndrome, particularly endocrinology. Insulin resistance is a condition where cells become less responsive to insulin, leading to increased levels of blood glucose, giving a pathway towards type 2 diabetes and cardiovascular disease. Obese patients typically present with increased levels of free fatty acids, which may disrupt insulin signaling and suppress glucose uptake in tissues. Moreover, the chronic inflammatory state of obesity, characterized by increased adipose tissue release of pro-inflammatory cytokines, enhances insulin resistance through interference with insulin receptor signaling. Such a multifaceted relationship indicates that not only does obesity lead to insulin resistance but it also leads the way to the development of other metabolic dysfunctions characteristic of the metabolic syndrome, once again highlighting the need for targeted intervention in this at-risk population. In the study of this relationship, it is well to remember comorbid conditions such as PCOS, which typically occur with obesity and insulin resistance. PCOS has been recognized as one of the most prevalent endocrine diseases found in women of childbearing age and has been implicated in several metabolic derangements, including insulin resistance. While not all women with PCOS are obese, those who are at an increased risk for the development of insulin resistance and related metabolic issues. Therapy for PCOS often involves attempts at weight loss, which can enhance insulin sensitivity as well as overall metabolic function. A lifestyle regulated by diet and exercise not only targets PCOS symptoms but also addresses the root insulin resistance, and thus underscores the vital connection between endocrinological wellbeing, obesity, and metabolic disease (Ghazeeri et al., 2021). Moreover, the concomitant presence of obstructive sleep apnea (OSA) with obesity and insulin resistance further entangles the picture of the metabolic syndrome. OSA is common in the population of obesity and tends to come with unwanted effects on metabolic health, so it is a two-way relationship where metabolic disease increases the signs of sleep apnea but also the disorder might cause further worsening of metabolic dysfunction. Increased insulin resistance in OSA can lead to more difficulty in glucose regulation, hence increasing the risk for type 2 diabetes. The interconnectivity of these conditions renders the treatment of a holistic management plan essential in addressing both metabolic and sleep disorders. Through weight loss and improved metabolic factors, clinicians can significantly abate the impact of both obesity and insulin resistance, allowing for increased intervention to treat obesity comorbidities like OSA and their long-term impact on disease outcomes (Arble et al., 2018).

9.4.1. Mechanisms of Insulin Resistance

The etiology of insulin resistance (IR) is a multifactorial process of physiological mechanisms, predominantly added to by obesity. Central to the process is enhanced excess adipose tissue, which deranges the usual milieu of hormones and metabolism. This derangement occurs primarily through pro-inflammatory cytokines secreted from adipocytes, leading to disruption of insulin signaling pathways. In particular, the induction of pro-inflammatory cytokines such as tumor necrosis factor-alpha (TNF-α) and interleukin-6 (IL-6) inhibits insulin receptor function, suppressing glucose uptake in peripheral tissues. Secondly, free fatty acid lipotoxicity to muscle and liver cells can trigger cellular dysfunction, adding to insulin resistance. As with higher rates of obesity, it is increasingly crucial to understand the mechanisms, particularly as a direct factor in type 2 diabetes and other metabolic disease development, justifying the need to examine insulin resistance within the broader framework of metabolic syndrome (Corrao et al., 2024). The relationship between metabolic syndrome and insulin resistance also complicates treatment approaches in managing obesity-induced conditions. Metabolic syndrome, as characterized by clustering of factors such as hypertension, dyslipidemia, and hyperglycemia, predisposes to cardiovascular disease and chronic kidney disease (Lin et al., 2024). Insulin resistance is the central feature in this syndrome, eliciting elevated blood glucose and lipid profiles that exacerbate the condition. The mechanistic relationship between metabolic syndrome and insulin resistance reveals how improper glucose and fat metabolism may trigger a cycle of deteriorating health consequences. An awareness of such interactions is important to healthcare professionals as it guides the way in treatment, such as lifestyle modification and drug therapy, to reverse the increasing epidemic of obesity and the consequent effects on the condition of systemic health (Lin et al., 2024). Another important sector in the treatment of insulin resistance relates to the role of pharmacological interventions, particularly novel therapies which specifically target such mechanisms. Novel improvement in drugs like Tirzepatide has proven to be effective in treating insulin resistance via the application of dual GLP-1 and GIP receptor agonism. Through increased insulin secretion, coupled with reduced glucagon release, these agents not only improve glycemic control in patients with type 2 diabetes but also induce weight loss and fat mass loss in obese individuals (Corrao et al., 2024). These therapeutic progresses underscore the value of multimodal treatment of obesity and metabolic comorbidities. Lastly, the pharmacologic management of insulin resistance with new alternative drugs, alongside lifestyle change, could potentially decrease considerably the burden of disease induced by obesity and metabolic syndrome and hence deserve greater interest and investment in the field (Corrao et al., 2024) (Figure 9.11).

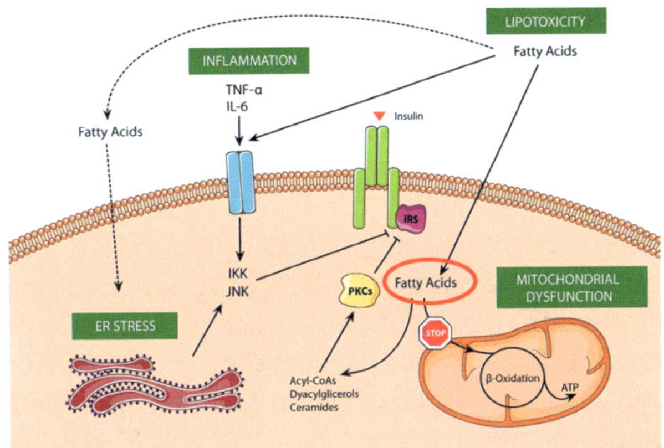

Figure 9.11. Mechanisms of insulin resistance.

Source: https://www.researchgate.net/profile/Josep-Villena/publication/260644291/figure/fig1/AS:392385440829447@1470563387318/Fig-1-Mechanisms-of-insulin-resistance-Several-mechanisms-have-been-identified-to.png.

9.4.2. Consequences of Insulin Resistance on Health

The actions of insulin resistance extend far beyond deranged glucose metabolism and have profound impacts on overall health in addition to risk for developing numerous chronic diseases. Insulin resistance is the decreased sensitivity of the body's tissue to insulin, which subsequently leads to a compensatory hyperinsulinemia that has a tendency to propagate inflammatory processes. Inflammation is most notably observed in obesity, with aberrant adipocytes secreting pro-inflammatory cytokines that further blemish insulin signaling. Thus, the risk of developing metabolic syndrome—a syndrome consisting of conditions like hypertension, dyslipidemia, and abdominal obesity—rises. Notably, the prevalence of metabolic syndrome among obese individuals indicates the far-reaching health outcomes of insulin resistance, including cardiovascular disease and type 2 diabetes (João, 2024). Hence, understanding of the multifaceted consequences of insulin resistance is instrumental to designing beneficial interventions and treatments. Besides, insulin resistance has also been strongly associated with the pathogenesis of polycystic ovary syndrome (PCOS), which is seen in a significant percentage of women of childbearing age. The relationship between insulin resistance and PCOS is distinguished by an array of changes in health status, including weight increase, menstrual dysfunction, and metabolic deviations. Research has shown that women with PCOS tend to experience concomitant insulin resistance, which causes them to have high risks of suffering from type 2 diabetes and cardiovascular diseases. The PCOS complications such as metabolic syndrome, obesity, and non-alcoholic fatty liver disease (NAFLD) explain the need for early diagnosis and treatment (Karolina et al., 2024). Thus, the management of insulin resistance not only prevents symptoms of PCOS but also prevents associated comorbidities. Insulin resistance has consequences beyond the physical realm, into the psychological, where patients who have this condition experience mental illness. The chronic nature of insulin resistance, particularly where it is found with obesity and metabolic syndrome, most often leads to loss of quality of life. Psychiatric problems such as depression and anxiety are often seen, which are compounded by the stress and stigma of obesity. In addition, the inflammatory mediators of insulin resistance are also implicated in the pathophysiology of these affective disorders, resulting in a vicious cycle that can also make it more difficult to treat. Hence, overall management strategies that address both physical and mental health parameters are a requirement in patients with insulin resistance and related ailments. Recognition of this overall problem is essential for improving patient outcomes and quality of life in the target group (Figure 9.12).

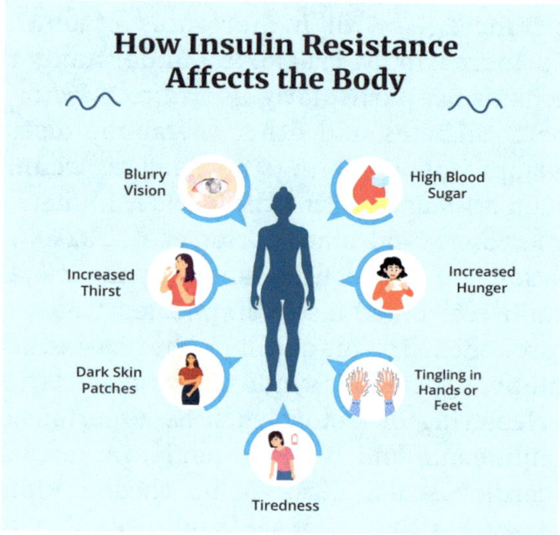

Figure 9.12. How insulin resistance affects the body?

Source: https://images.everydayhealth.com/images/seo-graphic-content-initiative/how-insulin-resistance-affects-the-body.png?sfvrsn=4fed0586_3.

9.4.3. Role of Weight Loss in Improving Insulin Sensitivity

The relationship between weight reduction and insulin sensitivity is a critical field of investigation within the framework of obesity and models of metabolic syndrome. Insulin resistance, one of the identifying elements of metabolic syndrome, appears when adipose tissue increases, and this leads to alterations in hormone signaling and inflammatory responses. Weight loss even to the level of 5.0% has been reported to play a significant role in increasing insulin sensitivity in individuals with obesity. The findings indicate that individuals who achieve such declines are likely to have lower scores of insulin resistance, along with other decreases in CVD risk factors of obesity, highlighting the significance of body weight control in the maintenance of metabolic health. As a first intervention, focus on sustainable weight loss is essential not just for blood glucose improvement, but also for global metabolic function and thus the removal of long-term metabolic syndrome risks (Yamakage et al., 2024). Various dietary interventions enable the attainment of effective weight loss and improved insulin sensitivity. For example, detox diets like the ketogenic diet and intermittent fasting have been found to have promising results in promoting weight loss and improving metabolic markers. Intermittent fasting regimens like the 16/8 regimen allow for lower caloric intake with adaptability, leading to remarkable improvement in insulin sensitivity. In addition, ketogenic diets induce rapid weight loss by inducing a state of ketosis where the body utilizes fats instead of carbohydrates as fuel. This process has widespread implications for insulin dynamics, with reduced carbohydrate intake alleviating the demand for insulin and hence enabling better glycemic control. These diets offer practical but varied solutions to obesity, but personalized strategies are necessary to maximize effectiveness and durability (Nicholas et al., 2024). Moreover, the long-term implications of weight loss maintenance on insulin sensitivity cannot be overstated. Evidence supports that weight losses of 7.5% or more may be even more valuable in terms of metabolic well-being. Beyond mere calorie restriction, enhanced insulin sensitivity is accompanied by improved lipid profiles, reduced inflammation, and better cardiovascular function. All of these benefits only help to highlight the need for weight loss interventions as part of overall treatment protocols for individuals with obesity and metabolic syndrome. With the advance of further research shedding light on the biological mechanisms underpinning such associations, practitioners increasingly become empowered to tailor interventions that not only provide for weight reduction but also promote sustaining advantages in terms of health, finally reshaping the discipline of obesity management (Yamakage et al., 2024).

Test Your Knowledge

1. How does excess adipose tissue contribute to the development of insulin resistance at the cellular level?
2. How does weight loss improve insulin sensitivity, and what physiological changes are observed in glucose metabolism as a result?

9.5. Psychological and Social Factors

Learning Outcome

1. Explain the psychological impact of obesity
2. Identify the socioeconomic factors contributing to obesity
3. Define the stigma and discrimination related to obesity

The interaction between psychological factors and obesity is complex and nuanced, influencing not only the onset but also the course of metabolic syndrome. In accordance with research, individuals under tremendous stress or depression may find comfort in food and thus end up consuming more food and gaining weight. Particularly in adolescents, elevated triglyceride levels have correlated with increased depressive behavior and consequently signify that emotional distress may enhance metabolic risk through physiological pathways. These correlations emphasize the inclusion of mental health in obesity treatments because unresolved psychological issues can perpetuate a vicious cycle of unhealthy eating and resultant weight gain. Besides, socioeconomic status (SES) is also of utmost importance; individuals from lower SES backgrounds have greater stressors that perpetuate psychological distress, again highlighting the interactive relationship between obesity and mental health in metabolic syndrome (Michael et al., 2017). In addition, the social context also has a substantial influence on the perception of obesity and metabolic syndrome. Social stigmatization accompanied by weight can create loneliness and low self-esteem, which aggravate the psychological burden of obesity. Social pressure may deter individuals from getting medical care or engaging in community support networks aimed at addressing their health conditions. In addition, social support or its absence can affect food and exercise behavior choice. Individuals with strong support tend to adhere to lifestyle changes, while those without support may experience more difficulties in dealing with obesity and its associated metabolic risks. It is thus necessary to attend to the social and psychological dimensions of obesity when designing comprehensive treatment plans with a goal of improving health outcomes and well-being (Michael et al., 2017). Additionally, there are some medical conditions such as polycystic ovary syndrome (PCOS) that demonstrate the interplay between obesity, metabolic health, and psychological and social factors. Females with PCOS usually have unique physical and psychologic challenges, including increased anxiety and depression, which contribute to their weight control issues. These psychological problems usually affect not only their metabolic health but also their social functioning, leading to interpersonal problems and quality of life concerns. Integrative wellness-based treatments that combine both physical and psychological aspects have been suggested to enhance their well-being. These holistically guided approaches can enable PCOS women to cope better with the subtleties of the condition, necessitating inter-disciplinary management of obesity and metabolic syndrome in endocrinological practice.

9.5.1. Psychological Impact of Obesity

The psychological consequences of obesity constitute a complex issue and include a range of emotional and cognitive reactions that usually disrupt the quality of life in people with obesity. Obese individuals tend to experience loneliness and low self-esteem as a result of internalized stigma and stigmatization stereotypes about their bodies. This psychological stress can lead to illnesses like depression and anxiety, both of which have been linked to obesity in countless studies. The interplay between psychology and obesity becomes a vicious circle: one will become an emotional eater in trying to deal with psychological distress, thereby contributing to weight gain. With obesity continuing to be regarded as a critical public health concern, comprehension of these psychological factors is becoming essential in order to create effective treatment strategies that not only treat the physical but also the mental conditions. Moreover, how obesity, psychological health, and metabolic syndrome connect with each other illustrates the interdependencies that exist in these diseases. It has been established through studies that gut microbiota (GM) is a critical determinant of obesity-associated metabolic dysregulation, which in turn brings about metabolic dysregulation and inflammation. Such physiological changes may also sustain psychological disturbances, which further form a vicious cycle and complicate prevention and intervention. The psychological anguish related to obesity could lead to a higher reliance on drug therapies for weight loss, with its own psychologic implications, as seen in the effects of obesity drugs approved for treatment (Rodrigo et al., 2024). Thus, psychological wellness needs to be included in any global approach in the treatment of obesity and its related metabolic syndromes. Highlighting the need to treat mental aspects of obesity, doctors are urged to incorporate mental health screening in routine treatment protocols. Understanding that unhealthy eating habits, alcohol use, and other alcohol-related issues, fueled by both mental health and gut microbiota, are drivers of obesity (Pillai et al., 2024), allows for an integrated understanding of the causes and dimensions of obesity. Innovative treatment programs, such as cognitive-behavioral treatment and mindfulness-based treatments, can allow patients to implement healthier coping mechanisms and improve dietary and exercise adherence. This synergistic treatment not only targets the physical features of obesity but also highlights the essential role of mental health treatment in sustaining weight loss in the long term. By integrating the psychological and physiological aspects of obesity, medical practitioners can facilitate a more streamlined, patient-centered model of care that will promote healthy long-term outcomes (Figure 9.13).

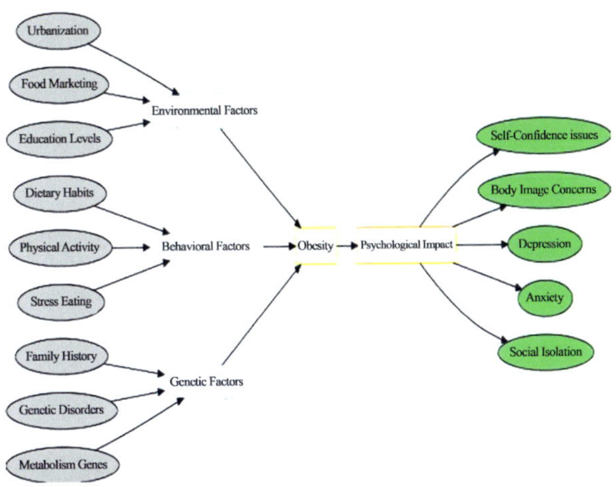

Figure 9.13. The psychological impact of obesity.

Source: https://www.researchgate.net/profile/Tarek-Cheriff-Boumadjen/publication/381608707/figure/fig1/AS:11431281254032844@1718996225114/The-Psychological-Impact-of-obesity.jpg.

9.5.2. Socioeconomic Factors Contributing to Obesity

The growing obesity trend in the modern world has raised considerable interest, with particular emphasis on socioeconomic determinants of this multifactorial disease. Economic insecurity tends to come before food insecurity, which coercively leads to the consumption of cheaper, high-calorie foods that are typically high in sugars and unsaturated fats. These types of eating patterns not only lead to weight gain but also pose challenges in achieving healthy options, contributing to metabolic syndrome and other ailments. Lower SES correlates with limited access to good care and health education, forming a poor diet and poor health cycle. A familiarity with the intersection of socioeconomic and obesity is critical, particularly within the realm of metabolic syndromes' correlation with acute diseases such as diabetes and cardiovascular disease, which most frequently target economically disadvantaged populations (Mary et al., 2023). Furthermore, the built environment is a critical factor in influencing food intake alongside the amount of physical activity among different socioeconomic groups. Urban communities often exhibit extreme disparities in access to food, so that poor communities may lack access to grocery stores with fresh foods, hence promoting reliance on convenience stores with lots of unhealthy foods. In addition, safe recreational spaces for exercising are typically underdeveloped in these communities, deterring individuals from maintaining an exercising lifestyle. This shortage of infrastructure, in addition to perpetuating obesity, is even making it more difficult to reverse the trend. Socioeconomic consequences extend beyond personal choice; they are symptoms of systemic inequalities that must be remedied through broader public health interventions concerned with access to food and urban planning aimed at promoting healthy living among vulnerable groups (Mary et al., 2023). The role of education as a socioeconomic factor only contributes to the multi-faceted nature of the obesity phenomenon. Limited education is connected with low health literacy, which affects one's understanding of nutritional information and health effects of obesity. Limited education can lead to poor comprehension of dietary habits, weight management, and the associated health effects of obesity, including metabolic syndrome. Interventions to increase nutritional education are able to address these disparities but tend to be underfunded and underrepresented in low socioeconomic communities. Notably, the combination of education with community-based interventions can result in a better educated population that is able to make healthier lifestyles, thereby leading to lower obesity rates and enhanced public health outcomes (Lin et al., 2021) (Figure 9.14).

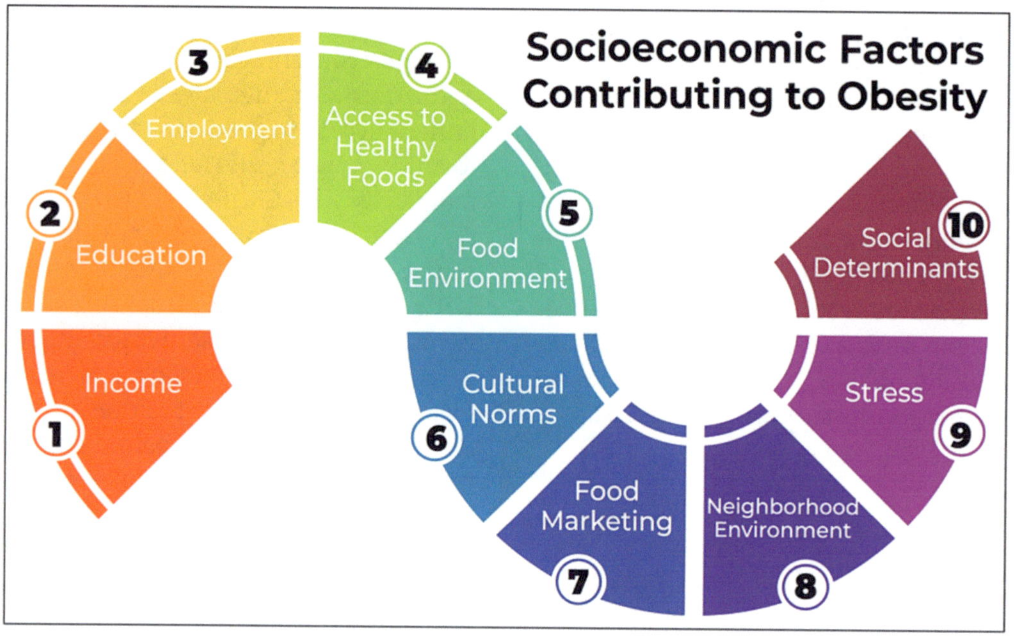

Figure 9.14. Socioeconomic factors that contribute to obesity.

Source: https://assets.cureus.com/uploads/figure/file/920723/article_river_4364b810cb1511ee92dcb144def4d8b0-Figure_2-5-.png.

9.5.3. Stigma and Discrimination Related to Obesity

The so-called obesity stigma is an essential barrier to effective healthcare delivery and communication with patients. Individuals who are obese are not only subject to social stigmatization but also to stigmatization in healthcare. Internalization of societal stigma potentially enhances shame and leads to avoiding sought medical care. Fundamentally, the prejudiced attitude in society fosters a cycle of viciousness in which patients who are obese delay or forgo crucial health interventions, hence worsening health inequalities. Being a critical part of endocrinology, understanding the impact of stigma on obese patients can assist healthcare providers in modifying their practice. This is particularly pertinent because effective treatment for concomitant metabolic syndromes depends on patient adherence to lifestyle change and medication regimes, which can be undermined by adverse self-perceptions and social prejudice. In addition, the impact of obesity stigma operates not only at the level of the individual but also extends to broader societal attitudes and policy. When stigma is deep-seated in cultural narratives, it can cause systemic prejudice to affect public health policy, funding, and public health education on obesity and metabolic syndrome. The lexicon of weight-weighted words is usually used to signal judgment and bias, rather than objective indices of health, thus misleading public perception of obesity as an individual flaw instead of a complex health condition with multiple determinants. This disinformation prevents promotion and establishment of awareness and enabling environments promoting healthier lifestyle choices. By illuminating the intricate interweaving dynamics between stigma, discrimination, and determinants of health, endocrinology can more convincingly advocate for comprehensive approaches that address obesity's causes in addition to its metabolic comorbidities. Knowledge of the intersectionality of obesity stigma with other social identities is what further deepens the understanding of discrimination within healthcare environments. Research indicates that individuals in stigmatized groups, including ethnic and racial minorities, have double the stigma both in their weight and identity. This two-tier level of discrimination has the potential to significantly impede access to care and equitable treatment outcomes, leading to higher rates of prevalence of metabolic syndromes in these populations. Secondly, medical practitioners must also recognize their biases and how these can affect their clinical decisions, leading to misdiagnosis and inappropriate treatment regimens. It has been found that health professionals have negative stereotypes towards fat individuals, which can lead to a lack of empathy or condescending behaviors during consultations. Such observations make it imperative to introduce training programs aimed at inculcating cultural competence and sensitivity toward patients experience in order to result in enhanced endocrinological treatment (Barber et al., 2018; Defreyne et al., 2019) (Figure 9.15).

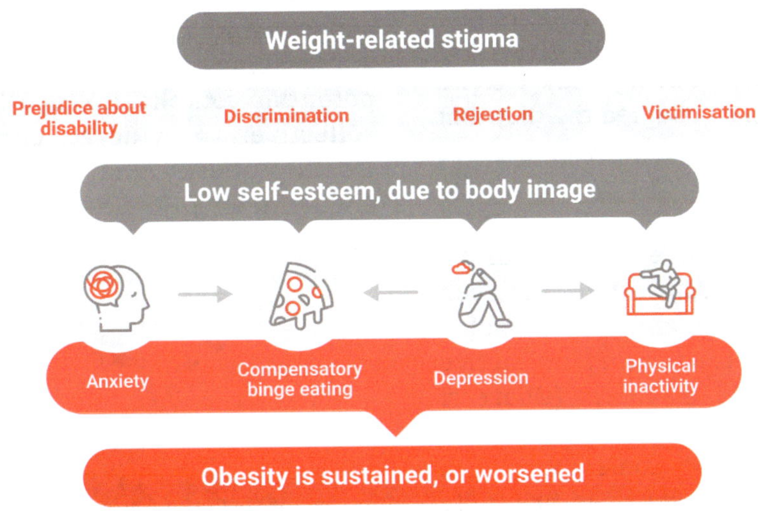

Figure 9.15. Weight-related stigma.

Source: https://uk.lilly.com/metabolic/assets/images/graphic_stigma.svg.

Test Your Knowledge

1. What are the common psychological effects of obesity on individuals, including risks for depression, anxiety, and low self-esteem?
2. How does weight-based stigma and discrimination in healthcare?

9.6. Treatment and Management Strategies

Learning Outcome

1. Explain the lifestyle interventions: diet and exercise
2. Discuss the pharmacological treatments for obesity
3. Identify the surgical options for severe obesity

Effective management and treatment of metabolic syndrome and obesity are both multifaceted in that they require lifestyle modification, medical treatment, and surgery. Lifestyle intervention, either by diet or physical activity, is the cornerstone of therapy. It has been shown through research that caloric restriction and exercise-induced weight loss improves insulin sensitivity and cardiovascular function in addition to reducing body weight. For instance, the addition of a healthy diet that minimizes saturated fat intake with a focus on healthy carbohydrates can automatically alleviate symptoms associated with metabolic syndrome. Such food interventions focus on breaking the complex associations between obesity, insulin resistance, and overall global metabolic health, demonstrating an active measure in curing these disorders (Ghazeeri et al., 2021). Where lifestyle modification is insufficient, pharmacotherapy comes into action. Such drugs as metformin, which is primarily used for the control of diabetes, have also proven effective against obesity and metabolic disorders. More modern anti-obesity drugs could also help with weight loss and lowering risk factors for metabolic syndrome. Drug selection should consider the general health status of the patient, side effects, and comorbidities. For instance, patients with Cushing's syndrome may require specialized approaches that involve targeting cortisol excess, bearing in mind the condition's potential to enhance metabolic syndrome and raise mortality risk (Biller et al., 2016). Thus, inclusion of pharmacotherapy in a broader regimen of management can add further improvements in outcomes. Surgery may become viable in certain situations as a treatment method that is particularly effective in patients who are obese and resistant to conservative management methods. Bariatric surgery has been shown to have excellent results in promoting weight loss and alleviating obesity-related comorbidities, like type 2 diabetes and hypertension. These procedures, including gastric bypass and sleeve gastrectomy, induce weight loss by a modification of the anatomy of the gastrointestinal tracts leading to diminished caloric intake and increased metabolic activity. However, candidates for surgery should be duly evaluated to ensure that they understand the risks and benefits of these procedures. It is essential that these patients get constant support and follow-up following surgery for maintaining weight loss and managing any potential complications. All these strategies collectively provide an entire paradigm for treating obesity and metabolic syndrome in endocrinology (Figure 9.16).

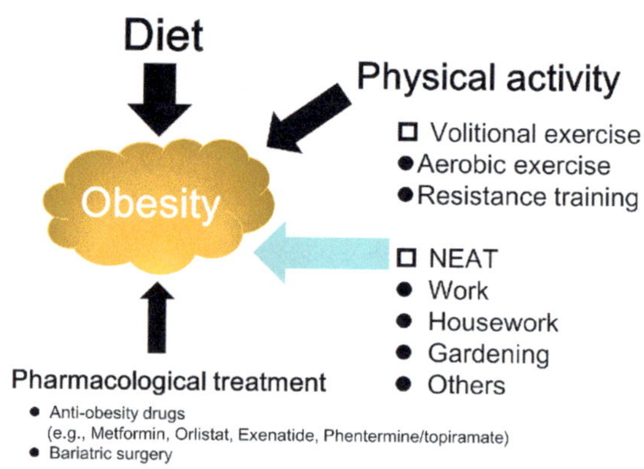

Figure 9.16. Obesity is treated with diet, physical activity, and pharmacologic therapy.

Source: https://www.researchgate.net/profile/Hidetaka-Hamasaki/publication/315366031/figure/fig1/AS:559809561927680@1510480408941/Obesity-is-treated-with-diet-physical-activity-and-pharmacologic-therapy-Diet-appears.png.

9.6.1. Lifestyle Interventions: Diet and Exercise

Lifestyle interventions, or eating and exercise, are the key contributions toward response to the mounting obesity epidemic and its attendant health costs. A multi-pronged approach for successful treatment of obesity includes change in diet and exercise on a regular basis. Restriction of caloric intake with balanced hypocaloric diets has been shown to induce significant weight loss, irrespective of the specific macronutrient focus. This adaptability makes it possible to formulate long-term, individualized eating habits which result ultimately in greater adherence and long-term success. The addition of exercise cannot be overestimated, with aerobic training being the most effective intervention for decreasing fat mass, particularly when combined with resistance training utilized to construct lean body mass. Thus, a shared emphasis on diet and physical activity emerges as a synergistic approach to managing obesity and its metabolic outcomes in clinical practice (Busetto et al., 2015). Translating formal lifestyle interventions in clinical practice is usually resource- and logistically intensive. However, innovative solutions are now possible, such as web-based behavioral interventions, which provide a readily accessible structure for weight control in primary care (Donkin et al., 2015). A recent randomized trial demonstrates that the combination of web-based diet advice with various forms of nurse support, either home-based or face-to-face, additionally enhances weight loss results. The participants who were involved in the structured program lost more mean weight than those receiving normal diet advice alone. Further, the cost-effectiveness of such an intervention additionally adds to its viability as a pragmatic intervention for population-level obesity management. By prioritizing digital interventions, health professionals can reach more and better offer customized support to weight management issues sufferers (Bradbury et al., 2016). Lifestyle therapy for obesity management and metabolic syndrome risk factor reduction is effective through the promotion of behavior change to achieve weight loss and maintenance. Treatment of the inner psychological problems with cognitive behavior therapy (CBT) can also prove highly beneficial in helping individuals alter unhealthy eating behaviors and sedentary lifestyle. CBT treatment empowers the patients to identify triggers and develop coping mechanisms, thereby promoting long-term compliance to a healthy lifestyle. Moreover, the comprehensive management of obesity includes a multidisciplinary array of practitioners to make sure that the patients are treated comprehensively for their physical as well as psychological health. Now that clinicians realize obesity to be a complex disease and not merely a behavioral disorder, the emphasis on holistic lifestyle interventions will certainly gain momentum, thus improving overall patient outcomes and quality of life in people with obesity and metabolic syndrome (Busetto et al., 2015).

9.6.2. Pharmacological Treatments for Obesity

Obesity, characterized by an excess of fat mass, is a multifactorial illness that makes a major contribution to metabolic syndrome pathogenesis. Drug therapy aimed at obesity attempts to modify pathophysiologic mechanisms of weight gain and the resultant health effects of this process. Various classes of anti-obesity drugs work through the mechanisms of inhibiting hunger, enhancing satiety, or raising energy expenditure. For instance, medications such as orlistat inhibit fat absorption in the gut, while others, e.g., phentermine-topiramate, affect central neurotransmitters to reduce hunger. These pharmacologic interventions represent a valuable alternative for patients who have not lost considerable weight with lifestyle changes alone, particularly when it comes with comorbidities of diabetes and hypertension that frequently accompany metabolic syndrome. The landscape of obesity pharmacotherapy has evolved significantly in recent years with the newer class of drugs exhibiting greater efficacy and safety profiles. For example, GLP-1) receptor agonists, whose therapeutic uses have historically been limited to diabetes management, have come into focus due to their weight loss benefit. Agents like liraglutide not only facilitate weight loss but also enhance glycemic control, thereby addressing several key features of metabolic syndrome simultaneously. The additive effect is one of the factors that can result in a more comprehensive treatment regimen for patients with both obesity and endocrine dysregulation. The effectiveness of these drugs is also enhanced with dietary restriction and exercise, providing a synergistic regimen that responds to the multifactorial etiology of obesity. Despite the promise of pharmacotherapy, its limitations must be recognized as well as the necessity of monitoring. Side effects, including gastrointestinal distress and potential cardiovascular risks, necessitate careful patient selection and follow-up. Moreover, long-term weight loss maintenance on drug therapy remains an unresolved issue; the majority of patients will regain weight after drug discontinuation. This emphasizes the importance of adjunctive behavioral intervention in conjunction with pharmacotherapy. In relation to endocrine health, particularly in situations like Cushing's syndrome, comorbid conditions must be treated through sophisticated and personalized care in order to decrease the devastating effects of obesity-induced endocrine disorders, as seen in studies that cite the high mortality and morbidity of endocrine imbalance (Biller et al., 2016; Bisschop et al., 2014).

9.6.3. Surgical Options for Severe Obesity

Surgery has emerged as a central intervention in the therapy of severe obesity, especially when conservative therapy has failed. Even with lifestyle modification and pharmacotherapy, medical management may be inadequate in patients with a body mass index (BMI) of greater than 40, as well as those complicated by co-morbid conditions such as type 2 diabetes mellitus and hypertension. Surgical techniques, including bariatric surgery, such as gastric bypass, sleeve gastrectomy, and adjustable gastric banding, facilitate extensive weight loss and improvement in metabolic function. Gastric bypass, for example, alters the mechanism of digestion by creating a small pouch of the stomach and rerouting the intestine, not only restricting food intake but also impacting hormonal messages regarding hunger and fullness. This way, surgical procedures handle not just weight loss but also overall endocrine issues of metabolic syndrome, significantly enhancing patient outcomes in the long term. The decision to take surgical intervention into account should include an in-depth evaluation of the patient's condition and a sound awareness of the risks and benefits present. Preoperative workups can include nutrition therapy, psychological assessment, and medical fitness testing to prepare the patient and minimize complications. A continued strong need exists for postoperative follow-up, as dietary and lifestyle changes are critical in ongoing weight maintenance. Further, psychological effects of adapting to extreme changes in body image and lifestyle can affect ultimate success. Evidence indicates that patients involved with multidisciplinary teams, such as dietitians, psychologists, and endocrinologists, following surgery experience better weight maintenance and improvement in obesity comorbidity. Therefore, attaining a holistic and integrated process maximizes the efficiency of severe obesity surgery treatments. Long-term post-bariatric surgery follow-up indicates promising benefits, particularly regarding metabolic well-being. Many patients observe such conditions, such as type 2 diabetes, hyperlipidemia, and hypertension, improving or resolving post-operatively. Implication of post-surgical changes in endocrine levels, such as ghrelin and peptide YY, is important in the modulation of the regulation of appetite and metabolic function. These changes bring the junction between surgical procedures and endocrine status to the forefront of the management of obesity. Moreover, knowledge of the possibility of weight regain and the necessity for continued surveillance is paramount to achieving metabolic stability. By employing surgical methods in conjunction with extensive endocrinological care, clinicians can guide the trajectory of obesity and associated syndromes, ultimately ensuring healthier prospects for individuals involved (Figure 9.17).

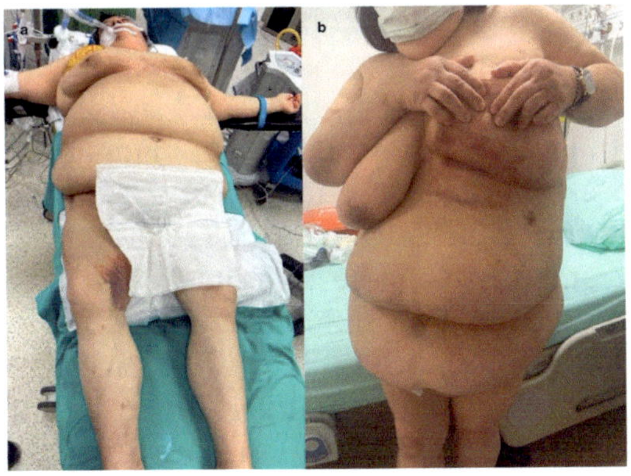

Figure 9.17. Female patient with morbid obesity. (a) On the operating table before surgery; and (b) standing on the fourth postoperative day.

Source: https://www.researchgate.net/publication/373522735/figure/fig3/AS:11431281213162717@1702962664099/Female-patient-with-morbid-obesity-a-On-the-operating-table-before-surgery-b-seen.tif.

Test Your Knowledge

1. What dietary modifications are most effective in managing obesity and metabolic syndrome?
2. How does regular physical activity contribute to weight loss and improved insulin sensitivity in individuals with obesity or metabolic syndrome?
3. What are the commonly prescribed pharmacological agents for obesity management?

SUMMARY

The outcome of the obesity and metabolic syndrome research identifies an important public health problem that contributes to several interwoven themes of endocrinology. While obesity rates across the world keep rising, their contribution to metabolic syndrome has become all the more significant. The condition is characterized by a cluster of metabolic disturbances like insulin resistance, dyslipidemia, and hypertension, all of which contribute to increased cardiovascular risk. Understanding the underlying mechanisms of these relationships is at the heart of planning and developing effective interventions and treatment programs. Furthermore, emerging data on the role of inflammatory markers such as leptin and adiponectin contribute importantly to understanding the pathophysiology of these diseases, as evidenced in reports indicating that hs-CRP, leptin, and adiponectin are significant predictors of cardiovascular disease risk in children (Stroescu et al., 2018). In addition to the traditional risk factors of metabolic syndrome and obesity, current studies lay significant emphasis on the microbiota-gut-brain axis. This intricate system not only demonstrates the way gut function influences metabolic activity but also demonstrates correlations with neuropsychiatric disorders. Because the gut microbiome interacts with host systems through more than one mechanism, including modulation of the immune system and release of neurotransmitters, it is an integral part in obesity and metabolic syndrome complications (John et al., 2019). Being aware of this interaction provides a multidisciplinary direction of management and prevention. Gut microbiota modification could give emerging therapeutic methods beyond drug treatments and dietary modification. Finally, the consequences of such results necessitate addressing obesity and metabolic syndrome from a multidisciplinary perspective to be effectively managed. Public health must prioritize preventative healthcare with the implementation of nutritional counseling, mental health services, and encouraging exercise while considering the growing role of gut microbiota intervention. Future research must seek to investigate the bidirectional interaction of gut-brain communication and its impact on metabolic health. By integrating knowledge from various disciplines, e.g., endocrinology, nutrition, and microbiology, an integrated framework can be formed to tackle these interconnected issues. Such an integrated approach is imperative to avert the dangers of obesity and metabolic syndrome and eventually result in improved health status for the populations at risk.

The relationship of obesity and metabolic syndrome is of critical significance to the practice of endocrinology, particularly in the management of tightly coupled disorders such as polycystic ovary syndrome (PCOS). The 2023 International Evidence-based Guidelines offer significant information on PCOS evaluation and treatment, which often co-occurs with obesity. These guidelines address 254 pieces of advice to facilitate evidence-based care, highlighting the connection between hormonal derangement and metabolic derangement in patients with PCOS. Significant revisions are directed towards recognizing more integrative metabolic risk factors for insulin resistance and obesity-related cardiovascular disease, which exacerbate women's challenges in PCOS. This connection highlights the need for coordinated care techniques that address both obesity and endocrine imbalance to improve overall health outcomes for affected individuals (Helena et al., 2023; Teede et al., 2023). In addition, the 2023 guidelines emphasize the necessity of increased educational sessions for health care providers and the presentation of evidence-based patient information. The persistent evidence-practice differences in PCOS management demonstrate the challenges faced in clinical practice, particularly in patients with concomitant obesity. Appreciating the heterogeneity of metabolic disorders in obesity, these guidelines support improved care models and shared decision-making that respect patients individual preferences. By fostering a holistic appreciation of the relationship between endocrine disorders and obesity, healthcare practitioners can facilitate active patient engagement with treatment strategies and ultimately achieve more meaningful health outcomes. These coordinated approaches are particularly important in the treatment of the psychosocial aspects of obesity and metabolic syndrome, which are often overlooked but account for patients' quality of life (Helena et al., 2023; Teede et al., 2023). In addition, the recommendations prioritize lifestyle modifications that guarantee emotional health and quality of life among patients with PCOS and obesity. Recommendations highlight the role of a healthy lifestyle not only for weight management but also as an integral part of comprehensive healthcare. Integration of mental health treatment with evidence-based medical treatment is critical in managing the multifaceted health issues of obesity and metabolic syndrome. Stigma surrounding weight in healthcare settings is also essential to intervene against because it can disrupt the therapeutic alliance between providers and patients. By promoting evidence-based management practices that ensure both physical and mental well-being, endocrinologists are able to enhance patient engagement and adherence to therapy, thereby generally improving control of obesity and its metabolic syndromes in clinical practice (Helena et al., 2023; Teede et al., 2023).

KEY TERMS FROM THIS CHAPTER

- Acute diseases
- Adipose tissue functions
- Cardiovascular risk
- Cholesterol levels
- Drug therapy
- Endocannabinoid signaling
- Endocrine dysregulation
- Environmental determinants
- Gastrointestinal tracts
- Glucocorticoid reactivation
- Insulin dynamics
- Insulin sensitivity
- Metabolic activity
- Metabolic function
- Adipose tissue
- Bisphenol A (BPA)
- CBC-derive inflammation indexes
- Clinical diagnostic indices
- Dyslipidemia
- Endocrine disruptors
- Energy homeostasis
- Gastric bypass
- Genetic data
- Inflammatory process
- Insulin resistance
- Ketogenic diets
- Metabolic control
- Metabolic markers

CRITICAL THINKING QUESTIONS

1. **Which of the following hormones is most involved in long-term regulation of body weight by signaling satiety to the hypothalamus?**
   a. Ghrelin
   b. Insulin
   c. Leptin
   d. Cortisol
2. **Which of the following is NOT one of the diagnostic criteria for metabolic syndrome according to the NCEP ATP III guidelines?**
   a. Elevated waist circumference
   b. High HDL cholesterol
   c. Elevated blood pressure
   d. Elevated fasting glucose
3. **How does visceral fat most directly contribute to insulin resistance?**
   a. By storing excessive glucose
   b. By secreting anti-inflammatory cytokines
   c. By releasing free fatty acids and pro-inflammatory cytokines
   d. By increasing insulin production
4. **Which psychological factor is most strongly associated with increased risk of obesity due to emotional eating behaviors?**
   a. Narcissism
   b. Anxiety and depression
   c. Obsessive-compulsive disorder
   d. Mania
5. **Which of the following is considered the cornerstone of effective obesity management?**
   a. Bariatric surgery
   b. Pharmacotherapy
   c. Hormone replacement therapy
   d. Lifestyle modification including diet and physical activity

Short Answer Questions

1. What hormonal and cellular mechanisms contribute to the development of obesity, particularly the roles of leptin, ghrelin, and adipose tissue inflammation?
2. What is the definition of metabolic syndrome, and what are the diagnostic criteria according to the American Heart Association (AHA) or other major guidelines?
3. How do endocrine-disrupting chemicals (EDCs) such as BPA and phthalates interfere with hormonal regulation and contribute to obesity and metabolic syndrome?
4. What is the relationship between obesity—particularly visceral fat—and the development of insulin resistance at the cellular level?
5. How do psychological factors such as chronic stress, depression, and weight stigma contribute to the onset or persistence of obesity?
6. How do socioeconomic status and environmental factors influence the prevalence of obesity and metabolic syndrome in different populations?

Answers to Critical Thinking Questions

1. (c) 2. (b) 3. (c) 4. (b) 5. (d)

REFERENCES

1. Abacı, A., Abalı, S., Adal, E., et al. (2015). Turner syndrome and associated problems in Turkish children: A multicenter study. https://core.ac.uk/download/227057395.pdf (accessed on 22nd July 2025).
2. Alves, J. V. C. (2024). Obesity relationship, metabolic syndrome and insulin resistance. *Health and Society*. https://www.semanticscholar.org/paper/6980a5fccb4c3c54f79e6e24a06f9d18f072e348 (accessed on 22nd July 2025).
3. Ameer, B., et al. (2018). Pediatric obesity: Influence on drug dosing and therapeutics. https://core.ac.uk/download/155271623.pdf (accessed on 22nd July 2025).
4. Annagur, A., Annagur, B., Beck, A., Benson, S., Cronin, C., Dennett, K., Dowdy, A., et al. (2018). Polycystic ovary syndrome across the life span of women: A wellness-based integrative intervention. https://core.ac.uk/download/213088882.pdf (accessed on 22nd July 2025).
5. Arble, D. M., & Framnes, S. N. (2018). The bidirectional relationship between obstructive sleep apnea and metabolic disease. https://core.ac.uk/download/213087655.pdf (accessed on 22nd July 2025).
6. Atkin, S. L., David, R., Gooderham, N. J., et al. (2015). Increased expression of circulating miRNA-93 in women with polycystic ovary syndrome may represent a novel, non-invasive biomarker for diagnosis. https://core.ac.uk/download/151157243.pdf (accessed on 22nd July 2025).
7. Aubert, C., Busetto, L., Butz, D., Kenyon, C. J., Contreras, A., Cowley, M., et al. (2003). Transgenic amplification of glucocorticoid action in adipose tissue causes high blood pressure in mice. https://core.ac.uk/download/20448745.pdf (accessed on 22nd July 2025).
8. Barber, T. M. (2018). Is obesity a disease? https://core.ac.uk/download/153326270.pdf (accessed on 22nd July 2025).
9. Biller, B. M. K., Colao, A., De Martino, M. C., et al. (2016). Complications of Cushing's syndrome: State of the art. https://core.ac.uk/download/54532161.pdf (accessed on 22nd July 2025).
10. Bisschop, P. H., Dieguez, C., Fernandez-Mallo, D., et al. (2014). Estradiol regulates brown adipose tissue thermogenesis via hypothalamic AMPK. https://core.ac.uk/download/29151222.pdf (accessed on 22nd July 2025).
11. Blumberg, B., & Egusquiza, R. J. (2020). Environmental obesogens and their impact on susceptibility to obesity: New mechanisms and chemicals. https://core.ac.uk/download/287622280.pdf (accessed on 22nd July 2025).
12. Bonin, C., Bonora, E., Dall'Alda, M., et al. (2013). Divergences in insulin resistance between the different phenotypes of the polycystic ovary syndrome. https://core.ac.uk/download/55800175.pdf (accessed on 22nd July 2025).
13. Bradbury, K. J., Byrne, C. D., Davoudianfar, M., et al. (2016). An internet-based intervention with brief nurse support to manage obesity in primary care (POWeR+): A pragmatic, parallel-group, randomized controlled trial. https://core.ac.uk/download/46558293.pdf (accessed on 22nd July 2025).
14. Bujalska, I. J., Darimont, C., Ermolieff, J., et al. (2008). A novel selective 11β-hydroxysteroid dehydrogenase type 1 inhibitor prevents human adipogenesis. https://core.ac.uk/download/pdf/19305.pdf (accessed on 22nd July 2025).

15. Busetto, L., Fried, M., Micic, D., et al. (2015). European guidelines for obesity management in adults. https://core.ac.uk/download/53528633.pdf (accessed on 22nd July 2025).

16. Carmina, E., Gnessi, L., Lanzolla, G., et al. (2017). Androgens and hypertension in men and women: A unifying view. https://core.ac.uk/download/98336137.pdf (accessed on 22nd July 2025).

17. Carrel, A. L., Cronk, C. E., Durkin, M. S., et al. (2009). Environment and obesity in the National Children's Study. https://core.ac.uk/download/213082314.pdf (accessed on 22nd July 2025).

18. Castro, M. C., Castrogiovanni, D. C., Francini, F., et al. (2016). Chronic glucocorticoid-rich milieu and liver dysfunction. https://core.ac.uk/download/159291096.pdf (accessed on 22nd July 2025).

19. Chait, A., & den Hartigh, L. J. (2020). Adipose tissue distribution, inflammation and its metabolic consequences, including diabetes and cardiovascular disease. *Frontiers in Cardiovascular Medicine, 7.* https://doi.org/10.3389/fcvm.2020.00022 (accessed on 22nd July 2025).

20. Choi, D. S., Yoo, H. J., Kang, H. J., Seo, J. A., Lim, K. I., Choi, K. M., Kim, N. H., et al. (2009). Prevalence of sarcopenia and sarcopenic obesity in Korean adults: The Korean Sarcopenic Obesity Study (KSOS). https://core.ac.uk/download/pdf/288318.pdf (accessed on 22nd July 2025).

21. Corrao, S., Pollicino, C., Maggio, D., Torres, A., & Argano, C. (2024). Tirzepatide against obesity and insulin-resistance: Pathophysiological aspects and clinical evidence. *Frontiers in Endocrinology, 15.* https://www.semanticscholar.org/paper/a418745014d572b796466df2f60d6d50c2b929aa (accessed on 22nd July 2025).

22. Cryan, J. F., O'Riordan, K. J., Cowan, C. S. M., Sandhu, K. V., Bastiaanssen, T. F. S., Boehme, M., Codagnone, M. G., et al. (2019). The microbiota-gut-brain axis. *Physiological Reviews, 99,* 1877–2013. https://doi.org/10.1152/physrev.00018.2018 (accessed on 22nd July 2025).

23. Defreyne, J., Iwamoto, S. J., Motmans, J., et al. (2019). Health considerations for transgender women and remaining unknowns: A narrative review. https://core.ac.uk/download/237010802.pdf (accessed on 22nd July 2025).

24. Ghazeeri, G., Hmedeh, C., Hmedeh, et al. (2021). Nutritional management in polycystic ovary syndrome: Challenges and opportunities. https://core.ac.uk/download/161103740.pdf (accessed on 22nd July 2025).

25. Harris, C. A., Lee, R. A., & Wang, J. C. (2018). Glucocorticoid receptor and adipocyte biology. https://core.ac.uk/download/323081126.pdf (accessed on 22nd July 2025).

26. Jakubowska-Kowal, K. M., Skrzynska, K., & Gawlik-Starzyk, A. (2024). Treatment and complications of PCOS in adolescents–what's new in 2023? *Frontiers in Endocrinology, 15.* https://www.semanticscholar.org/paper/c27675d49448ca052c14b115909be0739d12f0b1 (accessed on 22nd July 2025).

27. Janesick, A., Janesick, A., Mantovani, A., Mantovani, A., Suvorov, A., Cohn, B. A., Angle, B. M., et al. (2015). Parma consensus statement on metabolic disruptors. https://core.ac.uk/download/42131375.pdf (accessed on 22nd July 2025).

28. Kerna, N. A., Ngwu, D. C., Jomsky, B. M., Holets, H. M., Nnake, I., Jeremiah, S. M., Flores, J. V., et al. (2024). Impact of detox diets on obesity and metabolic syndrome: Implications for weight loss, metabolic health, and clinical practice. *European Journal of Medical and Health Research.*

https://www.semanticscholar.org/paper/01f269e93474f57262ba3e3e1ac4358a02325381 (accessed on 22nd July 2025).

29. Kyrou, I., & Weickert, M. O. (2010). Clinical problems caused by obesity. https://core.ac.uk/download/46324.pdf (accessed on 22nd July 2025).

30. Lane, H. (2020). Shift work: Gut health and metabolic disease. https://core.ac.uk/download/322850892.pdf (accessed on 22nd July 2025).

31. Li, Y., Chang, Y., Li, H., Li, F., Zou, Q., Liu, X., Chen, X., et al. (2024). Inflammation mediates the relationship between diet quality assessed by healthy eating index-2015 and metabolic syndrome. *Frontiers in Endocrinology, 15.* https://www.semanticscholar.org/paper/ddede709eddf096282ed7610696e2bb7d31914ba (accessed on 22nd July 2025).

32. Lin, L., Pan, X., Feng, Y., & Yang, J. (2024). Chronic kidney disease combined with metabolic syndrome is a non-negligible risk factor. *Therapeutic Advances in Endocrinology and Metabolism, 15.* https://www.semanticscholar.org/paper/0ec2a40066e278a95afed81e57b7bdacc0bad614 (accessed on 22nd July 2025).

33. Lin, X., & Li, H. (2021). Obesity: Epidemiology, pathophysiology, and therapeutics. *Frontiers in Endocrinology, 12.* https://doi.org/10.3389/fendo.2021.706978 (accessed on 22nd July 2025).

34. Lombardo, J. F., Poiset, S. J., Burke, S. E., Shah, M., Doyle, L. A., Harrison, A. S., Nowak Choi, K., et al. (2024). The impact of obesity on acute skin toxicity from radiation treatment for breast cancer: Opportunities to predict and address. *Endocrinology, Metabolism and Nutrition.* https://www.semanticscholar.org/paper/e2b657614429f3c5453321dff3b0ef5b4c6793d5 (accessed on 22nd July 2025).

35. Mantovani, G., Bastepe, M., Monk, D., De Sanctis, L., Thiele, S., Usardi, A., Ahmed, S. F., et al. (2018). Diagnosis and management of pseudohypoparathyroidism and related disorders: First international consensus statement. *Nature Reviews Endocrinology, 14*, 476–500. https://doi.org/10.1038/s41574-018-0042-0 (accessed on 22nd July 2025).

36. Marjani, A., & Moghasemi, S. (2012). The metabolic syndrome among postmenopausal women in Gorgan. https://core.ac.uk/download/52204779.pdf (accessed on 22nd July 2025).

37. Marra, A., Bondesan, A., Caroli, D., & Sartorio, A. (2024). Complete blood count (CBC)-derived inflammation indexes are useful in predicting metabolic syndrome in adults with severe obesity. *Journal of Clinical Medicine, 13.* https://www.semanticscholar.org/paper/8375261139e90f97d3d33b6d0f6fc24186faaa58 (accessed on 22nd July 2025).

38. Michael, J. R. (2017). The relations of metabolic syndrome to anxiety and depression symptoms in children and adults. https://core.ac.uk/download/84397711.pdf (accessed on 22nd July 2025).

39. Milewicz, A., Jedrzejuk, D., Lwow, F., Dunajska, K., Laczmanski, L., & Tworowska-Bardzinska, U. (2009). Are endocannabinoid type 1 receptor gene (CNR1) polymorphisms associated with obesity and metabolic syndrome in postmenopausal Polish women? https://core.ac.uk/download/pdf/288906.pdf (accessed on 22nd July 2025).

40. Moreira, R. O., Valério, C., Hohl, A., Moulin, C., Moura, F., Trujilho, F. R., Gerchman, F., et al. (2024). Pharmacologic treatment of obesity in adults and its impact on comorbidities: 2024 update and position statement of specialists from the Brazilian Association for the Study of Obesity and Metabolic Syndrome (Abeso) and the Brazilian Society of Endocrinology and Metabolism

(SBEM). *Archives of Endocrinology and Metabolism, 68*. https://www.semanticscholar.org/paper/73e34a33f33af64e4113d7fe322cb5b5e970a6e6 (accessed on 22nd July 2025).

41. Pillai, S. S., Gagnon, C. A., Foster, C., & Ashraf, A. (2024). Exploring the gut microbiota: Key insights into its role in obesity, metabolic syndrome, and type 2 diabetes. *The Journal of Clinical Endocrinology and Metabolism, 109*, 2709–2719. https://www.semanticscholar.org/paper/318f2e4572f2676fa97af845537abdfeb8e29e6e (accessed on 22nd July 2025).
42. Rinella, M. E., & Sookoian, S. (2023). From NAFLD to MASLD: Updated naming and diagnosis criteria for fatty liver disease. *Journal of Lipid Research, 65*, 100485–100485. https://doi.org/10.1016/j.jlr.2023.100485 (accessed on 22nd July 2025).
43. Shen, X., Yang, L., Liu, Y., Zhang, X. H., Cai, P., Huang, J., & Jiang, L. (2023). Associations between urinary iodine concentration and the prevalence of metabolic disorders: A cross-sectional study. *Frontiers in Endocrinology, 14*. https://www.semanticscholar.org/paper/e4fdb11931de28573890670d03d933aefd725531 (accessed on 22nd July 2025).
44. Speiser, P., Arlt, W., Auchus, R. J., Baskin, L. S., Conway, G. S., Merke, D. P., Meyer-Bahlburg, H. F. L., et al. (2018). Congenital adrenal hyperplasia due to steroid 21-hydroxylase deficiency: An Endocrine Society* clinical practice guideline. *The Journal of Clinical Endocrinology & Metabolism, 103*, 4043–4088. https://doi.org/10.1210/jc.2018-01865 (accessed on 22nd July 2025).
45. Stroescu, R., Mărginean, O., Bizerea, T., Gafencu, M., Voicu, A., & Doroș, G. (2018). Adiponectin, leptin and high sensitivity C-reactive protein values in obese children–Important markers for metabolic syndrome? *Journal of Pediatric Endocrinology and Metabolism, 32*, 27–31. https://doi.org/10.1515/jpem-2018-0378 (accessed on 22nd July 2025).
46. Teede, H. J., Tay, C., Laven, J., Dokras, A., Moran, L. J., Piltonen, T., Costello, M., et al. (2023). Recommendations from the 2023 international evidence-based guideline for the assessment and management of polycystic ovary syndrome. *European Journal of Endocrinology, 189*(2), G43–G64. https://www.semanticscholar.org/paper/5f184245355fb8df2cd2fa605c6573cac46c5721 (accessed on 22nd July 2025).
47. Teede, H., Tay, C., Laven, J., Dokras, A., Moran, L., Piltonen, T., Costello, M., et al. (2023). Recommendations from the 2023 international evidence-based guideline for the assessment and management of polycystic ovary syndrome. *The Journal of Clinical Endocrinology and Metabolism, 108*, 2447–2469. https://www.semanticscholar.org/paper/7eca8753e20c2430964ffa100b6c597b2eeba54b (accessed on 22nd July 2025).
48. Wang, H., Zhang, Z., Zou, L., Zhang, J., Jia, Z., Zhao, L., Han, X., et al. (2024). Peripheral artery disease mediating the effect of metabolic syndrome related diseases on lower limb ulcers: Mendelian randomization analysis. *Frontiers in Endocrinology, 15*. https://www.semanticscholar.org/paper/54119076086ca96ff77882cc313a50bcc3b2788d (accessed on 22nd July 2025).
49. Yamakage, H., Jo, T., Tanaka, M., Kato, S., Hasegawa, K., Masuda, I., Matsuhisa, M., et al. (2024). Five percent weight loss is a significant 1-year predictor and an optimal 5-year cut-off for reducing the number of obesity-related cardiovascular disease risk components: The Japan Obesity and Metabolic Syndrome Study. *Frontiers in Endocrinology, 15*. https://www.semanticscholar.org/paper/41bd1bb6e4189ef35278a892867a443436697465 (accessed on 22nd July 2025).

50. Younes, V. (2024). The role of specific nutrients and pollutants with endocrine activity on fertility in women. https://core.ac.uk/download/620848711.pdf (accessed on 22nd July 2025).

51. Zong, X., Bovet, P., & Xi, B. (2022). A proposal to unify the definition of the metabolic syndrome in children and adolescents. *Frontiers in Endocrinology, 13*. https://www.semanticscholar.org/paper/7a42fb67bcdabb0378de5de1e1864abb496bc9fb (accessed on 22nd July 2025).

BONE AND MINERAL METABOLISM

10

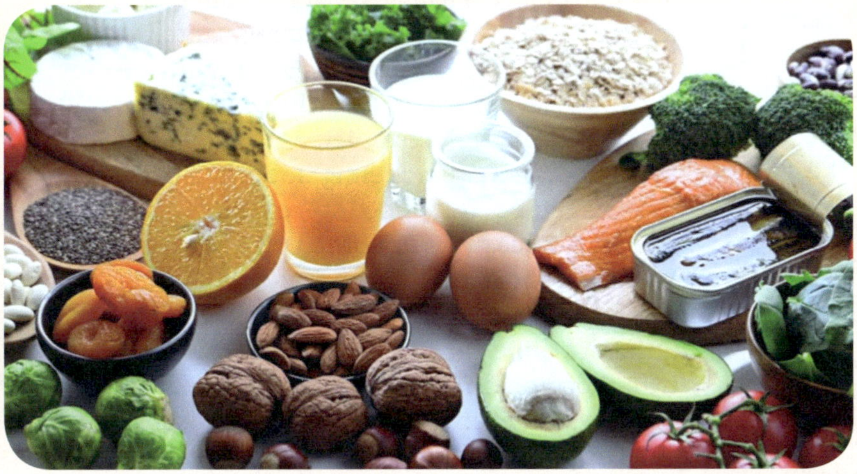

LEARNING OBJECTIVES

After studying this chapter, you will be able to:

1. Understand the anatomy of bone;
2. Describe the mineral composition of bone;
3. Focus on hormonal regulation in the maintenance of bone and mineral metabolism;
4. Explain the bone remodeling process;
5. Discuss the relationship between nutrition and bone health;
6. Deal with disorders of bone and mineral metabolism.

Introduction

The intricate processes that control mineral and bone metabolism are critical to maintain skeletal integrity as well as overall physiological homeostasis. This question emerges against the backdrop of the increasing incidence of conditions related to bone integrity, such as osteoporosis and osteomalacia. Despite the fact that bone is a structural framework, it is a dynamic tissue liable to continuous remodeling by the activity of osteoblasts and osteoclasts. It is governed by multiple factors, such as hormones, nutrition, and exercise, emphasizing the need for an integral approach to bone health. As a population grows older, the need to maintain bone density and mineral homeostasis becomes more exigent. Hence, it is worthwhile to study the biological and biochemical processes of bone metabolism as well as the intricate mechanisms for their disturbance in view of organizing preventive interventions and therapeutic approaches against bone disorders. Deficiency or surplus of the requisite minerals, such as calcium and phosphorus, can lead to serious metabolic disturbances, such as bone density and strength. The interaction among these minerals, mediated to a great extent by hormones like parathyroid hormone (PTH) and vitamin D, is responsible for calcium homeostasis. When the body perceives alterations in levels of minerals, it triggers the compensatory mechanisms to try to re-equilibrate. But underlying conditions like subclinical thyroid disease can further confuse these mechanisms. Evidence suggests that subclinical hyperthyroidism and hypothyroidism can adversely affect bone metabolism, with possible elevation of fracture risk and decrease in mineralization. Moreover, the clinical significance of these thyroid derangements has remained controversial, with management guidelines still discordant. While discussing the complexity of mineral effects on bone, it is clear that an understanding of these dynamics is crucial to defining effective treatment protocols.

With ongoing research comes the need for holistic guidelines on bone and mineral metabolism. So far, literature emphasizes the importance of determining individual differences in metabolism, with an individualized prevention and treatment method suggested. Interventions can be through lifestyle modification, dietary changes, and drug therapy to correct mineral imbalance.

In addition, the realization of the effect of other diseases on bone metabolism, as presented by Suh et al. (2015, p. 246), brings to the fore the need for interdisciplinary collaboration among healthcare professionals. Following Mach et al. (2019; pp. 111–188), the development of consensus guidelines can empower clinicians to make informed decisions based on evidence, thereby promoting improved patient outcomes. Lastly, the advancements made in our understanding of bone and mineral metabolism not only enhance skeletal health but also contribute to the overall discourse on human health and longevity.

Definition of Bone and Mineral Metabolism

Understanding bone and mineral metabolism is key to appreciating the physiological processes that regulate skeletal health. Bone metabolism involves the dynamic processes of bone building and breakdown, which are quite tightly regulated by osteoblasts and osteoclasts, respectively. Mineral metabolism involves the control of minerals the body requires, particularly calcium and phosphorus, which are significant elements in bone structure. This metabolic interaction is what assists in keeping the strength of the skeletal system intact and allows it to adapt to various physiological demands. The ongoing process of bone remodeling not only maintains the structure but also stores and releases minerals necessary for other bodily functions, such as those required by the endocrine system to maintain homeostasis. Several factors influence bone and mineral metabolism, varying from hormonal regulation to nutritional status and physical exercise. The important hormones, such as parathyroid hormone (PTH), calcitonin, and vitamin D, play a very significant role in the regulation of the body's level of calcium. For instance, PTH increases serum calcium by inducing bone resorption and enhancing intestinal absorption of calcium. On the other hand, vitamin D has a function in optimal gastrointestinal mineral absorption and aids in proper bone mineralization. Epidemiological literature suggests that inadequate vitamin D status leads to impaired bone density and increased fracture risk, and hence, there is a need to maintain adequate levels of minerals for overall skeletal function. Further, lifestyle habits such as regular weight-bearing activity contribute to increased bone density, with ease of adaptation and resistance to change with age. Clinically, bone and mineral metabolism measurement is critical in the diagnosis and management of disease conditions such as osteoporosis and renal osteodystrophy. Dual-energy X-ray absorptiometry (DXA) is recognized as the gold standard for the assessment of bone mineral density and can be expressed in unambiguous diagnostic criteria through T-scores and Z-scores. A comprehension of discordance between the scores can detect underlying health complications, particularly in relation to age, gender, and body mass index. Studies have indicated that a great difference between T-scores and Z-scores can be present, which shows the complexity of bone measurement in diverse populations (Heidari et al., 2025). Therefore, with the application of advanced diagnostic tools and understanding of the metabolic bone and mineral pathways, prevention and treatment of metabolic bone diseases are vital to eventually enhancing patient care and outcomes (Figure 10.1).

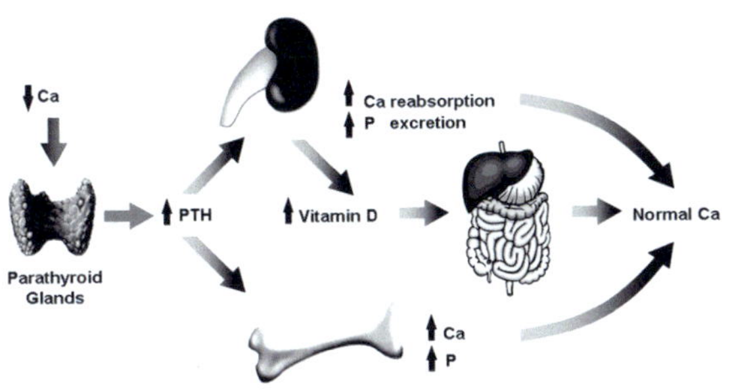

Figure 10.1. Mineral metabolism in healthy individuals.

Source: https://www.researchgate.net/profile/Marlies-Noordzij/publication/23803379/figure/fig1/AS:667214344622080@1536087704128/Mineral-metabolism-in-healthy-individuals.jpg.

Importance of Bone Health

Bone health is more than mere structural support to the human body; it is also deeply related to total metabolic function and general health. Bone serves as a storage site for essential minerals, such as calcium and phosphorus, and is also involved in the regulation of mineral homeostasis. As a person ages, the balance between bone resorption and bone formation may be disrupted and, therefore, result in conditions such as osteoporosis. This disparity highlights the need for optimal nutrition supply for sustained bone density throughout life. Optimizing bone health is also necessary not only to avoid fractures but also to support important body functions. The interrelated nature of bone health with other aspects of health highlights the need for comprehensive measures focusing on diet intake, lifestyle modification, and preventive health habits to achieve a healthier population. It is very important to recognize the determinants of bone health, particularly among those prone to mineral imbalance. Such a mineral that directly influences bone metabolism is magnesium (Mg). It has been suggested by the scientific community that maintaining proper Mg homeostasis is essential, particularly in chronic kidney disease (CKD) patients who typically have bone complications. CKD patients often experience disturbances such as hyperphosphatemia and secondary hyperparathyroidism, conditions that can be mitigated with appropriate Mg supplementation. Although the supplementation enhances the growth of bones, it also assists in normal mineralization, thus affirming the multifunctional role of Mgs in halting bone abnormalities. Overcoming the issues noted above through targeted interventions significantly improves clinical responses, emphasizing the value of mineral management in bone health. Inuit populations provide a solid basis for the comprehension of bone mineral content (BMC) and its relationship with skeletal health. BMC, particularly in Inuit populations, has been proven by studies to increase to its highest level during young adult years and progressively decline later in life. Research shows the resistance of BMC in the groups, but concurrently also being vulnerable to aging-related risks, as they stand a chance of developing osteoporosis. It is valuable to understand differences in BMC across various populations to tailor bone health strategies to certain requirements. Above all, the imperative of ongoing research into exploring more specific factors influencing BMC, including diet and exercise, remains indispensable. This ongoing pursuit of knowledge can shed more light on the health of the bones and their management in various populations, further fueling discussions on the pivotal place held by the minerals in bone metabolism and general health.

10.1. Anatomy of Bone

Learning Outcome

1. Explain the types of bone tissue;
2. Understand bone structure and function;
3. Discuss the role of bone marrow.

Anatomically, bone tissue is made up of a complex structure comprising cells, organic matrices, and mineral elements that act as both a structural support and an active organ involved in mineral metabolism. The three primary cell components are osteoblasts, osteocytes, and osteoclasts, each playing distinct roles different from others concerning bone formation, upkeep, and resorption. The osteoblasts produce the organic matrix, primarily collagen and non-collagenous proteins, which impart structural strength. When these cells become embedded in the matrix, they become osteocytes, which are responsible for signaling and bone homeostasis. Osteoclasts, however, are multinucleated cells responsible for the degradation of bone tissue to produce free minerals such as calcium and phosphorus into the bloodstream, which are necessary for the body's mineral balance. Understanding the interplay of these cell components is key to appreciating how bone reacts to various physiological demands, particularly under the influence of mechanical loading that adjusts its structure and function. Mechanical stress greatly affects bone anatomy, triggering the bone to adapt in such a way as to maintain skeletal system integrity. Mechanotransduction is the process by which bone cells convert mechanical stimulation into biochemical signals, thereby enabling mineral metabolism and bone remodeling. For instance, osteocytes can detect mechanical load through the activation of signaling pathways, such as the Wnt/Lrp5 pathway, which regulate bone resorption and formation. Research indicates that mechanical stress imposed on the teeth by orthodontic treatment can trigger a multifaceted cascade of cellular signaling leading to alveolar bone remodeling. The Wnt signaling pathway, functioning in osteocytes, is involved in mediating these mechanotransduction events and showing the dynamic function of bone under biomechanical forces (Ahn et al., 2025). This adaptability is not only critical for bone density preservation but also for establishing optimized levels of phosphate and calcium within the body, which are vital for various physiological functions. It is also further illustrated by the physical response of bone to different environmental stresses, e.g., microgravity. Investigations indicate that mechanical loading alterations, such as those experienced with travel to space, result in significant bone composition and density alterations. Specifically, regions of bone can experience demineralization or aberrant mineralization patterns due to the removal of gravitational forces, as indicated by documented effects on the heelbone and skull (Arnaud et al., 2025). Ground-based models have validated these findings, showing that unloading induces reversible but transient changes in bone structure, which is evidence for the high plasticity of bone tissue. This knowledge is crucial not only about the mechanism of mineral metabolism in the skeleton but also about future therapeutic strategies for preventing the adverse effects of disuse or microgravity on skeletal conditions.

10.1.1. Types of Bone Tissue

An understanding of bone tissue types is important to comprehend the complex process of bone and mineral metabolism. Bone tissue is typically divided into two broad categories:

cortical bone and trabecular bone. Cortical bone or compact bone is a hard outer layer of bones that serves as a framework. This bone is extremely organized, with osteons or Haversian systems being close-packed, which provides strength and stiffness.

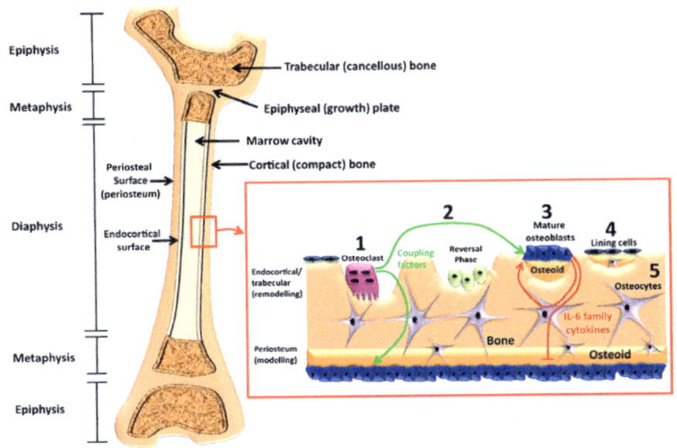

Figure 10.2. Structure of trabecular and cortical bone.

Source: https://www.researchgate.net/publication/318641668/figure/fig1/AS:960355207479326@1605977932550/Structure-of-trabecular-and-cortical-bone-the-process-of-bone-remodeling-and-cellular.gif.

By contrast, trabecular bone, also referred to as cancellous or spongy bone, is found primarily at the ends of long bones and within the centers of others and has a porous texture, facilitating metabolic processes such as mineral exchange. The distinctive architecture of these bone types is not just crucial for structural integrity but also for the regulation of various body processes, like mineral storage and the regulation of calcium, the inherent pillars of mineral and bone metabolism.

The physiological differences between cortical and trabecular bone are pertinent in the most important respect to bone disease and health. Due to its dense structure, cortical bone has a lower metabolic rate, providing mechanical stability, while trabecular bone is more active and responsive to metabolic changes. Trabecular bone, for instance, makes quick adaptation to stress and mechanical load through processes such as bone remodeling, with osteoblasts and osteoclasts remodeling the bone matrix continuously (Figure 10.2).

Research has shown that a dysfunction in this remodeling process has been associated with conditions such as osteoporosis, which is defined by decreased bone mass and increased susceptibility to fractures. In addition, physiologic adaptation to mechanical loading is particularly visible in trabecular bone, where mineralization rates are greater under loaded conditions, reflecting the considerable interdependence of mechanical forces and bone tissue type in the overall scenario of mineral metabolism (Tran et al., 2025).

Furthermore, bone tissue types also interact with other physiological and environmental factors, including hormonal influences and nutrition, in a complicated manner. Hormones such as parathyroid hormone (PTH) and calcitonin powerfully influence bone remodeling, influencing the equilibrium between osteoblast and osteoclast activity. Nutritional factors, particularly calcium and vitamin D, are critical to cortical and trabecular bone integrity. Notably, the absence of these nutrients has been found to impact mineralization, underscoring dietary practices and bone alignment. Moreover, pathological mechanisms that disrupt hormone regulation can significantly alter the structure and density of these tissues and, by extension, undermine their functionality in metabolizing minerals. Such knowledge of bone tissue types and their respective functions is pivotal in developing targeted interventions for clinical populations, particularly those affecting mineral metabolism (Ajbage et al., 2025) (Figure 10.3).

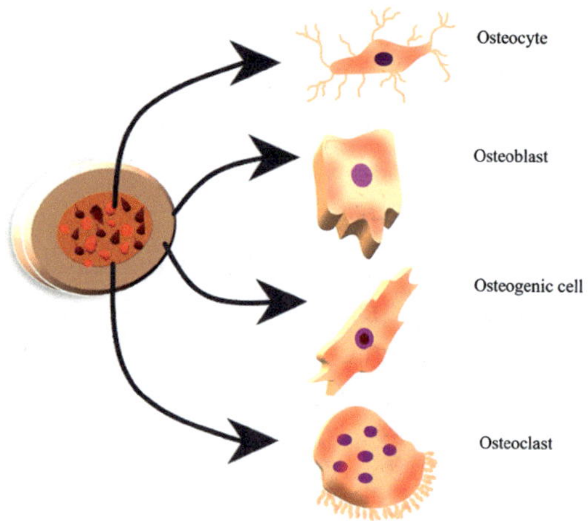

Figure 10.3. Bone tissue has four types of cells: Osteocyte, osteoblast, osteogenic cells, and osteoclast.

Source: https://www.researchgate.net/profile/Suresh-Kumar-Anandasadagopan/publication/367221370/figure/fig3/AS:11431281171482273@1688177890499/Bone-tissue-has-four-types-of-cells-osteocyte-osteoblast-osteogenic-cells-and.png.

10.1.2. Bone Structure and Function

Bone's intricate structure is required to facilitate its multitude of functions, such as the maintenance of mineral homeostasis within the body. Comprising primarily of a collagen fiber-dense matrix and hydroxyapatite crystals that have been mineralized, bone tissue provides strength along with flexibility. The duality serves to allow bones to withstand colossal forces while at the same time being lightweight enough to support movement. In addition, bone tissue is a dynamic living tissue that continually undergoes remodeling by the activities of bone formation and resorption, which allows it to be responsive to mechanical stress and to heal micro-damage. Osteoblast-osteoclast-osteocyte interaction towards each other suggests the dynamic nature of bone metabolism. Through this redesign, bone is a reservoir for phosphate and calcium, which are essential hormones regulated by parathyroid hormone (PTH) and vitamin D to create mineral balance in the body (Khundmiri et al., 2016, pp. 561–601). Apart from providing structural support, bone is important in the protection of internal organs and locomotion. Axial skeleton, which includes skull, vertebral column, and rib cage, serves to cover and shield the brain, spinal cord, and organs of the thorax. The appendicular skeleton enables movement and agility, as seen with limbs. Bone-to-bone articulation at joints and leverage from the attachment of muscles are necessary for effective movement. In addition, bones serve as a storage for minerals essential in physiological processes; bone homeostasis disturbances may result in severe clinical conditions. Studies emphasize that both vitamin D and PTH regulate mineral metabolism, controlling calcium and phosphate levels critical in the normal process of bone formation and repair.

Their regulatory functions are not only concerned with mineral homeostasis but hold far-reaching implications for overall health, including cardiovascular function (Damm et al., 2014, pp. 249–272). Central to the understanding of bone biology is an understanding of the cellular signaling pathways governing bone structure and function. The activation of various cellular pathways, such as calcineurin in skeletal muscle, is a testament to the complex interactions between bone and muscle physiology. The role of calcineurin, a calcium-calmodulin-activated phosphatase, in fiber-type-specific expression points to its role in determining the development of the muscle in response to bone movement. The interaction between muscle and bone points to the concept of mechanotransduction, whereby mechanical stress on bones triggers molecular responses that strengthen bones and make them more resilient. Besides, bone and muscle function interaction is reflected in the modulation of hormones such as PTH and vitamin D, underlining their significance not just in mineral homeostasis but also in musculoskeletal adaptation to functional demands. Knowledge of these connections enhances the concept of bone health and its impact on overall well-being (Khundmiri et al., 2016, pp. 561–601) (Figure 10.4).

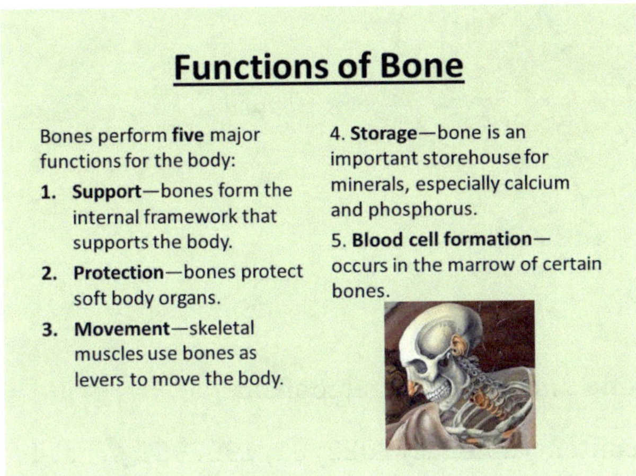

Figure 10.4. Functions of bone.

Source: https://images.slideplayer.com/14/4284436/slides/slide_3.jpg.

10.1.3. Role of Bone Marrow

Bone marrow plays a critical role in bone and mineral metabolism, the major site for hematopoiesis, and storage of principal cell types involved in bone maintenance and bone remodeling. Osteoblasts, which are the bone-producing cells involved in forming the bone matrix and allowing for the deposition of minerals, arise from mesenchymal stem cells within the marrow. In addition to osteoblasts, bone marrow contains osteoclasts, which are necessary to dissolve bones and thus maintain a controlled turnover of bone tissue.

The regulation is important for the maintenance of skeletal integrity and mineral homeostasis. Dysregulation of different functions of bone marrow can lead to metabolic bone disorders such as osteoporosis, and it therefore contributes importantly to the general health of the bone and mineral balance in the body. Furthermore, the role of oxidative stress in bone marrow has been of great interest, particularly with respect to its influence on bone quality and density. Studies indicate that nuclear factor erythroid 2-related factor 2 (Nrf2) is a vital master regulator for oxidative responses and influences bone metabolism, particularly in the context of postmenopausal osteoporosis. Nrf2 deficiency has also been linked with increased oxidative stress in cells of bone marrow origin, enhancing osteoclastic activity with further bone resorption. This shifts the bone remodeling equilibrium toward catabolism and thus leads to a reduction in trabecular bone density. These findings highlight the intersection of oxidative stress and bone marrow health, proposing a site for therapeutic intervention to ensure bone health during periods of heightened oxidative demands (Alcaraz et al., 2025). The effect of exogenous stress, such as simulated microgravity, also represents a fundamental challenge to the function of bone marrow as well as to overall mineral homeostasis. Model studies of hind-limb unloading have demonstrated that long-term unloading results in defective osteoprogenitor cell function and reduced osteoblast mineralization. Although nitric oxide supplementation has been viewed as a countermeasure for mitigating bone loss in microgravity, its efficacy remains questionable. This implies that the regulation of nitric oxide within the bone marrow may not be sufficient to normalize bone metabolism in the presence of altered mechanical loading. Hence, comprehension of the complex role of bone marrow in mineral metabolism goes beyond cellular existence to include reactions to environmental changes, which ultimately impact skeletal well-being (Tran et al., 2025) (Figure 10.5).

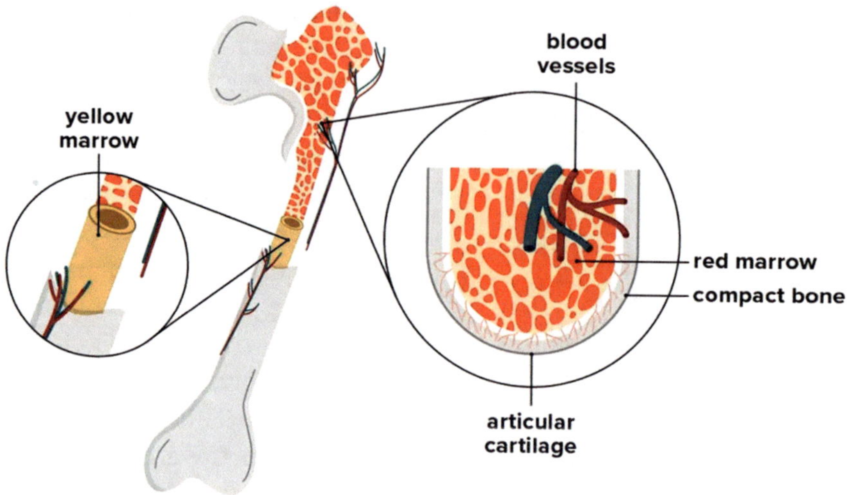

Figure 10.5. Bone marrow plays a critical role in bone and mineral metabolism.

Source: https://i0.wp.com/post.healthline.com/wp-content/uploads/2022/01/1907952_What-Is-Bone-Marrow-and-What-Does-It-Do-01.jpg?w=1155&h=1997.

Test Your Knowledge

1. What are the main types of bone tissue?
2. What are the key components of a long bone's structure, including the diaphysis, epiphysis, periosteum, and medullary cavity?
3. What types of bone marrow exist, and how does bone marrow contribute to hematopoiesis and fat storage?

10.2. Mineral Composition of Bone

Learning Outcome

1. Discuss key minerals involved in bone health;
2. Explain the role of calcium in bone metabolism;
3. Understand the importance of phosphorus and magnesium.

The inorganic structure of bone is characterized primarily by the hydroxyapatite, a crystalline phase derived from calcium phosphate. Hydroxyapatite constitutes approximately 70% of dry bone weight and contributes most to imparting strength and stiffness to the skeleton. Hydroxyapatite's arrangement in the organic matrix, primarily collagen, enables bones to withstand numerous mechanical loads while still retaining a certain amount of flexibility. A balance between organic and mineral elements is necessary in maintaining general bone integrity. In the bone-formation model, there is also a complex interaction between the osteoclasts, which resorb the bone in remodeling activity, and the osteoblasts, which secrete the organic matrix. This kind of dynamic balance is necessary to compensate for bone to mechanical stress and supply sufficient mineral content based on physiological demands. Other than hydroxyapatite, bone also comprises other minerals that are somehow related to its structure and function. Magnesium, sodium, and carbonate ions exist in the matrix of the bone and play an important role in controlling the physical properties of bone. Not only do these minerals contribute to some extent to the general process of mineralization, but they also play a role in controlling acid-base balance within the bone environment. Current research indicates that eating patterns have a great influence on the accessibility of these minerals, and therefore can contribute to changes in bone strength and density. This connectedness of bone nutrition and mineralization is highlighted in contemporary nutrigenomics studies, which have revealed that excess or deficiency of minerals might have a transgenerational effect on bone health and metabolism and, eventually, the susceptibility to diseases like osteoporosis and fracture risk (Michael et al., 2025). New imaging technologies, such as micro-computed tomography (μCT), have radically shifted the exploration of bone mineral content and structure. μCT allows high-resolution three-dimensional reconstructions of bone samples to be produced in a manner that images the microarchitecture and mineral density to characterize bone quality. Through the measurement of parameters such as trabecular thickness and porosity, researchers can study how diet and hormonal fluctuation affects bone metabolism and mineralization. In particular, these newer imaging techniques permit exploration of the relationship between mineral makeup and pathologies leading to degeneration or loss of bone, which enables early detection and intervention procedures. Since public bone health is becoming increasingly a public health concern, understanding how mineral makeup responds to extrinsic and intrinsic stimuli will be essential to developing effective treatments and prevention strategies for bone diseases (Iriê et al., 2018, pp. 227–238).

10.2.1. Key Minerals Involved in Bone Health

The bone's health is dependent on a variety of essential minerals that result in the strength and function integrity of its structure. The most common minerals found in bone, phosphorus and calcium, are the most effective ones in forming hydroxyapatite, the complex mineral which provides bones with strength and stiffness. Calcium, which comprises approximately 99% of the total content of calcium in bone, is not only necessary for bone formation but also for the preservation of bone density throughout life. Phosphorus, with calcium, contributes to the bone matrix, enhancing its strength and functional capacity. Their deficiency causes diseases such as osteoporosis, which is manifested by diminished bone mass and increased fragility. Therefore, adequate consumption of calcium and phosphorus is essential for healthy bones, especially during growth periods and in postmenopausal women, who are most vulnerable to mineral deficiencies. In addition to calcium and phosphorus, trace minerals also play a significant role in bone metabolism. Magnesium, for instance, contributes to bone health in the process of bone mineralization and in the promotion of parathyroid hormone regulation that is key to calcium homeostasis. Findings indicate that magnesium deficiency may undermine bone mineralization and formation, deviating from optimal metabolic pathways. Similarly, copper plays a significant role in collagen synthesis and cross-linking of collagen molecules in the bone matrix, effectively consolidating the bone. Besides this, manganese is being noted for its multi-dimensional function in the bone remodeling process, where it modulates the activity of osteoblasts and osteoclasts, pivotal cells whose function is that of bone formation and resorption, respectively. A complete understanding of these trace minerals, as well as their combined mechanism, is crucial for the development of preventive strategies for bone maintenance. New findings point out the interconnection between lipid metabolism and bone density, contributing to the nuance of the important minerals of this category. For instance, Duchenne muscular dystrophy patients exhibit severe disturbances of lipid profiles that are related to decreased bone mineral density, as per Wang et al. (2025). It would seem, based on these findings, that there is a complex interaction whereby hypertriglyceridemia and remnant cholesterol have adverse impacts on bone. Moreover, manganese, as a trace element, enables both osteoblast and osteoclast functions to occur, which is essential for maintaining skeletal system integrity. Manganese has been found to impact the RANK/RANKL/OPG signaling pathway, which plays a critical role in osteoclastogenesis regulation, thus being critical to mineral metabolism. Understanding how these minerals behave in various metabolic processes will enhance our ability to prevent and treat diseases affecting the skeleton, and in so doing, achieve optimal bone health.

10.2.2. Role of Calcium in Bone Metabolism

Calcium has a fundamental role in bone metabolism as the predominant mineral constituent of bone for bone architecture. Almost 99% of body calcium is deposited in bones and teeth, and thus it is important to maintain bone density and strength. Bone remodeling is a continuous process that has a delicate balance between osteoblast activity, which is responsible for bone deposition, and osteoclasts for the resorption of bone. This equilibrium is significant, as decreased calcium levels will enhance the increased activity of osteoclasts relative to that of osteoblasts, making the bones weaker and giving rise to diseases such as osteoporosis. Further, dietary calcium is utilized in the formation of bone-forming proteins that contribute to health, pointing to the role of nutritional supply in enhancing maximum bone metabolism and overall bone welfare. The interaction between vitamin K and calcium is particularly important since these two nutrients work synergistically in their function to make bone stronger. Vitamin K is needed for the synthesis of proteins, such as osteocalcin, which play a crucial role in binding calcium into the bone matrix, hence facilitating mineralization. Age-related diseases have been linked to deficiencies of these nutrients, leading to impaired bone homeostasis and increased fracture risk. Research highlights the importance of combining calcium-rich foods, such as dairy products and leafy green vegetables, with sufficient vitamin K to provide adequate mineralization and bone strength.

The dietary synergy demonstrates how a deficiency of one or both of these nutrients can have a detrimental effect on calcium's function in bone metabolism, suggesting the importance of a balanced nutritional regimen for the prevention of bone-related ailments. Moreover, the complex interconnection of vascular health with bone metabolism demands major aspects in relation to calcium homeostasis. Growing evidence points to the fact that some pathological conditions, for instance, CKD, lead to calcification of vascular tissue, which diminishes bone mineralization and formation. For instance, calcified vascular cells have been shown to inhibit calcium crystal formation in osteoblast-like cells, further destabilizing bone metabolism dynamics. This evidence points towards the multifaceted aspect of bone health, in which factors beyond normal metabolic processes, like vascular mineralization, also play a role in the overall bone strength. Appreciation of these interactions is significant for the development of integrative approaches to enhancing bone health and mitigating the impact of diseases of aging and other metabolic conditions, with priority being given to escalated research in this critical area (Mace et al., 2025; Mahajan et al., 2025) (Figure 10.6).

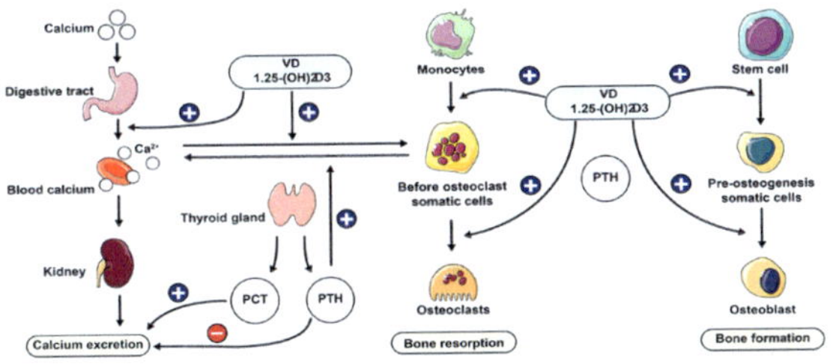

Figure 10.6. Role of calcium-regulating hormones in bone metabolism. [PCT: Procalcitonin; and PTH: parathyroid hormone].

Source: https://www.researchgate.net/figure/Role-of-calcium-regulating-hormone-in-bone-metabolism-PCT-Procalcitonin-PTH_fig1_383056416#:~:text=Role%20of%20calcium%2Dregulating%20hormone%20in%20bone%20metabolism.

10.2.3. Importance of Phosphorus and Magnesium

Phosphorus and magnesium are significant minerals that play crucial roles in bone and mineral metabolism, which have an impact on the overall skeletal health and function. Phosphorus is a significant mineral in the body, with a majority of it found in bones and teeth in the form of hydroxyapatite, which imparts structural hardness.

Moreover, phosphorus is involved in the energy transfer through adenosine triphosphate (ATP) and is a core component of nucleic acids with effects on cellular metabolism and signaling pathways. Magnesium, on the other hand, acts as a cofactor for over 300 enzymatic processes, like bone remodeling and the synthesis of nucleotides.

The interaction not only is credited with optimal bone mineralization but also assists in the maintenance of normal homeostatic processes, and thus, they are essential for the maintenance of skeletal integrity with time. Either a deficiency of phosphorus or magnesium has serious impacts on health, particularly in terms of bone density and strength. Inadequate phosphorus may lead to decreased bone mineralization, resulting in osteomalacia in adults or rickets in children. Similarly, magnesium deficiency has also been implicated in increasing the likelihood of osteoporosis since it is involved in ensuring appropriate calcium equilibrium in bones and activating osteoblasts to produce new bones. Surprisingly, research has shown that an imbalance of minerals between these minerals becomes secondary to one another's deficiencies, sustaining advanced pathophysiologic conditions.

Therefore, an adequate dietary supply of phosphorus and magnesium becomes essential to prevent such disorders and promote optimal bone health, particularly important in ageing populations predisposed to bone disease. The physiological actions of phosphorus and magnesium extend beyond the bone system to affect other functions, including kidney function. Abundant quantities of minerals may become a reason for disorders like the development of kidney stones, in this case, the calcium oxalate stones, because they affect levels of urinary saturation.

An overabundance of phosphorus has been known to result in hyperparathyroidism and increase calcium levels, and may enhance the likelihood of stone formation (Alelign et al., 2018, pp. 1–12). Moreover, the interdependence between these minerals necessitates an organized approach in supplementation because a surplus in one leads to the other's deficiency (Kumar et al., 2020, p. 2179). A better understanding of the role of phosphorus and magnesium in bone and mineral metabolism is necessary in order to set optimal dietary guidelines and therapeutic protocols for enhancing bone health and mineral disorder prevention (Figure 10.7).

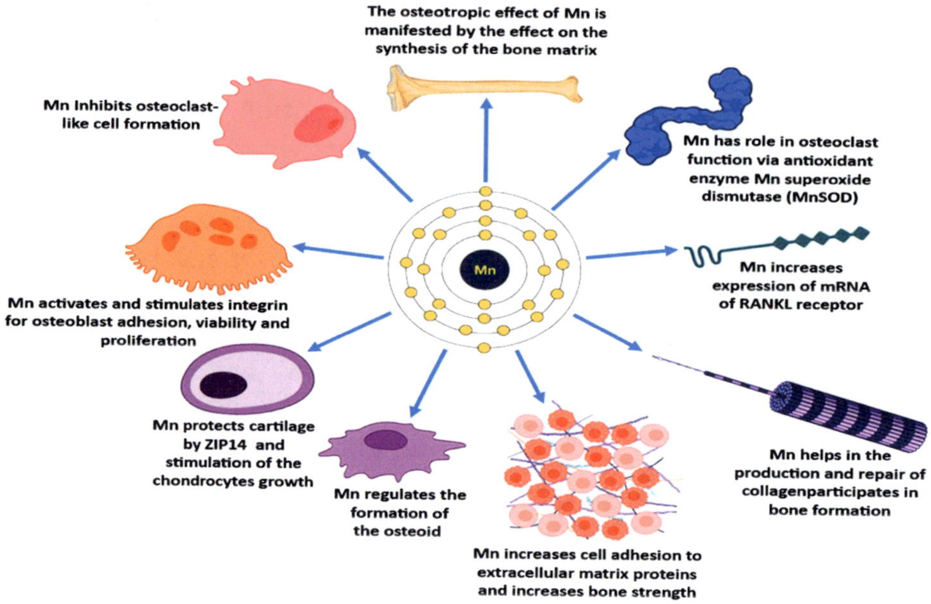

Figure 10.7. The role of manganese (Mn) in bone cellular and molecular functions.

Source: https://www.mdpi.com/jcm/jcm-13-04679/article_deploy/html/images/jcm-13-04679-g001.png.

Test Your Knowledge

1. What are the primary minerals that make up the mineral matrix of bone?
2. How does calcium contribute to bone strength and remodeling, and what hormones regulate calcium balance in the body?
3. How can imbalances or deficiencies in calcium, phosphorus, or magnesium affect bone density?

10.3. Hormonal Regulation

Learning Outcome

1. Explain the role of parathyroid hormone (PTH);
2. Discuss the function of calcitonin;
3. Understand the influence of vitamin D on bone metabolism.

Hormonal regulation is the key process of bone and mineral metabolism maintenance, and it is most importantly conducted by the interaction of several hormones controlling bone remodeling and calcium balance. The most important hormones in this aspect are parathyroid hormone (PTH), calcitonin, and vitamin D. PTH has the primary function of elevating the levels of serum calcium by stimulating osteoclastic activity, and bone resorption ensues, with an increase in intestinal and renal calcium absorption as well. Calcitonin, however, has the function of reducing blood calcium levels by inhibiting osteoclast activity, thereby promoting bone formation. The function performed by vitamin D is equally significant since it allows the guts to absorb calcium, thereby contributing to mineral adequacy for use in bone. This hormonal balance is critical because any disruption could result in disorders such as osteoporosis or hypercalcemia, pointing to the finicky nature of hormonal regulation of bone quality. These hormones' functioning is even made more complex by extrinsic factors, such as dietary supply and physiological states like lactation or aging. For instance, during lactation, as it has increasingly been recognized in recent years, there is an increased demand for calcium that exceeds the hormonal accommodation typically available to the body. This is particularly true in milking dairy cattle, in which hormonal reactions may fall behind the chaotic fluctuations of milking demands for calcium. It has been established through studies that by maximizing the dietary components to facilitate calcium metabolism, incidences of diseases like hypocalcemia can be reduced by a wide margin. Specifically, methods such as minimizing dietary cation–anion difference (DCAD) have been proposed to enhance absorption of calcium and prevent transient hypocalcemia at calving, which is widespread, suggesting the need to couple measures of nutritional control with hormonal control to maintain bone and mineral health (Lopez et al., 2025). Beyond rudimentary mineral metabolism, such hormonal interactions have broader implications, affecting overall health and resistance to disease. Conservative hormonal regulation not only supports structural integrity in bone but also influences metabolic activities essential for growth and tissue repair. Disruptions within this regulation can have disastrous implications, particularly during states of increased demand, such as pregnancy and lactation, in which there are dynamic changes in calcium and mineral requirements. An understanding of the complexity of such hormonal relationships is essential to design effective therapy in veterinary medicine as well as human medicine. More understanding of such mechanisms can enable better nutritional advice and treatment courses, ultimately yield stronger bone health and eliminate the risks inherent with hormonal imbalance (Ajbage et al., 2025).

10.3.1. Role of Parathyroid Hormone (PTH)

The parathyroid hormone (PTH) plays a crucial role in the regulation of calcium and phosphorus metabolism, with an important role to play in bone integrity. Released by the parathyroid glands, PTH facilitates the mobilization of calcium from bone into blood and hence increases the serum level of calcium when it falls below physiological levels. It is achieved through stimulation of osteoclasts, which enhance bone resorption. As the level of PTH rises, the hormone binds to its receptors on the osteoblasts, leading to subsequent RANKL synthesis, which is a cytokine that promotes osteoclast formation. This delicate mechanism, catalyzed by PTH, plays a critical role in normal skeletal development and the sustenance of normal bone growth, preventing conditions such as osteoporosis in which bone resorption is so pronounced that bones are deficient in their number, highlighting the importance of this hormone in mineral and bone metabolism. In addition to its direct effect on bone, PTH also plays a part in affecting renal handling of calcium and phosphorus. PTH enhances distal convoluted tubule reabsorption of calcium and phosphate excretion through its action on the proximal tubules. This combined effect helps to keep serum calcium levels as it controls phosphate levels, an important function for overall mineral balance. Interestingly, its synergism with other hormones, such as vitamin D, emphasizes its role in mineral metabolism. Vitamin D enhances calcium and phosphate levels from the intestine, showing a synergistic role in maintaining bone integrity. Dysregulation of PTH can also result in disrupting this balance, leading to hyperparathyroidism or hypoparathyroidism, with clinical consequences ranging from bone fragility to organ calcification, and demonstrating the significance of PTH in the broader context of bone health. More recent evidence has also implicated PTH in the pathogenesis of bone metastases, particularly in malignancies such as breast cancer. The binding of PTH with type 1 PTH receptors and extracellular calcium-sensing receptors within the bone microenvironment establishes a complex feedback loop that can hasten metastasis-induced osteolysis. New studies indicate that cancer cells hijack the normal signaling pathways of PTH to stimulate bone resorption in addition to feeding tumor growth to establish a vicious cycle. Elucidating these mechanisms not only reveals PTH's intricate role in bone and mineral homeostasis but also provides new avenues for therapy. Manipulation of these pathways could provide new prospects for the therapy of bone-related metastasis-related complications, emphasizing the therapeutic potential of modulating PTH signaling in clinical therapy (Wang et al., 2025; Fear et al., 2025) (Figure 10.8).

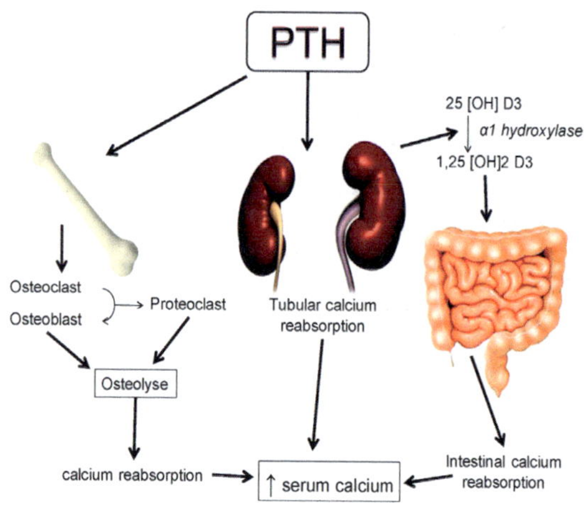

Figure 10.8. Mechanisms of action of parathyroid hormone.

Source: https://www.researchgate.net/publication/342298993/figure/fig1/AS:905831528796160@1592978474089/Mechanisms-of-action-of-parathyroid-hormone.ppm.

10.3.2. Function of Calcitonin

Calcitonin, the parafollicular cell secretory hormone of the thyroid gland, is an important regulator of calcium homeostasis and bone metabolism. Primarily acting to inhibit osteoclastic function, calcitonin effectively reduces bone resorption, the process by which bone tissue is broken down, releasing calcium into the bloodstream. Such inhibition of osteoclast function is contrary to the effect of parathyroid hormone (PTH), which causes bone resorption and elevation in blood calcium levels. As a result, calcitonin plays a pivotal role in the regulation of eucalcemia, ensuring calcium levels remain within a physiological range necessary for various bodily processes, including neuromuscular function and blood clotting. The intricate interplay between calcitonin and the other hormones, such as PTH, underscores the regulatory complexity of bone metabolism and identifies calcitonin's crucial function in the maintenance of skeletal integrity and mineral homeostasis. Calcium also plays, in addition, a vital role in osteoblasts by controlling their activity and function, an insight with therapeutic implications. Calcitonin has been suggested in recent studies to enhance the activity of osteoblasts in a way that "stimulates bone matrix synthesis and potentially increases bone density." This two-part mechanism of bone suppression and bone facilitation situates calcitonin in the middle of the dynamic bone remodeling process. Bone remodeling, in turn, is regulated by a fine-tuned interplay of various factors ranging from local signals by cytokines and growth factors to systemic signals like calcitonin and estrogen. Being aware of this intricate regulatory system can account for the disease pathology in bone disorders such as osteoporosis, wherein there is a disturbance between the resorption and the formation, leading to weakened bone structure and increased susceptibility to fracture (Florêncio-Silva et al., 2015, pp. 1–17). In addition to its functions in bone metabolism, calcitonin also possesses emergent functions in total mineral homeostasis, particularly in the metabolic disorder of CKD. In CKD patients, deranged calcium and phosphate metabolism can form vascular calcification, which contributes further to cardiovascular disease risk. Research has indicated that calcitonin is a potential therapeutic agent in inhibiting such processes by maintaining calcium levels stable and suppressing the toxic action of excess phosphate on vascular smooth muscle cells. Vascular calcification can be caused by elevated calcium and phosphate through multiple mechanisms, such as apoptosis and differentiation of vascular smooth muscle cells into bone-like cells (Shanahan et al., 2011, pp. 697–711). Thus, discovering calcitonin's multifaceted functions not only consolidates its position in bone and mineral metabolism but also offers avenues for novel treatment methods concerning bone as well as cardiovascular health.

10.3.3. Influence of Vitamin D on Bone Metabolism

The action of vitamin D on bone metabolism is of utmost significance, as the secosteroid hormone plays a central role in calcium absorption and bone mineralization. Proper levels of vitamin D are required to facilitate regular bone mineral density (BMD). People, particularly older individuals, usually present with sub-optimal vitamin D status that has been described by an increased prevalence of osteoporosis—a disease of high morbidity and high healthcare cost. It has long been established that a lack of vitamin D can lead to rickets in children and osteomalacia in adults. Given that these diseases directly impact bone health, it is essential to determine the role of vitamin D in preventing bone diseases. Therefore, actions to increase vitamin D in risk groups are a major aspect of maintaining skeletal integrity and decreasing fracture risk, a serious issue in geriatric populations. In addition, the interaction of vitamin D with muscle function is evidence of its relevance to bone health. Current studies have shown the potential for vitamin D supplementation to increase muscle mass and, therefore, lower the occurrence of falls among the elderly, one of the primary reasons for fracture incidence. Such evidence suggests a role for vitamin D not only in contributing to skeletal structure but also in affecting functional capacity in the musculoskeletal system. The classic presentation of vitamin D deficiency disorders, such as rickets, is usually muscle weakness, which implies a multi-dimensional aspect to its function in health. Further, the action of vitamin D extends into the area of inflammation since it is possible for pro-inflammatory cytokines to exert a negative effect on bone metabolism. Hence, through a variety of mechanisms, including muscle function and immunomodulation, vitamin D plays a key role in the prevention of fractures and overall bone health, particularly in the elderly (Abrahamsen et al., 2025). Recent studies have also shed light on the regulatory pathways of phosphate metabolism and their interaction with vitamin D, with a growing focus on a complex endocrine feedback mechanism that regulates bone homeostasis. The discovery of Fibroblast growth factor-23 (FGF23) and its role in phosphate metabolism has brought new insight into the interaction between vitamin D and bone metabolism. Specifically, vitamin D regulates the expression of FGF23, with FGF23 acting to modulate calcium and phosphate balance. This carefully controlled interaction is critical to maintaining healthy bone metabolism, for disruption can lead to pathologies such as osteoporosis. The function of vitamin D in the control of FGF23 secretion is a significant development in the research on bone health. What this study indicates is that optimization of vitamin D levels not only enhances systemic levels of calcium and phosphate but may also mitigate risks of complications from bone disease, further validating the central role of vitamin D in the broader context of bone and mineral metabolism (Clinkenbeard et al., 2025) (Figure 10.9).

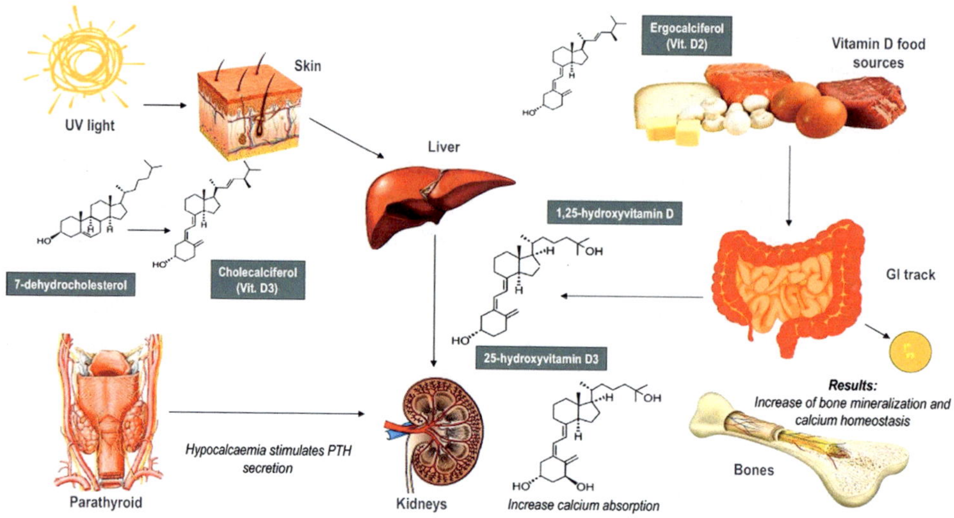

Figure 10.9. The role of vitamin D in bone metabolism.

Source: https://www.researchgate.net/publication/348446042/figure/fig1/AS:11431281256565039@1719546624460/The-role-of-vitamin-D-in-bone-metabolism.jpg.

Test Your Knowledge

1. How does parathyroid hormone (PTH) regulate blood calcium levels, and what is its effect on bone resorption?
2. What is the role of calcitonin in calcium homeostasis, and how does it counteract the effects of PTH?
3. How do PTH, calcitonin, and vitamin D work together to maintain calcium and phosphate balance in the blood and bones?

10.4. Bone Remodeling Process

Learning Outcome

1. Understand osteoblasts and osteoclasts;
2. Explain the stages of bone remodeling;
3. Describe factors affecting bone remodeling.

Bone remodeling is a dynamic, multi-staged process essential to the structure and metabolic health of the bone tissue. The continuous process involves two basic cellular processes: osteoblast-mediated bone formation and osteoclast-mediated bone resorption. In normal adults, these are precisely coordinated to balance constant bone mass while altering bone based on mechanical loading and metabolic demand. The hormonal components, such as the parathyroid hormone and calcitonin, also play significant roles in regulating osteoclastic and osteoblastic activities. Understanding this balance is essential, as an imbalance results in pathological conditions such as osteoporosis, where bone mineral density is lost and the risk of fracture is increased. A deep understanding of bone remodeling, therefore, lies at the foundation of the creation of therapeutic interventions aimed at enhancing bone health and the control of metabolic bone disease. Current studies have revealed the part played by dipeptidyl peptidase 4 (DPP-4) in the process of bone remodeling, in which its multi-faceted function has been seen beyond glucose metabolism. The entero-endocrine-osseous axis demonstrates that DPP-4 activity is also inversely linked with bone mineral density, such that higher levels of DPP-4 can lead to poorer bone integrity. DPP-4 exerts its action through various gastrointestinal substrates, namely glucose-dependent insulinotropic polypeptide (GIP), which has been revealed to stimulate bone formation. In contrast, some substrates of DPP-4, such as pancreatic peptide YY and neuropeptide Y, have the potential to cause bone resorption. This intricate relationship indicates the importance of learning more about the mechanisms involved in DPP-4 in bone metabolism. By demystifying these mechanisms, researchers can possibly design targeted interventions for osteoporosis and fractures, bringing new light to therapeutic possibilities in disorders of bone and mineral metabolism (Pechmann et al., 2025). Furthermore, vitamin D3 has emerged as the major contributor to bone remodeling, in particular, in orthodontics. It has been purported that vitamin D3 drives osteoblast activity and enhances bone mineralization, which ultimately leads to enhanced tooth movement in orthodontic therapy. It targets RANKL expression that plays a critical role in osteoclast differentiation and function, thereby inducing an optimal process of bone remodeling. This relationship illustrates vitamin D3's anabolic function in the overall context of bone metabolism. Because orthodontic tooth movement also relies heavily on successful alveolar bone remodeling, its use may actually add to optimal treatment outcomes. Future research, however, is necessary to establish optimal dosing and delivery strategies to maximize the use of its therapeutic benefits. Lastly, the finding of vitamin D3's synergistic actions with hormones in bone remodeling will further enhance orthodontics and bone health (Zamanian et al., 2024, pp. 3164–3176).

10.4.1. Overview of Osteoblasts and Osteoclasts

This dynamic balance of bone metabolism is regulated with utmost complexity by two differentiated cell forms: osteoblasts and osteoclasts. Osteoblasts are cells that make bone from mesenchymal stem cells and are responsible for synthesizing the bone matrix and its mineralization. They secrete collagen and other proteins that build the structural framework of bone and, simultaneously, control the mineral deposition by the action of osteocalcin and bone morphogenetic proteins. By enabling the formation of new bone tissue, osteoblasts play a crucial role in skeletal stability as well as in response to mechanical loading. Significantly, osteoblast activity is regulated by various factors, among which hormonal signals from vitamin D are significant, which bind to nuclear receptors of osteoblasts, ultimately influencing bone health and mineral metabolism (Li et al., 2025). Opposing osteoclasts are multinucleated and large cells responsible for bone resorption, which break down the bone matrix. Osteoclasts are derived from hematopoietic stem cells and play a critical function in regulating the body's calcium and phosphate balance by resorbing mineralized bone. It is essential not only for bone structural integrity but also to permit the continuous process of remodeling that enables bone to respond to mechanical stress and repair injury. The activity of osteoclasts is controlled by signaling molecules, including receptor activator of nuclear factor kappa-B ligand (RANKL) and osteoprotegerin, that control their differentiation and activation. Therefore, any imbalance in osteoclast or osteoblast activity has the potential to result in diseases such as osteoporosis, emphasizing the significant role these cells play in overall bone and mineral metabolism (Wang et al., 2025). Both osteoblasts and osteoclasts, although collaborating to achieve homeostasis in the skeletal system, bear wide-ranging clinical implications when their function is dysregulated. The balance between the bone-forming functions of osteoblasts and the bone-resorbing function of osteoclasts is essential to maintaining bone strength and density. For example, age, hormonal change, and nutritional deficiency can disrupt the balance, leading to excessive bone resorption and decreased formation, characteristic of osteoporosis. Recent work has also provided insight into the role of osteoblast-derived factors in controlling osteoclast function, with a description of a sophisticated intercellular communication network. Lastly, a distinct understanding of osteoblasts and osteoclasts enables us to design meaningful therapeutic strategies that are capable of fixing pathologic imbalances responsible for various metabolic bone diseases so that therapy of conditions like osteoporosis can be enhanced (Wang et al., 2025) (Figure 10.10).

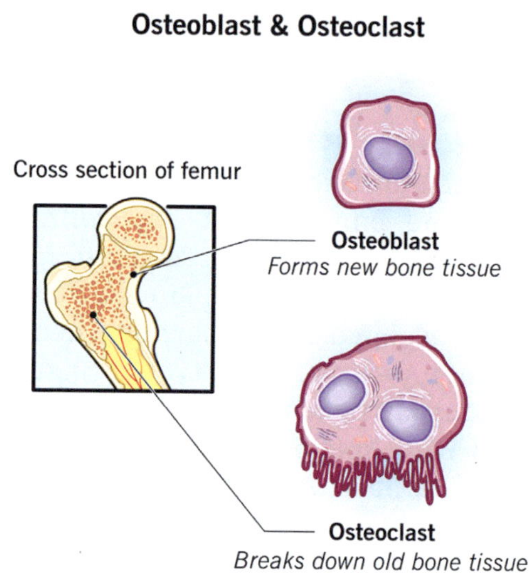

Figure 10.10. Illustration of osteoblast and osteoclast.

Source: https://my.clevelandclinic.org/-/scassets/images/org/health/articles/24871-osteoblast-osteoclast.

10.4.2. Stages of Bone Remodeling

Bone remodeling is an active and continuous process that maintains bone strength and mineral homeostasis throughout an individual's life. It is a carefully regulated sequence of events involving bone resorption and formation, primarily mediated by osteoclasts and osteoblasts, respectively.

The remodeling cycle can be subdivided into three principal phases: activation, resorption, and formation. During the activation stage, a number of signaling molecules, like hormones and cytokines, trigger the recruitment of osteoclast precursors to bone areas that require remodeling. This stage is fundamental to the subsequent stages because it creates the platform for productive bone resorption, which ensures the removal of old or damaged bone matrix. During resorption, activated osteoclasts bind to the bone surface, forming a tight compartment in which they release large volumes of acids and proteolytic enzymes to lyse the mineralized matrix. It not only performs the area for new bone formation but also plays a critical role in releasing minerals such as calcium and phosphate into the circulation, maintaining systemic mineral equilibrium.

A mismatch at this level can encourage pathological conditions, such as osteoporosis, characterized by excessive loss of bones. Furthermore, studies report that localized factors, for example, elevated FGF-23 and reduced osteocalcin levels, are able to stimulate resorption in conditions such as CKD, hence compromising bone structure as is witnessed in type 2 diabetic patients (Lu et al., 2025). Finally, the formation stage is marked by the transition from bone resorption to new bone deposition by osteoblasts.

This culminates in the manufacture of new bone matrix that becomes increasingly mineralized. Proper coordination of osteoclast and osteoblast activities is necessary to ensure that bone turnover occurs effectively without loss of bone density. Dysregulation of this balance, particularly in the case of altered environmental conditions such as microgravity, produces changes in osteoprogenitor cell proliferation and differentiation and results in changes in the quantity and quality of bone formed (Tran et al., 2025). Knowledge of the phases of bone remodeling is core to the development of targeted treatments for metabolic bone disease to enhance bone status in different populations (Figure 10.11).

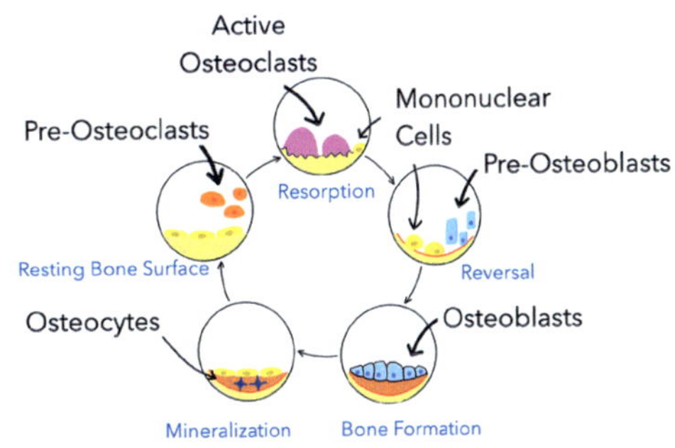

Figure 10.11. Stages of the bone remodeling cycle.

Source: https://www.researchgate.net/publication/355409690/figure/fig1/AS:1080850917666832@1634706348419/Stages-of-the-bone-remodeling-cycle.png.

10.4.3. Factors Affecting Bone Remodeling

Bone remodeling is a dynamic and continuous process of resorption and formation, and is regulated by a number of intrinsic and extrinsic factors. Hormonal regulation is an important part of the intrinsic factors, e.g., parathyroid hormone (PTH) and calcitonin, which directly regulate osteoclast and osteoblast activity, respectively, and thus control the rates of bone resorption and formation. In addition, sex hormones such as testosterone and estrogen have been reported to contribute towards bone density through the promotion of osteoblast activity and suppression of osteoclast function. Loss or decrease of these hormones, as in the case of women during menopause, is likely to promote bone resorption and cause osteoporosis. Hence, information about hormonal control of bone remodeling is helpful in appreciating the pathophysiological underpinnings of various bone diseases and the potential directions for therapeutic intervention. Another key controller of bone remodeling is mechanical loading because bones respond to the imposed loading stress. Mechanostat theory suggests that bones sense mechanical strain and modulate bone density and material properties of the structure in response to alterations in load. Repetitive weight-bearing stimuli stimulate osteoblast activity, leading to the formation of bone, while a sedentary lifestyle may induce bone demineralization. Skeletal loading adaptation is controlled through signaling pathways, including the Wnt/β-catenin pathway, which has been shown to be stimulated by mechanical stress. This interaction indicates that lifestyle elements, such as exercise, are necessary for the maintenance of peak bone density, particularly in high-risk individuals for compromised bone mass and high fracture risk. Lastly, nutrition contributes significantly to bone remodeling and mineral homeostasis, asserting the need for a well-balanced lifestyle. Adequate intake of major nutrients such as calcium, vitamin D, and protein is required to maintain bone health. Calcium is needed for mineralization of bone, whereas vitamin D enhances calcium absorption from the intestine and bone remodeling processes. Furthermore, more recent evidence suggests that obesity may have a detrimental effect on bone through endocrine and inflammatory pathways. Sedentary obese individuals' sera have been found to suppress the function of osteoblasts and disrupt bone homeostasis, and therefore, nutritional remodeling of body composition and physical exercise may positively affect bone remodeling activities. Hence, nutritional interventions, in combination with lifestyle changes, have a crucial role to play in the management of bone health and metabolic bone diseases in diverse populations (Ajbage et al., 2025; Baldari et al., 2025) (Figure 10.12).

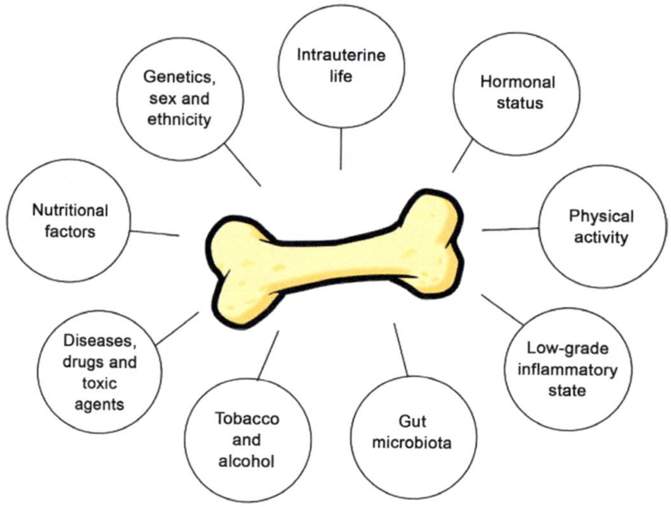

Figure 10.12. Factors influencing bone formation during childhood and adolescence.

Source: https://www.researchgate.net/profile/Pilar-Codoner-Franch/publication/327913924/figure/fig1/AS:747315405021184@1555185285905/Factors-influencing-bone-formation-during-childhood-and-adolescence.jpg.

Test Your Knowledge

1. What are the roles of osteoblasts and osteoclasts in bone remodeling?
2. What are the major stages of the bone remodeling cycle, from activation to formation?

10.5. Nutritional Factors

Learning Outcome

1. Explain dietary sources of essential minerals in maintaining bone and mineral metabolism;
2. Understand the impact of vitamin D on mineral absorption;
3. Discuss the role of protein in bone health.

The interplay between nutrition and bone is significantly controlled by various components of the diet required to ensure effective mineral metabolism. Calcium, in particular, plays a key function in the processes of bone resorption and deposition. The foods of the dairy group are traditionally associated with their calcium abundance, but a number of dietary strategies are aimed at regulating calcium metabolism more effectively. For example, accurate control of the dietary cation–anion difference (DCAD) has been shown to enhance calcium clearance from the blood. By inducing systemic acidosis through dietary adjustment, bone resorption and intestinal calcium absorption can be increased. Such nutritional interventions are also crucial, as in the case of lactation of milk cows, where the consumption of calcium is astronomically high, and thus conditions like hypocalcemia are developed if not managed (Lopez et al., 2025). This shows the importance of meal planning to prevent deficiencies that may impact the health of bones. Another essential nutrient to the maintenance of bone and mineral metabolism is vitamin D, which has been in the spotlight for its role beyond calcium homeostasis. The presence of a vitamin D receptor in the muscle cell indicates its potential impact on skeletal muscle integrity, exerting a direct effect on muscle proliferation and differentiation. This interaction between vitamin D, bone, and muscle is particularly important in populations with chronic conditions, such as CKD, where the interrelated nature of muscle and bone conditions is impaired. Observational studies have confirmed that deficiency levels of 25-hydroxyvitamin D in serum correlate with severe skeletal outcomes, such as decreased bone mineral density and increased risk of fractures (Bover et al., 2025). Thus, the maintenance of adequate vitamin D either by diet or supplements can be important in the enhancement of musculoskeletal health and the avoidance of weakening of bone structure. Additionally, the establishment of the synergistic effects of nutritional components holds true for the establishment of their total effects on health. The case of vitamin D and calcium helps illustrate how nutrition assists in the mutual reinforcement of each other's effect on bone health. For instance, the bioavailability of calcium is greatly increased in the presence of adequate vitamin D to facilitate proper absorption and usage by the body. Accordingly, interventions aimed at addressing calcium and vitamin D levels in food consumption are required, particularly among populations at risk of deficiency, such as older patients or those with insufficient sun exposure. Besides, dietary strategy optimization can help in the better understanding of the modulation of bone metabolism, the reduction of the burden of osteoporosis, and other resultant diseases. Evaluation of these food components in terms of bone and mineral metabolism only confirms the need for multidisciplinary dietary advice, ensuring maximum skeletal health throughout life.

10.5.1. Dietary Sources of Essential Minerals

Trace mineral food sources play a significant role in maintaining mineral and bone metabolism. Calcium, magnesium, and phosphorus are part of the architecture and structure of bone. Milk food products, green leafy vegetables, and fortified foods are some of the richest food sources of calcium that occupy a significant amount of the recommended daily amount. Magnesium, needed for activation of vitamin D and for mineralization of the bones, is found in nuts, whole grains, and legumes. Phosphorus, which helps calcium to form hydroxyapatite, the mineral content of the bone, exists in animal protein, milk products, and certain nuts. Their interaction and balance are the secrets of healthy skeletal well-being, stressing the need for a nutrient-dense diet. While the focus is often on macrominerals like phosphorus and calcium, trace minerals also impact bone and mineral metabolism significantly. Trace minerals such as zinc, copper, and manganese are involved in various biochemical processes that promote bone integrity. Zinc, for instance, is involved in regulating osteoblasts and osteoclasts, cells responsible for bone development and breakdown, respectively. Dietary sources of zinc are meat, shellfish, legumes, and seeds. Less commonly referred to, copper supports the formation of collagen and connective tissue, and its insufficiency can cause some impairment of bone health. Manganese supports the development of bone and cartilage, and the best foods to obtain this nutrient are nuts, whole cereals, and leafy green vegetables. The importance must be recognized in these trace elements as part of a holistic plan for bone health, with the understanding aimed at attaining adequate intake of minerals from a diversified food source. The most recent studies bring to attention the link between dietary minerals and oral health, in particular that of periodontal disease with bone health implications. Current studies emphasize the significance of minerals in inflammation and immune response, underscoring their importance over traditional bone health markers. Calcium, for example, is important in the preservation of alveolar bone supporting the teeth, while some mineral diets may influence the progression of periodontal disease. Therefore, a diet rich in minerals and minerals alone not only contributes to skeletal well-being but also oral well-being and reduces inflammatory disease. This intricate interaction between food sources for basic minerals and their multi-roles in not just bone metabolism but in health as a whole mirrors the critical need for ongoing research and public health measures aimed at mineral-rich eating habits (Anonymous et al., 2025; Battino et al., 2025) (Figure 10.13).

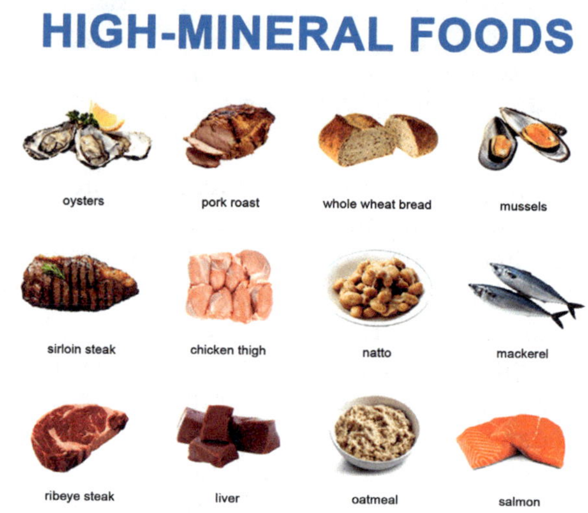

Figure 10.13. High mitral food.

Source: https://optimisingnutrition.com/wp-content/uploads/2023/11/image-93.png.

10.5.2. Impact of Vitamin D on Mineral Absorption

Vitamin D is pivotal in the intestinal absorption of essential minerals, particularly calcium and phosphorus, essential for maintaining bones and mineral metabolism. As a fat-soluble vitamin, it facilitates the intestinal absorption of calcium by stimulating calcium-binding protein production, enhancing the effectiveness of mineral absorption in the gastrointestinal tract. This process emphasizes the physiological significance of vitamin D in regulating optimal levels of calcium, which are not only essential to bone density but also to neuromuscular transmission and cardiovascular stability. Vitamin D deficiencies have been indicated to compromise calcium absorption and may lead to a number of disorders, including osteomalacia and osteoporosis, which shows the vitamin's vital role in mineral homeostasis as it relates to skeletal health. The consequences of inadequate vitamin D status are particularly evident in populations at risk of bone and mineral disease. CKD is a case in point, where the kidneys are an essential component of the conversion of vitamin D to its active form, calcitriol, which is the key to calcium absorption. They have also been discovered in research to be often associated with disturbances in phosphorus and calcium metabolism in patients with CKD, leading to a condition referred to as CKD-mineral and bone disorder (CKD-MBD) (Dod et al., 2025).

CKD-MBD has the potential to exacerbate bone fragility and also enhance the risk of cardiovascular complications, which necessitates initial action on vitamin D supplementation and bone health monitoring. The relationship between vitamin D status and mineral absorption not only illustrates the role of the nutrient in bone health but also calls attention to its importance in more general metabolic functions. In addition to its influence on calcium absorption, vitamin D influences the metabolism of other critical minerals, such as magnesium. Magnesium is a critical part of bone formation and function, but absorption and homeostasis can be disrupted in individuals who are suboptimally vitamin D-replete. This interaction is more relevant in the context of bariatric surgery, which disrupts nutrient intake and absorption. Operations like Roux-en-Y gastric bypass (RYGB) often lead to deficiencies of not just fat-soluble vitamins like vitamin D, but also minerals like magnesium (Aaseth et al., 2025). Maintaining a proper amount of vitamin D is crucial for preventing these deficiencies and their consequent complications, thereby highlighting the intricate interrelationship between vitamin D and mineral absorption as a core feature of good bone and mineral metabolism control.

10.5.3. Role of Protein in Bone Health

The role of protein in the development of optimum bone health is increasingly recognized as an essential component of bone and mineral metabolism. Proteins are an integral component required for the skeleton, assisting in the synthesis of bone matrix proteins, primarily collagen, which forms the bulk of the bones organic composition. Adequate protein intake has been associated with increased bone mineral density (BMD), a factor relevant in the prevention of fractures, particularly in the elderly. Moreover, proteins influence the activity of osteoblasts and osteoclasts, the cells that are active in bone remodeling, and therefore are actively involved in bone turnover. This regulation of bone homeostasis places emphasis on the requirement of an adequate diet with excessive protein consumption to ensure skeletal integrity, particularly in populations susceptible to osteoporosis and other metabolic bone diseases. Protein thus emerges as a key nutrient in the bone health paradigm. Furthermore, the relationship between protein consumption and calcium metabolism buttresses the function of protein in bone health. Calcium is an important bone-building mineral and has been theorized by certain research to be enhanced by sufficient levels of protein to enhance gut calcium absorption, as well as a favorable calcium balance. This mechanism is particularly relevant in the elderly, as calcium retention can become impaired, thus raising the risk of fractures. Because protein and calcium are synergistic nutrients for bone, inadequate protein not only compromises the structural quality of bones but also reduces the process of mineralization as a whole. In addition, nutritional recommendations increasingly encourage a balance between adequacy for protein and foods rich in calcium to achieve maximum bone mineral content, emphasizing the need for a synergistic, integrated strategy for nutrition from nutrient interactions rather than single foods. Recent findings have also revealed that the interaction between protein, fat, and muscle tissue has the potential to influence bone health, as evidenced by diseases like non-alcoholic fatty liver disease (NAFLD). Bone mineral density and muscle loss, with increased incidence of NAFLD, illustrate how metabolic disease influences skeletal strength. The potential interplay between osteoporosis, sarcopenia, and metabolic disturbance underscores the importance of maintaining adequate protein intake to support not only muscular health but also bone metabolism. Such interdependence only serves to point towards the necessity for addressing holistic dietary regimens, and not specific nutrients, in the instance of intervention into bone health. With these connotations, a well-balanced diet plan with proper protein intake can be a preventive factor against metabolic bone diseases such as osteoporosis and enhance overall bone and mineral metabolism health (Ajbage et al., 2025; Chiesa et al., 2025) (Figure 10.14).

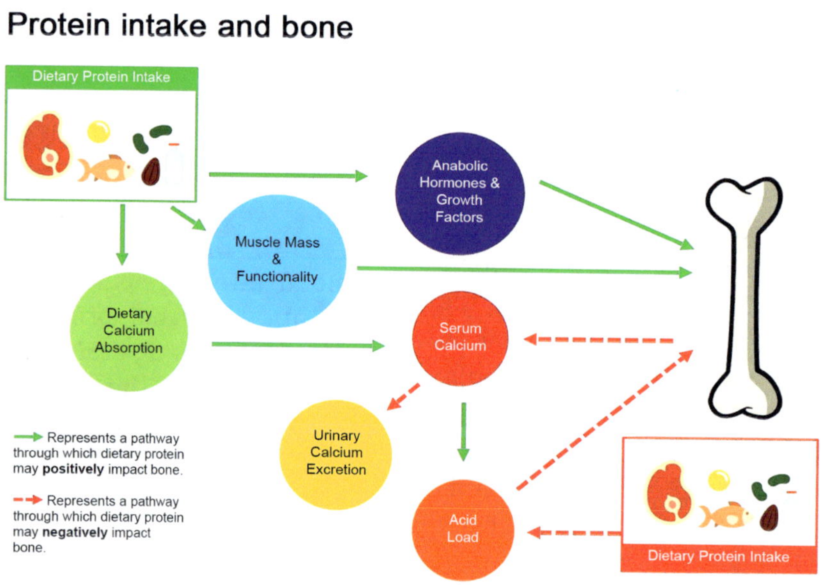

Figure 10.14. Protein intake and bone.

Source: https://static.wixstatic.com/media/a27d24_796a9a4057a24efd865725fbf2be37e3~mv2.png/v1/fill/w_1000,h_722,al_c,q_90,usm_0.66_1.00_0.01/a27d24_796a9a4057a24efd865725fbf2be37e3~mv2.png.

Test Your Knowledge

1. What are the primary dietary sources of calcium, phosphorus, and magnesium, and how do these minerals contribute to bone strength?
2. How does vitamin D facilitate the absorption of calcium and phosphorus from the gastrointestinal tract?
3. Why is adequate calcium intake throughout life critical for preventing bone loss?

10.6. Disorders of Bone and Mineral Metabolism

Learning Outcome

1. Describe osteoporosis and its implications;
2. Understand rickets and osteomalacia disorders;
3. Explain hyperparathyroidism and its effects.

Mineral and bone metabolism disorders are a group of conditions that cause derangement of the complex interaction between bone mineralization, resorption, and mineral homeostasis. These conditions may generate significant skeletal complications that are manifestations of alterations in bone density as well as structural characteristics. Osteoporotic fracture caused by decreased bone mineral content is one of the most common diseases, which is often asymptomatic until fracture ensues. These intricacies are then further added to by a number of risk factors that include aging, hormonal imbalances, and co-morbid chronic diseases such as CKD. Hence, understanding these intricate mechanisms is important for the effective prevention and management of bone-related complications. As the population grows, aged disorders of bone and mineral metabolism are also on an increasing trend, which requires ongoing research and clinical development in this field. The role of alkaline phosphatases (APs) in bone metabolism illustrates the delicate balance in normal bone dynamics. While APs are essential to the process of mineralization in bones, activity must be strictly regulated since excessive levels are dangerous, with possible adverse impacts like calcification of blood vessels. The complexity of APs is compounded in CKD, where changes in mineral metabolism can contribute to an increased risk of cardiovascular disease. Furthermore, the emerging awareness of the presence of multiple isoforms, such as the bone-specific alkaline phosphatase, is to make us realize the promise for isoform-specific treatments with the capacity to modulate AP activity. Healthcare providers and scientists are beginning to realize the prognostic value of AP levels in the settings of bone turnover and cardiovascular disease, putting these enzymes in the driver's seat of CKD-Mineral and Bone Disorder (CKD-MBD) treatment decision-making (Aguilar et al., 2025). Subsequent studies investigating the gut microbiota's influence on bone health have illuminated yet another level of intricacy in disorders of bone and mineral metabolism. The normobiosis theory, in which healthy microbial communities predominate, is opposite to dysbiosis, a state that may lead to many metabolic disorders, including bone health disorders. Recent evidence points to the fact that dietary prebiotic intake, which selectively stimulates growth of healthy gut flora, may enhance calcium absorption and, thus, promote bone mineral density. This interaction emphasizes the potential of nutritional intervention as a therapeutic modality in susceptible populations for bone metabolism disorders, particularly in susceptible populations prone to imbalanced gut microbiota. The interaction among diet, gut microbiota, and systemic physiological effect is a novel and exciting field of research that has the potential to lead to innovative treatment options for bone and mineral metabolism disorders while reinforcing the importance of integrated preventive strategies for health (Meheust et al., 2025).

10.6.1. Osteoporosis and Its Implications

The effects of osteoporosis extend far beyond the bone framework, as it significantly affects overall health and quality of life. Osteoporosis, a condition characterized by low bone mineral density (BMD), is a major fracture risk factor, particularly in postmenopausal women and older people. The findings of a study involving 300 patients indicated a startling 33.7% incidence of osteoporosis in the lumbar spine and 16.7% in the femoral neck. These figures indicate the seriousness of the situation, as each fracture can lead to long-term harm such as chronic pain, immobility, and dependency on caregivers. Additionally, osteoporosis is not just a physical condition; it has significant psychological effects, with patients developing a fear of falling and hence subsequent fractures, resulting in anxiety and depression. Therefore, understanding the multifactorial etiology of osteoporosis is crucial for developing effective treatment modalities and preventive interventions. When examining the pathophysiology of osteoporosis, consideration of the factors leading to low BMD is important. Several factors, including age, sex, and body mass index (BMI), are significant determinants of bone health. The relationship between bone density and aging has been precisely defined; with age, the rate of bone resorption is generally greater than bone formation, leading to significant losses in density. The above study indicated a strong correlation of BMI and age with BMD values and reaffirmed that low BMI, more frequently seen in the elderly, causes increased bone loss. Intervention efforts need to take note of these findings and not only respond to individualized assessment of bone condition but also provide lifestyle and dietary support tailored to optimize BMD. Intervention against these risk factors is necessary to reduce the disease burden of osteoporosis. Prevention strategies for osteoporosis are going to need to be multifaceted, including lifestyle modifications, pharmacologic therapies, and public health initiatives. Keeping weight-bearing activity and following a diet rich in calcium and vitamin D are part and parcel of osteoporosis prevention. Moreover, public education campaigns about awareness and the causes of osteoporosis can lead to early screening and interventions in high-risk populations. Pharmacologic treatment may involve bisphosphonates and other medications that are able to inhibit bone loss and BMD acquisition. Following the evidence indicating prevention at early stages for patients at high risk, the clinician must give importance to routine screening with BMD for patients over a certain age or those with previous risk factors. With the implementation of these recommendations, the overall public health impacts of osteoporosis are prevented, finally resulting in stronger bones in populations (Figure 10.15).

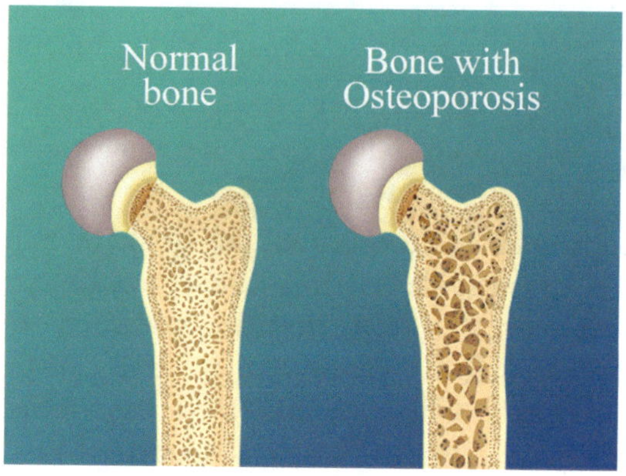

Figure 10.15. Bone with osteoporosis.

Source: https://medigramhospital.com/uploads/blogs/1684503081-osteoporosis-doctor%20in%20saharanpur.png.

10.6.2. Rickets and Osteomalacia

Two important disorders are osteomalacia and rickets, which illustrate the importance of normal bone and mineral metabolism, particularly the roles of phosphate and vitamin D. Rickets is found in children and is related to abnormal mineralization of developing bones, leading to skeletal deformity and growth retardation. The disorder arises primarily due to a deficiency of vitamin D, which regulates calcium consumption and phosphate homeostasis. As deficiency in vitamin D has become more prevalent in certain sections, individuals with limited sunshine exposure and the elderly, knowledge of the risk factors and physiological repercussions has become increasingly important in reducing disease burden in the contemporary era (Diamond et al., 2025). Osteomalacia, which has the same etiology as rickets but typically occurs in adults, causes bone fragility and increased vulnerability to fractures, highlighting the importance of maintaining sustained vitamin D and mineral sufficiency throughout the life cycle. The pathophysiology of osteomalacia and rickets demonstrates the fine balance of vitamin D, calcium, and phosphate in the development of strong bones. In both conditions, impaired mineralization occurs not only as a consequence of vitamin D deficiency but also due to other etiological factors such as nutritional deficiencies and genetic abnormalities influencing mineral metabolism. Another critical element in the knowledge about these disorders is the involvement of fibroblast growth factor-23 (FGF23), an endocrine mediator of phosphate homeostasis that has been the focus in recent studies. Changes in FGF23 regulation and expression can have extremely profound influences on inherited and acquired disorders of phosphate metabolism (Econs et al., 2025). This is evidence of the complexity of bone and mineral metabolism, which is essential in the formulation of effective therapeutic measures and preventive interventions to combat these debilitating diseases. Effective prevention and management of osteomalacia and rickets rely on the treatment of the etiology of deficiencies in vitamin D and minerals. Public health initiatives are increasingly aimed at raising awareness of the benefits of adequate exposure to the sun and vitamin D supplementation through diets, particularly in risk groups. As a substitute for inadequate sun exposure, supplementation is essential for those who cannot expose themselves adequately to the sun, for example, the elderly or those with specific diseases. According to the revised recommendations, prevention of deficiency occurs with 400 IU/d vitamin D per day, and the higher doses are recommended in patients with established vitamin D deficiency (Diamond et al., 2025). In addition, further research on the molecular processes within phosphate metabolism, particularly the role of FGF23, is important in the development of new treatment modalities for rickets and osteomalacia-affected patients, thereby determining the need for a multi-modal strategy in the management of bone (Figure 10.16).

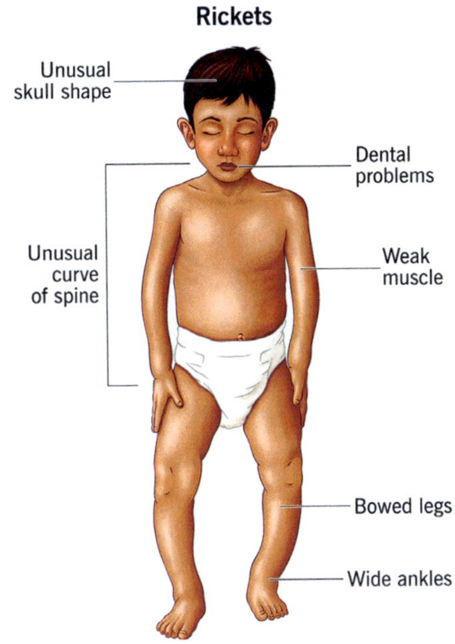

Figure 10.16. Illustration of rickets.

Source: https://my.clevelandclinic.org/-/scassets/images/org/health/articles/22459-rickets.jpg.

10.6.3. Hyperparathyroidism and Its Effects

Hyperparathyroidism, with hypersecretion of parathyroid hormone (PTH), profoundly influences mineral and bone metabolism. In primary hyperparathyroidism, hyperfunction of a parathyroid gland may cause hypermobilization of calcium from the bone through its demineralizing effects and high fracture risk. Hyperparathyroidism not only interferes with bone structure but also mineral homeostasis, predisposing to hypercalcemia and hypophosphatemia. The relationship between high levels of PTH and bone metabolism is also of particular significance, as long-term high exposure to PTH can lead to osteitis fibrosa cystica, a condition characterized by massive alterations in bone tissue. With compromised bone health, the patients can develop symptoms of skeletal pain and enhanced fragility, thereby showing the clinical relevance of early diagnosis and treatment of hyperparathyroidism. Furthermore, secondary hyperparathyroidism (SHPT) is usually established due to renal insufficiency or CKD, wherein the body's regulatory mechanisms become stimulated due to low serum calcium and increased phosphate levels. The condition reflects the body's attempt to maintain mineral balance, but with inappropriate PTH secretion against deranged kidney function. The action of SHPT is multi-faceted: not only does it lead to abnormalities in bone metabolism, including elevated bone resorption, but it also contributes to vascular calcification and cardiovascular disease. Restriction in dietary phosphate, supplemented with adequate calcium and vitamin D, is commonly recommended to manage SHPT and avoid its adverse effects on mineral and bone metabolism (Bargagli et al., 2025). However, the efficacy of these nutritional regimens remains under investigation. Pharmacologic management of hyperparathyroidism has come to rely more on calcimimetics, such as cinacalcet, which assist in lowering PTH concentrations and improving calcium homeostasis in patients with SHPT. Clinical trials demonstrate cessation of such treatment raises serum PTH, calcium, and novel biomarkers of CKD -mineral and bone disorder (CKD-MBD) significantly (Ruderman et al., 2025). Cinacalcet withdrawal is also linked with negative clinical outcomes, including fractures and cardiovascular events, indicating the central role effective pharmacotherapy must play in the control of hyperparathyroidism. As researchers continue to explore long-term management strategies, the implications of hyperparathyroidism on patients' overall health and the importance of individualized therapeutic approaches are becoming increasingly apparent. These findings highlight the need for a comprehensive understanding of hyperparathyroidism's effects on bone and mineral metabolism to optimize patient care (Figure 10.17).

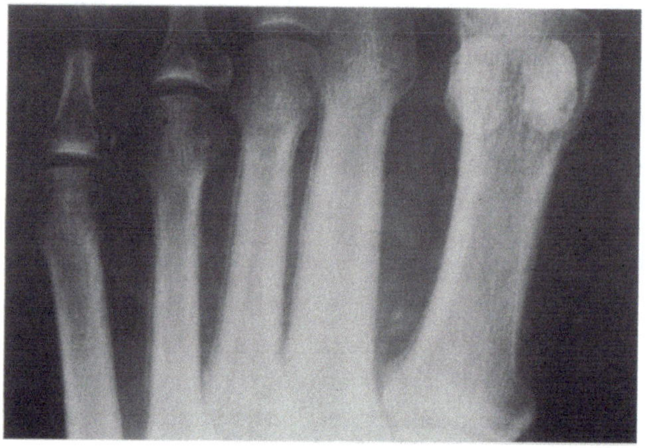

Figure 10.17. Subperiosteal new bone formation in hyperparathyroid bone disease.

Source: https://www.researchgate.net/profile/Neveen-Hamdy/publication/19251521/figure/fig4/AS:339522580697090@1457959899848/Sub-periosteal-new-bone-formation-in-hyperparathyroid-bone-disease-Note-the-periosteal.png.

Test Your Knowledge

1. What are the key risk factors for developing osteoporosis, and how does the condition affect bone density and fracture risk?
2. What are the causes and clinical differences between rickets (in children) and osteomalacia (in adults), and how are they related to vitamin D deficiency?

SUMMARY

The science of bone and mineral metabolism is at the core of understanding the complexity of skeletal disease and health. The intricate dynamic interaction between various minerals, particularly calcium, phosphorus, and magnesium, not only decides bone density but also the metabolic status of patients with chronic conditions. Notably, measurement of serum magnesium in CKD patients reveals an alarming trend toward dysregulation of magnesium as the disease progresses. As shown by current evidence, the prevalence of hypomagnesemia and hypermagnesemia grows in CKD stages G3-G5, representing a direct correlation with disorders of mineral metabolism, specifically CKD-MBD. These trends validate the necessity of routine monitoring of magnesium levels in clinical practice for ensuring timely interventions and minimization of late stages of CKD risks (Cao et al., 2025, pp. 1847–1856). Complemented with traditional approaches, new therapies such as Traditional Chinese Exercise (TCE) are effective adjuncts to the treatment of bone health, especially for postmenopausal osteoporosis patients. Meta-analysis results prove that involvement with TCE not only enhances mineral density of bone but also enhances patients' quality of life in general by enhancing balance and reducing pain. However, the study also revealed no variations in biochemical markers of bone metabolism, further clouding the waters of non-pharmacologic therapies. While TCE presents an encouraging substitute, the clinical significance demands a careful consideration of how such treatments fit into overall bone metabolism strategies. Integrating treatment from both drug and lifestyle domains can offer a clearer view of how to best treat the multifaceted nature of mineral metabolism disorders (Li et al., 2025). Ultimately, the available research concludes that there is an urgent need for an integrated approach in managing mineral and bone metabolism. With chronic diseases such as CKD becoming increasingly prevalent, healthcare providers must highlight patient education, dietary modification, and lifestyle modifications alongside pharmacotherapy. Understanding the interaction of main minerals maximizes the effectiveness of treatment, leading to better outcomes in high-risk patient groups for bone-related complications. With additional research, greater emphasis will be needed to develop individually tailored treatment programs to optimize skeletal health and address the complexities of mineral metabolism diseases. This comprehensive strategy not only will enhance clinical practice but will further our knowledge of the biofeedback mechanisms that regulate bone health and set the stage for future development of treatment methods.

The intricate relationship between bone and mineral metabolism is of utmost importance in maintaining overall health. One of the foundations of this relationship is harmony among various minerals, hormones, and biological processes that maintain bone health. Osteogenesis-osteoclastogenesis balance is of critical significance; any disruption can lead to the development of conditions such as osteoporosis or osteopenia. The bone microenvironment is greatly influenced by extracellular matrices and several signaling pathways, which, in combination, control osteoblast and osteoclast functions. Moreover, new evidence for the way in which dietary components affect mineral absorption, such as calcium and phosphorus, further supports the preeminent place of nutrition in bone health. Such new knowledge underlines those genetic and environmental factors—food lifestyle among them—are prime regulators of bone density and processes of mineralization. The role of the gut microbiota in bone and mineral homeostasis has gained increasing attention in the past decade. Studies show that a well-balanced gut microbiome is able to effectively control the absorption of minerals and influence inflammatory responses, thereby maintaining bone integrity and health. More precisely, the concept of normobiosis pictures a perfect state of gut microbial balance in relation to functional support of positive metabolic activity, e.g., the stimulation of certain microbial populations favorable to mineral absorption. Conversely, dysbiosis can induce a condition of equilibrium disruption with detrimental impacts on metabolic activity and the potential to contribute to long-term diseases. Studies have shown that prebiotic food ingredients are able to selectively stimulate advantageous populations of bacteria, for example, bifidobacteria, which have been shown to be powerfully associated with enhanced calcium intake and, by consequence, increased bone mineral content (Meheust et al., 2025). This illustrates the central significance of gut health in optimizing bone metabolism and managing linked disorders. Chronic kidney disease (CKD) is especially difficult in mineral and bone metabolism, leading to diseases such as hyperphosphatemia and secondary hyperparathyroidism. Elevated levels of fibroblast growth factor 23 (FGF23) have been identified as independent markers for cardiovascular morbidity in patients with CKD, illustrating the systemic nature of mineral imbalance. Therapeutic interventions for phosphate level regulation and anemia management are important here. Auryxia®, as a new agent with the dual capability of a phosphate binder and iron supplement, exhibits a newer approach to robust management of these complications (Bino et al., 2025). Clinical trials highlight its potential effectiveness in relieving mineral disturbances, which reflects its possible use in targeted therapies to improve outcomes among patients. The combined understanding of the impact of CKD on mineral and bone metabolism eventually underscores the necessity of multimodal clinical management strategies in promoting skeletal health.

KEY TERMS FROM THIS CHAPTER

- Adenosine triphosphate (ATP)
- Bone alignment
- Bone measurement
- Bone remodeling
- Calcium homeostasis
- Cellular existence
- Chronic kidney disease (CKD)
- Dysregulation
- Gastrointestinal mineral absorption
- Hormonal regulation
- Inflammatory disease
- Metabolic bone diseases
- Mineral homeostasis
- Musculoskeletal adaptation
- Bone abnormalities
- Bone marrow
- Bone metabolism
- Bone-producing cells
- Calcium-binding protein production
- Cellular pathways
- Diagnostic tools
- Environmental stresses
- Hormonal change
- Hyperphosphatemia
- Meal planning
- Micro-computed tomography (μCT)
- Mineral pathways
- Nutritional deficiency

CRITICAL THINKING QUESTIONS

1. Which of the following structures is primarily responsible for producing new bone tissue?

a. Osteoclasts

b. Osteoblasts

c. Chondrocytes

d. Osteocytes

2. What is the most abundant mineral found in bone tissue?

a. Potassium

b. Sodium

c. Calcium

d. Magnesium

3. Which sequence correctly represents the bone remodeling cycle?

a. Resorption → Activation → Formation → Resting

b. Formation → Resorption → Activation → Resting

c. Resting → Formation → Activation → Resorption

d. Activation → Resorption → Formation → Resting

4. Which nutrient is essential for calcium absorption in the intestines?

a. Vitamin C

b. Vitamin D

c. Vitamin A

d. Vitamin K

5. Which condition is characterized by reduced bone density and an increased risk of fractures?

a. Osteoporosis

b. Osteoarthritis

c. Osteopetrosis

d. Rickets

Short answer Questions

1. What are the structural components of a typical long bone (e.g., diaphysis, epiphysis, periosteum), and how do compact and spongy bone differ in structure and function?
2. Which minerals are essential for bone structure, and how do calcium, phosphorus, and magnesium contribute to bone strength and integrity?
3. How do parathyroid hormone (PTH), calcitonin, and vitamin D work together to maintain calcium and phosphate balance in the body?
4. What are the stages of the bone remodeling cycle, and how do osteoblasts and osteoclasts coordinate bone resorption and formation?
5. How do dietary factors such as calcium, vitamin D, and protein intake influence bone health across the lifespan?
6. What is the role of vitamin D in enhancing intestinal absorption of calcium and phosphate, and how does deficiency impact bone metabolism?
7. What are the causes and consequences of osteoporosis and osteomalacia, and how are they diagnosed and managed?

Answers to Critical Thinking Questions

1. (b) 2. (c) 3. (d) 4. (b) 5. (a)

REFERENCES

1. Aaseth, J., & Alexander, J. (2023). Postoperative osteoporosis in subjects with morbid obesity undergoing bariatric surgery with gastric bypass or sleeve gastrectomy. *Nutrients.* https://www.semanticscholar.org/paper/3c6ac38a3b87c804ca6d418875d3adf182f4723d (accessed on 22nd July 2025).
2. Abrahamsen, B., Adachi, J. D., Adams, J. E., Agrawal, S., Albagha, O. M. E., Aloia, J. F., Armas, L. A. G., et al. (2010). Vitamin D and bone health; potential mechanisms. *MDPI.* https://core.ac.uk/download/pdf/8669791.pdf (accessed on 22nd July 2025).
3. Aghaei, M., Bazrafshan, H. R., Qorbani, M., et al. (2013). Bone mineral density in Iranian patients: Effects of age, sex, and body mass index. https://core.ac.uk/download/52205455.pdf (accessed on 22nd July 2025).
4. Aguilar, A., Benito, S., Bover, J., et al. (2018). Alkaline phosphatases in the complex chronic kidney disease-mineral and bone disorders. *Springer Science and Business Media LLC.* https://core.ac.uk/download/153367114.pdf (accessed on 22nd July 2025).
5. Ahn, Y., Balemans, W., Cui, Y., Fu, H. D., Gong, Y., Harris, S. E., Leupin, O., et al. (2019). Osteocytes and mechanical loading: The Wnt connection. *Wiley.* https://core.ac.uk/download/323269749.pdf (accessed on 22nd July 2025).
6. Ajbage, J. O., Heijsters, G., Politis, C., Salem, et al. (2015). Coronectomy of deeply impacted lower third molar: Incidence of outcomes and complications after one-year follow-up. *Stilus Optimus.* https://core.ac.uk/download/55765860.pdf (accessed on 22nd July 2025).
7. Alcaraz, M. J., Brines, R., Cuadrado, A., et al. (2014). Effects of Nrf2 deficiency on bone microarchitecture in an experimental model of osteoporosis. *Hindawi Limited.* https://core.ac.uk/download/208516037.pdf (accessed on 22nd July 2025).
8. Alelign, T., & Petros, B. (2018). Kidney stone disease: An update on current concepts. *Advances in Urology, 2018*, 1–12. https://doi.org/10.1155/2018/3068365 (accessed on 22nd July 2025).
9. Anonymous, & White, C. L. (2025). Detection and treatment of mineral nutrition problems in grazing sheep. https://core.ac.uk/download/pdf/6377290.pdf (accessed on 22nd July 2025).
10. Arnaud, S. B., & Morey-Holton, E. (2025). Skeletal responses to spaceflight. https://core.ac.uk/download/pdf/42812904.pdf (accessed on 22nd July 2025).
11. Baldari, C., Bimonte, V. M., Di Luigi, L., et al. (2016). Physical activity and hypocaloric diet recover osteoblasts homeostasis in women affected by abdominal obesity. *Springer Science and Business Media LLC.* https://core.ac.uk/download/80310762.pdf (accessed on 22nd July 2025).
12. Bargagli, M., Arena, M., Naticchia, A., Gambaro, G., Mazzaferro, S., Fuster, D., & Ferraro, P. M. (2021). The role of diet in bone and mineral metabolism and secondary hyperparathyroidism. *Nutrients.* https://www.semanticscholar.org/paper/149e0013a8d7da3bad5681d4ad4b5488409f1dbc (accessed on 22nd July 2025).
13. Battino, M., Bullon, P., Giampieri, F., et al. (2016). A systematic review on the implication of minerals in the onset, severity and treatment of periodontal disease. *MDPI AG.* https://core.ac.uk/download/161255425.pdf (accessed on 22nd July 2025).

14. Benavides Damm, T., & Egli, M. (2014). Calcium's role in mechanotransduction during muscle development. *Cellular Physiology and Biochemistry, 34*, 249–272. https://doi.org/10.1159/000356667 (accessed on 22nd July 2025).

15. Bino, A., Ganz, T., & Salusky, I. B. (2019). Mechanism of action and clinical attributes of Auryxia® (Ferric Citrate). *eScholarship, University of California*. https://core.ac.uk/download/323076204.pdf (accessed on 22nd July 2025).

16. Bover, J., Carrero, J. J., Molina, P., Ureña Torres, P., Chauveau, P., & Mazzaferro, S. (2017). Vitamin D, a modulator of musculoskeletal health in chronic kidney disease. *Wiley*. https://core.ac.uk/download/153367338.pdf (accessed on 22nd July 2025).

17. Cao, Y. P., Zhu, L. P., Ge, H. J., Zhang, R. Q., Chen, R. J., Yuan, B., & Shi, W. J. (2025). Impact of serum magnesium levels on mineral-bone metabolism in non-dialysis-dependent chronic kidney disease. *Risk Management and Healthcare Policy, 18*, 1847–1856. https://www.semanticscholar.org/paper/187a49af896f844ee0f3cbe92d073f0b68928644 (accessed on 22nd July 2025).

18. Chiesa, C., Donini, L. M., Lenzi, A., et al. (2017). Non-alcoholic fatty liver disease connections with fat-free tissues: A focus on bone and skeletal muscle. *Baishideng Publishing Group Inc*. https://core.ac.uk/download/98335830.pdf (accessed on 22nd July 2025).

19. Clinkenbeard, E. L., & White, K. E. (2016). Systemic control of bone homeostasis by FGF23 signaling. *Springer Science and Business Media LLC*. https://core.ac.uk/download/84831873.pdf (accessed on 22nd July 2025).

20. Diamond, T. H., Eisman, J. A., Mason, R. S., et al. (2004). Vitamin D in Australia: Issues and recommendations. *The Royal Australian College of General Practitioners*. http://hdl.handle.net/10536/DRO/DU:30002479 (accessed on 22nd July 2025).

21. Díaz-Tocados, J. M., Lloret, M. J., Domínguez-Coral, J. D., Tinoco Aranda, A. P., Fayos de Arizón, L., Massó Jiménez, E., Bover, J., et al. (2025). Magnesium balance in chronic kidney disease: Mineral metabolism, immunosuppressive therapies and sodium-glucose cotransporter 2 inhibitors. *International Journal of Molecular Sciences*. https://www.semanticscholar.org/paper/a8967907aa6500b1600068d0fe4b07dac23d9355 (accessed on 22nd July 2025).

22. Dod, K., Vandna, V., & Thakur, R. (2024). A comprehensive analysis: Prevalence of metabolic bone disease in chronic kidney disease through biochemical profiling. *International Journal of Scientific Research*. https://www.semanticscholar.org/paper/46e865e04b7dbc2fb6d6ca9f4fd27fcd96d3e572 (accessed on 22nd July 2025).

23. Econs, M. J., Hum, J. M., & White, K. E. (2014). Hypophosphatemic rickets: Revealing novel control points for phosphate homeostasis. *Springer Science and Business Media LLC*. https://core.ac.uk/download/46961948.pdf (accessed on 22nd July 2025).

24. Fear, A. L. (2005). *Pre- and Pro-Biotics May Improve Mineral Absorption and Retention in The Growing Male Rat: A Thesis Submitted in Partial Fulfilment of The Requirements for The Degree of Master of Science in Nutritional Science at Massey University, Turitea, Palmerston North, New Zealand. Massey University*. https://core.ac.uk/download/154947106.pdf (accessed on 22nd July 2025).

25. Florêncio-Silva, R., da Silva Sasso, G. R., Sasso-Cerri, E., Simões, M. J., & Cerri, P. S. (2015). Biology of bone tissue: Structure, function, and factors that influence bone cells. *BioMed Research International, 2015*, 1–17. https://doi.org/10.1155/2015/421746 (accessed on 22nd July 2025).

26. Heidari, B., Khashayar, P., Larijani, B., et al. (2014). Dual energy X-ray absorptiometry diagnostic discordance between Z scores and T scores in a young Iranian population. *Tehran University of Medical Sciences*. https://core.ac.uk/download/46560053.pdf (accessed on 22nd July 2025).

27. Iriê, M. S., Rabelo, G. D., Spin-Neto, R., Dechichi, P., Borges, J. S., & Soares, P. B. F. (2018). Use of micro-computed tomography for bone evaluation in dentistry. *Brazilian Dental Journal, 29*, 227–238. https://doi.org/10.1590/0103-6440201801979 (accessed on 22nd July 2025).

28. Khundmiri, S. J., Murray, R. D., & Lederer, E. D. (2016). PTH and vitamin D. *Comprehensive Physiology, 6*, 561–601. https://doi.org/10.1002/cphy.c140071 (accessed on 22nd July 2025).

29. Kumar, A., Cabral-Pinto, M. M. S., Chaturvedi, A. K., Shabnam, A. A., Subrahmanyam, G., Mondal, R., et al. (2020). Lead toxicity: Health hazards, influence on food chain, and sustainable remediation approaches. *International Journal of Environmental Research and Public Health, 17*, 2179. https://doi.org/10.3390/ijerph17072179 (accessed on 22nd July 2025).

30. Li, L., Wang, Y., & Fan, T. (2024). Efficacy of traditional Chinese exercise on postmenopausal osteoporosis: A systematic review and meta-analysis. *Journal of Orthopedic Surgery and Research*. https://www.semanticscholar.org/paper/788b073762531c2a6125e1115e942eb0d3db7546 (accessed on 22nd July 2025).

31. Li, Y., Zhao, P., Jiang, B., Liu, K., Zhang, L., Wang, H., Tian, Y., et al. (2023). Modulation of the vitamin D/vitamin D receptor system in osteoporosis pathogenesis: Insights and therapeutic approaches. *Journal of Orthopedic Surgery and Research*. https://doi.org/10.1186/s13018-023-04320-4 (accessed on 22nd July 2025).

32. Mace, M., Gravesen, E., Nordholm, A., Egstrand, S., Morevati, M., Ølgaard, K., & Lewin, E. (2022). The calcified vasculature in chronic kidney disease secretes factors that inhibit bone mineralization. *JBMR Plus*. https://www.semanticscholar.org/paper/e3554521db5619dc5017380a0032f4f3e465c718 (accessed on 22nd July 2025).

33. Mach, F., Baigent, C., Catapano, A. L., Koskinas, K. C., Casula, M., Badimón, L., Chapman, M. J., et al. (2019). 2019 ESC/EAS Guidelines for the management of dyslipidemias: Lipid modification to reduce cardiovascular risk. *European Heart Journal, 40*, 111–188. https://doi.org/10.1093/eurheartj/ehz455 (accessed on 22nd July 2025).

34. Mahajan, P., & Katoch, S. (2022). Vitamin K: A micro-nutrient with new perspective. *International Journal of Scientific Research in Science and Technology*. https://www.semanticscholar.org/paper/cc5eb2ca3c0200c76b8f418436282cc6711fdf57 (accessed on 22nd July 2025).

35. Martin-Tereso Lopez, J., & Verstegen, M. W. A. (2011). A novel model to explain dietary factors affecting hypocalcaemia in dairy cattle. https://core.ac.uk/download/pdf/29230002.pdf (accessed on 22nd July 2025).

36. Meheust, A., McCartney, A. L., Neyrinck, A. M., Balsari, B., Ben, B., Stahl, B., Watzl, B., et al. (2010). Prebiotic effects: Metabolic and health benefits. *Cambridge University Press (CUP)*. https://core.ac.uk/download/9368.pdf (accessed on 22nd July 2025).

37. Pechmann, L. M., Pinheiro, F. I., Andrade, V., & Moreira, C. (2024). The multiple actions of dipeptidyl peptidase 4 (DPP-4) and its pharmacological inhibition on bone metabolism: A review. *Diabetology & Metabolic Syndrome*. https://www.semanticscholar.org/paper/d5927860e4627658eb1c987cfdde465c40ae5001 (accessed on 22nd July 2025).

38. Ribeiro, A. L., Silva, A. P., Bacchetta, J., Bernheim, J., Block, G., Daya, N., Desjardins, L., et al. (2020). FGF23-klotho axis as predictive factors of fractures in type 2 diabetics with early chronic kidney disease. *Elsevier BV*. https://core.ac.uk/download/288958484.pdf (accessed on 22nd July 2025).

39. Ruderman, I., Smith, E., Toussaint, N., Hewitson, T., & Holt, S. (2018). Longitudinal changes in bone and mineral metabolism after cessation of cinacalcet in dialysis patients with secondary hyperparathyroidism. *BMC Nephrology*. https://www.semanticscholar.org/paper/9dd2c2d79a107e9a36d4c2807d33e5c2a731976d (accessed on 22nd July 2025).

40. Shanahan, C. M., Crouthamel, M. H., Kapustin, A., & Giachelli, C. M. (2011). Arterial calcification in chronic kidney disease: Key roles for calcium and phosphate. *Circulation Research*, *108*, 697–711. https://doi.org/10.1161/circresaha.110.234914 (accessed on 22nd July 2025).

41. Skjøth, J. B., Hagens, T. M., Fleischer, I., Laursen, M., & Andersen, S. (2025). Bone mineral content among Inuit–A systematic review of data. *International Journal of Circumpolar Health*. https://www.semanticscholar.org/paper/8b9f4e5d38c5b022083601b56c9ab95c4017c833 (accessed on 22nd July 2025).

42. Suh, S., & Kim, D. K. (2015). Subclinical hypothyroidism and cardiovascular disease. *Endocrinology and Metabolism*, *30*, 246. https://doi.org/10.3803/enm.2015.30.3.246 (accessed on 22nd July 2025).

43. Taskozhina, G., Batyrova, G., Umarova, G., Issanguzhina, Z., & Kereyeva, N. (2024). The manganese–bone connection: Investigating the role of manganese in bone health. *Journal of Clinical Medicine*. https://www.semanticscholar.org/paper/6893e6efd2d6cf8b847d0c0dbef71e10f6aeeb2a (accessed on 22nd July 2025).

44. Tran, L. (2015). The role of nitric oxide in skeletal simulated microgravity response. *SJSU ScholarWorks*. https://core.ac.uk/download/70426315.pdf (accessed on 22nd July 2025).

45. Wang, B., & Yang, Y. (2018). PTH1R-CaSR cross talk: New treatment options for breast cancer osteolytic bone metastases. *Jefferson Digital Commons*. https://core.ac.uk/download/213444641.pdf (accessed on 22nd July 2025).

46. Wang, G., Meng, Y., Ouyang, W., Zhao, C., & Zhao, W. (2023). Effect of pilose antler polypeptide on the mechanism of bone homeostasis in osteoporosis. *Frontiers in Medicine*. https://doi.org/10.3389/fmed.2023.1289843 (accessed on 22nd July 2025).

47. Wang, Y., Chang, Y., Zhang, P., Zheng, Z., Ai, X., Zhang, S., & Wu, S. (2025). Association between triglycerides and remnant cholesterol levels and spine bone mineral density in Duchenne muscular dystrophy. *Lipids in Health and Disease*. https://www.semanticscholar.org/paper/c414507f13327e0c70cf0d890d06b95210d4bccc (accessed on 22nd July 2025).

48. Williams, M. B., & Watts, S. A. (2019). Current basis and future directions of zebrafish nutrigenomics. *Genes & Nutrition*. https://doi.org/10.1186/s12263-019-0658-2 (accessed on 22nd July 2025).

49. Zamanian, M., Golmohammadi, M., Vadiyan, F. V., Almulla, A. A., Vadiyan, D. E., Morozova, N. S., Alkadir, O., et al. (2024). A narrative review of the effects of vitamin D3 on orthodontic tooth movement: Focus on molecular and cellular mechanisms. *Food Science & Nutrition*, *12*, 3164–3176. https://www.semanticscholar.org/paper/c82bab6526f94ce829c7bd0f3c4a2778d47ea239 (accessed on 22nd July 2025).

ENDOCRINE HYPERTENSION

11

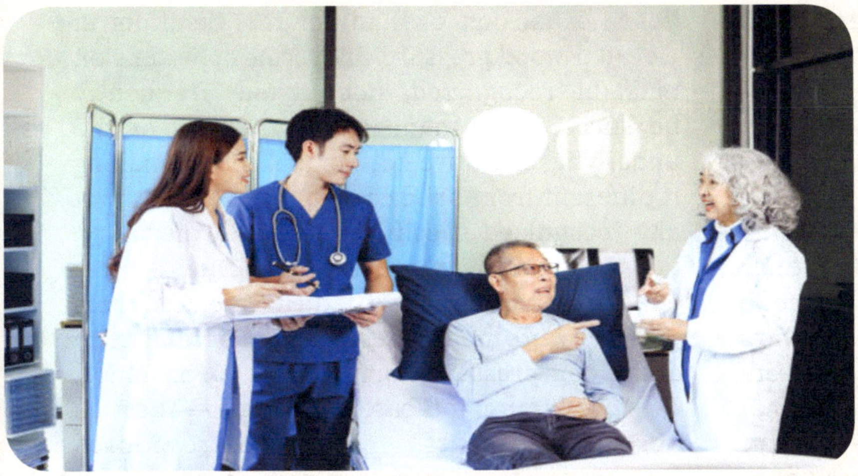

LEARNING OBJECTIVES

After studying this chapter, you will be able to:

1. Understand the types of endocrine hypertension;
2. Discuss the pathophysiology of endocrine hypertension;
3. Focus on the diagnosis of endocrine hypertension;
4. Deal with effective management of endocrine hypertension;
5. Describe complications associated with endocrine hypertension.

Introduction

Hypertension is a major global health issue, affecting millions and causing several cardiovascular diseases. Out of its many etiologies, endocrine hypertension has become noticeable because of its multifaceted pathophysiological mechanisms that tend to overlap with tumor biology. In particular, this condition develops as a consequence of excessive hormone secretion by endocrine glands, which in turn may cause major health problems. Endocrine hypertension is a group of conditions, like primary aldosteronism, Cushing's syndrome, and pheochromocytoma, which are all marked by specific dysregulations in hormones that require a complex understanding for a proper diagnosis and treatment. For this reason, the identification of the association between hormonal imbalance and hypertension is important for designing targeted therapy and enhancing patient outcomes in clinical care. Incidence of primary aldosteronism, identified as one of the most prevalent causes of secondary hypertension, underscores the importance of early diagnosis and treatment. Even so prevalent, the results of studies reveal a disconcerting trend of underdiagnosis in these patients. As described in more recent studies, Endocrine Society guidelines established in 2016 for screening primary aldosteronism remain unfulfilled, accompanied by a concomitant loss of diagnostic and therapeutic potential. The consequences of such a lack of monitoring are significant, as early diagnosis can significantly enhance the prognosis and welfare of patients. Given the difficulty of controlling hypertension in the face of elevated levels of aldosterone, medical professionals must approach with the utmost significance exhaustive screening methods in dealing with patients showing difficult-to-control hypertension, based on recent clinical evidence regarding the subject matter (Ruiz-Sánchez et al., 2024). Other than primary aldosteronism, other endocrine paraneoplastic syndromes (ePNS) carry their own unique complexities in terms of hormone secretion as well as hypertension. ePNS occurs when neoplastic cells inappropriately secrete hormones, leading to disturbances in normal physiology that present clinically as a broad array of clinical manifestations, including hypertension. Ectopic Cushing's syndrome and paraneoplastic acromegaly are two examples of how malignancies can cause severe endocrine disturbances, complicating the overall scenario. Against these facts, clinicians must be vigilant for incipient ePNS when assessing hypertensive patients. Furthermore, knowledge of the interaction between cancer pathology and hormone control can potentially enhance diagnostic utility and therapeutic efficacy in patients in whom conventional hypertension management is a failure, as emphasized by current literature (Quiroz-Aldave et al., 2025). This intersection of oncology and endocrinology is an essential borderland in the ongoing pursuit to effectively control endocrine hypertension.

Definition of Endocrine Hypertension

Endocrine hypertension is a term used to describe increased blood pressure as a result of endocrine disturbances, particularly those related to endocrine disorders. This type of hypertension is typically triggered by inappropriate production of certain hormones like catecholamines, aldosterone, cortisol, and other endocrine regulators. Hyperaldosteronism, Cushing's syndrome, and pheochromocytoma are excellent illustrations of endocrine dysfunction manifesting as hypertension. Under such conditions, hyper-secretion of hormones such as aldosterone increases sodium retention and hence expansion of fluid volume, resulting in elevated blood pressure. Endocrine hypertension must be recognized, since it may frequently be successfully managed by reversal of the underlying causative hormonal disorder, making it different from primary hypertension without any recognized specific etiology. Furthermore, the cross-talk between the endocrine system and hypertension points to the tremendous role played by hormonal messages in vascular tone and blood pressure homeostasis. For instance, overproduction of catecholamines—such as adrenaline—elicits physiological responses that cause vasoconstriction and elevated heart rates. The catecholamine-driven response also worsens the hypertensive condition. In addition to these hormones, the renin-angiotensin-aldosterone axis (RAAS) plays a key role in both the body's fluid homeostasis and the control of blood pressure. Dysregulation of this axis leads to hypertension and is a common condition in diseased states such as kidney disease or heart failure. In conclusion, understanding of the endocrinological foundation of hypertension illuminates the pathogenesis of its cause and directs treatment specifically aimed at the etiology. Moreover, effective endocrine hypertension treatment depends on appropriate diagnosis and familiarity with the various endocrine disorders involved. Diagnosis is most often obtained by assessing hormone concentrations in urine or blood to detect dysregulations. Imaging studies, such as CT scans or MRIs, may also be employed to detect tumor-secreting excess hormones, further determining the cause of hypertension. Treatment once diagnosed involves surgical interventions and pharmacologic therapy aimed at normalizing hormone levels. Pharmacologic therapies such as mineralocorticoid receptor antagonists can exert action over the excess action of aldosterone, while surgery can be required in cases involving the presence of adrenal tumors. Such targeted treatment highlights the importance of a comprehensive understanding of endocrine hypertension, as successful treatment is often feasible through correcting the specific hormonal imbalance present (Jennifer et al., 2021; Mary et al., 2023) (Figure 11.1).

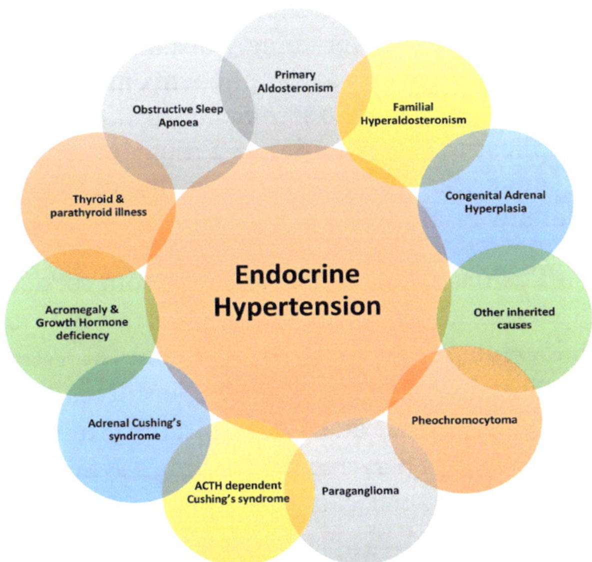

Figure 11.1. Illustration of endocrine hypertension.

Source: https://ars.els-cdn.com/content/image/3-s2.0-B9780323961202000224-mmc01-01-9780323961202.jpg.

Importance of Understanding Endocrine Hypertension

Endocrine hypertension is important to comprehend due to its distinct nature based on primary hypertension as it results from discernible hormonal imbalance. Secondary hypertension of this nature, although less common, can result from the likes of primary aldosteronism, Cushing syndrome, and pheochromocytoma, among others. The uncommon etiology of endocrine hypertension requires a specific diagnostic approach. Accurate identification of the etiology can lead to customized treatment regimens that not only cure hypertension but reverse it as well. By using advanced diagnostic methods, such as liquid chromatography-tandem mass spectrometry, clinicians are able to measure low-level hormones accurately, thus improving patient outcomes in this multicausal disease (Courcelles et al., 2024). In addition, an entire comprehension lessens the chances of misdiagnosis, allowing on-time interventions that significantly influence the patient's health. Treatment for endocrine hypertension is also a reflection of the necessity for ongoing research into its associated biomarkers and therapy strategies. With each increasing knowledge of endocrine illness, new strategies and technologies, particularly through omics approaches, have emerged that hold hopeful avenues for diagnosis as well as treatment. These methods enhance our ability to identify novel biomarkers and targets for therapy, which are crucial in light of the multifactorial pathogenesis of endocrine hypertension (Courcelles et al., 2024). Furthermore, understanding the mechanisms involved may present new sources for developing efficient therapies targeting not only hypertension signs but also the underlying hormonal dysregulations. Thus, continual studies in this field can improve the overall quality of care for patients and reduce the cardiovascular effects of untreated secondary hypertension. Importantly, the impact of endocrine hypertension on health in general cannot be overlooked. The prolonged exposure to elevated blood pressure as a result of endocrine imbalance can lead to life-threatening complications like cardiovascular disease, stroke, and kidney failure. As has been established in many studies, appropriate treatment and early diagnosis of endocrine hypertension can diminish these risks and improve patients quality of life considerably. This emphasizes that clinicians should be very suspicious of patients with hypertension, especially in atypical presentations. By fostering a synergistic perception of endocrine hypertension, doctors are in a position to introduce early treatment programs that combat the hypertension as well as the underlying endocrine causes simultaneously, leading to better cardiovascular health and optimal patient outcomes over the long term. Understanding of the intricacy of the disease is necessary in order to achieve successful treatment as well as intervention, highlighting the synergy between endocrinology and hypertension management in achieving whole care for patients.

11.1. Types of Endocrine Hypertension

Learning Outcome

1. Describe primary hyperaldosteronism;
2. Understand the relationship between Cushing's syndrome and endocrine hypertension;
3. Explain pheochromocytoma.

Endocrine hypertension is a general classification of several different types, each with a cause derived from the specific imbalance of hormones in the body. One of the primary types is primary aldosteronism (PA), and its cause is an excess production of the hormone aldosterone. It significantly affects mineral balance by stimulating sodium retention and potassium elimination, which increases blood volume and leads to hypertension. PA is associated with an augmented prevalence in subjects with severe hypertension and is generally asymptomatic, so awareness and screening are crucial to effective management. The typical clinical presentation is elevated aldosterone with suppressed renin activity, but hypokalemia—a characteristic marker—is found in a minority of patients, reflective of the diagnostic challenge as well as treatment modalities of endocrine hypertension (Tjandra et al., 2025). Another important reason for endocrine hypertension is pheochromocytoma, a rare tumor of chromaffin cells that secretes catecholamines. These chemicals can cause paroxysmal spells of hypertension, accompanied by symptoms of palpitations, headache, and sweating. Pheochromocytoma-associated hypertension may be malignant and resistant to control, requiring a multidisciplinary team approach to its treatment. Diagnosis is typically by measurement of free plasma metanephrines or 24-hour urinary catecholamines, with imaging studies employed for tumor localization. With curable potential, early pheochromocytoma detection is crucial to minimize cardiovascular complications and improve patient outcomes in endocrine disease-associated hypertension (Tjandra et al., 2025).

Cushing's syndrome resulting from cortisol hypersecretion is another significant type of endocrine hypertension. This condition can be caused by a variety of different causes, including adrenal adenomas, pituitary tumors, or ectopic ACTH secretion. Cushing's syndrome hypercortisolemia causes weight gain, insulin resistance, and hypertension through several mechanisms, with increased vascular sensitivity to catecholamines. Elevated cortisol not only contributes to causing hypertension through fluid retention but also has a direct effect on endothelial function. Clinical diagnosis is also often performed by 24-hour urinary free cortisol measurement, late-night salivary cortisol level, and low-dose dexamethasone suppression tests. As in all forms of endocrine hypertension, diagnosis of Cushing's syndrome is crucial to ensure effective therapeutic interventions and improve the quality of life of those afflicted (Tovkai et al., 2024).

11.1.1. Primary Hyperaldosteronism (Conn's Syndrome)

Of the numerous etiologies of endocrine hypertension, Primary Hyperaldosteronism, or Conn's Syndrome, stands out due to its prevalence and distinctive pathophysiologic mechanisms. The condition is characterized by hypersecretion of aldosterone by adrenal adenomas or hyperplasia. The resulting hyperaldosteronism is induced by increased sodium retention, decreased potassium, and resultant hypertension. Clinically, the patient presents with hypertension and hypokalemia of significant severity, which can lead to muscle weakness and arrhythmia. Diagnosis of Conn's Syndrome is based on a detailed assessment of clinical symptoms, electrolytes, and advanced imaging diagnostics that facilitate differentiation of adrenal malignancies from benign hyperaldosteronism states (Pedro et al., 2025). Treatment of Primary Hyperaldosteronism involves multidirectional treatment, and treatment is based on the etiology of hyperaldosteronism. Surgical intervention, in the context of laparoscopic adrenalectomy, is an option in those instances wherein adrenal adenomas are present, leading to great relief from hypertension and correction of metabolic abnormalities. In those instances, wherein surgery is not an option or in bilateral adrenal hyperplasia, drug therapy is the first consideration. Mineralocorticoid receptor antagonists, such as spironolactone and eplerenone, are the gold standard for pharmacological treatment, being able to reverse the effects of aldosterone and mitigate hypertensive complications. In broad summaries, initiation of therapy highlights the significance of early diagnosis and appropriate treatment in avoiding the long-term cardiovascular complications of poorly controlled hypertension (Tarrazona et al., 2024). Despite separate treatment regimens, the diagnosis of primary hyperaldosteronism is difficult to a great extent due to its non-specific clinical features. The fatigue, headache, and palpitations can lead to misdiagnosis or delayed initiation of therapy because they are manifested by more common diseases. Furthermore, the insidious onset of hypokalemia may be undetected in simple laboratory investigations, prompting clinicians to underestimate the likelihood of aldosteronism in patients with hypertension. A high suspicion index, along with diligent laboratory workup, is thus warranted to diagnose the condition in a timely fashion. The increased awareness among clinicians regarding the impact of Primary Hyperaldosteronism not only highlights its position in the picture of endocrine hypertension but also establishes the tone for improved patient outcomes with specific interventions (Pedro et al., 2025) (Figure 11.2).

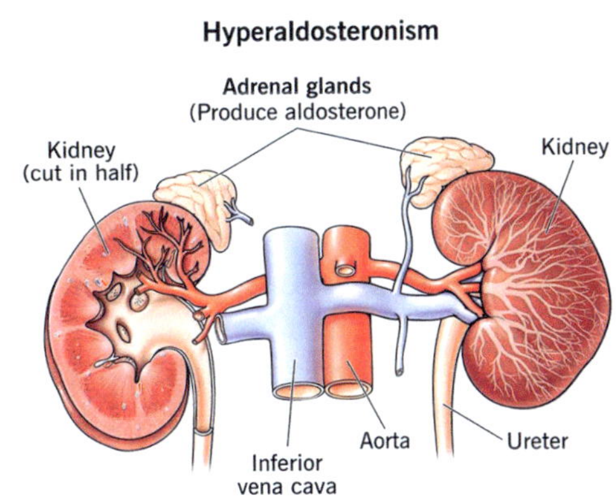

Figure 11.2. Hyperaldosteronism illustration.

Source: https://my.clevelandclinic.org/-/scassets/images/org/health/articles/16448-hyperaldosteronism-illustration.

11.1.2. Cushing's Syndrome

The multifaceted interaction of Cushing's Syndrome with endocrine hypertension serves to emphasize the complexity of hormonal equilibrium in the human organism. Cushing's Syndrome, through its production of excess cortisol, can induce a range of metabolic disturbances, one of which is hypertension.

The excess cortisol leads to sodium retention, elevated vascular volume, and increased sensitivity to catecholamines, which all contribute to increasing blood pressure. Besides, the syndrome may be etiologically caused by many etiologies, such as adrenal adenomas or ectopic ACTH production, complicating the clinical image by potentially hiding the characteristic presentation of hypercortisolism. With the variations in presentation, a diagnosis of Cushing's Syndrome becomes necessary for maximal control of hypertension because untreated cases may result in severe cardiovascular complications, hence increasing morbidity and mortality among those with the condition (Jennifer et al., 2023). Therapy of Cushing's Syndrome involves multidimensional treatment, particularly for its hypertensive effect. Therapy may include surgery or drug therapy aimed at suppressing cortisol secretion. Notably, low-dose ketoconazole has been an acceptable choice for a selected group of patients, with the potential to normalize cortisol production and consequently blood pressure (Jennifer et al., 2023). This drug therapy may be in the form of a minimally invasive procedure for the resistant patients. Practitioners must, however, be watchful of treatment-resistant hypertension, which is often severe in Cushing's Syndrome patients. This kind of status complicates the entire treatment program of the patient and may call for multiple antihypertensive medications to achieve effective blood pressure, particularly for high-risk populations like African Americans. Awareness of the subtle features of Cushing's Syndrome and hypertension uncovers important considerations for clinicians. Follow-up must be regular because the risk of developing treatment-resistant hypertension accumulates with chronicity of hypercortisolism. Diagnostic evaluation must also encompass screening for common comorbid diseases of Cushing's, such as obstructive sleep apnea and chronic kidney disease. Such a comorbid disease may exacerbate the hypertensive burden and should not be overlooked. In addition, patient education on lifestyle variables is critical since weight control, diet modification, and exercise each have an impact on cortisol levels and blood pressure individually. Finally, a combined, multidisciplinary evaluation that addresses both endocrine dysfunction and hypertension will best optimize clinical outcomes in patients with Cushing's Syndrome (Figure 11.3).

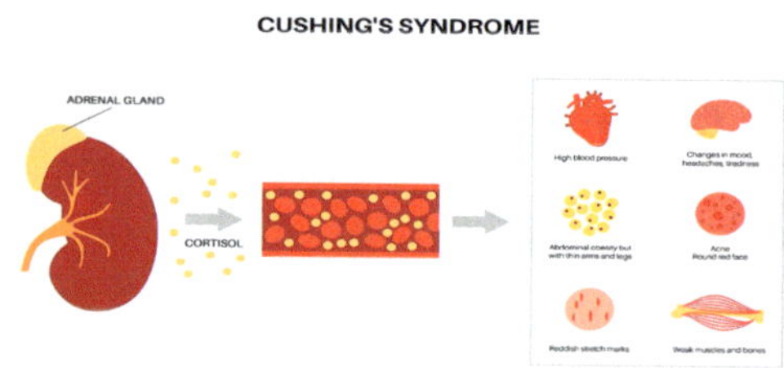

Figure 11.3. Cushing's syndrome (hypercortisolism).

Source: https://www.sog.com.sg/wp-content/uploads/2023/04/SOG-cushings-syndrome.jpg.

11.1.3. Pheochromocytoma

Pheochromocytoma is an endocrine tumor arising from the neuroendocrine family of tumors that occurs infrequently in adrenal gland chromaffin cells and plays a significant role in secondary hypertension as part of endocrine disorders. Pheochromocytoma is characterized by the excessive production of catecholamines, primarily epinephrine and norepinephrine, which lead to episodic or persistent hypertension. Clinical presentation of pheochromocytoma can be misleading, with symptoms such as palpitations, headache, and diaphoresis. Since these symptoms can mimic those of other diseases, diagnosis is a significant challenge. Moreover, the difficulty of diagnosing pheochromocytoma is compounded in pregnancy, where physiological changes render it hard to interpret hormonal alterations and hemodynamic data. As underscored in recent literature, understanding of adrenal tumors, namely pheochromocytomas, in pregnancy is crucial because improper management would result in harmful outcomes for both mother and fetus (Marisa et al., 2022). Pregnancy may be complicated by the development of pheochromocytoma, which also endangers the mother and fetus with severe maternal and fetal complications. The endocrine changes in pregnancy are capable of masking the symptoms of excess catecholamines, thereby making diagnosis more difficult to prompt. Because diagnosis of pheochromocytoma has been based primarily on biochemical laboratory testing and imaging in the past, the physicians also face additional obstacles based on the risk of contraindication of such tests in pregnancy. Even the normal increases in cortisol levels and aldosterone levels in pregnancy are capable of misleading the diagnosis of hypersecretion of adrenal neoplasms like pheochromocytomas. This is an aspect that calls for a good degree of clinical suspicion from clinicians, the necessity for tailored diagnostic approaches that consider the special physiological status of pregnant patients (Alison et al., 2020). Management plans in pheochromocytoma during pregnancy are focused on minimizing maternal and fetal risk and effectively treating the underlying hormonal disorder. In most cases, surgery is considered to be the treatment of choice, especially when the blood pressure is not adequately controlled with medical treatment. Timing is critical; the second trimester has been noted as the best time for the correction by surgery since it poses less risk of miscarriage and preterm labor compared to the first and third trimesters. Multidisciplinary treatment by endocrinologists, obstetricians, and anesthesiologists is required for the preoperative, intraoperative, and postoperative management of the affected patients. Moreover, careful monitoring of catecholamine and blood pressure is also imperative throughout pregnancy to enable both the mother and the baby to achieve an optimal outcome despite this complex endocrinopathy (Alison et al., 2020) (Figure 11.4).

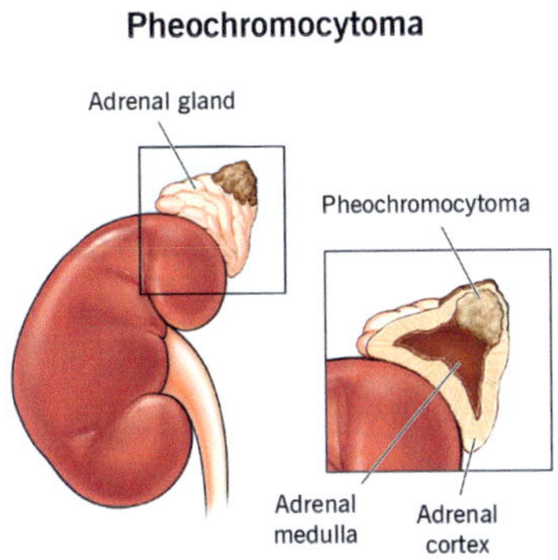

Figure 11.4. Pheochromocytoma.

Source: https://my.clevelandclinic.org/-/scassets/images/org/health/articles/23373-pheochromocytoma.

Test Your Knowledge

1. What is the underlying hormonal abnormality in primary hyperaldosteronism?
2. How does excess cortisol in Cushing's syndrome contribute to the development of hypertension?
3. What are the classic symptoms of pheochromocytoma?

11.2. Pathophysiology of Endocrine Hypertension

Learning Outcome

1. Describe mechanisms of hormonal regulation of blood pressure;
2. Understand the impact of excess hormones on vascular resistance;
3. Discuss the role of the renin-angiotensin-aldosterone system (RAAS).

The pathophysiology of endocrine hypertension is multifactorial, mainly through alterations in hormone secretion leading to deficient homeostatic regulation of blood pressure. Of the various endocrine diseases, primary hyperaldosteronism, involving mainly the excessive secretion of aldosterone by the adrenal cortex, is noteworthy because of its role in the development of hypertension. The elevated level of aldosterone leads to retention of sodium, augmented water reabsorption, and expansion of blood volume, which accounts for hypertension. Moreover, the pathophysiological consequence of this excess hormone extends beyond sodium retention. The ensuing hypernatremia and consequent effects may also cause cardiovascular remodeling, leave ventricular hypertrophy, and increase vascular resistance, also contributing to the maintenance of hypertension. Understanding the intricate signal transduction pathways underlying the action of aldosterone is important, as it highlights the potential for developing targeted therapeutic strategies that specifically counter the hormone's effects on blood pressure regulation. Another significant endocrine cause of hypertension is the production of hypercortisol, which most commonly occurs in Cushing's syndrome. Cortisol influences cardiovascular function in a way that promotes vascular reactivity and sodium retention, hence increasing blood pressure. In these cases, the participation of the sympathetic nervous system becomes more evident. Hypercortisolism can directly stimulate sympathetic nervous activity and exacerbate blood pressure dysregulation. Research has shown that Cushing's syndrome patients typically present with heightened sympathetic activity, which correlates with a myriad of cardiovascular risks. Therefore, the goal in correcting the underlying hypercortisolism is not just to restore normal endocrine function, but also to mitigate the concomitant hypertensive impacts. The interdependent nature of these systems underlines the complexity of endocrine hypertension and the necessity of an integrated approach for successful control. The dialogue between the autonomic nervous system and hormones occupies the center of the pathophysiology of endocrine hypertension. The sympathetic nervous system has been put in the spotlight of research as the key to the development of hypertension, a return of attention following several decades of relative neglect.

The accurate quantitation of sympathetic nerve discharge and its connection to blood pressure regulation has demonstrated that dysregulated activity of the sympathetic nervous system is an important contributor to the perpetuation of high blood pressure in patients. This action is particularly significant with the accompaniment of oversecretion of adrenal hormones, such as catecholamines.

These hormonal disturbances not only increase blood pressure but also induce vascular alterations that provide the basis for the progression of hypertensive disease. This fresh understanding of the mechanism of sympathetic activation in endocrine hypertension, along with hormonal drives like those detailed by Murray et al. (2024), adds fuel to the argument for exploring novel therapies with the ultimate purpose of restoring homeostatic balance and damping the trajectory of hypertension.

11.2.1. Mechanisms of Hormonal Regulation of Blood Pressure

In endocrine hypertension, mineralocorticoid receptor (MR) action in vascular smooth muscle cells (SMCs) is one of the key mechanisms in the control of blood pressure. With advancements in molecular technology in recent times, researchers have been able to selectively knockout SMC-MR in mouse models, thereby shedding light on the finer functions of the receptors in the regulation of the cardiovascular system. Activation of SMC-MR contributes to the regulation of vasomotor tone and blood pressure through various mechanisms, such as the alteration of calcium channels and angiotensin II type-1 receptors. These mechanisms contribute to vasoconstriction and myogenic tone that can increase systemic blood pressure, ultimately influencing the overall hypertensive phenotype of most patients. Moreover, the effect of SMC-MRs on gene expression could explain its function in vascular remodeling and other cardiovascular diseases, emphasizing the significance of this hormone receptor in understanding endocrine hypertension and corresponding pathology, such as heart failure and vascular calcification (Nicholas et al., 2024). Furthermore, hormone participation in blood pressure regulation also extends beyond immediate receptor mechanisms to gene and epigenetic regulation of blood pressure control. Dr. Lewis K. Dahls seminal work elucidated critical interrelationships between renal function, sodium, and hypertension that implicated genetic predispositions heavily in hormonal adaptation. Genome-wide association studies have identified numerous genetic variants associated with hypertension, indicating that blood pressure regulation is a quantitative trait influenced by multiple biological and environmental factors. These results have clarified how particular mutations and changes in gene expression can lead to an increase in blood pressure, indicating a management of hypertension that is of a multidimensional nature, requiring both genetic information and hormonal information (Pandey, 2024). Lastly, in the hormonal model of blood pressure regulation, it is most crucial to understand how systemic hormones modulate local vascular responses. Aldosterone-type hormones are critical in sodium and water retention, and thus, blood volume and pressure. In addition, the interaction between vasodilatory and vasoconstrictive stimuli is crucial to attaining homeostasis.

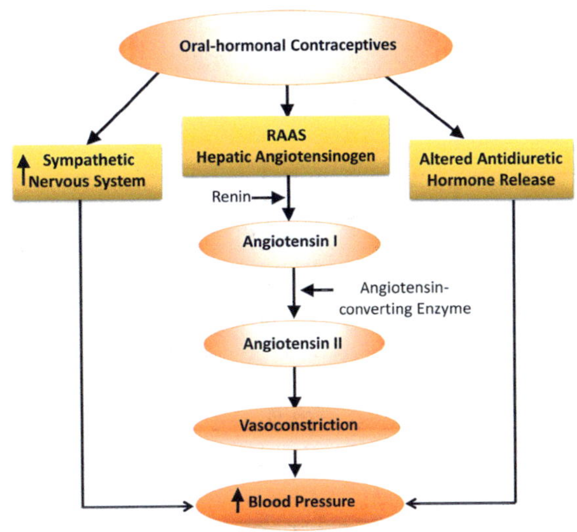

Figure 11.5. A schematic of the mechanism by which oral hormonal contraceptives elevate blood pressure. [RAAS: Renin-angiotensin-aldosterone system].

Source: https://www.researchgate.net/publication/380822525/figure/fig3/AS:11431281291103291@1731922170944/A-schematic-of-mechanism-of-oral-hormonal-contraceptives-in-elevating-blood-pressure.jpg.

Hormonal dysregulation, including aldosterone overproduction or vascular tissue sensitivity to vasodilators, may be a contributory cause of hypertension. Finally, the complex and multifactorial mechanisms of hormone and receptor action must be taken into account when therapeutic targets are available in the management of endocrine hypertension.

Investigations targeting intervention of such pathways potentially have the potential to improve cardiovascular disease outcome, particularly in individuals with resistant hypertension. As more is known about these complex systems, it provides new avenues for the treatment of hypertension that are both effective and personalized (Figure 11.5).

11.2.2. Impact of Excess Hormones on Vascular Resistance

Excess hormones' action on vascular resistance is one of the main factors in endocrine hypertension. Adrenaline, cortisol, and aldosterone are among the hormones that affect vascular tone through contraction and relaxation of the smooth muscles of the blood vessels. For instance, an excess of catecholamines leads to vasoconstriction, which is a result of elevated blood pressure. Such a hyperactive reaction is common in chronic stress diseases, where activation of the sympathetic nervous system produces perpetually high levels of adrenaline. It can thus increase peripheral vascular resistance, leading to hypertension over time. Moreover, the pathophysiological mechanisms behind the alterations involve complex cascades of signaling, like the activation of the mitogen-activated protein kinase (MAPK) cascades that transmit cellular response to inflammation and stress, thus enhancing vascular reactivity and resistance (Chen et al., 2017). Research on glucocorticoids' action presents more proof of their ability to enhance vascular resistance. Elevated cortisol levels could also enhance sodium retention through renal mechanisms, with augmented blood volume and consequent elevated arterial pressure. The link indicates how hormonal imbalance skews physiological homeostasis and leads to chronic hypertension. The following augmentation of vascular resistance due to elevated levels of glucocorticoids can further be attributed to endothelial dysfunction, which ablates vasodilatory responses. This interaction between inflammatory processes and hormones is indeed crucial, since chronic inflammation can feed back onto hormonal regulation in a manner that sustains a loop of vascular injury and increased resistance. Effective management of the hypertensive conditions may thus potentially require addressing not only the treatment of the excess hormone but also the contributory inflammation and its downstream mechanisms (Elliott et al., 2014). The clinical relevance of hormone-induced increased vascular resistance is profound, with significant implications for patient management. The mechanisms through which hormones adjust vascular tone allow clinicians to make evidence-based therapeutic interventions. Therefore, the therapeutic use of antihypertensive drugs can be complemented by interventions to counteract hormone levels or block their action. These can include lifestyle modifications to reduce stress or pharmacological treatments specifically that inhibit the pathological over-signaling pathways produced by hyper-reactive hormones. Furthermore, understanding these interactions can also enhance preventative medical care against developing conditions such as diabetes and metabolic syndrome, which are often highly interconnected with hormone deregulation. With a complete realization of both vascular physiology and hormonal effects, practitioners can manage endocrine hypertension's barriers optimally and improve outcomes in patients (Chen et al., 2017).

11.2.3. Role of Renin-Angiotensin-Aldosterone System (RAAS)

The RAAS has a crucial role in maintaining blood pressure and electrolyte balance, hence being a critical factor in the pathogenesis of endocrine hypertension. The system is activated upon low blood pressure or in the case of decreased sodium chloride delivery to the tubules of the kidney and causes the release of renin from the juxtaglomerular cells of the kidneys. This enzyme converts liver-synthesized angiotensinogen to angiotensin I. Angiotensin I is then converted to angiotensin II by angiotensin-converting enzyme (ACE), mainly in the lungs. Angiotensin II is a potent vasoconstrictor that raises blood pressure and stimulates the adrenal glands to secrete aldosterone, which causes sodium retention and hence increased blood volume, all underlining the pathophysiology of hypertension. Aside from its direct effects on vascular tone and fluid balance, angiotensin II also influences other endocrine systems, thereby potentiating the hypertensive response. For instance, it has been shown to release hormones such as cortisol, which would, in turn, potentially enhance sodium retention and increase vascular reactivity. Furthermore, the RAAS has an inherent link with other hormonal systems such as the natriuretic peptide system and sympathetic nervous system, constituting an interaction network that governs cardiovascular homeostasis. Disruption of this system potentially leads to chronic hypertension and accompanying cardiovascular complications. Recent studies also further elucidate this interaction, with data on the role of vitamin D signaling as a suppressor regulator of RAAS, and vitamin D deficiency perhaps enhancing RAAS activation and exaggerating blood pressure rise in patients (Latic et al., 2022). RAAS antihypertensive drug therapy has increasingly played a critical role in clinical practice, especially with the development of ACE inhibitors, ARBs, and direct renin inhibitors. These medications effectively interrupt the cascade initiated by renin, and consequently, prevent angiotensin II production and its pressor effect. This type of therapy has been immensely effective in lowering blood pressure, preventing cardiovascular events, and improving outcomes among hypertensive patients. However, the heterogeneity of patient response to RAAS inhibitors emphasizes the importance of personalized medicine approaches in the treatment of hypertension. Recent studies are investigating the intricacies of peptide modulation of hormone signaling, as seen in the progress of peptide drug development (Wang et al., 2022). Such emergent knowledge indicates the promise of new therapies possibly targeting RAAS members strategically to more efficiently cure endocrine hypertension (Figure 11.6).

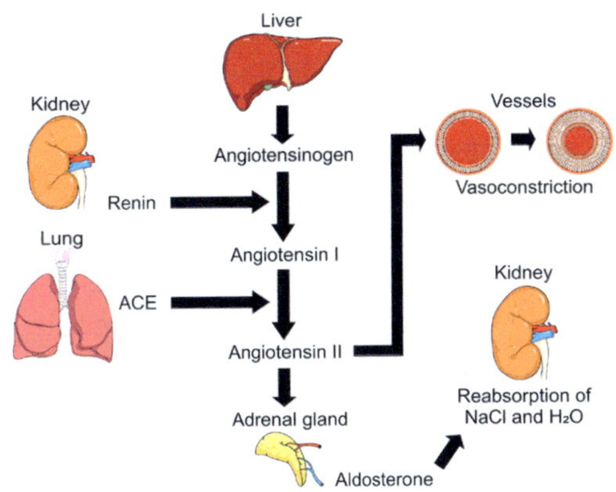

Figure 11.6. Representation of renin-angiotensin-aldosterone system (RAAS)

Source: https://www.researchgate.net/publication/357836725/figure/fig3/AS:11431281187871069@1694449873768/Representation-of-Renin-Angiotensin-Aldosterone-System-RAAS-Regulation-mechanism-of.tif.

Test Your Knowledge

1. How do hormones such as aldosterone, cortisol, and catecholamines influence blood pressure under normal physiological conditions?
2. In what ways do excess cortisol, aldosterone, or catecholamines increase systemic vascular resistance, leading to hypertension?
3. What is the role of the renin-angiotensin-aldosterone system (RAAS) in maintaining blood pressure and fluid balance?

11.3. Diagnosis of Endocrine Hypertension

Learning Outcome

1. Describe clinical symptoms and signs associated with endocrine hypertension;
2. Understand laboratory tests and imaging techniques for the diagnosis of endocrine hypertension;
3. Discuss differential diagnosis in hypertensive disorders.

Endocrine hypertension, an important secondary hypertension category, is diagnosed with the accurate knowledge of its etiologic hormonal origins. Cushing's syndrome, primary aldosteronism, and pheochromocytoma are frequent disorders that induce hypertension through excess hormone overproduction. Most crucial hints are resistant raised blood pressure and unaccountable hypokalemia, especially in primary aldosteronism. The aldosterone-to-renin ratio is particularly valuable in screening for these conditions, with a ratio greater than 200 serving as a critical diagnostic cutpoint. Further, the stratification of patients based on clinical presentation and specific hormone levels enables targeted diagnostic testing, enhancing treatment in endocrine hypertensives (Naruse et al., 2022). In the case of suspected primary aldosteronism, confirmation of hyperaldosteronism is required. This can be followed by a series of confirmatory studies, like saline infusion tests, oral sodium loading, or adrenal vein sampling for lateralization analysis. Confirmatory studies help to distinguish between the diagnosis of unilateral adenomas and bilateral hyperplasia, ultimately guiding treatment decisions toward surgical therapy versus medical therapy. The adrenal function diagnosis in patients with possible adrenal masses also has to include precise hormonal evaluations. This would involve measuring cortisol, ACTH, and other steroid precursors to establish the specific pathophysiology that underlies the hypertension (Fa Mßnacht et al., 2020). Additionally, in the diagnosis of paraganglioma and pheochromocytoma, measurement of plasma-free or urinary-fractionated metanephrines is necessary. These biochemical measurements offer robust screening techniques given the excess of catecholamines in the tumors. The diagnosis is made clinically significant by the presence of symptoms like episodic hypertension, tachycardia, and other manifestations related to catecholamines. Imaging modalities such as CT and MRI aid in localizing these tumors and predicting their metastatic potential, thus deciding the multidisciplinary treatment approach required for endocrine hypertension patients. With advancing research, standards continue to renew diagnostic processes and treatment strategies, demonstrating the interaction between evidence-based medicine and individualized patient care (Fa Mßnacht et al., 2020).

11.3.1. Clinical Symptoms and Signs

The clinical presentation and signs of endocrine hypertension are intricate, typically originating from a hormone imbalance that affects fluid balance and vascular tone. The patients typically present with classically diagnosed hypertension in the form of elevated readings of blood pressure. In addition to this basic symptom, patients may develop secondary signs such as persistent headaches, visual disturbances, and palpitations. Their presence may signal underlying endocrine disease, such as primary hyperaldosteronism or pheochromocytoma, leading to severe hypertension due to peripheral vasculature exposure to excess adrenal hormone. Such clinical features are critical to identify early for effective treatment, as uncontrolled hypertension can lead to end-organ damage. In particular, the relationship between the symptoms and patients' clinical histories can lead healthcare providers to assign appropriate diagnostic tests and treatment modalities of endocrine-related hypertension. A different key characteristic in diagnosing endocrine hypertension is identifying some symptoms with which particular hormonal dysfunctions are associated. For instance, patients with pheochromocytoma may present with paroxysmal syndromes of hypertension accompanied by sweating, pallor, and anxiety, secondary to catecholamine release. Conversely, hyperaldosteronism patients would typically exhibit hypokalemia, leading to muscle weakness and fatigue, among other clinical signs of importance for mineralocorticoid excess. These symptomatologies are not only employed as diagnostic clues but also highlight the necessity for a thorough evaluation of the patient, including a comprehensive physical examination and laboratory investigation. The clinicians must be observant during their clinical assessments, as subtle clinical findings go a long way in establishing the diagnosis of endocrine hypertension secondary to these conditions, thereby providing avenues for early treatment and improved outcomes in patients. Aside from the typical presentations, all endocrine hypertension is accompanied by other comorbidities, which further narrow down the clinical presentation. Obesity, metabolic syndrome, and cardiovascular illnesses are able to accumulate with hormonal imbalances and further exacerbate hypertension. The interaction of endocrine diseases with such comorbid conditions poses a challenge to doctors who must disentangle the cause of symptoms resulting from endocrine disease or those resulting from coexisting medical conditions. Furthermore, there is evidence that dysregulated hormone levels may directly influence the vascular endothelium, potentially causing dysfunctional endothelium, as is presented in COVID-19 and other chronic illnesses. Thus, the treatment of endocrine hypertension must be balanced, taking into account not only the urgency of the effects of hormonal excess but also their impact on overall vascular status and patient well-being, highlighted by Mary et al. (2023) and Varga et al. (2020) (Figure 11.7).

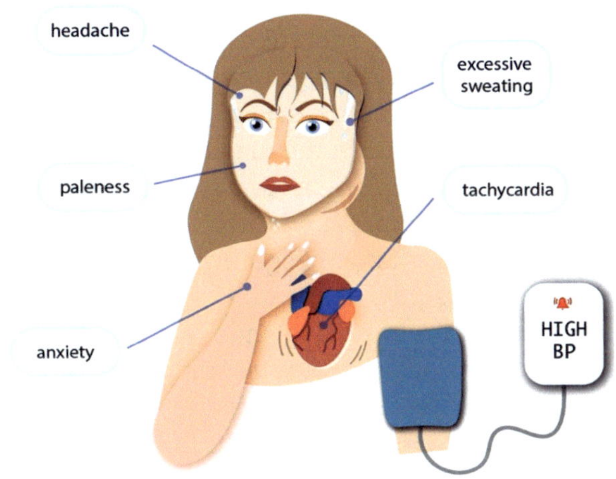

Figure 11.7. Symptoms of pheochromocytoma.

Source: https://www.endocrineharmony.sg/wp-content/uploads/2024/12/Symptoms-of-Pheochromocytoma.png.

11.3.2. Laboratory Tests and Imaging Techniques

Endocrine hypertension is to be diagnosed through an exhaustive method that encompasses laboratory investigations as well as specific imaging modalities. Among the key laboratory studies is the measurement of plasma renin activity and aldosterone concentration, which play a crucial role in the regulation of blood pressure along with body fluid balance. Disequilibrium in these hormones may indicate disorders such as primary hyperaldosteronism or pheochromocytoma, which are both secondary etiologies for hypertension. Additionally, measurement of serum electrolytes, particularly potassium, can provide critical diagnostic information because hyperaldosteronism is typically associated with hypokalemia. Utilizing these laboratory tests in combination with imaging studies increases diagnostic specificity. For instance, imaging studies, including computed tomography (CT) or magnetic resonance imaging (MRI), may be used to image adrenal glands and thereby help identify potential adenomas or tumors that induce hypertension. Imaging techniques play an essential role in the evaluation of patients who are thought to have endocrine hypertension. Of them, adrenal gland imaging is of great importance in the diagnosis of illnesses such as pheochromocytoma, aldosterone-producing adenomas, and Cushing's syndrome. High-resolution imaging equipment, such as CT scans, enables physicians to identify structural variations in the adrenal glands that can disrupt the hormone balance. Additionally, ultrasound can be used to assess the kidneys and their associated vascular pathways for pathology that may lead to hypertension, such as renal artery stenosis. Percutaneous biopsies can also be facilitated by sophisticated imaging modalities as needed, providing valuable diagnosis confirmation. When accompanied by full laboratory tests, imaging studies effectively complement clinicians' diagnostic roles for endocrine-related hypertensive diseases. Advances in laboratory techniques and imaging technology have enhanced early diagnosis and treatment of endocrine hypertension. Recent technologies like high-performance liquid chromatography for the measurement of catecholamines or plasma metanephrines are significant in diagnosing conditions like pheochromocytoma, whose clinical presentation is based on episodic hypertension. Moreover, the incorporation of functional imaging techniques, like PET, can unveil metabolic disturbances of endocrine hypertension. Using a multimodal approach combining both laboratory observation and advanced imaging tools, clinicians are now capable of formulating more targeted treatment plans. These new technologies promise a time in the not-too-distant future when patient-specific management plans will become more feasible, potentially improving patient outcomes for endocrine hypertension at the same time as improving the quality of care provided (Figure 11.8).

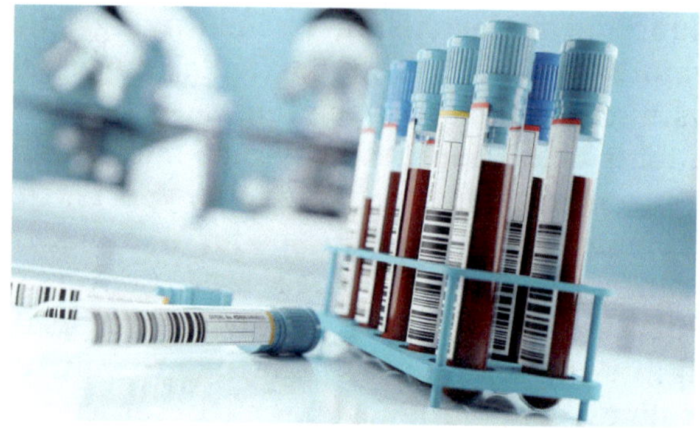

Figure 11.8. Laboratory tests for endocrine hypertension focus on identifying hormonal imbalances that cause high blood pressure.

Source: https://www.sog.com.sg/wp-content/uploads/2023/04/SOG-endocrine-hypertension-diagnosis-1024x623.jpg.

11.3.3. Differential Diagnosis from Other Hypertensive Disorders

Differential diagnosis of hypertensive disorders is essential in distinguishing endocrine hypertension from other hypertensive disorders, i.e., primary hypertension and hypertensive disorders of pregnancy. Endocrine hypertension most commonly arises due to the underlying hormonal imbalance as a result of diseases like pheochromocytoma, primary hyperaldosteronism, or Cushing's syndrome. Proper identification is established through a detailed examination of clinical history, laboratory tests, and imaging. For example, the hyperaldosteronism suspected patients and patients with gestational hypertension may present with metabolic alkalosis and hypokalemia to be differentiated from patients who have gestational hypertension and do not have such electrolyte imbalances. Besides, the multifactorial etiology of hypertensive diseases demands careful clinical evaluation to avoid misdiagnosis and direct appropriate management measures accordingly, which is the essence in view of the increasing maternal risks associated with hypertensive disorders in pregnancy as observed in recent studies (Mawulorm et al.,

2024). In hypertensive conditions, the distinction of chronic hypertension from gestational or preeclampsia becomes important, especially in pregnant women. Chronic hypertension is hypertension that is already present pre-pregnancy or develops before 20 weeks of gestation, while gestational hypertension occurs later than this. In the context of differential diagnosis, the absence of clinical signs typical of preeclampsia, for example, proteinuria or extreme headache, tends to assist in classifying chronic hypertension. Nonetheless, it is essential that clinicians remain vigilant in observation, as changes in conditions such as preeclampsia have significant implications for maternal and fetal outcomes. The new evidence on the link between hypertensive disorders of pregnancy and cardiovascular death highlights the need for accurate differential diagnosis, since a raised risk remains well into the postpartum period (Lee et al., 2024). In addition, incorporating patient history and family history into the process of differential diagnosis can provide valuable insights when considering endocrine hypertension. Familial hyperaldosteronism, for example, predisposes to early-onset hypertension, while secondary hypertension from thyroid disease may have characteristic metabolic profiles. On the part of the practitioner, awareness of these genetic and familial elements is worth everything in arriving at accurate diagnoses. Furthermore, measurement of hormonal levels and dynamic suppressive tests will segregate the etiology of hypertension and will differentiate such disorders from endocrine-independent etiologies. Through advances in the endocrinology field, there is a requirement for ongoing research to refine diagnostic parameters and offer patients individualized treatment guidelines that address the underlying cause of their elevated blood pressure to improve general health outcomes (Mawulorm et al., 2024) (Figure 11.9).

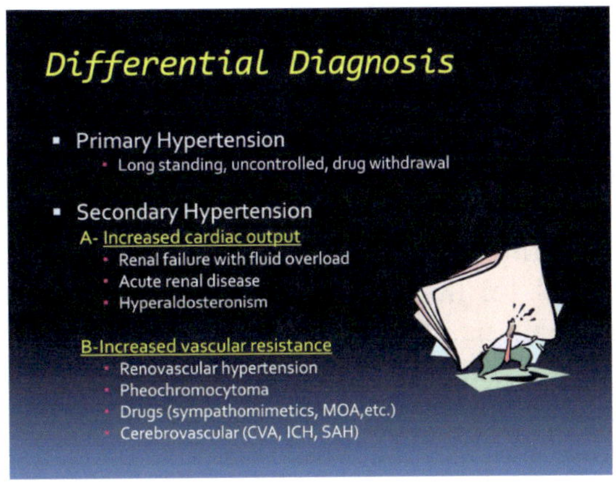

Figure 11.9. Differential diagnosis.

Source: https://image1.slideserve.com/2240586/differential-diagnosis-l.jpg.

Test Your Knowledge

1. What are the key clinical symptoms and signs that may suggest an underlying endocrine cause of hypertension?
2. What specific hormonal blood and urine tests are used to diagnose endocrine hypertension?

11.4. Treatment Options

Learning Outcome

1. Explain how pharmacological interventions play a crucial role in managing endocrine hypertension;
2. Discuss about surgical approaches to managing endocrine hypertension;
3. Focus on lifestyle modifications in the management of endocrine hypertension.

Effective control of endocrine hypertension necessitates a multi-disciplinary approach that often includes surgical, medical, and adjunctive therapy tailored specifically to the underlying pathology. Surgical management is particularly effective in situations such as primary hyperaldosteronism, in which adrenalectomy can be very beneficial in alleviating hypertension. With acromegaly patients, for instance, transsphenoidal surgery has been useful in relieving pressure from pituitary tumors and reducing levels of growth hormone and hence stabilizing blood pressure. Studies indicate that while surgical procedures can yield high levels of improvement, they may not necessarily result in full resolution and thus must be followed up with additional medical care for optimal regulation of hormone levels and also of blood pressure (Hasni et al., 2024). It is thus common for the surgical operation to be complemented with therapies to control hormones in an integrative solution for the management of endocrine hypertension. Pharmacologic treatment is essential in managing endocrine hypertension, particularly when surgery is not adequate or even possible. Such patients are usually treated with several antihypertensives in combination with drugs specifically tailored to inhibit faulty hormonal pathways. For instance, somatostatin receptor ligands (SRLs) were employed to manage hypertension in acromegaly through inhibition of the secretion of growth hormone, and new medications like pasireotide are now available for those not responding to standard treatments (Hasni et al., 2024). Newer therapies targeting various mechanisms for the renin-angiotensin system, the sodium-glucose cotransporter 2, and the nonsteroidal mineralocorticoid receptor antagonists offer additional mechanisms to treat hypertension. Because resistance to conventional antihypertensive drugs is so prevalent in patients with endocrine disorders, these novel pharmacologic agents play a key role in maximizing outcomes and tailoring therapy to the patient's specific requirements. Besides surgery and pharmacologic treatment, patient education and behavioral modification are important components of managing endocrine hypertension. Educating patients regarding the need to follow prescribed regimens and the potential impact of weight management, salt intake, and physical activity can enhance the overall efficacy of treatment. In addition, monitoring and intervening on the basis of a patient's response to the therapeutic regimen is crucial for long-term control of blood pressure. The interaction between patient participation and reinforcement of ongoing management has the potential to lead to improved health outcomes. With evolving research, the incorporation of new therapeutic modalities addressing both hormonal and hemodynamic aspects of endocrine hypertension will continue to fine-tune treatment paradigms with the ultimate aim of enhancing the quality of life in affected patients.

11.4.1. Pharmacological Interventions

Pharmacotherapy plays a significant role in the treatment of endocrine hypertension, particularly when lifestyle changes are insufficient. Various classes of antihypertensive drugs are employed, including diuretics, beta-blockers, ACE inhibitors, and calcium channel antagonists, which all target different mechanisms of high blood pressure. In cases with hypertension that accompany endocrine diseases like hyperaldosteronism or pheochromocytoma, specific therapies such as mineralocorticoid receptor blockers are necessary. These personalized therapies address the root hormonal disarrays causing worsening of hypertension and thus enhance the overall treatment strategy. Effective pharmacologic management addresses not just blood pressure reduction but also the limitation of long-term cardiovascular consequences of untreated hypertension, favoring the use of personalized therapeutic programs based on patient-related conditions and outcomes. Treatment of endocrine hypertension's multifactorial etiology requires a comprehensive insight into the involved pathophysiologic mechanisms. For instance, obesity is an immediate risk factor for various cardiovascular disorders, including hypertension, and demands targeted pharmacological treatments in conjunction with non-pharmacological interventions (Khachatryan et al., 2024). Interactions among body weight, metabolic syndrome, and hypertension may complicate treatment regimens. Recent studies report the effectiveness of diet and weight loss alone, such as DASH and Mediterranean diets, to augment pharmacological regimens, enhancing their efficiency in lowering blood pressure.

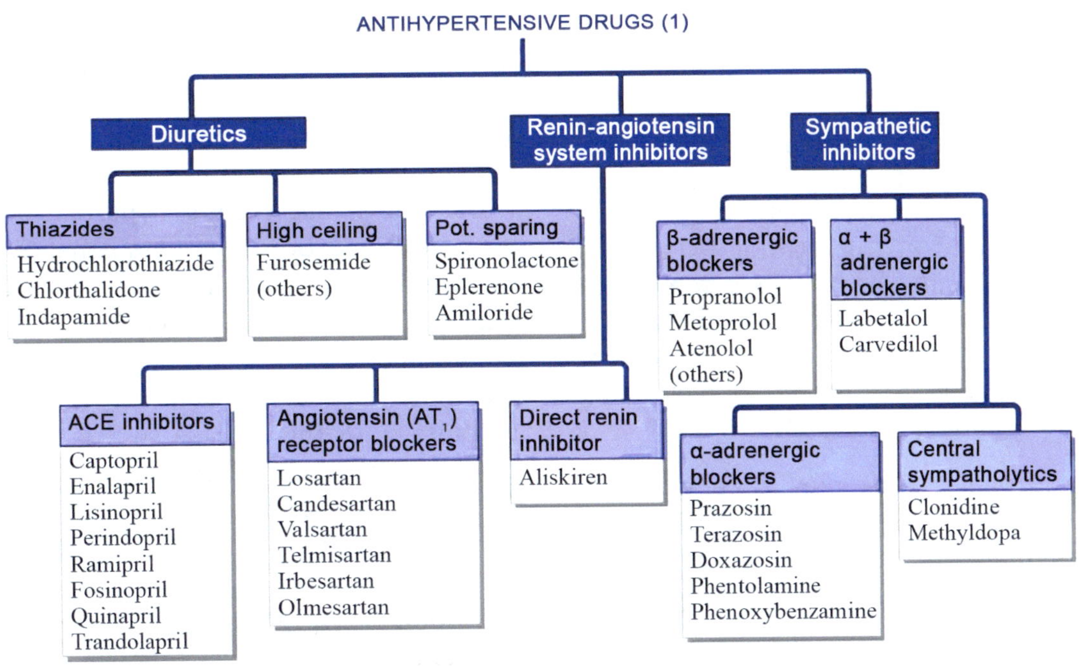

Figure 11.10. Antihypertensive drugs.

Source: https://pharmacyfreak.com/wp-content/uploads/2023/10/Antihypertensive-drugs-1.webp.

Overall, this highlights the importance of a multidisciplinary system in combining lifestyle interventions and pharmacological treatment, so that complex patient profiles receive extensive care tailored to their individualized needs. While traditional antihypertensive medications remain prevalent, the newest developments in treatment options, such as renal denervation, bring new promise for resistant hypertension patients. Approved by the FDA, this treatment is performed through ablating renal sympathetic nerves, taking a neurogenic approach to addressing hypertension (Jennifer et al., 2024). Clinical trials established that renal denervation could provide substantial reductions in blood pressure, specifically in individuals who had been insufficiently responsive to lifestyle changes and conventional pharmacotherapy. The safety profile at this time is promising, yet further investigation is indicated to define long-term outcomes and characterize the patient populations that are most likely to benefit from this treatment. As the treatment of hypertension becomes more subtle, the incorporation of complex therapy with basic pharmacologic regimens reinforces the dynamic nature of the treatment of endocrine hypertension and the necessity of ongoing research and patient management to optimize treatment regimens (Figure 11.10).

11.4.2. Surgical Approaches

Surgical treatment of endocrine hypertension can offer curative therapy for judiciously selected patients, particularly those with a delineable underlying etiology. Primary hyperaldosteronism, pheochromocytoma, and Cushing's syndrome are some conditions that might need surgical intervention to restore normal blood pressure levels by correcting abnormal hormone production.

The adrenal glands play a central role in the secretion of blood pressure-regulating hormones; therefore, their removal by surgery in cases of hyperfunction not only targets the focal point of disease but has the potential to reverse or greatly alleviate hypertension. In addition, early diagnosis and surgical intervention minimize the risk of severe end-organ damage, as demonstrated by the rise in cardiovascular complications and renal failure in untreated patients (Borozan et al., 2025). These interventions are priceless, as they change the therapy of endocrine hypertension from a largely pharmacologic practice to one that can be effective in addressing the underlying cause. Other than adrenal disease, surgery may also be applied in renal-related disorders that evoke endocrine hypertension. For instance, surgical interventions utilized to correct renal artery stenosis may be effective in improving the blood pressure control significantly in subjects with secondary hypertension. These procedures not only treat the hypertension but also prevent further complications, such as end-organ damage. In addition, the area of surgical techniques encompasses newer technology such as laparoscopic adrenalectomy, which is useful with faster recovery and reduced morbidity compared to open surgery. The utilization of minimal invasive techniques has increased the number of surgical alternatives for endocrine hypertension, and it currently presents a less frightening alternative for clinicians and patients (Dell, 2024). As the realization of surgical efficacy evolves, utilization of the interventions is of greater significance in the worldwide management of hypertension. While surgery unquestionably offers benefits, proper selection of patients is the key to optimal outcomes. Endocrine hypertensive patients must be thoroughly evaluated to identify the patient most likely to benefit from surgery compared to those with the disease sufficiently treated by the application of medical interventions. Considering patient-specific variables such as age, comorbidities, and overall health status is crucial while planning treatment. Surveillance algorithms integrating surgical methods with maintenance of medical therapy can provide a continuum of care that changes over time to suit the patients' needs. As the clinician's setting matures towards precision medicine, clinicians are initiated to remain updated on innovations in surgical techniques and their applicability to patient outcomes (Borozan et al., 2025). These innovations provide room for a less overt treatment model for endocrine hypertension, contrasting the benefits of surgical procedures with patient-specific care strategies (Figure 11.11).

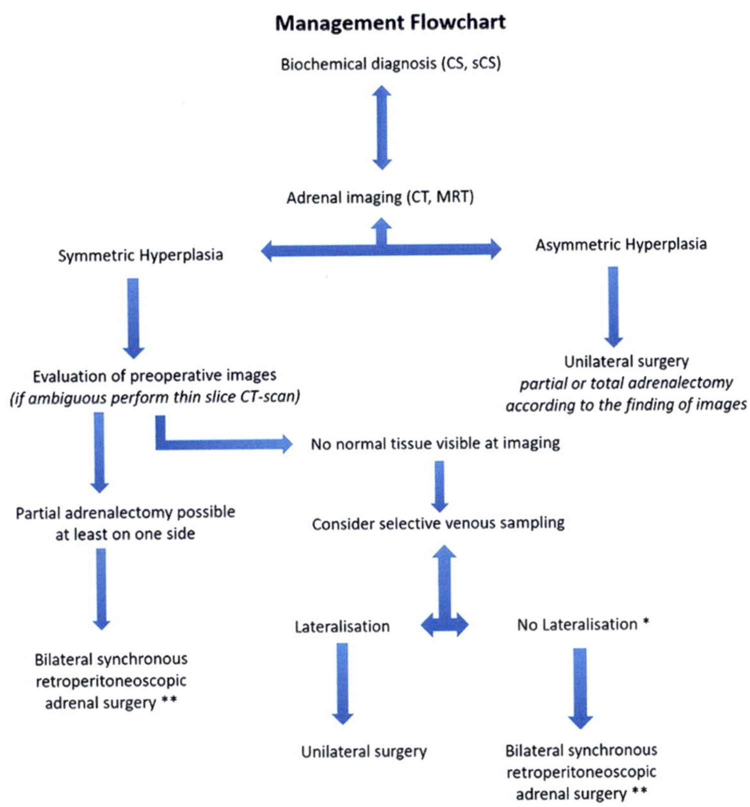

Figure 11.11. Flowchart outlining the management approach and surgical decision-making strategy. Consider observation for asymptomatic patients with subclinical Cushing syndrome (*). If possible, prefer cortical-sparing surgery on the left side (**).

Source: https://www.researchgate.net/publication/314126920/figure/fig3/AS:960133697904653@1605925120683/Flow-chart-outlining-the-management-approach-and-surgical-decision-making-strategy.gif.

11.4.3. Lifestyle Modifications

Lifestyle adjustments have become a key component of managing endocrine hypertension, which in many instances controls therapeutic interventions in addition to medical interventions. Lifestyle adjustments typically entail alterations in dietary habits, improvements in exercise, and reductions in stress. Adhering to a low-sodium and potassium-rich diet can have a significant impact on blood pressure and vascular health as a whole. In terms of emphasizing fruits, vegetables, whole grains, and fats, it is beneficial not just for weight control but also serves to counteract the comorbid diseases associated with high blood pressure. Apart from this, as suggested in several studies, individuals with regular aerobic exercise demonstrate substantial improvement in sustaining both blood pressure and metabolic factors, which lies at the center of controlling endocrine-related hypertensive diseases (Alexander et al., 2022). In addition to diet and exercise interventions, changes in behavior have been found to be essential to the attainment of long-term results. The use of formal self-monitoring techniques encourages active participation in one's health care. A daily record of food intake, activity, and measuring blood pressure allows individuals to see patterns and contributors to their status. Furthermore, developing support groups, either through group therapy or community initiatives, can maximize adherence to lifestyle changes. Feeling responsible, coupled with increased motivation through such joint efforts, is highly advantageous for people who have health issues. Indeed, the integration of life-style change is essential; not only does it cure symptoms of endocrine hypertension, but it also promotes general well-being, highlighting the multidimensional nature of effective interventions in health management (Alexander et al., 2022). The implementation of lifestyle change stretches further than transient relief of symptoms, with an impact on long-term effects on health from endocrine hypertension. As studies show, those individuals who successfully introduce lasting changes to lifestyle manage to attain significantly lowered levels of cardiovascular risk factors and thereby enhance the quality of their life. Notably, this is particularly critical in the management of widespread conditions such as obesity, which is often accompanied by endocrine hypertensive disorders. Interventions for weight management, such as encouraging exercise and healthy eating, address not only hypertension but also prevent the attendant complications of diabetes and dyslipidemia. Therefore, experts must bring these combined approaches to the forefront to respectfully manage endocrine hypertension within a more effective and holistic healthcare strategy beyond simplistic reliance on drugs alone to foster a better continuum of healthy lifestyles among those at risk or already affected (Alexander et al., 2022).

Test Your Knowledge

1. What classes of medications are used to manage hypertension caused by endocrine disorders?
2. What are the key considerations in monitoring patients after surgery for endocrine hypertension to ensure resolution and prevent recurrence?

11.5. Complications Associated with Endocrine Hypertension

Learning Outcome

1. Understand the intersection of endocrine hypertension and cardiovascular risks;
2. Discuss renal implications in the context of endocrine hypertension;
3. Explain the impact on quality of life with endocrine hypertension.

The intricate interaction between endocrine hypertension and its associated complications heightens a region of great concern within endocrinology. Endocrine hypertension, often precipitated by diseases such as primary hyperaldosteronism and Cushing's syndrome, has the potential to result in a variety of adverse health consequences. The individuals experiencing high blood pressure due to overproduction of hormones are likely to experience cardiovascular complications, including left ventricular hypertrophy and heart failure. Such complications are not sporadic events; rather, they trigger a cascade of health events that aggressively disable quality of life. Consequently, the disabling effects of endocrine hypertension can result in increased morbidity and mortality, and thus early intervention and long-term management strategies need to be implemented to consider such risks. Moreover, the metabolic effects of endocrine hypertension can't be overlooked. Patients with conditions like polycystic ovary syndrome (PCOS) typically exhibit a range of complications, including insulin resistance and obesity, which are exacerbated by hypertension. The interplay of these metabolic derangements has the potential to raise the risk for subsequent complications, including type 2 diabetes and dyslipidemia, particularly among patients with PCOS, where endocrine dysregulation adds to impaired metabolic status. As proposed by recent studies, hormonal imbalances and obesity can be addressed by utilizing specific nutritional treatment to achieve sizeable improvement in metabolic and hypertensive status, as determined in studies highlighting the efficacy of dietetic control of such complications (Kang, 2025). Furthermore, an inflammatory response that is typical of endocrine disease increases the risk for cardiovascular disease. An activated inflammatory state can potentially contribute to the change in arterial function and structure and is most pivotal in hypertension pathogenesis. This favors the investigation of the underlying mechanisms that sustain the interrelationship between low-grade chronic inflammation and increased blood pressure. For instance, dietary interventions, such as the DASH diet, have been shown to be encouraging in bringing about alterations in inflammatory markers and improving both hormonal and metabolic profiles in PCOS patients (Zohrabi et al., 2023). Thus, management of inflammatory pathways, along with the best possible control of endocrine hypertension, is of paramount importance to a complete treatment regimen, ultimately encouraging improved patient outcomes and reducing the occurrence of secondary complications.

11.5.1. Cardiovascular Risks

In exploring the connection between endocrine hypertension and cardiovascular risks, it should be remembered that in addition to the specific cardiovascular effects considered here, elevated blood pressure overall brings with it greater overall cardiovascular consequences. Hypertension is an uncontested risk factor for a wide variety of cardiovascular events, including heart attack, stroke, and heart failure. The presence of endocrine disorders, such as primary hyperaldosteronism or Cushing's syndrome, can exacerbate hypertension, resulting in a sharp increase in cardiovascular morbidity and mortality. New evidence has shown a synergistic interaction between metabolic diseases and cardiovascular health, and adipose tissue dysfunction at the core of promoting hypertension and subsequent cardiovascular complications. By addressing these underlying endocrine impairments, practitioners are able to diminish resulting cardiovascular risk factors substantially and potentially improve patient outcomes and quality of life in patients who have hypertension (Mary et al., 2023). The fact that hypertensive patients often have comorbidities makes management of cardiovascular risk all the more complex. Endocrine-derived variables such as insulin resistance and dyslipidemia have synergistic effects on increasing cardiovascular risk profiles, calling for a multidisciplinary treatment approach. For example, patients with both dyslipidemia and hypertension experience an additive effect leading to increased risk for adverse cardiovascular events. Further, the growing body of research emphasizes the correlation between nonalcoholic fatty liver disease (NAFLD) and cardiovascular risk in the hypertensive group. Because these patients also carry other metabolic diseases, early discovery and management of such conditions are of paramount significance in reducing cardiovascular risk from endocrine hypertension (Varga et al., 2020). Multidisciplinary therapeutic strategies involving lifestyle, drug, and interventional therapy are required to maximize cardiovascular outcomes among this high-risk population. In addition to the direct repercussions of hypertension and its metabolic complications, the evolving clinical situation of infectious illnesses such as COVID-19 also emphasizes cardiovascular risks of endocrine hypertension. The endothelial damage caused by endocrine disease has the potential to make an individual predisposed to serious complications of viral infection. Studies indicate that COVID-19 has a propensity to exacerbate preexisting cardiovascular disease and lead to endotheliitis, resulting in increased cardiovascular morbidity. This interaction signifies the immediate and secondary pathways through which endocrine hypertension can exert its influence on cardiovascular health. It thus necessitates vigilant cardiovascular follow-up and control in the context of these patients. As we are increasingly confronted with the challenge of hypertension from the endocrinological viewpoint, it increasingly becomes evident that the resolution of these interconnected disease states is of prime importance if we are to ameliorate patient outcomes and care (Varga et al., 2020) (Figure 11.12).

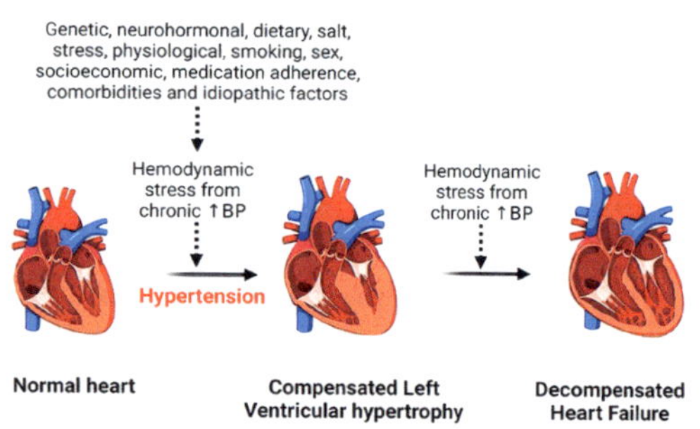

Figure 11.12. Effect of chronic hemodynamic stress on the heart.

Source: https://www.researchgate.net/publication/371685758/figure/fig1/AS:11431281168881900@1687159234819/Effect-of-chronic-hemodynamic-stress-on-the-heart-Chronic-hypertension-resulting-from.tif.

11.5.2. Renal Implications

Renal presentations in the context of endocrine hypertension are sophisticated, and thus a sophisticated understanding of how endocrine derangements affect renal function is necessary. Hormonal derangement, particularly for aldosterone and angiotensin II, plays an essential role in regulating renal hemodynamics and electrolyte balance. Stimulation of the RAAS by the existence of hypertension can potentially lead to increased vascular resistance and impaired renal perfusion. Thus, such changes may contribute to secondary hypertension, ischemic nephropathy, and eventual renal failure unless treated. The realization of such dynamics takes support in improved management methods that are aimed at preventing long-term renal damage, and the emphasis is on early identification and intervention in the hypertensive population, especially those with indicative features of renal insufficiency or other related dysfunctions. The effect of antiphospholipid syndrome (APS) on renal health exemplifies the multifaceted relationship between endocrine elements and renal pathophysiology. APS subjects often form renal artery and vein thrombosis, resulting in renal function loss. The disease, despite its complications in diagnosis due to the multifaceted nature of presentation, often results in hypertension, proteinuria, and renal insufficiency, according to research findings on aPL-nephropathy (aPL-N) (Hoxha et al., 2025). Pathogenic processes include antiphospholipid antibody-mediated thrombotic and inflammatory pathways to the renal vasculature. The complications underscore the need for clinicians to exercise both clinical wisdom and state-of-the-art diagnostic techniques in the treatment of endocrine hypertension with suspected APS. Management of the underlying pathophysiology with appropriate therapy is crucial for the best patient outcome and preservation of renal function. Renal artery stenosis (RAS) is another dangerous condition that deserves attention due to its etiologic contribution to the development of renovascular hypertension (RVH). Pathophysiology of RAS is marked by decreased renal perfusion, which activates the RAAS and causes secondary hypertension and subsequent nephropathy (Shao et al., 2025). While treatment modalities have shifted—from medical therapy to procedures like renal artery stenting—the dilemma persists regarding the most effective treatment modalities. Recent evidence, for instance, from the HERCULES trial, has demonstrated notable reductions in blood pressure following stenting, particularly in individual patient subsets (Shao et al., 2025). However, patient selection and optimization of these therapies remain controversial, highlighting the requirement for additional investigation to maximize therapy. Thus, therapy of RAS not only improves blood pressure control but also overall renal function and avoids long-term endocrine hypertension-related complications (Figure 11.13).

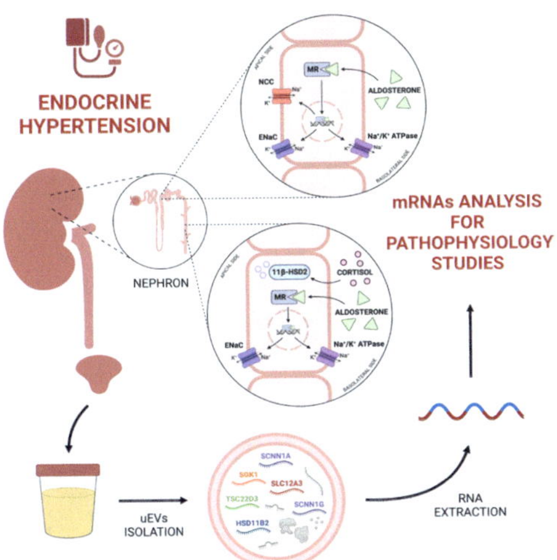

Figure 11.13. Renal implications in the context of endocrine hypertension are multifaceted, necessitating a thorough understanding of how hormonal imbalances affect renal function.

Source: https://images-provider.frontiersin.org/api/ipx/w=1200&f=png/https://www.frontiersin.org/files/Articles/1155011/fendo-14-1155011-HTML-r1/image_m/fendo-14-1155011-g001.jpg.

11.5.3. Impact on Quality of Life

The prevalence of endocrine hypertension has measurable effects on quality of life (QoL) for individuals who experience it. Endocrine disorders such as primary aldosteronism or pheochromocytoma, which cause elevated blood pressure, can initiate a constellation of physical symptoms such as headaches, tiredness, and risk of cardiovascular events.

Adding the physical symptoms to the stress and psychological burden of managing a chronic illness, these factors have a strong effect to detract from an individual's sense of well-being. These are usually communicated to the patient by them as reduced capacity for physical or social activity, leading to depression and isolation. The support systems and treatment plan must be developed by the healthcare providers, keeping in mind both psychosocial factors as well as the medical treatment; the holistic impact of endocrine hypertension must be considered (Jennifer et al., 2021).

Moreover, endocrine hypertension is also treated by complex medication regimens and lifestyle changes that can further compromise QoL. Antihypertensive medications can inflict side effects upon patients, including dizziness or gastrointestinal distress, which can interfere with medication compliance. The never-ending cycle of frequent visits to physicians for monitoring and follow-up can also result in stress or feelings of anxiety that consume mental well-being.

This is added for patients with comorbidities as they would be confronted with the problem of integrating various treatment regimens. Hence, its holistic provision by interprofessional teams of endocrinologists, dietitians, and mental health professionals becomes pertinent to alleviate the patient's burden and optimize their overall QoL (Kirchhof et al., 2016). Moreover, quality of life assessment of endocrine hypertensive patients must incorporate not only clinical and physiological determinations but also the patients' subjective experiences of daily life. Scales of emotional, social, and physical function may prove highly useful in a patient population to determine how the condition impinges on the lives of patients. Interventions that incorporate both lifestyle modification and psychological counseling have been proven through research to achieve dramatic QoL improvements. Engagement of patients in shared decision-making for their treatment is found to empower them and enhance adherence to health-related behavior. Ultimately, by taking into account the multifaceted impact of endocrine hypertension on QoL, clinicians can better individualize interventions that address the whole spectrum of patient needs so that treatment is not only confined to blood pressure control but also improves overall life satisfaction and disease outcome (Jennifer et al., 2021).

Test Your Knowledge

1. How does endocrine hypertension increase the risk of cardiovascular complications?
2. What are the effects of prolonged endocrine hypertension on kidney function, and how can it lead to chronic kidney disease?
3. How can the symptoms and complications of endocrine hypertension affect a patient's daily functioning and psychological well-being?

SUMMARY

In reviewing endocrine hypertension, it is apparent that endocrine hypertension represents a significant intersection of hormonal deregulation and cardiovascular disease. Hormonal action, including aldosterone and catecholamines, is fundamental; they can result in sustained increases in blood pressure as well as increased risk of cardiovascular events. Significantly, studies have shown that patients with hypertension tend to present with comorbid diseases that exacerbate their condition, indicating the need for comprehensive treatment protocols. A knowledge of the nuances of endocrine control is important for healthcare providers, given its direct connection to diagnosis and treatment protocol, indicating the need for a complete understanding of patient history in treating endocrine-related hypertension effectively. In addition, the importance of clinical practice is vast in terms of potential impact because effective control of endocrine hypertension may profoundly affect outcome. Clarification of pathophysiologic mechanisms present allows rational therapeutic approaches, which can include lifestyle intervention and drug therapy according to specific needs. In addition, comorbid conditions' relation to poor outcome suggests screening for endocrine illness in hypertensive patients regularly. Accordingly, integrative models of care that include endocrinology and cardiology have the potential to be extremely helpful to manage this multi-factorial disorder. With a high level of evidence supporting the productivity of such models, there is a need for healthcare organizations to commit to facilitating their implementation to enhance care delivery. Ultimately, ongoing research into the pathophysiology of endocrine hypertension continues to reveal novel therapeutic targets. As highlighted by other studies, managing risk factors such as obesity and diabetes along with hypertension is crucial in a bid to improve prognosis. The COVID-19 pandemic has also illustrated the vulnerability of the hypertensive population, particularly those with other comorbidities, as reflected by their increased mortality rates (Grasselli et al., 2020; Guan et al., 2020). Thus, there is a need to strive more for public health education on prevention and early intervention strategies. In conclusion, awareness of the multifactorial nature of endocrine hypertension will enable healthcare practitioners to combat this silent public health disorder effectively, ultimately improving the quality of life and care in affected patients.

In conclusion of the key aspects of endocrine hypertension, it is essential to appreciate its severity and various hormonal mechanisms controlling blood pressure. One of the key conditions underlying secondary hypertension is primary aldosteronism (PA), the most prevalent endocrine origin of secondary hypertension. Primary aldosteronism can lead to chronic hypertension and carries serious cardiovascular implications when untreated. Research has identified that PA continues to be underdiagnosed, and this necessitates enhanced vigilance among clinicians. This needs to be followed through with better educational practices in medical school, as consensus among experts implies recognition of PA should be incorporated into the evaluation of hypertensive patients. This data could prompt timely interventions, ultimately transforming patient outcomes for hypertension treatment, illustrating the importance of effectively closing knowledge gaps in clinical practice (Ryan et al., 2025). Furthermore, management strategies for endocrine hypertension must incorporate not only pharmacotherapy but also surgical interventions in the final analysis. For instance, in cases where the hypertension arises as a direct consequence of adrenal tumors or hyperplasia, interventions such as adrenalectomy can yield excellent outcomes in the management of blood pressure. Moreover, guidelines have emphasized the importance of thoroughly considering patients who develop progressive pulmonary hypertension, thereby establishing optimal practices for intervention. Interventions such as atrial septal defect and lung transplant are central to treatment consideration, particularly for non-responders to conventional therapies. Such strategies reflect a holistic response to treatment-resistant cases, reflective of flexible and robust clinical practice that places emphasis on patient-focused care (Ryan et al., 2025). Lastly, proactive screening of endocrine-related causes and ongoing education on hypertension are needed. Reinforcing medical training courses with newer evidence and management regarding endocrine hypertension will help promote improved awareness and clinical practice. Specialists recommend training medical students in necessary epidemiological data portraying how awareness regarding PA in patients with hypertension is vital, with emphasis on a diagnostic approach paradigm shift. Such aggressive treatment not only assists in the management of endocrine hypertension complexity but also aligns with broader public health goals to reduce morbidity with uncontrolled hypertension. With this emergent awareness cultivated within the medical community, we can expect continued improvement in treatment paradigms, which ultimately translates to improved health outcomes in patients with endocrine hypertension (Widjaja et al., 2024).

KEY TERMS FROM THIS CHAPTER

- Adrenal tumors
- Aldosterone-producing adenomas
- Angiotensin-converting enzyme (ACE)
- Arterial pressure
- Biochemical laboratory testing
- Cardiovascular complication
- Cardiovascular morbidity
- Disease-associated hypertension
- Dysregulated activity
- Endocrine hypertension
- Epigenetic regulation
- Hormone aldosterone
- Hypertensive complications
- Hypokalemia
- Inflammatory processes
- Aldosterone levels
- Anesthesiologist
- Antihypertensive medications
- Bilateral adrenal hyperplasia
- Blood pressure control
- Cardiovascular diseases
- Catecholamines
- Disequilibrium
- Endocrine dysfunction
- Endothelial damage
- Glucocorticoids
- Hormone secretion
- Hypertensive conditions
- Individualized treatment guidelines
- Interventional therapy

CRITICAL THINKING QUESTIONS

1. **Which of the following is NOT a common type of endocrine hypertension?**
   a. Primary hyperaldosteronism
   b. Pheochromocytoma
   c. Cushing's syndrome
   d. Essential hypertension
2. **What is the main pathophysiological mechanism behind primary hyperaldosteronism causing hypertension?**
   a. Excess catecholamine secretion leading to vasoconstriction
   b. Excess cortisol causes sodium retention and volume expansion
   c. Excess aldosterone causes sodium retention and potassium excretion
   d. Increased thyroid hormone causes increased cardiac output
3. **Which of the following is the gold standard test for diagnosing pheochromocytoma?**
   a. Plasma free metanephrines measurement
   b. 24-hour urinary cortisol
   c. Serum aldosterone-to-renin ratio
   d. Dexamethasone suppression test
4. **What is the first-line management for primary hyperaldosteronism?**
   a. Beta-blockers
   b. Corticosteroid replacement therapy
   c. Surgical removal of adrenal adenoma or mineralocorticoid receptor antagonists
   d. Calcium channel blockers
5. **Which of the following is a common complication of untreated endocrine hypertension?**
   a. Pulmonary fibrosis
   b. Left ventricular hypertrophy and heart failure
   c. Osteoporosis
   d. Peripheral neuropathy

Short Answer Questions

1. What are the common types of endocrine hypertension, and which hormones are involved in each type?
2. How does primary hyperaldosteronism lead to hypertension? Describe the underlying pathophysiology.
3. Explain the role of pheochromocytoma in causing endocrine hypertension.
4. What diagnostic tests are used to differentiate between the various causes of endocrine hypertension?
5. How is endocrine hypertension diagnosed through biochemical and imaging studies?
6. What are the main principles in the effective management of primary hyperaldosteronism?

Answers to Critical Thinking Questions

1. (b) 2. (c) 3. (a) 4. (c) 5. (b)

REFERENCES

1. Affinati, A. H., & Auchus, R. (2020). Endocrine causes of hypertension in pregnancy. *Gland Surgery*, *9*(1), 69–79. https://www.semanticscholar.org/paper/0e4caf7fe8185c7fe91f333369c90c3b2a5801ec (accessed on 22nd July 2025).
2. Angelidi, A. M., Stefanakis, K., Chou, S. H., Valenzuela-Vallejo, L., Dipla, K., Boutari, C., Ntoskas, K., et al. (2024). Relative energy deficiency in sport (REDs): Endocrine manifestations, pathophysiology and treatments. *Endocrine Reviews*. https://www.semanticscholar.org/paper/76d59d9e1c1e0ee1d5d6c171b55850a6d5d9c146 (accessed on 22nd July 2025).
3. Bartz-Kurycki, M. A., Dream, S. Y., & Wang, T. S. (2022). Surgical treatment of adrenal tumors during pregnancy. *Reviews in Endocrine & Metabolic Disorders*, *24*, 107–120. https://www.semanticscholar.org/paper/ded31995cfcefac427637084f946c95477a1b8b5 (accessed on 22nd July 2025).
4. Borozan, S., Kamrul-Hasan, A., Shetty, S., & Pappachan, J. M. (2025). Approach to endocrine hypertension: A case-based discussion. *Current Hypertension Reports*, *27*. https://www.semanticscholar.org/paper/9a137979e239bce04aad622aa6bbf2d52dc41963 (accessed on 22nd July 2025).
5. Camarda, N. D., Ibarrola, J., Biwer, L. A., & Jaffe, I. (2024). Mineralocorticoid receptors in vascular smooth muscle: Blood pressure and beyond. *Hypertension*, *81*, 1008–1020. https://www.semanticscholar.org/paper/727c9dd264670141fc7a2fad7a8f3840a0fee91a (accessed on 22nd July 2025).
6. Chen, L., Deng, H., Cui, H., Fang, J., Zuo, Z., Deng, J., Li, Y., et al. (2017). Inflammatory responses and inflammation-associated diseases in organs. *Oncotarget*, *9*, 7204–7218. https://doi.org/10.18632/oncotarget.23208 (accessed on 22nd July 2025).
7. Cluett, J. L., Blazek, O., Brown, A. L., East, C., Ferdinand, K. C., Fisher, N. D. L., Ford, C. D., et al. (2024). Renal denervation for the treatment of hypertension: A scientific statement from the American Heart Association. *Hypertension*, *81*, e135–e148. https://www.semanticscholar.org/paper/f927a92812c153c1b71e6e9154adcb19dd423c95 (accessed on 22nd July 2025).
8. Coleman, R. D., Cohen, S. P., Eghtesady, P., Grady, R. M., Morales, D. L. S., Hayes, D., Ruminjo, J. K., et al. (2025). Summary for clinicians: Clinical practice guideline on interventional strategies for children with progressive pulmonary hypertension despite optimal therapy. *Annals of the American Thoracic Society*. https://www.semanticscholar.org/paper/561c6dff128a15d4f3491578351cefbb9bd5922a (accessed on 22nd July 2025).
9. Courcelles, L., Stoenoiu, M., Haufroid, V., Lopez-sublet, M., Boland, L., Wauthier, L., Beauloye, C., et al. (2024). Laboratory testing for endocrine hypertension: Current and future perspectives. *Clinical Chemistry*. https://www.semanticscholar.org/paper/21078ee49b2112bb5dc51b0bff296b44a4e00f5a (accessed on 22nd July 2025).
10. Dell'Atti, L. (2024). Current treatment options for erectile dysfunction in kidney transplant recipients. *Sexual Medicine Reviews*. https://www.semanticscholar.org/paper/3eb722145a351ada0ef9725ba392e85e70115164 (accessed on 22nd July 2025).
11. Denu, M. K. I., Shankara, S. B., Shao, C., Tak, K., Do, K., & Kovell, L. C. (2024). Abstract P107: Training for home blood pressure monitoring among women with a diagnosis or risk factors for hypertensive disorders of pregnancy. *Hypertension*. https://www.semanticscholar.org/paper/7f3bbb8f4175912ad62467dd439267c8fc2a3687 (accessed on 22nd July 2025).

12. Elliott, P., Anastasakis, A., Borger, M. A., Borggrefe, M., Cecchi, F., Charron, P., Hagège, A., et al. (2014). 2014 ESC Guidelines on diagnosis and management of hypertrophic cardiomyopathy. *European Heart Journal, 35*, 2733–2779. https://doi.org/10.1093/eurheartj/ehu284 (accessed on 22nd July 2025).

13. Esler, M. D., Osborn, J. W., & Schlaich, M. (2024). Sympathetic pathophysiology in hypertension origins: The path to renal denervation. *Hypertension*. https://www.semanticscholar.org/paper/92ed443d759b53efcfd50b9e9d0d9c51e1f4e180 (accessed on 22nd July 2025).

14. Faßnacht, M., Assié, G., Baudin, E., Eisenhofer, G., de la Fouchardière, C., Haak, H. R., de Krijger, R. R., et al. (2020). Adrenocortical carcinomas and malignant phaeochromocytomas: ESMO–EURACAN Clinical Practice Guidelines for diagnosis, treatment and follow-up. *Annals of Oncology, 31*, 1476–1490. https://doi.org/10.1016/j.annonc.2020.08.2099 (accessed on 22nd July 2025).

15. Flack, J., Buhnerkempe, M. G., & Moore, K. T. (2024). Resistant hypertension: Disease burden and emerging treatment options. *Current Hypertension Reports, 26*, 183–199. https://www.semanticscholar.org/paper/a268a53723a0ca76b9c3bbef50d1fba6ae4e7626 (accessed on 22nd July 2025).

16. Grasselli, G., Zangrillo, A., Zanella, A., Antonelli, M., Cabrini, L., Castelli, A., Cereda, D., et al. (2020). Baseline characteristics and outcomes of 1591 patients infected with SARS-CoV-2 admitted to ICUs of the Lombardy Region, Italy. *JAMA, 323*, 1574. https://doi.org/10.1001/jama.2020.5394 (accessed on 22nd July 2025).

17. Guan, W., Liang, W., Zhao, Y., Liang, H., Chen, Z., Li, Y., Liu, X., et al. (2020). Comorbidity and its impact on 1590 patients with COVID-19 in China: A nationwide analysis. *European Respiratory Journal, 55*, 2000547. https://doi.org/10.1183/13993003.00547-2020 (accessed on 22nd July 2025).

18. Guzmán Ramos, P. J., & Shiel, R. E. (2025). Hyperaldosteronism (Conn's syndrome) in cats. *In Practice*. https://www.semanticscholar.org/paper/b08c67764fb1e4ee09d9483695517f6e5e8ec7c3 (accessed on 22nd July 2025).

19. Hasni, Y., Nouira, S., El Fekih, H., Thabet, M., Ssafi, W., Thabet, N., Halloul, I., et al. (2024). Management strategies for mixed GH and prolactin-secreting macroadenomas following surgical failure: A case report. *Journal of Innovations in Medical Research*. https://www.semanticscholar.org/paper/675902c6358b9beb71c1f5b016a6b9a894969b68 (accessed on 22nd July 2025).

20. Hatfield, J. S., Godar, C. M., Vietor, N. O., Hoang, T. D., & Shakir, M. (2023). FRI266 Medical management of Cushing's syndrome caused by primary bilateral macronodular adrenal hyperplasia (PBMA) with low dose of ketoconazole. *Journal of the Endocrine Society, 7*. https://www.semanticscholar.org/paper/0c9b88c049b24c7f939cba860b824569463009d6 (accessed on 22nd July 2025).

21. Hoxha, A., Del Prete, D., Condonato, I., Martino, F. K., Lovisotto, M., Nalesso, F., & Simioni, P. (2025). Perspective on renal involvement in antiphospholipid syndrome: Implications for diagnosis, pathogenesis, and treatment. *Journal of Clinical Medicine, 14*. https://www.semanticscholar.org/paper/7a7d4cdc7ae8699d5a33286728ccb67ebca930e1 (accessed on 22nd July 2025).

22. Kang, X. (2025). The prognostic value of serum prolactin (PRL), testosterone (T), follicle-stimulating hormone (FSH), and luteinizing hormone (LH) and inflammatory markers in obese patients with polycystic ovary syndrome after treatment with clomiphene citrate, antihypergly. *Journal of Medical Biochemistry*. https://www.semanticscholar.org/paper/7e051e487445b87e82c73008f8fc736e406f29f7 (accessed on 22nd July 2025).

23. Khachatryan, M. T., Zhernakova, J. V., Blinova, N. V., & Chazova, I. (2024). Study of various dietary interventions in patients with hypertension and metabolic syndrome. *Systemic Hypertension*. https://www.semanticscholar.org/paper/5fe63ea8bbd1c95c0556bda373a7898441382d69 (accessed on 22nd July 2025).

24. Kirchhof, P., Benussi, S., Kotecha, D., Ahlsson, A., Atar, D., Casadei, B., Castellà, M., et al. (2016). 2016 ESC Guidelines for the management of atrial fibrillation developed in collaboration with EACTS. *European Heart Journal, 37*, 2893–2962. https://doi.org/10.1093/eurheartj/ehw210 (accessed on 22nd July 2025).

25. Konstantinidis, C., Zachariou, A., Evgeni, E., Çayan, S., Boeri, L., & Agarwal, A. (2025). Recent advances in the diagnosis and management of retrograde ejaculation: A narrative review. *Diagnostics, 15*. https://www.semanticscholar.org/paper/920b2a3a92eb95b3d8baaa3b977fb79fddb041a1 (accessed on 22nd July 2025).

26. Lai, J. C., Tandon, P., Bernal, W., Tapper, E. B., Ekong, U. D., Dasarathy, S., & Carey, E. J. (2021). Malnutrition, frailty, and sarcopenia in patients with cirrhosis: 2021 practice guidance by the American Association for the Study of Liver Diseases. *Hepatology, 74*, 1611–1644. https://doi.org/10.1002/hep.32049 (accessed on 22nd July 2025).

27. Latic, N., & Erben, R. G. (2022). Interaction of vitamin D with peptide hormones with emphasis on parathyroid hormone, FGF23, and the renin-angiotensin-aldosterone system. *Nutrients, 14*, 5186. https://doi.org/10.3390/nu14235186 (accessed on 22nd July 2025).

28. Lee, R., Brandt, J., Joseph, K. S., & Ananth, C. (2024). Pregnancy-associated mortality due to cardiovascular disease: Impact of hypertensive disorders of pregnancy. *Pediatric and Perinatal Epidemiology*. https://www.semanticscholar.org/paper/028b558f66bb01fd9b3e29bd8ecb6cfbc7a19198 (accessed on 22nd July 2025).

29. Leung, A. K. C., Wong, A. H. C., & Hon, K. L. E. (2022). Childhood obesity: An updated review. *Current Pediatric Reviews, 20*, 2–26. https://doi.org/10.2174/15733963186662208010932 25 (accessed on 22nd July 2025).

30. Lyon, A. R., López-Fernández, T., Couch, L. S., Asteggiano, R., Aznar, M. C., Bergler-Klein, J., Boriani, G., et al. (2022). 2022 ESC Guidelines on cardio-oncology developed in collaboration with the European Hematology Association (EHA), the European Society for Therapeutic Radiology and Oncology (ESTRO) and the International Cardio-Oncology Society (IC-OS). *European Heart Journal, 43*, 4229–4361. https://doi.org/10.1093/eurheartj/ehac244 (accessed on 22nd July 2025).

31. Naruse, M., Katabami, T., Shibata, H., Sone, M., Takahashi, K., Tanabe, A., Izawa, S., et al. (2022). Japan Endocrine Society clinical practice guideline for the diagnosis and management of primary aldosteronism 2021. *Endocrine Journal, 69*, 327–359. https://doi.org/10.1507/endocrj.ej21-0508 (accessed on 22nd July 2025).

32. Odion-Omonhimin, L. O., Marwizi, F. M., Chive, M., Obasi, N. B., Akinrinmade, A. O., Obitulata-Ugwu, V. O., Victor, F., et al. (2022). Etiology and management of treatment-resistant

hypertension in African American adults ≥18 years: A literature review. *Cureus, 14.* https://www.semanticscholar.org/paper/fbc74f5bf18904ddaaf8dd634d770582499360a3 (accessed on 22nd July 2025).

33. Pandey, K. (2024). Genetic and epigenetic mechanisms regulating blood pressure and kidney dysfunction. *Hypertension (Dallas, Tex.: 1979), 81*, 1424–1437. https://www.semanticscholar.org/paper/faba2a954979ed783ae8bdf68c5d5afb03740700 (accessed on 22nd July 2025).

34. Quiroz-Aldave, J., Suarez-Rojas, J., Gamarra-Osorio, E., Rivera-Fabián, K., Durand-Vásquez, M., Concepción-Urteaga, L., Paz-Ibarra, J., et al. (2025). Paraneoplastic endocrine syndromes: A contemporary overview. *Expert Review of Endocrinology & Metabolism, 20*, 51–62. https://www.semanticscholar.org/paper/a53546b4f6d1baec927980ebf3d6937a8b68f44f (accessed on 22nd July 2025).

35. Rinella, M. E., Neuschwander-Tetri, B. A., Siddiqui, M. S., Abdelmalek, M. F., Caldwell, S. H., Barb, D., Kleiner, D. E., et al. (2023). AASLD Practice Guidance on the clinical assessment and management of nonalcoholic fatty liver disease. *Hepatology, 77*, 1797–1835. https://doi.org/10.1097/hep.0000000000000323 (accessed on 22nd July 2025).

36. Ruiz-Sánchez, J. G., Fernández Sánchez, Á., Cárdenas-Salas, J., Fernández-Cagigao, Y., Alegre Bellassai, E. R., Rossello, M. G., Fernandez-Fernandez, B., et al. (2024). Primary aldosteronism prevalence enhanced by strict adherence to 2016 Endocrine Society guidelines: Insights from an endocrine hypertension unit. *Journal of Hypertension, 42*, 1813–1822. https://www.semanticscholar.org/paper/cdcf458ee847a95cf23bd081562a243f0efa40eb (accessed on 22nd July 2025).

37. Shao, C., Chi, G., Li, F., Ren, H., Zhang, L., Yang, J., Wang, B., et al. (2025). Impact of renal artery stenosis on renovascular hypertension and the therapeutic role of renal artery stenting: A comprehensive review. *Kidney & Blood Pressure Research.* https://www.semanticscholar.org/paper/a572d1902ff86b333eaff9e2d98a719cfcf881b3 (accessed on 22nd July 2025).

38. Tarrazona-Dominisac, R. T., Lantican, M., & Aragon, J. B. (2024). 7697 Co-existing overt Cushing syndrome and primary aldosteronism secondary to unilateral adrenal adenoma. *Journal of the Endocrine Society, 8.* https://www.semanticscholar.org/paper/14362c4c81e8b85731e7763f24b81f9937bb1422 (accessed on 22nd July 2025).

39. Tjandra, M., Moningkey, S. I., & Lim, H. (2025). The influence of the severity of obstructive sleep apnea on the incidence of hypertension. *Medicinus.* https://www.semanticscholar.org/paper/b6c5893996fd56e425883b6bf3b520de267a45e0 (accessed on 22nd July 2025).

40. Tovkai, O., Grossman, A., Yuzvenko, T., & Pankiv, V. (2024). Primary aldosteronism and cardiovascular risk. *Clinical Endocrinology and Endocrine Surgery.* https://www.semanticscholar.org/paper/53c88312c735a7df31c1be42f14c1f9d97523661 (accessed on 22nd July 2025).

41. Varga, Z., Flammer, A. J., Steiger, P., Haberecker, M., Andermatt, R., Zinkernagel, A. S., Mehra, M. R., et al. (2020). Endothelial cell infection and endotheliitis in COVID-19. *The Lancet, 395*, 1417–1418. https://doi.org/10.1016/s0140-6736(20)30937-5 (accessed on 22nd July 2025).

42. Wang, A., Chang, H., Luo, D., Wang, H., Lv, H., Yu, W., & Wang, F. (2025). From imaging techniques to laboratory tests: A multimodal stratification for varicocele-associated decreased semen quality. *Basic and Clinical Andrology, 35.* https://www.semanticscholar.org/paper/613db066fd196f00a2cfd505bbe9aa81bea1590f (accessed on 22nd July 2025).

43. Wang, L., Wang, N., Zhang, W., Cheng, X., Yan, Z., Shao, G., Wang, X., et al. (2022). Therapeutic peptides: Current applications and future directions. *Signal Transduction and Targeted Therapy, 7.* https://doi.org/10.1038/s41392-022-00904-4 (accessed on 22nd July 2025).
44. Widjaja, J., Yang, J., & Harrison, J. (2024). Improving diagnosis of primary aldosteronism through education: A modified Delphi study to identify key learning points. *Therapeutic Advances in Chronic Disease, 15.* https://www.semanticscholar.org/paper/4d938fd5084c92362a12d1b026b25d66f0850eaf (accessed on 22nd July 2025).
45. Zohrabi, T., Sheikhha, M. H., Jambarsang, S., Nadjarzadeh, A., Aflatoonian, A., & Mozaffari-Khosravi, H. (2023). Effect of dietary approaches to stop hypertension, and standard diets with and without curcumin on interleukin-1 alpha, 5-alpha reductase gene expressions, and androgenic and glycemic profile in polycystic ovary syndrome women undergoing *in vitro* fertilization treatment: A study protocol. *International Journal of Reproductive Biomedicine, 21,* 433–442. https://www.semanticscholar.org/paper/f34bb71df6cfc1155928fafcb31f49208eabafaa (accessed on 22nd July 2025).

HORMONES OF THE GASTROINTESTINAL TRACT AND LIVER

12

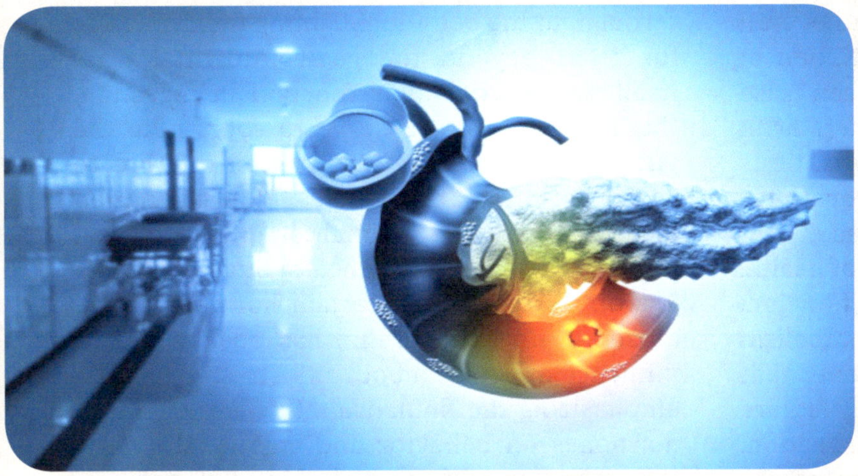

LEARNING OBJECTIVES

After studying this chapter, you will be able to:

1. Understand the gastrointestinal tract;
2. Discuss the key hormones of the gastrointestinal tract;
3. Focus on hormonal regulation of appetite;
4. Describe hormones produced by the liver;
5. Deal with the interaction between gut hormones and liver function;
6. Explain clinical implications of hormonal dysregulation within the gastrointestinal tract and liver.

Introduction

The intricate interaction between hormones in the liver and the gastrointestinal tract plays a vital role in keeping various physiological activities that are important in preserving homeostasis. Gastrin, secretin, and cholecystokinin are produced by enteroendocrine cells and play a regulatory role in digestion processes such as gastric acid, bile, and pancreatic enzyme secretion. These hormones are not only facilitators of digestion but also have roles in more widespread physiological regulation of metabolism, influencing hunger, satiety, and balance of energy. Understanding this complex hormonal landscape is central, as derangements in hormone secretion or function can lead to states of disease, such as obesity, diabetes, and gastrointestinal illness, and thus underscore the need for comprehensive research in this area to uncover therapeutic targets. In concert with endocrine signaling, more current research has also emphasized the gut microbiota's function of regulating hormonal responses and gut health. The microbiome engages in a complex interplay with host hormones to facilitate nutrient metabolism and the formation of metabolites that further regulate endocrine functions. For instance, short-chain fatty acids (SCFAs) produced by bacterial fermentation have been shown to regulate the release of hormones such as glucagon-like peptide-1 (GLP-1), an important hormone involved in glucose homeostasis as well as control of appetite. By describing such interactions, researchers can better understand the relationship between gut health, regulation of hormones, and overall metabolic processes because dysregulation of these significant hormonal pathways can arise due to imbalances within the microbiota (Martin et al., 2020). Beyond that, the implications of dysregulation in gastroenteric hormones extend well beyond metabolic diseases and implicate countless systemic outcomes of health. Endocrine disorders can influence liver function, considering the liver's critical role in metabolism and detoxification. For instance, hormones that stimulate bile secretion and help emulsify fats are a crucial part of lipid digestion and absorption. Moreover, the liver metabolizes and processes numerous hormones, creating a feedback system that can impact levels throughout the body. This interrelatedness draws attention to the necessity of an integrated learning approach to the hormones of the gastrointestinal system and liver, since the intricate cross-talk between these systems has the potential to unveil new knowledge regarding prevention and disease management strategies (Balali et al., 2021).

Definition of Hormones in the Gastrointestinal Tract and Liver

Hormones that are released in the gastrointestinal (GI) tract and liver play a significant role in the regulation of various physiological activities, primarily related to digestion and metabolism. Such hormones are released by specific cells, which are strategically located along the GI tract, e.g., the stomach, intestines, and pancreas, or even within the liver. A few examples of such hormones are gastrin, secretin, cholecystokinin, and insulin. Each of these hormones has a specific function; gastrin, for instance, stimulates gastric acid release, and secretin causes the release of bicarbonate from the pancreas. They work together to enable maximum food digestion, absorption of nutrients, and energy homeostasis. The nuanced interaction of these hormonal messages is of paramount significance not only to gastrointestinal well-being but also to overall metabolic equilibrium throughout the body, highlighting their intrinsic functions beyond the gastrointestinal tract itself. Aside from their function in digestion, these hormones also serve to coordinate the gut with the brain, an association referred to as the gut-brain axis at times. This association highlights the way hormonal communication can impact not only physical health but also mental health. The release of certain hormones, such as serotonin and ghrelin, has been noted to influence appetite, mood, and stress response, emphasizing the immense influences of the GI hormones on behavior and emotional health. Dysregulation of these hormones can also lead to several disorders, including obesity, anorexia, and anxiety, which demonstrate the endocrine profile of the GI tract is strongly linked to states of psychological and overall health. Therefore, understanding hormonal activities in the GI tract and the liver is very significant for the development of integrative treatment approaches to many states of health, including those within the spectrum of chronic diseases. The liver, often referred to as the body's metabolic hub, also produces hormones that act in concert with the gastrointestinal system's hormones. In particular, the liver produces insulin-like growth factors that stimulate cell growth and metabolism. The factors play a role in maintaining control of several of the body's metabolic operations, including glucose homeostasis, lipid metabolism, and protein synthesis. Furthermore, the liver is also involved in detoxification, where hormonal interaction influences the body's response to drugs and hormones themselves. The newly emerged field of microbiota research also proves the interaction between metabolic control and gut hormones, e.g., gut microbiota have been shown to regulate hormones such as GLP-1, which plays a part in insulin sensitivity and food consumption (Hou et al., 2022). With the advancement of research, the importance of knowing the balance of hormones in both the liver and GI tract becomes increasingly evident, unveiling complex pathways that determine health and disease overall (Visseren et al., 2021) (Figure 12.1).

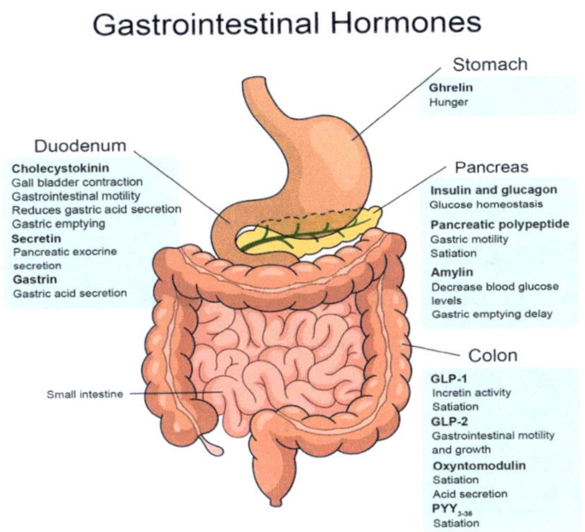

Figure 12.1. Gastrointestinal hormones.

Source: https://www.shutterstock.com/image-vector/gastrointestinal-hormones-including-their-origins-600w-2469250541.jpg.

Importance of Hormonal Regulation in Digestion

The intricate process of hormone regulation in digestion plays a crucial role in maintaining homeostasis in the gastrointestinal (GI) tract. Hormones released by the endocrine cells of the GI tract regulate various physiological processes, including the release of digestive enzymes, maintenance of gut motility, and regulation of appetite and energy balance. For instance, the hormone gastrin stimulates the release of gastric acid for the digestion of proteins, while secretin and cholecystokinin regulate the release of bile and pancreatic juices needed for fat emulsification. These endocrine signals not only maximize the effectiveness of digestion but also enable the GI tract to dynamically respond to dietary changes. The interaction between these hormones ensures optimal use of the nutrients by the body, highlighting the role of hormonal control as a fundamental component of gastrointestinal integrity and intrinsic metabolic function. Another significant component of hormonal control is the interaction between energy metabolic hormones and gastrointestinal hormones, particularly in obesity and metabolic disease. Studies have shown that the gut secretes over 30 hormones that have a direct impact on appetite control and the metabolic pathways of glucose and lipid metabolism. For instance, ghrelin, also known as the hunger hormone, stimulates appetite, while peptide YY and GLP-1 stimulate satiety and enhance insulin secretion. This complex hormonal conversation is crucial to maintain energy homeostasis; disruption of this balance can contribute to obesity and related disorders, like non-alcoholic fatty liver disease (NAFLD). By knowing these mechanisms, scientists are currently developing interventions that will disrupt these hormonal loops, revealing potential therapeutic approaches to obesity and metabolic health (Parkhomenko et al., 2019; Sonne, 2021). Additionally, the involvement of bile acids in hormonal control has become of interest because of their dual roles as digestive constituents and metabolic signal molecules. Previously thought to be valued mainly for their role in fat digestion, bile acids are now recognized for their ability to regulate glucose metabolism and energy expenditure. Activation of the nuclear farnesoid X receptor (FXR) by bile acids enhances several metabolic functions, including glucose and lipid metabolism. The regulatory interaction underscores the significance of bile acid enterohepatic circulation in metabolic homeostasis and suggests bile acids of therapeutic value for metabolic disorders like type 2 diabetes. Hence, hormonal regulation of digestion not only ensures effective use of nutrients but also has a significant function in being a crucial interface in the solution of broader metabolic health issues, once again illustrating the significance and complexity of gastrointestinal hormones in human physiology (Sonne, 2021).

12.1. Overview of the Gastrointestinal Tract

Learning Outcome

1. Explain the anatomy and function of the gastrointestinal tract;
2. Discuss the role of hormones in digestive processes;
3. Understand the interaction between the gastrointestinal tract and the liver.

The gastrointestinal system is a complicated and integral process for nutrient breakdown and absorption. Consisting of a long tube that begins with the mouth and ends with the anus, the gastrointestinal system is divided into regions that each serve a unique role in the digestive process. The oral cavity and salivary glands initially begin to break down food mechanically, while enzymes begin chemical digestion. After this, the food goes through the esophagus and into the stomach, where gastric juices further break it down into chyme. The chyme goes into the small intestine, a critical site of nutrient uptake, with the help of the presence of the liver and pancreas. The coordinated actions of hormones such as gastrin and secretin are essential in regulating these processes, indicating the intricate interaction between gut organs and hormonal signals that regulate function along this pathway. While chyme moves through the small intestine, the intricate architecture of the intestinal wall, through villi and microvilli, offers maximum surface area for absorption. Here, vitamins, nutrients, and minerals are transferred from the lumen into the blood, where they are transported to other tissues for utilization. Secretion of hormones such as cholecystokinin and GLP-1 plays a crucial role in the stimulation of secretions of digestive enzymes and the release of bile, hence facilitating fat and nutrient absorption. Balance and composition of gut microbiota also play significant roles in the function of this region of the gastrointestinal tract. Recent research has revealed that changes in microbiota can impact metabolic processes and contribute to a wide range of diseases, as documented in existing literature. This literature provides insight into the molecular mechanisms by which gut microbes influence host metabolism and immunity (Willem et al., 2022).

Once digested, the remaining unabsorbed residues enter the large intestine, where water and electrolytes are absorbed, hence producing feces. The large intestine serves not only to squeeze the waste but also as a habitat for a dense microbiome that is an important determinant of disease and health. Experiments have shown that toxins and heavy metals can poison the microbiome with harmful health consequences. For instance, heavy metal exposure, including lead and cadmium, has been proven to inhibit digestive functions and cause oxidative stress, indicating the potential hazard of environmental pollutants (Balali et al., 2021). The efficiency and operation of the gastrointestinal tracts are thus strongly influenced by intrinsic hormonal management and environmental factors, which highlight the importance of complete knowledge on its operation in complete human health.

12.1.1. Anatomy and Function of the Gastrointestinal Tract

The gastrointestinal system, a very convoluted and intricately organized organ system, is tasked with digestion, absorption, and regulating hormones. It is divided into a handful of well-differentiated regions, including the esophagus, stomach, small intestine, large intestine, and anus, all of which contribute to the overall digestive process.

Their structure is specialized to optimize their special functions, such as mechanical disruption of food by peristalsis in the esophagus and chemical digestion in the stomach. In the small intestine, the absorption area is optimized by villi and microvilli for efficient uptake of nutrients.

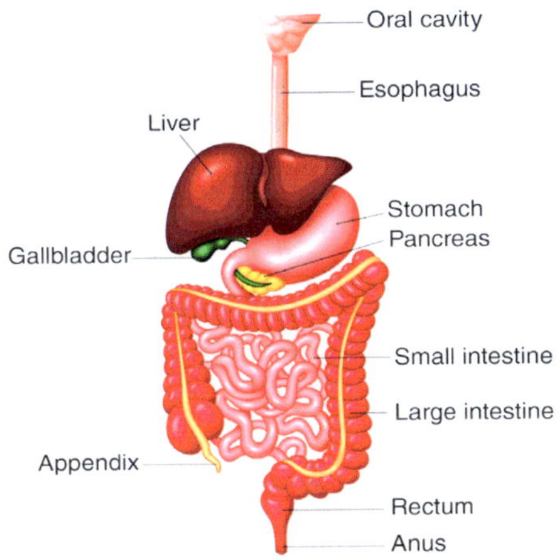

Figure 12.2. Gastrointestinal tract.

Source: https://cdn1.byjus.com/wp-content/uploads/2017/12/Gastrointestinal-Tract.png.

The hormones released by the EECs regulate functions like appetite, nutrient absorption, and intestinal motility. Importantly, more recent evidence confirms that most EECs have basal processes known as neuropods, expanding their function beyond hormone secretion. The EECs can directly communicate with enteric nerves via neuropods, hence enhancing their ability to sense and respond to alterations in the gastrointestinal tract (Rodger, 2019). This multifaceted role of EECs is a critical intersection between neural control and hormonal regulation, emphasizing their function in maintaining gut homeostasis. One such example of the enteric central nervous system cross-talk is vagal influence. The vagus nerve is the main component of the parasympathetic nervous system, which mediates brain-to-gut and gut-to-brain communication.

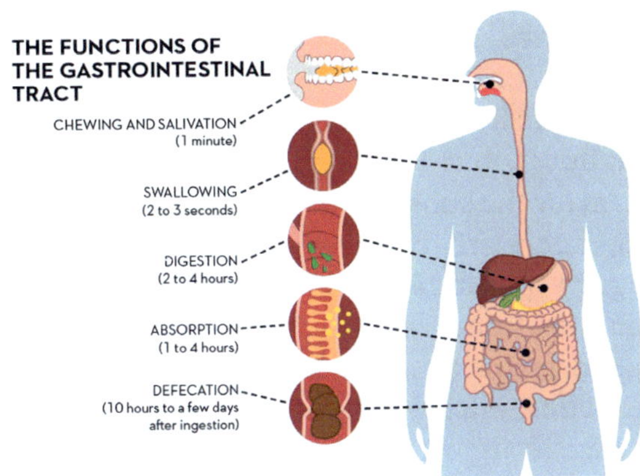

Figure 12.3. The functions of gastrointestinal tract.

Source: https://www.alimentarium.org/sites/default/files/media/image/2016-05/alm_esa_corps_en_fonctions_tube_0.jpg.

It plays an important regulatory role in digestion. It conveys afferent information from the gut to the brain, and reciprocally, information regarding the operation of the digestive organs can influence mood, immunity, and overall health. In addition, vagus nerve stimulation has been proposed as an experimental treatment for gastrointestinal and mental disease, leveraging its ability to augment vagal tone and modulate the body's stress response.

This demonstrates the interconnectedness of gut function and hormonal regulation, illustrating how hormonal signals can influence not only digestive processes but also broader physiological reactions in the entire body (Figure 12.3).

12.1.2. Role of Hormones in Digestive Processes

The subtle interaction of hormones used in digestive processes plays a vital role in homeostasis regulation of the gastrointestinal (GI) tract. Hormones such as gastrin, secretin, and cholecystokinin (CCK) guide the physiologic responses required for efficient digestion. Gastrin, for instance, is released primarily due to food consumption, stimulating gastric acid secretion and gastric motility. Not only does it aid in food breakdown, but it also prepares the digestive system for the subsequent processes of digestion. Also, secretin, released in the duodenum, triggers pancreatic bicarbonate secretion, which buffers the introduction of gastric acids into the small intestine. This hormonal interaction maximizes the digestive milieu for enzymatic digestion, and the importance of hormonal regulation in the formation of the digestive milieu is thereby highlighted. Digestive hormones' action is solely secretory; they have the ability to facilitate communication between the gut and the brain through the gut-brain axis. Their interaction with digestion doesn't just limit itself to influencing digestion but also to appetite and metabolic signals. CCK, for example, released upon stimulation by fatty food residue, not only contracts the gallbladder and releases pancreatic enzymes but also initiates satiety signals to the brain so that it regulates the intake of food. The dynamic feedback of these hormonal messages is indicative of the way the gastrointestinal tract reacts to the nutritional content of food. An awareness of the varied impact of such hormones indicates their role in not just digestive well-being but also within the broad scheme of metabolic syndrome, linking digestive pathology to obesity and type 2 diabetes, which emphasizes the regulatory role of such hormones across the body. Besides, gut microbiota interacts with these hormones, imposing another level of complexity on digestion control. Gut bacteria have been implicated in the modulation of the release of such hormones as ghrelin and peptide YY (PYY) by recent studies, which play a crucial role in hunger and satiation. Evidence emerging from studies reveals that short-chain fatty acids produced from gut microbiota have the ability to activate receptors of hormone signal transduction pathways, hence modulating energy homeostasis and metabolism. This crosstalk between microbiota and intestinal hormones not only more precisely delineates digestive physiology but also suggests potential therapeutic targets for metabolic disorders due to gut dysbiosis. Through this intricate network of interactions, the future of our knowledge of the involvement of hormones in digestion can have significant consequences in the design of novel therapeutic strategies and in the optimization of overall gastrointestinal well-being, predicated largely on the variability and flexibility of the human body systems (Campanale et al., 2020; Willem et al., 2022) (Figure 12.4).

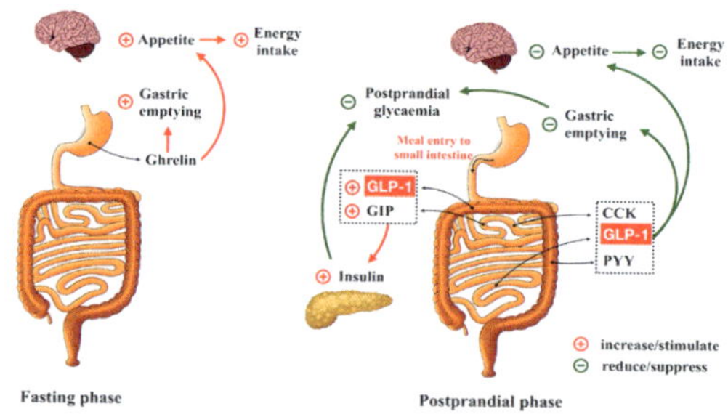

Figure 12.4. Role of gastrointestinal hormones in the regulation of gastric emptying, postprandial glycemia, and energy intake.

Source: https://www.researchgate.net/publication/327923530/figure/fig1/AS:11431281256093789@1719494622787/Role-of-gastrointestinal-hormones-in-the-regulation-of-gastric-emptying-postprandial.tif.

12.1.3. Interaction Between the Gastrointestinal Tract and the Liver

The interaction between the GI tract and the liver is vital to homeostasis maintenance as well as the regulation of many of the metabolic processes. This exchange is typically regulated by a complex mixture of hormones as well as signaling pathways between these two organs. The liver receives nutrient-rich blood from the GI tract via the portal vein so that hepatic function may be directly regulated depending on the character of the absorbed substances. This connection enables the liver to respond quickly to the body's current state of nutrition, playing a central role in digestion, metabolism, and detoxification. The gut-liver axis is also regulated by microbial metabolites and gut hormones, which manage liver function and general metabolic health. The intricate signaling pathways implicated are essential in both health and disease states, thereby making the interaction relevant to clinical practice and research (Yan et al., 2023). Hormones secreted by the GI tract greatly affect liver function, with specific reference to the control of metabolic functions such as glucose and lipid metabolism. For instance, eating releases hormones like GLP-1 and peptide YY (PYY) and has been shown to enhance insulin sensitivity and induce the secretion of insulin from the pancreas. These hormones have at the same time, direct effects on the liver through gluconeogenesis and lipogenesis control and therefore regulate metabolic homeostasis. In addition to this, the gut-derived short-chain fatty acids (SCFAs), formed through the fermentation of dietary fiber by gut microbiota, are brought into portal circulation and can have a systemic effect on energy metabolism. SCFAs participate in signaling pathways that mediate gene expression in liver cells, ultimately affecting lipid and carbohydrate metabolism (Bart et al., 2021). This intricate interaction of hormones portrays the vital role played by the GI tract in liver regulation and metabolic health. Immune function and inflammation regulation are also crucial roles played by the GI tract and liver interaction. The gut is an important site of immune function and harbors a large number of immune cells that interact with gut microbiota to maintain a healthy balance of immune response. This interaction is also connected to the liver through the gut-liver axis, where immune mediators and inflammatory signaling may influence hepatic physiology. Ligands from gut microbiota, such as SCFAs, have been identified to play important roles as modulators of this interaction with significant implications on metabolic disorders and liver disease. This communication between the gut and liver has been dysregulated in conditions like NAFLD and metabolic syndrome, and thus, understanding these interactions can shed light on new therapeutic strategies. Leveraging the understanding of the hormonal and immunological conversation between the liver and gut can potentially create specific treatments in metabolic and inflammatory disorders (Yan et al., 2023).

Test Your Knowledge

1. What are the major anatomical components of the gastrointestinal (GI) tract?
2. How do gastrointestinal hormones such as gastrin, secretin, and cholecystokinin (CCK) regulate digestive processes?

12.2. Key Hormones of the Gastrointestinal Tract

Learning Outcome

1. Describe gastrin and its role in gastric function;
2. Understand secretin and its influence on pancreatic secretion;
3. Explain cholecystokinin (CCK) and its effects on bile release.

Within the GI tract's complicated environment, several primary hormones play key roles in regulating digestive functions and maintaining metabolic homeostasis. One such hormone is ghrelin, which has the nickname the hunger hormone. Secreted predominantly by the stomach, ghrelin stimulates appetite and causes food intake by acting on the hypothalamus. It raises its level preprandially and lowers it postprandially, influencing energy balance. Furthermore, ghrelin has been implicated in the regulation of gastric secretion and motility, aiding in the digestion process. Understanding the mechanisms behind how ghrelin and similar hormones function is crucial to their classification as factors that control diet intake and potentially their role in obesity and metabolic disease, highlighting the importance of hormonal signaling in the gut. Another such critical hormone of the GI tract is the GLP-1, released by the intestines after food intake. GLP-1 plays a multifaceted function, not just stimulating the release of insulin from the pancreas but also inhibiting the release of glucagon, thereby contributing to glucose homeostasis. GLP-1 further slows down gastric emptying, thereby perpetuating the feeling of satiety after eating. Research in recent years has progressively highlighted the therapeutic role of GLP-1 analogues in the treatment of diabetes and obesity. The identification of GLP-1's dual role reflects the intricacy of the interplay between gastrointestinal hormones and metabolic regulation, highlighting their function in disease and health. Thus, clinical relevance to enhance GLP-1 signaling is gigantic, and understanding of the role of this hormone in metabolic regulation must be continued. Short-chain fatty acids (SCFAs) are another key element in gastrointestinal hormonal regulation, due to fiber fermentation by gut microbiota. SCFAs like acetate, propionate, and butyrate not only serve as a source of energy for colonocytes but also have a significant effect on systemic metabolism and the immune system. Their signaling function is not restricted to the intestine, but has effects on the liver through portal circulation, in which SCFAs have the ability to control gluconeogenesis and lipogenesis. Recent evidence uncovers that SCFA signaling is transduced by some G-protein-coupled receptors, exhibiting a high-level layer of hormonal interaction that regulates energy metabolism and inflammation. Dysregulation of SCFA production and signaling by diet has also been linked to disease conditions such as nonalcoholic fatty liver disease (NAFLD), again highlighting the importance of gastrointestinal health to maintain overall metabolic health. Knowledge about how SCFAs function can provide hints at discovering new therapeutic strategies for metabolic diseases and, therefore, is of utmost significance in the studies of gastrointestinal hormones (Bart et al., 2021; Tilg et al., 2020).

12.2.1. Gastrin and Its Role in Gastric Function

Gastrin, a key gastrointestinal hormone, plays a vital role in the regulation of gastric function. Released from gastric mucosal G cells, gastrin secretion is stimulated by the entry of food into the stomach, particularly proteins. The hormone exists primarily to stimulate parietal cell secretion of gastric acid, which is essential for protein digestion and nutrient absorption. Moreover, gastrin facilitates the proliferation of gastric epithelial cells, thus maintaining the integrity and nutrition of the gastric mucosa. The reciprocal dynamic between gastrin and gastric acid secretion emphasizes its importance in facilitating digestive processes and preventing gastrointestinal disorders such as ulcers and dyspepsia, both of which can be exacerbated by ectopic gastrin levels. Other than its stimulating function in gastric acid secretion, gastrin also plays a part in gastric motility.

By stimulating stomach muscle contraction, gastrin ensures that food becomes well mixed with gastric juices, thereby facilitating efficient digestion. The role of the hormone in gastric emptying is multifaceted; it could aid in regulating the rate at which chyme leaves the stomach and enters the duodenum for further digestion and absorption of nutrients. Gastrin release and its respective physiological effects must be regulated for efficient gastric function. Disruptions in this balance can lead to conditions such as gastritis or Zollinger-Ellison syndrome, highlighting the regulatory role of gastrin as a principal hormone of the gastrointestinal tract. Beyond the use of gastrin as a digestive hormone are the therapeutic applications, highlighted in research on peptide drug development. Advances in peptide modification and delivery have opened doors to explore gastrin's therapeutic potential in gastric disease. For instance, understanding the interactions between gastrins and other gastrointestinal hormones can lead to the development of new therapies for obesity and type 2 diabetes, such as advancements with hormones like GLP-1, which has been shown to exert broad metabolic actions, including inhibition of gastric emptying and modulation of satiation (Timo et al., 2019). This new generation of research confirms the significance of knowledge about gastrins in gastric physiology and their potential manipulation for therapeutic purposes, highlighting the significance of hormonal regulation in gastrointestinal function and health (Figure 12.5).

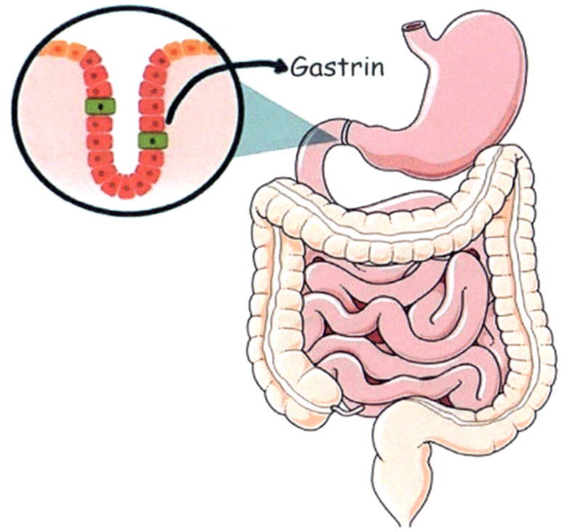

Figure 12.5. Gastrin illustration.

Source: https://www.yourhormones.info/media/dhukchz2/gastrin.jpg.

12.2.2. Secretin and Its Influence on Pancreatic Secretion

Secretin's function in the regulation of pancreatic secretion is a gem of gastroenterology physiology. Secretin, a peptide hormone produced in S cells of the duodenum, is released because of the acidity of chyme that enters the small intestine. Its primary function is to cause the pancreas to release a bicarbonate-rich fluid that neutralizes gastric acid, setting the optimal pH for enzymatic activity in the intestine. This is significant because the pancreas's secreted enzymes must be found in a slightly alkaline or neutral environment to be most effective. Secretin thus not only contributes to digestion by regulating the chemical environment but also contributes to the whole process of assimilation of nutrients, making its function in digestive health extremely essential. In addition, secretin influences pancreatic secretion through the stimulation of pancreatic acinar cell proliferation and survival, consequently enhancing glandular function (Figure 12.6).

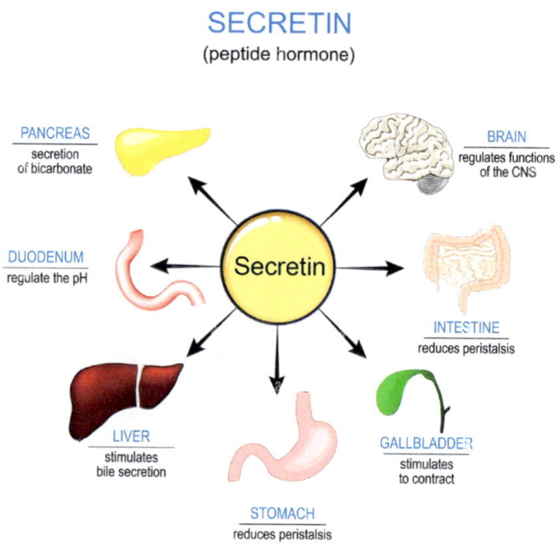

Figure 12.6. Secretin (peptide hormone).

Source: https://c8.alamy.com/comp/2RMEKD9/secretin-gastrointestinal-peptide-hormones-human-digestive-system-endocrine-system-vector-illustration-2RMEKD9.jpg.

Research indicates that secretin acts on the pancreas by attaching to specific receptors that start signaling cascades leading to increased synthesis and secretion of enzymes. This encompasses the control of water flow through the pancreatic ductal cells, crucial for the production of the enzymatic digestion fluid. Without secretin, the pancreas would be unable to produce sufficient secretions required for successful digestion, with the risk being malabsorption and nutrient deficiencies. Therefore, secretin's multifunctional activities underscore its function to keep the balance of digestive functions in the gut. Secretin's interaction with other gastrointestinal hormones serves further to augment its function in pancreatic secretion. Secretin, for instance, works in conjunction with cholecystokinin (CCK), another regulatory hormone, to maximize pancreatic enzyme secretion. When secretin preconditions the pancreas for the secretion of bicarbonate, CCK is the stimulant that causes the release of digestive enzymes in the presence of fats and proteins in the duodenum. Such a symbiotic behavior allows for a balanced digestive response, releasing enzymes at the right time as and when needed. Additionally, recent studies have indicated that secretin may have an impact on the release of incretin hormones like GLP-1, which are important for glucose homeostasis and appetite regulation (Timo et al., 2019). Therefore, an understanding of secretin's action on pancreatic secretion and its interaction with other hormones is of significant interest in comprehending the regulatory mechanisms of the gastrointestinal tract and in identifying therapeutic opportunities for digestive and metabolic disorders (Mark et al., 2013) (Figure 12.7).

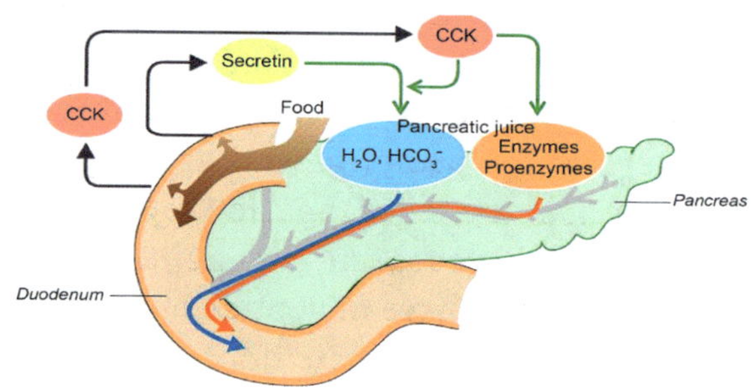

Figure 12.7. Pancreatic secretion.

Source: https://upload.medbullets.com/topic/106039/images/pancreatic%20secretions.jpg.

12.2.3. Cholecystokinin (CCK) and Its Effects on Bile Release

Cholecystokinin (CCK) is an important hormone in the complex physiology of the gastrointestinal tract, as it relates to the discharge of bile from the gallbladder. Discharged by the I cells of the duodenum, CCK is discharged most notably following the ingestion of fats and proteins. This discharge results in various physiological events, including the contraction of the gallbladder, enabling the bile to be discharged into the small intestine. The released bile acids not only promote emulsification and digestion of ingested lipids but also play a major role in nutrient uptake. The mode of action by which CCK works underscores its function, since it optimizes digestive capacity by delivering bile in harmony with food ingestion. Upon release, CCK binds to receptors present throughout the gastrointestinal tract, whose activation has several downstream consequences relevant to digestion. CCK's action is not just on the contraction of the gallbladder; it also acts on pancreatic exocrine secretory function to stimulate the release of digestive enzymes. Moreover, studies have shown that the shorter isoforms of CCK, such as CCK-8 and CCK-4, are absorbed into the gastrointestinal mucosa and carried into the liver through unique transport mechanisms. The shorter isoforms are metabolized and then secreted into bile and thus provide evidence of an increase in the availability of hormones within the digestive process (Ismair et al., 2001). This interaction sets CCK's critical balance between regulation of hormones and digestion, with additional implications for its role in directing digestive processes. CCK actions on the release of bile and overall digestive function are also altered by surgical rearrangement of the gastrointestinal anatomy. For instance, following Roux-en-Y gastric bypass (RGBY) surgery, the dynamics of bile acid release are altered, which has a far-reaching impact on the enterohepatic circulation. The increased absorption of bile acids in the postprandial state could be different because studies reveal that bile acids will no longer bind to food and hence bring about unexpected alterations in fat absorption and digestion (Javitt, 2018). These changes are reflective of the adaptive character of the gastrointestinal system to anatomical and physiological changes and are reasons for concern about how CCKs work in releasing bile, which can be modified post-surgery. Information regarding these interactions might be utilized to identify the correct design for therapeutic approaches to ensure optimal digestive efficiency among patients with altered gastrointestinal structures (Figure 12.8).

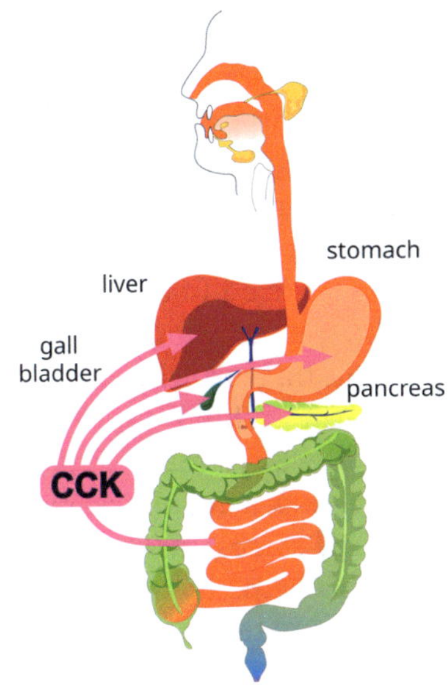

Figure 12.8. Effects of cholecystokinin on the gastrointestinal tract.

Source: https://upload.wikimedia.org/wikipedia/commons/thumb/8/83/Effects_of_CCK_on_the_gastrointestinal_tract.svg/800px-Effects_of_CCK_on_the_gastrointestinal_tract.svg.png.

Test Your Knowledge

1. What is the primary function of gastrin, and how does it regulate gastric acid secretion?
2. How is gastrin secretion controlled, and what stimuli increase or inhibit its release?
3. What are the main effects of cholecystokinin (CCK) on the gallbladder, pancreas, and satiety?

12.3. Hormonal Regulation of Appetite

Learning Outcome

1. Describe ghrelin and its role in hunger signaling;
2. Explain leptin and its effects on satiety;
3. Understand peptide YY (PYY) and its impact on food intake.

The intricate hormonal regulation of appetite is part and parcel of energy homeostasis, with several hormones that exist in an intercommunicating relationship to manage food intake and energy expenditure. The key hormones, such as ghrelin, leptin, and insulin, play a significant role in the regulation of signaling pathways to influence hunger and satiety. Ghrelin, released in the stomach, is also known as the hunger hormone, which provokes hunger by signaling in the hypothalamus. Conversely, leptin, which is released from adipose tissue, signals satiety and suppresses appetite, thus giving a feedback signal to the brain about energy stores. Insulin, released from the pancreas, also helps by sending a signal to the brain to cut down on appetite following consumption of food. In concert, these hormones exhibit a multifaceted interaction wherein not only is the availability of nutrients, but also a variety of hormonal signals, accountable for obtaining energy intake to expenditure balance, finally influencing long-term body weight control. Regulation of appetite by the hormones is greatly affected by the autonomic nervous system (ANS) through the mediation of dialogue between peripheral organs and the central nervous system (CNS). Gastrointestinal tract signals, including nutrient and hormonal signals, travel up via afferent vagus nerve pathways to terminate in hypothalamic regions that regulate feeding. Integration of these signals by the CNS controls appetite through both sympathetic and parasympathetic pathways, modulating systemic metabolic actions within various organs, including the pancreas and liver. As noted in recent studies, the connection not only ensures the availability of energy to meet demand but also plays a significant role in maintaining homeostasis at the organismal level, indicating the importance of the autonomic nervous system in controlling appetite and energy metabolism (Imai et al., 2021). Furthermore, short-chain fatty acids (SCFAs), produced by fermentation of dietary fiber in the gut, are found to play a vital role in maintaining appetite regulation. SCFAs such as acetate, propionate, and butyrate act as signaling molecules with effects on hormonal pathways involved in the regulation of appetite. They operate through G-protein-coupled receptors (GPCRs) of enteroendocrine cells to trigger the release of hormones like GLP-1 and peptide YY (PYY), both of which are known for their satiety-inducing potential. The production of SCFA underscores the interconnection between diet, intestinal microbiota, and hormonal regulation of hunger, ultimately to provide evidence for the fact that food habits have a strong influences on metabolic health (Bart et al., 2021). Knowledge of these mechanisms is crucial to the development of interventions intended to treat obesity and related metabolic disorders.

12.3.1. Ghrelin and Its Role in Hunger Signaling

The intricate relationship between hunger signaling and hormones is best described by the function of ghrelin, often referred to as the hunger hormone. The majority of ghrelin is secreted by the stomach and is an important mediator in stimulating appetite and energy homeostasis. Release is primarily induced by fasting and declines following food intake, arising as a feedback mechanism that regulates hunger and satiation. This dynamic process is important for homeostasis since it promotes individuals to seek food intake when their energy stores are low. Research has shown that elevated levels of ghrelin correspond to higher food consumption, highlighting its fundamental role in hunger signaling, as well as its potential role in the interpretation of metabolic syndrome and obesity disorders, in which ghrelin signaling would be disrupted (Fahed et al., 2022). In addition, ghrelin influences not just hunger but also various neural pathways that control energy balance. When released, ghrelin is carried to the hypothalamus, a part of the brain that helps regulate appetite, and binds to specific receptors. This attachment activates a chain of neurochemical events that enhance the drive for hunger. In addition, the action of ghrelin is not only to cause immediate food consumption, but also to have a role in the long-term maintenance of body weight. Emerging evidence points out that obese individuals can have defective ghrelin responses that contribute to their failure to lose weight.

As researchers delve deeper into these mechanisms, ghrelin's function in hunger signaling could open new therapeutic pathways for the prevention of obesity and its related health problems (Timo et al., 2021). The implications of studies on ghrelin are far-reaching, ranging from the development of anti-obesity drugs to the treatment of metabolic syndrome. With the long-term problem of managing obesity, the hormonal origin of hunger signaling is becoming more crucial. Ghrelin antagonists, for example, are being investigated as possible therapeutic agents that could modulate appetite and induce weight loss. But the intricacies of regulating appetite stand in the way, with ghrelin being only one of a number of hormones that work in this system. It is crucial that subsequent studies account for these interactions, especially when it comes to creating effective treatments for obesity that take advantage of knowledge about ghrelin's signaling mechanisms. Lastly, the crossroads of gastrointestinal hormones like ghrelin in the hunger signaling terrain are a central target for unraveling as we attempt to moderate the compounding public health crises linked with obesity and metabolic disease (Fahed et al., 2022) (Figure 12.9).

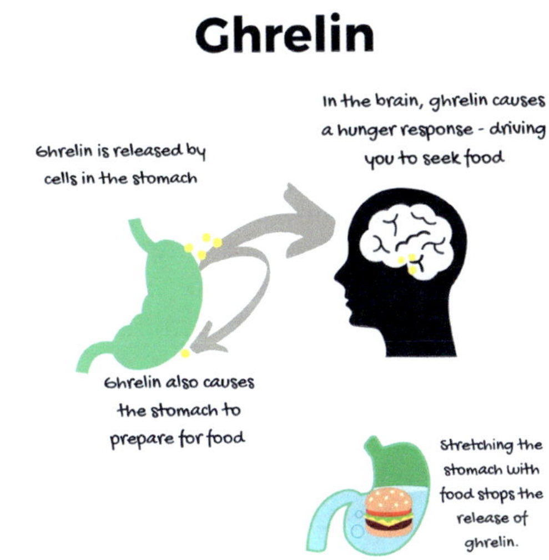

Figure 12.9. Ghrelin, often called the "hunger hormone," is a peptide hormone primarily produced by the stomach that plays a key role in signaling hunger to the brain.

Source: https://www.geneticlifehacks.com/wp-content/uploads/2015/10/Ghrelin-genes.jpg.

12.3.2. Leptin and Its Effects on Satiety

Leptin, predominantly produced by adipocytes, is a hormone that controls energy balance and regulates appetite through its action on satiety. The peptide hormone informs the hypothalamus of the amount of fat stored and thus informs the body how much energy is available for utilization. An elevated level of leptin typically indicates a sufficient energy reserve, leading to decreased food intake and increased energy expenditure. Conversely, reduced levels of leptin, typically found in states of energy deficit or in states of obesity, stimulate hunger and decrease metabolic rate. Through these control mechanisms, leptin governs feeding behavior, ensuring its role as a vital part of the complex cycle of hunger and metabolism, being vital to maintaining homeostasis within the gastrointestinal tract and affecting health. Several studies have highlighted the function of leptin in combating obesity and obesity comorbidities. However, the satiety-inducing role of leptin is lost due to resistance to leptin, a characteristic shared by the majority of obese individuals. The resistance can arise when the body compensates by developing resistance to the signals provided by leptin, typically leading to increased food intake despite raised circulating levels of the hormone. Experiments on the mechanisms of this resistance are critical, since knowledge about these mechanisms might reveal what obesity control strategies could work. By the investigation of the delicate equilibrium between leptin level and brain sensitivity to its message, researchers are now able to plan therapy with the goal of fixing leptin sensitivity, hence re-establishing a normal control of appetite and weight, domains of utmost interest in gastrointestinal hormone research. Also, the interaction between leptin and other satiety-regulating hormones, such as GLP-1 demarcates the intricate interplay involved in the regulation of satiety. While leptin plays a central role in communicating energy status, GLP-1, released from the gut following food consumption, contributes to the sense of fullness via slow gastric emptying and increased secretion of insulin. Therefore, the synthesis and secretion of these hormones act in concert to regulate hunger and energy homeostasis. Appreciation of the synergistic action of leptin and GLP-1 continues to shed light on obesity pathophysiology and the intricacy of appetite regulation. Such a multi-factorial process in appreciating hormone interaction highlights that treatment of obesity and obesity-related syndromes needs an overall approach, emphasizing the role of such hormones as leptin in the context of gastrointestinal health and metabolic homeostasis (Figure 12.10).

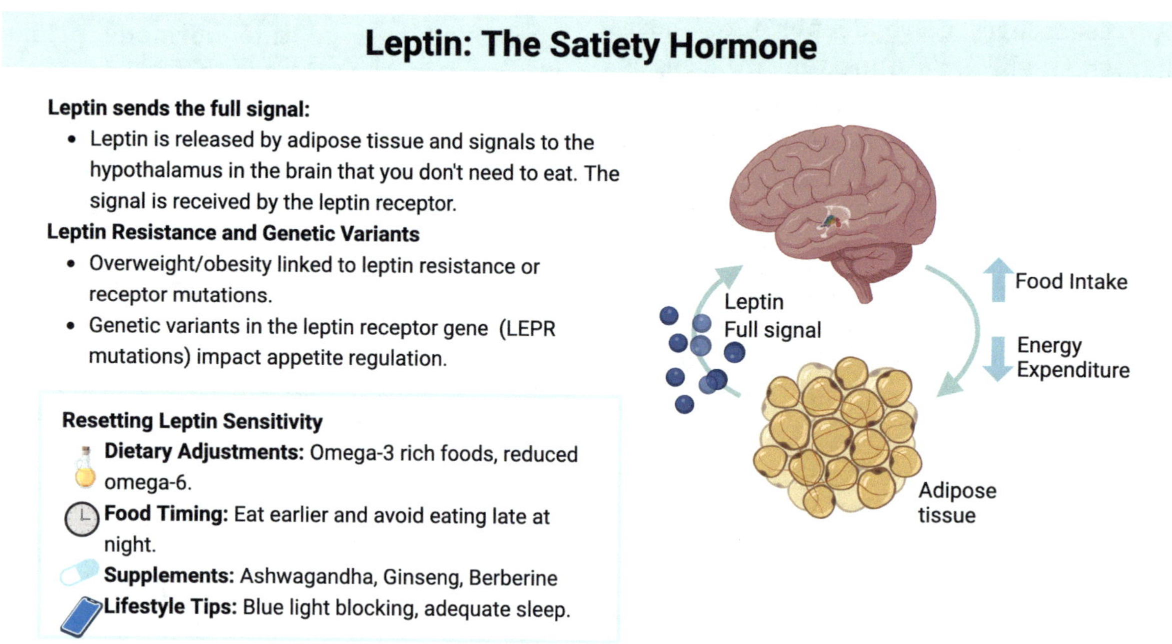

Figure 12.10. Leptin: The satiety hormone.

Source: https://www.geneticlifehacks.com/wp-content/uploads/2022/02/Leptin_-The-Satiety-Hormone.png.

12.3.3. Peptide YY (PYY) and Its Impact on Food Intake

Peptide YY (PYY) plays a key role in the regulation of food intake as a satiety hormone. Secreted by intestinal L-cells following the ingestion of nutrients, the level of PYY rises postprandially to provide the message of satiety to the central nervous system. It is effective through mechanisms that include neuropeptide Y (NPY) receptors, the majority of which are located in the hypothalamus, a key region in the regulation of appetite. Because PYY induces a feeling of satiation, it effectively suppresses the hunger impulse, thus fulfilling its role in the subtle balance of energy homeostasis. Changes in PYY levels are important because they can signal an individual's susceptibility to obesity, as poor responses can potentially lead to overeating and resultant weight gain. This understanding of the PYY mechanism makes it a potential target for therapy for weight control and other metabolic disease management, where appetite control is paramount.

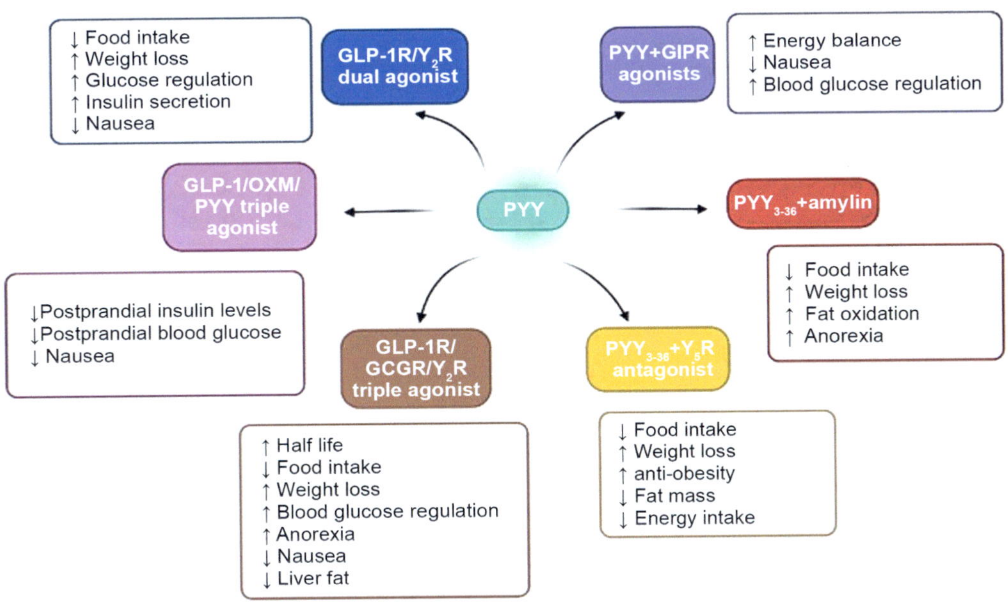

Figure 12.11. Peptide YY (PYY) plays a crucial role in regulating food intake, primarily functioning as an appetite suppressant.

Source: https://ars.els-cdn.com/content/image/1-s2.0-S0045206823004698-gr3.jpg.

For the complete appreciation of the action of PYY on food intake, it is important to know what it does with diet composition in its regulation. Diets rich in fat, for instance, have been shown to modulate PYY responses, with evidence for interaction between PYY and gut microbiota. It is indicated by evidence that certain dietary lipids have the potential to modulate the composition and function of gut microbiota, consequently affecting PYY secretion. Specifically, metabolic byproducts of gut microbiota, particularly short-chain fatty acids, have been found to enhance PYY production, bridging the nutritional fuel of foods and hormonal output. This interaction implies a complex regulatory mechanism whereby diet not only impacts concentrations of PYY but also places emphasis on the role of gut function in satiety and general metabolic processes. Such an understanding places even greater emphasis on the role of gut microbiota and food consumption in the development of successful weight management. In addition to regulation of appetite, the significance of PYY also extends to broader metabolic pathways, including lipid metabolism. It has been confirmed through research that PYY secretion influences blood lipid content and the total metabolism of lipids, as it performs a multi-functional role. The changes induced by PYY following food consumption can lead to changes in body fat composition, which are critical in order to prevent conditions like NAFLD and metabolic syndrome. In addition, the interaction of PYY with gut microbiota highlights the requirement to take into account how changes in systemic metabolism could change hormonal responses. By understanding these dynamics, scientists can better define how PYY influences food intake and metabolic health and thus begin the process of designing new diet and pharmacological interventions that are made possible by the interaction between hormones, diet, and gut microbiota, which is highlighted in the most recent literature involving gut physiology and health management (Mukherjee et al., 2020; Schoeler et al., 2019) (Figure 12.11).

Test Your Knowledge

1. What is the role of ghrelin in hunger signaling, and how does its secretion change with fasting and feeding?
2. What is Peptide YY (PYY), and how does it affect appetite and gastrointestinal motility after a meal?
3. How does leptin regulate satiety and energy balance, and which organ is primarily responsible for its production?

12.4. Hormones Produced by the Liver

Learning Outcome

1. Describe insulin-like growth factor (IGF) and its functions;
2. Explain the role of angiotensinogen in blood pressure regulation;
3. Understand the influence of hepcidin on iron metabolism.

The liver is also a key component of the endocrine system since it releases a variety of hormones important in maintaining metabolic homeostasis. Among these hormones, insulin-like growth factor 1 (IGF-1) is of significant relevance since it acts as an intermediary for the action of growth hormone (GH) and promotes the growth and development of tissues. IGF-1 is mainly synthesized in the liver and distributed via the bloodstream, impacting cellular functions such as differentiation, proliferation, and survival. Furthermore, its production is controlled by a myriad of factors, including nutrition and endocrine stimuli, establishing a dynamic interconnection between liver metabolism and overall body metabolism. The ability of the liver to produce and secrete IGF-1 suggests its central role in controlling growth and energy homeostasis, explaining the critical association between endocrine and metabolic processes in the body, which is waiting to be thoroughly investigated (Hou et al., 2022).

Another vital hormone secreted by the liver is angiotensinogen, the precursor to angiotensin I, which is significant to the regulation of blood pressure and fluid control. Angiotensinogen is secreted into the bloodstream, where it is hydrolyzed into angiotensin I by renin, which is a secreted enzyme from the kidneys. This change is a significant component of the renin-angiotensin-aldosterone system (RAAS), a highly developed system of hormones that regulates blood pressure and electrolyte homeostasis. The liver, therefore, has a major function in cardiovascular homeostasis through the production of angiotensinogen and hence regulation of the RAAS. Any impairment in any component of the system can lead to hypertension and other cardiovascular diseases. Given the liver's function of hormone production, like angiotensinogen, not only does it provide insights into its endocrine role but also sheds light on the far-reaching implications on cardiovascular disease and health (Ghosh et al., 2021). Further, the liver also synthesizes numerous critical proteins like thrombopoietin and hepcidin, both of which play significant systemic hormone-like impacts. Thrombopoietin is a critical regulator of platelet production in the bone marrow and thus hemostasis. Concurrently, hepcidin regulates the body's iron homeostasis by modulating dietary iron absorption and mobilization from stores.

Both these proteins highlight the liver's extensive endocrine activity, reflecting its significant role in the upkeep of not just metabolism but also hematological balance. The interaction with the hormones and gut further brings into focus the central role of the liver within the overall hormonal realm of influence, affecting a spectrum of physiological processes and reactions that necessitate further examination of their mechanisms and pathways (Hou et al., 2022).

12.4.1. Insulin-Like Growth Factor (IGF) and Its Functions

Insulin-like growth factor (IGF) plays a very significant role in growth and development, though primarily during childhood and adolescence, but also has an influence on various metabolic processes as well during adulthood. It is primarily produced in the liver, which can be stimulated by growth hormone, thus linking endocrine liver function to overall growth. IGF exerts its effects by binding to specific receptors on target cells, where it triggers signaling pathways responsible for increased cell growth, tissue growth, and survival. These effects make IGF not only essential for growth in the body's development but also for the maintenance of muscle mass and metabolic health in adults. Disturbance of IGF regulation has been linked to a number of conditions of ill health, such as obesity and diabetes, and thus the hormone takes on importance as a measure of metabolic well-being of the body and of potential involvement in aging and longevity, as reviewed in current literature (Guo et al., 2022). The biological effects of IGF are channeled primarily by the activation of the insulin receptor substrate (IRS) and subsequent activation of the phosphoinositide 3-kinase (PI3K) and mitogen-activated protein kinase (MAPK) cascades. The cascades are involved in the anabolic functions of protein synthesis and glucose utilization, and thus further link IGF to liver and gut vital activities. In addition, the action of IGF on other hormones, i.e., insulin, reinforces its action on energy metabolism and glucose homeostasis. The fine balance of IGF signaling is essential for normal growth, but on the other hand, the deregulation of IGF signaling has its adverse outcomes, including susceptibility to chronic diseases, i.e., cancer and metabolic syndromes. The connection of IGF with mechanisms involved in disease and inflammation also highlights the necessity for ongoing investigation into its diverse roles in health and disease (Hu et al., 2021).

Furthermore, the relationship between IGF, aging, and age-related disorders is an expanding area of concern for endocrinologists. As noted in recent studies, changes in IGF can influence aging and the onset of age-related disorders, like sarcopenia and osteopenia. The complex interaction of IGF with pathways like JAK/STAT underscores the importance of understanding how endocrine signals influence longevity and the well-being of older populations. Moreover, interventions modulating IGF signaling in the future provide therapeutic interventions enhancing healthy aging in the elderly, which alleviate the growing issues of aging populations. These discoveries about the intricate roles of IGF not only explain the functions of hormones but also open up new avenues for effective solutions of successful aging (Guo et al., 2022) (Figure 12.12).

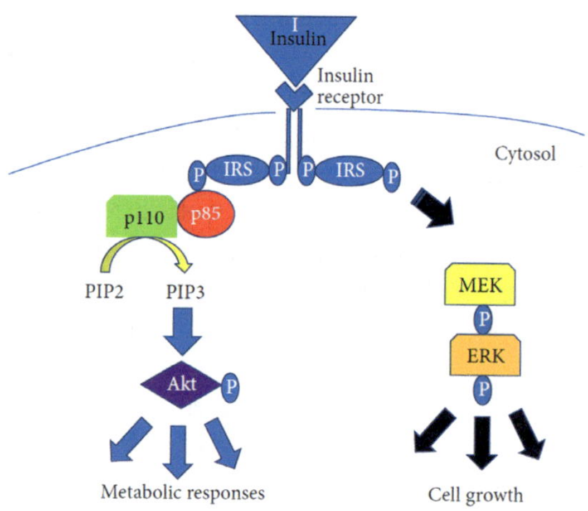

Figure 12.12. Insulin or insulin-like growth factor 1 (IGF-1) binds to its receptor and activates the receptor tyrosine kinase.

Source: https://www.researchgate.net/publication/235692012/figure/fig1/AS:1088996176334848@1636648329439/Insulin-or-insulin-like-growth-factor-1-IGF-1-binds-to-its-receptor-and-activates-the.jpg.

12.4.2. Angiotensinogen and Its Role in Blood Pressure Regulation

Angiotensinogen, a precursor protein that is synthesized mainly in the liver, is involved in the regulation of blood pressure through the RAAS. Secretion of renin from the kidneys on reduction in blood pressure or renal blood flow results in the transformation of angiotensinogen into angiotensin I. This inactive decapeptide is subsequently transformed into angiotensin II by the action of angiotensin-converting enzyme (ACE), which is mainly localized in the lung and vascular endothelium. Angiotensin II is a potent vasoconstrictor, which leads to blood vessel constriction and hence increases systemic vascular resistance, a critical mechanism for rising blood pressure. Thus, the production of angiotensinogen and its release are not only crucial for circulatory homeostasis but also for the investigation of the pathophysiology of hypertension and hypertension-related complications. Angiotensinogen levels are also controlled by many physiological and pathological stimuli ranging from gastrointestinal and hepatic hormonal stimulants to intracrines. For instance, hormones such as insulin and glucagon have been found to regulate the production of angiotensinogen, linking metabolic states with blood pressure regulation. In obesity and metabolic syndrome, which put people at risk for cardiovascular diseases, the levels of angiotensinogen tend to rise. Because such conditions create a constantly increasing issue worldwide, knowing the link between angiotensinogen production and its contribution to controlling blood pressure is now a priority. Emerging evidence suggests that dysregulation of angiotensinogen levels may enhance the hypertension and cardiovascular effects of hypertension, necessitating further study of the role of targeted therapies and interventions in the treatment of metabolic syndrome (Fahed et al., 2022). Considering the multifaceted interaction of angiotensinogen in the modulation of blood pressure, the existing body of evidence is exploring the role of therapeutic agents targeted at the RAAS pathway. For instance, angiotensin receptor blockers (ARBs) and ACE inhibitors are widely utilized in the clinic to act as counteragents against hypertension. Furthermore, the role of Angiotensin Converting Enzyme 2 (ACE2), which is an enzyme that counteracts the action of angiotensin II, has come into the spotlight with regard to how it influences both hypertension and COVID-19 pathophysiology (Arno et al., 2020). Understanding angiotensinogen's multifaceted activity shows the way in which interactions between hormones influence cardiovascular disease and health. Thus, a clear understanding of angiotensinogen, along with the complementary roles of gastrointestinal and liver hormones, is relevant to the development of effective treatment protocols for hypertension and related metabolic disorders (Figure 12.13).

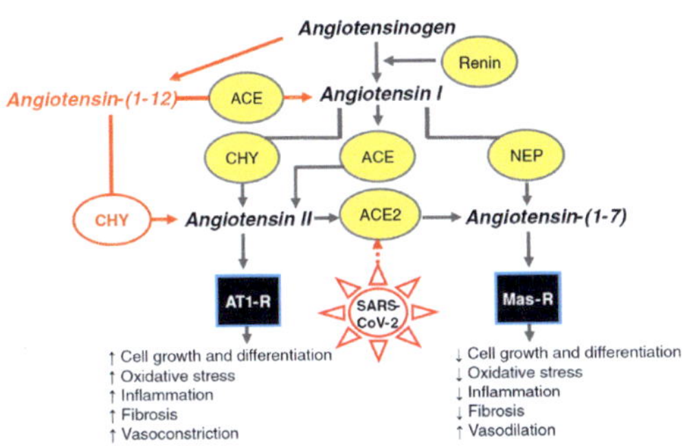

Figure 12.13. Overview of angiotensinogen products and their functions in the RAS.

Source: https://www.researchgate.net/profile/Sarfaraz-Ahmad-6/publication/343918536/figure/fig2/AS:962680701587457@1606532373559/Overview-of-angiotensinogen-products-and-their-functions-in-the-RAS-Angiotensinogen-is.png.

12.4.3. Hepcidin and Its Influence on Iron Metabolism

Hepcidin, which is primarily produced in the liver as a peptide hormone, is an important regulator of iron homeostasis. Its regulation is mediated by several parameters like iron levels, erythropoiesis, and inflammation. Elevated serum iron levels stimulate the production of hepcidin, leading to ferroportin internalization and degradation, an iron exporter restricted to enterocytes and macrophages. This process actually inhibits dietary iron absorption as well as prevents the mobilization of recycled iron from macrophages and reduces overall availability of iron in the circulation needed to maintain homeostasis. In contrast, inflammatory or anemia states trigger the reduction in hepcidin levels, increasing iron bioavailability by activating ferroportin and mobilizing stored iron, which ultimately supports erythropoiesis during periods of increased physiological demand (Pavord et al., 2019). Abnormality in the regulation of the hepcidin levels is associated with a number of iron metabolism diseases. In genetic disorders like hereditary hemochromatosis, HFE mutations disrupt the normal feedback loop that typically controls hepcidin production, leading to hyperabsorption and tissue iron accumulation. This tissue accumulation can result in very damaging organ damage, emphasizing the requirement for tight control of hepcidin levels to prevent overload. In addition, inflammatory diseases, for example, chronic infection and disease, will stimulate the production of hepcidin, producing anemia of inflammation. This condition is characterized by iron sequestration within macrophages and impaired mobilization from reserves, hence exhibiting an intricate interaction between hepcidin, iron sufficiency, and general well-being (Edward et al., 2018). The understanding of these processes has a significant contribution to the development of therapeutic approaches aimed at iron balancing. Apart from regulating iron metabolism, hepcidin's role also extends to being interconnected with metabolic pathways controlled by other hormones in the liver and gastrointestinal tract. To illustrate, insulin signaling has been shown to influence hepcidin expression, suggesting a connection between glucose homeostasis and iron homeostasis. As metabolic disorders rise all over the world, research into the interaction between these hormones is becoming increasingly relevant. Investigation into how hepcidin responds to nutrition, hormonal state, and pathophysiologic states will shed light on the more general importance of iron regulation in systemic disease and health. Thus, investigation into therapeutic interventions that modulate the activity of hepcidin may provide new avenues for the treatment of iron disorders and the optimal iron metabolism in various clinical conditions (Pavord et al., 2019) (Figure 12.14).

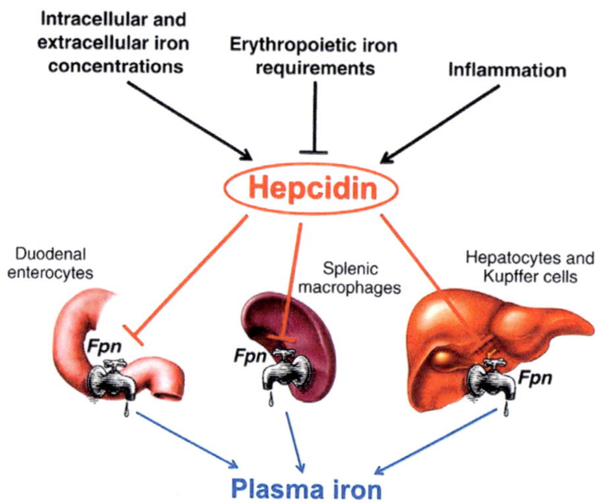

Figure 12.14. Regulation of iron balance.

Source: https://www.intechopen.com/chapters/79891.

Test Your Knowledge

1. What is Insulin-like Growth Factor (IGF), and how does it mediate the effects of growth hormone in the body?
2. What is the function of angiotensinogen in the renin-angiotensin-aldosterone system (RAAS)?

12.5. Interaction Between Gut Hormones and Liver Function

Learning Outcome

1. Understand the role of gut hormones in metabolic regulation;
2. Describe feedback mechanisms between the gut and liver;
3. Deal with implications for liver diseases and disorders.

The gut-hormone-liver axis plays a significant role in the explanation of metabolic disease and health. The gut-released hormones, such as GLP-1 and peptide YY (PYY), play direct roles in regulating glucose homeostasis, insulin secretion, and appetite. The hormones are secreted after food consumption and play a role in communication with the liver to control its functions. For instance, GLP-1 promotes the release of insulin and, simultaneously, inhibits glucagon release from the pancreas, leading to reduced hepatic glucose output. The dynamic interplay between these hormones and liver function underscores the delicate balance that maintains metabolic homeostasis, particularly in patients with metabolic disease. Disruption of this regulatory feedback can lead to conditions including insulin resistance and type 2 diabetes, and the study of these intricate interactions is crucial in both clinical and therapeutic applications. Bile acids, which are produced in the liver and secreted into the gastrointestinal tract, are another very important element in the interaction between gut hormones and liver function. In addition to their traditional role in fat digestion, bile acids are also signaling molecules that impact carbohydrate and lipid metabolism. They act on nuclear receptors such as Farnesoid X receptor (FXR) and G protein-coupled receptors (TGR5), whose actions regulate their activities on glucose homeostasis and energy expenditure. Disturbances in bile acid homeostasis have also been linked with metabolic diseases like obesity and type 2 diabetes, in which altered profiles of bile acids regulate gut hormone secretion. Recent evidence has indicated that reabsorption and secretion of bile acids as being able to control the secretion of gut hormones like GLP-1, illustrating a two-way communication between the liver and the gut that is essential in maintaining metabolic balance in the body (Wang et al., 2024). Moreover, interactions between gut hormone secretion and liver function are regulated by dietary influences and gut populations of microorganisms. A diet rich in saturated fats and sugar can have harmful effects on gut hormone secretion, leading to faulty liver function and vulnerability to metabolic disease. Simultaneously, gut microbiota have also been shown to play a considerable role in bile acid and hormone metabolism, which, in turn, affect the health of the liver. For example, changes in the gut microbial community can lead to modified bile acid metabolism and secretion of gut hormones, thereby affecting the function of the liver. The finding of these intricate mechanisms holds the promise for therapeutic interventions to normalize balance in gut-liver axes, which might lower the risk of metabolic disease among susceptible individuals (Krishna et al., 2024).

12.5.1. The Role of Gut Hormones in Metabolic Regulation

The interactive dynamics between gut hormones and metabolic control underscore the key function of these signaling molecules in modulating energy homeostasis and energy balance. On sensing nutrient ingestion, the gastrointestinal tract releases various gut hormones such as GLP-1 and peptide YY (PYY), which together play pivotal roles in appetite regulation and glucose metabolism. GLP-1 has also been demonstrated to enhance insulin secretion and suppress the secretion of glucagon, thereby creating a state of anabolic metabolism. Besides that, PYY is a suppressor of appetite, which signals satiety to the central nervous system and impacts energy intake. Control of these hormones is not simply a response to what has been eaten as food; their activity is also modulated by the gut microbiota, indicating complex crosstalk that exerts a significant impact on metabolic disease and overall well-being (Willem et al., 2022). Short-chain fatty acids (SCFAs), which are produced as a result of the fermentation of dietary fiber by the gut microbiota, are a critical area of intersection between gut health and metabolic regulation. These metabolites have been shown to increase the release of gut hormones like GLP-1 and PYY, and thereby amplify their effects on insulin secretion and appetite regulation. SCFAs exert their effects via G-protein-coupled receptors on enteroendocrine cells, finally causing downstream activation of signal pathways for metabolic activity. Further, SCFAs are believed to induce epigenetic changes that impact gene expression for metabolic processes (Bart et al., 2021). This reveals that nutritional consumption, particularly the intake of dietary fiber, plays a critical role in metabolic health, once again making the incorporation of nutrition imperative in the prevention and management of metabolic diseases. The multiple roles of gut hormones in metabolic regulation extend beyond energy homeostasis; they are also involved in the control of intestinal permeability and immunity. For instance, gut hormones have been implicated in maintaining the integrity of the intestinal barrier against the translocation of pathogens and toxins into the circulation. Furthermore, the interaction between the immune cells and the gut hormones plays a crucial role in modulating inflammation, particularly in conditions such as diabetes and obesity. The two-way interaction between metabolic function and the gut underscores the need for further research to better understand the mechanisms of gut hormones. Targeting the hormonal–microbial relationship may open up new ways to treat metabolic syndromes and gastrointestinal disorders (Willem et al., 2022) (Figure 12.15).

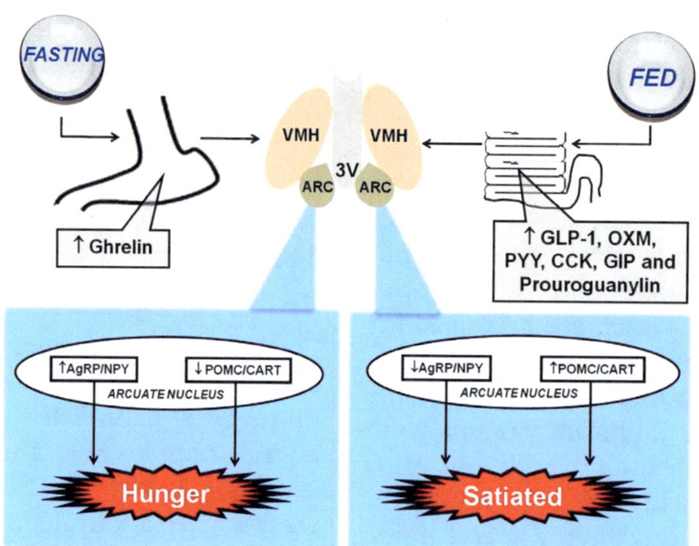

Figure 12.15. Role of gut hormones in the fasting (right) and postprandial (left) states.

Source: https://www.researchgate.net/profile/Ronaldo-Thomatieli-Santos/publication/223972153/figure/fig1/AS:202967325122560@1425402589006/Role-of-gut-hormones-in-fasting-right-and-postprandial-left-state-During-fasting.png.

12.5.2. Feedback Mechanisms Between the Gut and Liver

The gut-liver feedback mechanisms also make important contributions toward metabolic homeostasis. Communication between the two is primarily controlled by hormones and signaling molecules secreted by the two organs. The gut secretes a variety of hormones, such as gastrin, cholecystokinin (CCK), and GLP-1, that have primary actions on liver function. For instance, CCK triggers gallbladder contraction and bile salt secretion, both of which are essential for lipid digestion, while GLP-1 stimulates insulin secretion from the pancreas, contributing indirectly to liver metabolism. These hormones not only regulate digestion but also pass information on nutrient availability to the liver, facilitating adaptive mechanisms that are essential to energy balance and nutrient homeostasis (Kelly, 2004). Furthermore, the liver also plays its part in these feedback pathways by synthesizing and secreting a myriad of metabolites and hormones that influence gastrointestinal physiology. A prime example is the liver's secretion of insulin-like growth factor 1 (IGF-1), which has been reported to regulate gastrointestinal function and nutrient uptake. The liver also has a crucial role to play in the regulation of the metabolism of compounds like glucose and lipids, both of which are vital for energy homeostasis. By controlling the release of glucose into the circulation and regulating the hormonal signals from the gut, the liver establishes a complete feedback loop that ensures an efficient energy supply and utilization during digestion (Raguso et al., 2000). Recent studies highlight the emerging new role of gut-derived hormones in the regulation of liver function, thereby supporting the importance of feedback in this axis. Leptin, most noted for its role in controlling food intake, has been discovered to be present within various gastrointestinal tissues, showing its effects may be more energetic and not exclusively centered on energy balance, but also on the action on liver metabolism. This localization shows the intricacy of the gut-liver axis, where hormones not only provide signals on nutrient uptake but could directly affect hepatic function. Knowledge of these feedback mechanisms is critical towards the development of better therapeutic interventions for metabolic disease, and highlights the need to study in more detail the complex interactions between the liver and gut (Kelly, 2004; Raguso et al., 2000).

12.5.3. Implications for Liver Diseases and Disorders

Hormone interactions between the liver and gastrointestinal tract are also key to a large number of liver diseases and disorders. Hormone signaling imbalance can result in hepatic steatosis, which is typically a product of insulin resistance and metabolic derangement. Resistance has a direct link with hormonal factors such as glucagon and insulin, and these are key actors in glucose homeostasis and lipid metabolism. Such an interference with hormonal signaling not only increases fatty accumulation in the liver but also provokes inflammation and fibrosis, ultimately causing NAFLD. It is thus critical to know the mechanisms in a bid to develop interventions that can avert liver complications of metabolic syndrome and thus design targeted therapeutic interventions to reverse normal hormonal function and improve liver function. Furthermore, research has predominantly focused on the involvement of gut microbiota in liver pathophysiology, further stressing the importance of hormonal interactions. Dysbiosis, or microbial imbalance in the gut, can significantly influence liver status by controlling hormone levels and immunity. For instance, some bacteria in the gut have been identified to generate metabolites such as short-chain fatty acids that exert protective functions on the activity of the liver and control inflammation. Consequently, dysbiosis is revealed to lead to the production of pathogenic metabolites accountable for inducing liver damage and cirrhosis or hepatocellular carcinoma. A wider understanding of the gut-liver axis extends the discussion of hormonal implication to suggest that treatments enhancing gut microbiota health may have downstream impacts on liver disease, thus offering a multi-dimensional treatment strategy incorporating both hormonal and microbial influence on liver disease (Hou et al., 2022). Clinical approaches to treating liver disease increasingly utilize knowledge of the interactions between microbiota and hormones, paving the way for new therapeutic strategies. The current evidence is that manipulation of gut microbiota using dietary treatment or probiotics can stabilize the disrupted hormonal environment and produce improved metabolic results in patients with liver disease. For example, gut microbiota production of bile acids under some hormonal stimuli is crucial for the metabolism and digestion of lipids. Disruption of the pathway results in increased liver disease through lipid inflammation or deposition. This highlighted the value proposition for developing therapies that not only correct hormonal imbalance but also leverage the therapeutic properties of the gut microbiota to restore liver function. Understanding these intersecting pathways may ultimately offer more effective prevention and treatment strategies for liver disease and disorder (Willem et al., 2022).

Test Your Knowledge

1. How do gut hormones such as GLP-1 (glucagon-like peptide-1) and GIP (gastric inhibitory peptide) influence liver glucose metabolism?
2. What feedback mechanisms exist between gut-derived hormones and hepatic insulin sensitivity?
3. In what ways can dysregulation of gut hormones impact the development or progression of liver diseases?

12.6. Clinical Implications of Hormonal Dysregulation

Learning Outcome

1. Understand the effects of hormonal imbalances on gastrointestinal health;
2. Explain the relationship between hormones and metabolic syndrome;
3. Describe potential therapeutic approaches targeting hormones.

The clinical impact of hormonal dysregulation in the liver and gastrointestinal tract is widespread, influencing many metabolic processes and resulting in a considerable difference in health. Leptin and insulin are significant hormones that are responsible for energy regulation and control of hunger; however, their dysregulation can typically be observed in diseases like metabolic-dysfunction-associated steatotic liver disease (MASLD) (Jeysson et al., 2025). With the increasing strength of metabolic syndrome, the linkage between hormonal disorders and hepatic outcomes cannot be overstressed. Insulin-resistant patients tend to have adipose tissue dysfunction that results in hepatic fat deposition.

The progression from simple steatosis to more severe liver diseases such as non-alcoholic steatohepatitis (NASH) and even hepatocellular carcinoma implies taking steps towards normalization of hormonal equilibrium and metabolic correction at an early stage. In addition, the relationship between the gastrointestinal hormones and liver function offers a critical element of hormonal dysregulation. Hormones such as cholecystokinin (CCK), glucagon-like peptide-1 (GLP-1), and peptide YY (PYY) play a central role in regulating gastric emptying, gut motility, and metabolism. Dysregulation of such hormones can lead to altered nutrient absorption and exacerbate liver disease, and it is directly associated with the clinical presentation of obesity-related liver diseases such as MASLD (Jeysson et al., 2025). Gastrointestinal hormone modulation has been suggested by studies to hold promising therapeutic options towards preventing the obesity-liver disease association. Thus, an understanding of how hormonal dysregulation influences gastrointestinal physiology will be key to the development of measures that promote liver function and better patient outcomes in individuals with metabolic disorders.

The role of precision medicine has been highlighted in recent work in addressing hormonal dysregulation and its associated sequelae. Personalized treatment strategies incorporating an individual's hormonal topography, as well as clinical background and lifestyle variables, are important for maximizing therapeutic interventions. Detection of hormonal biomarkers and their correlation with the disease process can provide valuable insights into patient prognosis and the course of recovery. For instance, as seen in clinical studies in immune-related adverse events (irAEs) of gastrointestinal malignancies, fluctuations of hematological markers within therapy cycles can be predictive of incidence as well as recovery from complications. This underlines the necessity for the integration of hormonal assessment into standard clinical practice via multidisciplinary intervention to enhance the management of dysregulated liver and gastrointestinal tract hormones' related disorders.

12.6.1. Effects of Hormonal Imbalances on Gastrointestinal Health

Hormonal dysregulation may significantly disrupt gastrointestinal health, manifesting in a variety of physiological and psychological signs. Serotonin, typically termed a neurotransmitter, plays a significant role in the regulation of gut motility, so a deficiency or excess may cause conditions such as irritable bowel syndrome (IBS) or constipation. Additionally, peptide hormones such as insulin and glucagon regulate nutrient absorption and metabolism, which is crucial for gut integrity maintenance. Disturbance of these hormones can lead to gastrointestinal disease by disrupting the composition of gut microbiota, a process that has been emphasized in current studies on the role of microbiota in homeostasis and immune maintenance. Alteration in the balance of these microbes due to changes in the hormones can result in dysbiosis and potentially contribute to inflammation and different gastrointestinal diseases, reflecting the inter-relationship between gastrointestinal health and endocrine health (Hou et al., 2022). Stress and hormonal alterations, particularly with cortisol, also exacerbate gastrointestinal disease. The primary stress hormone cortisol tends to increase in the presence of physical or psychological stress, leading to dysfunctional digestion and alterations in gut flora. Elevation of cortisol chronically has been reported to disrupt the gut-brain axis by studies and can lead to ulcerative colitis and gastroesophageal reflux disease (GERD). Elevated cortisol has also been found to be associated with inflammation, which may exacerbate an underlying gastrointestinal condition or even cause it. These physiological responses highlight the significance of hormonal equilibrium in optimizing gastrointestinal function, showing how psychological stress can have significantly different effects on physical health (Visseren et al., 2021). Sex-hormonal differences, particularly involving estrogen and progesterone, also account for gender variations in gastrointestinal health. These changes in hormones during menstrual cycles, pregnancy, or menopause may lead to various gastrointestinal symptoms such as bloating, abdominal discomfort, and altered bowel habits (Figure 12.16).

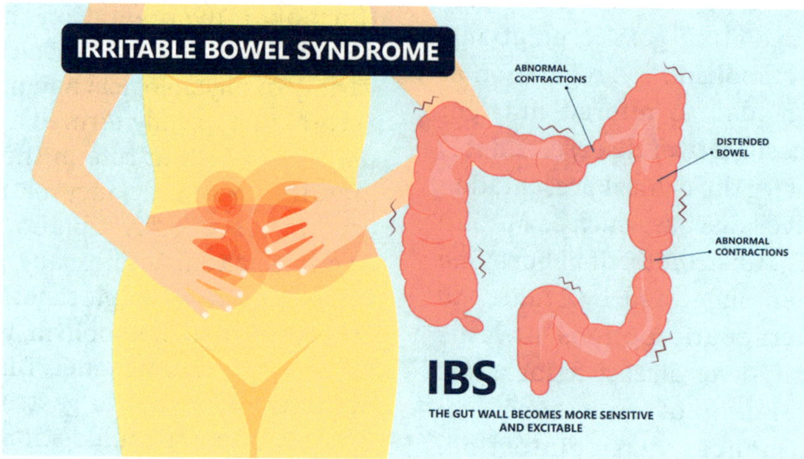

Figure 12.16. Irritable bowel syndrome (IBS).

Source: https://www.hmsmirdifhospital.ae/contents/uploads/media/irritable-bowel-syndrome.jpg.

For instance, premenstrual syndrome (PMS) and menopause are often exacerbated by a hormonal imbalance that may alter gut motility. This relationship suggests that perception and control of these hormonal alterations are important in the design of sound intervention strategies for women with gastrointestinal diseases. Interventions to balance these hormone levels might open new avenues for minimizing symptoms and enhancing GI well-being and ultimately, the quality of life of the affected parties (Hou et al., 2022) (Figure 12.17).

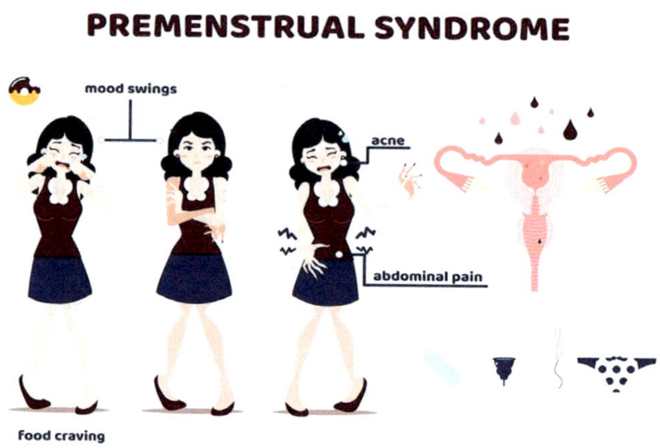

Figure 12.17. Premenstrual syndrome (PMS).

Source: https://i0.wp.com/www.gynsurgery.org/wp-content/uploads//pms-plan-to-reduce-symptoms-suffering.jpg.

12.6.2. Relationship Between Hormones and Metabolic Syndrome

When one analyzes the intricate interaction between metabolic syndrome and hormones, one is able to clearly see that hormone dysregulation is a key component of the etiology of this multifactorial condition. Metabolic syndrome is characterized by a cluster of metabolic disturbances that include obesity, insulin resistance, dyslipidemia, and hypertension. The gastrointestinal tract and the liver produce an array of hormones whose impact on metabolic functions is immense. For instance, hormones like GLP-1 and cholecystokinin (CCK) are involved in the regulation of appetite and glucose homeostasis, both of which are typically impaired in metabolic syndrome. Moreover, leptin and ghrelin—hormones that regulate satiety and hunger messages—have been reported to have perturbed levels in the obese, thereby increasing the risk of metabolic syndrome. Gut microbiota's influence on hormone levels definitely establishes its crucial function in metabolic disease and well-being. It has now been found that changes in the gut microbiome composition influence the secretion of gastrointestinal hormones involved in energy metabolism (Willem et al., 2022). For example, short-chain fatty acids produced by gut bacteria from fermentation of dietary fiber could enhance GLP-1 secretion, promoting insulin sensitivity and satiety. Further, gut microbiome dysbiosis has also been implicated as an instigator of inflammation, which can in turn cause disruption of endocrine activity and proceed to metabolic syndrome pathogenesis. With such interaction understood, this opens avenues for potential therapeutic intervention, such as using probiotics for re-balancing of the microbes and subsequent regulation of hormonal pathways important to metabolic status. The entire narrative concerning metabolic syndrome and hormone interaction calls for integral practice in prevention alongside treatment regimens. Consistent with the ESC Guidelines' advisories, clinicians must consider the biological basis of hormone functions when creating clinical interventions for metabolic syndrome (Visseren et al., 2021). This necessitates consideration of inter-individual differences in hormonal responses to food habits, exercise, and psychosocial factors. For instance, personalized nutrition plans according to hormonal feedback are likely to enhance metabolic performance. Additionally, new treatments with individualized targeting of hormonal signaling pathways, such as GLP-1 receptor agonists, possess potential in not only metabolic indicators but also general health outcomes in the case of metabolic syndrome. An in-depth comprehension of hormone-gut microbiota interactions is thus necessary for additional advancement in clinical practice in the effective management of metabolic syndrome.

12.6.3. Potential Therapeutic Approaches Targeting Hormones

The intricate hormonal interplay within the gastrointestinal tract and liver represents one of the explanations for the maintenance of metabolic homeostasis and, as such, represents a site of therapeutic intervention. Hormone modulation, particularly through agents that are able to modulate the secretion or activity of gastrointestinal hormones, including ghrelin, peptide YY, and GLP-1, presents new opportunities for intervention in metabolic disease. For instance, agents that increase GLP-1 levels are useful in enhancing insulin secretion and glycemic control in type 2 diabetic patients. This method illustrates the therapeutic potential of manipulating hormone action to achieve metabolic benefit and, by extension, encourages further research into such techniques with other hormones involved in the regulation of appetite and energy expenditure. Understanding the mechanism of how such hormones bring about their action will be essential to planning useful therapy for obesity and related metabolic disease. As an expansion of direct hormonal manipulation, the potential of natural products that modulate hormone secretion and action also needs to be addressed. Certain dietary components with bioactive molecules may beneficially modulate the intestinal flora with enhanced secretion and sensitivity of appetite-controlling and metabolism-controlling hormones. For example, polyphenols and polysaccharides found in most fruits and vegetables exhibit immunomodulatory activities with potential in modifying gut hormone levels and thus the regulation of metabolism. This suggests that dietary management in the form of adjunct therapies could provide functional benefits in obesity and type 2 diabetes control. The integration of such natural products into part of normal meals might exploit their hormone-modulating activities while encouraging an overall strategy for wellness. These strategies highlight the intersection of diet, hormones, and disease, and the results are new therapeutic modalities that leverage the intrinsic synergy of dietary components and hormonal regulation. Investigation of the biochemistry of hormone action presents promising therapeutic potential in the treatment of metabolic illnesses. Hormone-targeting drugs, such as those activating adenosine monophosphate-activated protein kinase (AMPK), can offer great benefit by enhancing insulin sensitivity and promoting weight loss. Activation of AMPK has been associated with improved glucose and lipid profiles, thereby contributing to the management of metabolic syndrome. Moreover, compounds like α-lipoic acid have been shown to be potential candidates in the activation of AMPK and, therefore, influence energy metabolism at the cellular level. Identification and synthesis of AMPK activators or other compounds have strong potential towards the prevention of comorbidities associated with obesity, i.e., cardiovascular disease and NAFLD. As increasingly more research illuminates the complex interactions of the hormonal milieu of the gastrointestinal tract and liver, emerging therapeutic strategies targeting these hormones will increasingly become important in the control of such metabolic states.

Test Your Knowledge

1. How do hormonal imbalances affect gastrointestinal function and motility?
2. What role do hormones like leptin, ghrelin, and insulin play in the development and progression of metabolic syndrome?

SUMMARY

The complex interrelationships between the gastrointestinal and liver hormones highlight their critical functions in homeostasis processes of the human body. These hormones control fundamental physiological functions, such as digestion, metabolism, and appetite regulation, which reflect their importance beyond digestive purposes. For instance, gastrin and cholecystokinin, in addition to participating in gastric motility and bile secretion, also belong to the global endocrine signaling pathway that regulates nutrient absorption and energy balance. It is essential to delineate these pathways to understand how deregulations contribute to the development of various gastrointestinal diseases and metabolic disorders. From such a knowledge base, future therapy that aims at balancing hormones and optimizing patient outcomes can be tailored. Apart from that, recent research has brought to light new facts about the role of hormones like ghrelin and leptin in hunger and energy homeostasis, thereby increasing our database on obesity and its complications. Hormonal interaction is a two-edged sword; it is primarily beneficial but can produce serious health consequences in the form of disturbances in these processes. For instance, a study presents a case of hypercalcemia with gastrointestinal stromal tumor. In this respect, elevated calcitriol due to hormonal activity of the tumor illustrates how some conditions can derange metabolic homeostasis via hormonal disturbances. The implication of such observation speaks for further investigation into the multifaceted roles of these hormones in diseased states, especially since they can prove beneficial in the formulation of targeted therapy in patients. Last, research into the hormonal physiology of the gut and liver calls for an integrated approach to research that combines clinical insight with basic science data. Tomorrow may hold promise in unmasking the molecular mechanisms of hormone secretion and action, as well as their interaction with various pathologies. The integration of hormonal studies into large-scale endocrine and metabolic research could uncover potential biomarkers for earlier diagnosis and customized treatment regimens. This integration is crucial to better understand diseases, like those indicated in work proposing hypercalcemia as a sign of specific gastrointestinal cancers, including gastrointestinal stromal tumors, and further enrich the field of endocrine research. A full comprehension of these hormone mechanisms will eventually equip healthcare professionals with the techniques to cure some of the most serious metabolic conditions that plague public health today.

The hormone analysis in the gastrointestinal tract and liver presents with a complex interaction of paracrine and endocrine signaling integral to metabolic homeostasis. Master hormones such as gastrin, cholecystokinin (CCK), and secretin control digestion and absorption of nutrients by modifying gastric acid secretion, bile, and pancreatic enzyme activity. In addition, the interaction of these hormones with several signaling pathways that influence the appetite and energy balance. Unraveling these hormone-regulated processes is important not only for the elucidation of basic physiological functions but also for the therapy of metabolic illnesses such as obesity and diabetes, where disruptions in hormone signal pathways form the basis of devastating complications. By unravelling these interactions, researchers aim to find possible therapeutic targets that can enhance metabolic health and clinical outcomes. New findings: molecular biology has demonstrated how microbiota of the gut can be implicated in hormone production and activity within the gut. Certain types of gut microbes have been indicated by some studies to modulate the secretion of significant hormones, such as incretins, indirectly affecting insulin sensitivity and glucose metabolism. This association highlights the importance of considering gut microbiota structure in evaluating hormone-related endpoints and therapeutic interventions for metabolic disorders. The microbiota-gut-brain axis makes things even more complicated in that gut hormones not only play a role in cognitive function and emotional reaction, but also emphasize an integrated approach to health with both the physiological and psychological factors. Progress here is raising new approaches to managing obesity and related disorders by microbial modulation. Furthermore, hormonal interactions between the liver and gastrointestinal tract involve the regulation of systemic energy balance and metabolism. Glucagon and insulin are just a few hormones that not only participate in glucose homeostasis but also carry vital information between these organs regarding energy storage and supply of nutrients. The liver's sensitivity to hormonal cues is central to the resolution of metabolic stress, and understanding this sensitivity will improve our knowledge of liver disease, including non-alcoholic fatty liver disease. It has been found that there is a close correlation between the metabolic function of the liver and hormonal milieu manipulated by diet and microbiota, highlighting the importance of profound knowledge of these interactions. Collectively, these results indicate the central roles played by hormones in the interactive gastrointestinal and hepatic systems and lay the foundation for subsequent studies aimed at improving metabolic health and disease regulation.

KEY TERMS FROM THIS CHAPTER

- Angiotensinogen
- Cholecystokinin
- Energy homeostasis
- Enteroendocrine cells
- Enzymatic activity
- Fat emulsification
- Gastric acid
- Gastric physiology
- Gastrointestinal anatomy
- Gastrointestinal hormones
- Gastrointestinal system
- Ghrelin antagonists
- Gut-brain axis
- Gut-liver axis
- Hormonal regulation
- Insulin-like growth factor (IGF)
- Autonomic nervous system (ANS)
- Electrolyte homeostasis
- Energy metabolism
- Enteroendocrine cells (EECs)
- Farnesoid X receptor (FXR)
- Gallbladder
- Gastric epithelial cells
- Gastroenterology physiology
- Gastrointestinal function
- Gastrointestinal integrity
- Gastrointestinal tract
- Gut hormones
- Gut-derived hormones
- Hormonal management
- Inflammatory signaling
- Lipid metabolis

CRITICAL THINKING QUESTIONS

1. **Which of the following hormones is primarily responsible for stimulating gastric acid secretion in the stomach?**
   a. Secretin
   b. Cholecystokinin (CCK)
   c. Gastrin
   d. Ghrelin
2. **What is the primary function of secretin in the gastrointestinal tract?**
   a. Stimulate insulin secretion
   b. Stimulate bile release from the gallbladder
   c. Stimulate bicarbonate secretion from the pancreas
   d. Increase appetite
3. **Which hormone is known as the "hunger hormone" and is primarily secreted by the stomach?**
   a. Leptin
   b. Ghrelin
   c. Peptide YY
   d. Insulin
4. **Which of the following is a hormone produced by the liver with a key role in regulating iron homeostasis?**
   a. Hepcidin
   b. Somatostatin
   c. Glucagon-like peptide-1 (GLP-1)
   d. Motilin
5. **Dysregulation of gut hormones like GLP-1 and insulin resistance in the liver is most commonly associated with which clinical condition?**
   a. Celiac disease
   b. Peptic ulcer disease
   c. Hemochromatosis
   d. Non-alcoholic fatty liver disease (NAFLD)

Short Answer Questions

1. What are the primary hormones produced by the gastrointestinal tract, and what are their main physiological functions?
2. How do hormones like ghrelin and peptide YY regulate appetite and satiety at the central and peripheral levels?
3. Which hormones are secreted by the liver, and how do they contribute to systemic metabolic regulation?
4. In what ways do gut hormones such as GLP-1 and CCK influence insulin secretion and glucose metabolism?
5. How does the enterohepatic circulation influence the hormonal communication between the gut and the liver?
6. How can alterations in gut hormone signaling contribute to the development or progression of non-alcoholic fatty liver disease (NAFLD)?
7. What therapeutic strategies are being developed or used to target gastrointestinal or hepatic hormones in metabolic or digestive disorders?

Answers to Critical Thinking Questions

1. (b) 2. (c) 3. (b) 4. (a) 5. (d)

REFERENCES

1. Balali-Mood, M., Naseri, K., Tahergorabi, Z., Khazdair, M. R., & Sadeghi, M. (2021). Toxic mechanisms of five heavy metals: Mercury, lead, chromium, cadmium, and arsenic. *Frontiers in Pharmacology, 12*. https://doi.org/10.3389/fphar.2021.643972 (accessed on 22nd July 2025).
2. Bourgonje, A. R., Abdulle, A. E., Timens, W., Hillebrands, J. L., Navis, G., Gordijn, S. J., Bolling, M. C., et al. (2020). Angiotensin-converting enzyme 2 (ACE2), SARS-CoV-2 and the pathophysiology of coronavirus disease 2019 (COVID-19). *The Journal of Pathology, 251*, 228–248. https://doi.org/10.1002/path.5471 (accessed on 22nd July 2025).
3. Breit, S., Kupferberg, A., Rogler, G., & Hasler, G. (2018). Vagus nerve as modulator of the brain–gut axis in psychiatric and inflammatory disorders. *Frontiers in Psychiatry, 9*. https://doi.org/10.3389/fpsyt.2018.00044 (accessed on 22nd July 2025).
4. Campanale, C., Massarelli, C., Savino, I., Locaputo, V., & Uricchio, V. F. (2020). A detailed review study on potential effects of microplastics and additives of concern on human health. *International Journal of Environmental Research and Public Health, 17*, 1212. https://doi.org/10.3390/ijerph17041212 (accessed on 22nd July 2025).
5. de Vos, W. M., Tilg, H., Van Hul, M., & Cani, P. D. (2022). Gut microbiome and health: Mechanistic insights. *Gut, 71*, 1020–1032. https://doi.org/10.1136/gutjnl-2021-326789 (accessed on 22nd July 2025).
6. Fahed, G., Aoun, L., Bou Zerdan, M., Allam, S., Bou Zerdan, M., Bouferraa, Y., & Assi, H. (2022). Metabolic syndrome: Updates on pathophysiology and management in 2021. *International Journal of Molecular Sciences, 23*, 786. https://doi.org/10.3390/ijms23020786 (accessed on 22nd July 2025).
7. Fitzsimons, E. J., Cullis, J. O., Thomas, W., Tsochatzis, E., & Griffiths, W. J. (2018). Diagnosis and therapy of genetic haemochromatosis (review and 2017 update). *British Journal of Hematology, 181*, 293–303. https://doi.org/10.1111/bjh.15164 (accessed on 22nd July 2025).
8. Ghosh, S., Whitley, C. S., Haribabu, B., & Jala, V. R. (2021). Regulation of intestinal barrier function by microbial metabolites. *Cellular and Molecular Gastroenterology and Hepatology, 11*, 1463–1482. https://doi.org/10.1016/j.jcmgh.2021.02.007 (accessed on 22nd July 2025).
9. Guo, J., Huang, X., Dou, L., Yan, M., Shen, T., Tang, W., & Li, J. (2022). Aging and aging-related diseases: From molecular mechanisms to interventions and treatments. *Signal Transduction and Targeted Therapy, 7*. https://doi.org/10.1038/s41392-022-01251-0 (accessed on 22nd July 2025).
10. Hou, K., Wu, Z. X., Chen, X. Y., Wang, J. Q., Zhang, D., Xiao, C., Zhu, D., et al. (2022). Microbiota in health and diseases. *Signal Transduction and Targeted Therapy, 7*. https://doi.org/10.1038/s41392-022-00974-4 (accessed on 22nd July 2025).
11. Hu, X., Li, J., Fu, M., Zhao, X., & Wang, W. (2021). The JAK/STAT signaling pathway: From bench to clinic. *Signal Transduction and Targeted Therapy, 6*. https://doi.org/10.1038/s41392-021-00791-1 (accessed on 22nd July 2025).
12. Hygum, K., Wulff, C., Harsløf, T., Boysen, A., Rossen, P., Langdahl, B., & Safwat, A. (2015). Hypercalcemia in metastatic GIST caused by systemic elevated calcitriol: A case report and review of the literature. *BMC Cancer, 15*. https://www.semanticscholar.org/paper/8baf79b78cf18b81dc929b1546c172033406b61c (accessed on 22nd July 2025).

13. Imai, J., & Katagiri, H. (2021). Regulation of systemic metabolism by the autonomic nervous system consisting of afferent and efferent innervation. *International Immunology, 34*, 67–79. https://doi.org/10.1093/intimm/dxab023 (accessed on 22nd July 2025).

14. Ismair, M., Stieger, B., Cattori, V., Hagenbuch, B., Fried, M., Meier, P., & Kullak-Ublick, G. (2001). Hepatic uptake of cholecystokinin octapeptide by organic anion-transporting polypeptides OATP4 and OATP8 of rat and human liver. *Gastroenterology, 121*, 1185–1190. https://www.semanticscholar.org/paper/81e8971f6c7d4a1e294c3d82f82adef1a1791f44 (accessed on 22nd July 2025).

15. Javitt, N. (2018). Fasting and postprandial serum bile acids after RYGB surgery. *Scandinavian Journal of Gastroenterology, 53*, 1425–1426. https://www.semanticscholar.org/paper/2b4d362868fac9595892592eef9c5c39963aab12 (accessed on 22nd July 2025).

16. Kelly, L. (2004). *Essentials of Human Physiology for Pharmacy*. https://www.semanticscholar.org/paper/4219f4edcfbeb281dc54006ce947a2795fbfb510 (accessed on 22nd July 2025).

17. Lee, I. (2011). Adenosine monophosphate kinase activator α-lipoic acid: A promising therapeutic agent for metabolic syndrome? *Journal of Diabetes Investigation, 2*, 241–242. https://www.semanticscholar.org/paper/b7e0e77e4ab1b5ddc9044fa7d16f877e75fe1f83 (accessed on 22nd July 2025).

18. Li, K., Wang, S., Qu, W., Ahmed, A. A., Enneb, W., Obeidat, M. D., Liu, H. Y., et al. (2024). Natural products for Gut-X axis: Pharmacology, toxicology and microbiology in mycotoxin-caused diseases. *Frontiers in Pharmacology, 15*. https://www.semanticscholar.org/paper/ec730da9b74e564b91b232b153104b189c91081e (accessed on 22nd July 2025).

19. Liddle, R. A. (2019). Neuropods. *Cellular and Molecular Gastroenterology and Hepatology, 7*, 739–747. https://doi.org/10.1016/j.jcmgh.2019.01.006 (accessed on 22nd July 2025).

20. Martin-Gallausiaux, C., Marinelli, L., Blottière, H. M., Larraufie, P., & Lapaque, N. (2020). SCFA: Mechanisms and functional importance in the gut. *Proceedings of The Nutrition Society, 80*, 37–49. https://doi.org/10.1017/s0029665120006916 (accessed on 22nd July 2025).

21. Mejía-Guzmán, J. E., Belmont-Hernández, R. A., Chávez-Tapia, N. C., Uribe, M., & Nuño-Lámbarri, N. (2025). Metabolic-dysfunction-associated steatotic liver disease: Molecular mechanisms, clinical implications, and emerging therapeutic strategies. *International Journal of Molecular Sciences, 26*. https://www.semanticscholar.org/paper/4c63d1bff27c7cfbe5c3091c5eb3445a0a04f186 (accessed on 22nd July 2025).

22. Mukherjee, A., Lordan, C., Ross, R. P., & Cotter, P. D. (2020). Gut microbes from the phylogenetically diverse genus *Eubacterium* and their various contributions to gut health. *Gut Microbes, 12*, 1802866. https://doi.org/10.1080/19490976.2020.1802866 (accessed on 22nd July 2025).

23. Müller, T. D., Blüher, M., Tschöp, M. H., & DiMarchi, R. D. (2021). Anti-obesity drug discovery: Advances and challenges. *Nature Reviews Drug Discovery, 21*, 201–223. https://doi.org/10.1038/s41573-021-00337-8 (accessed on 22nd July 2025).

24. Müller, T. D., Finan, B., Bloom, S. R., D'Alessio, D. A., Drucker, D. J., Flatt, P. R., Fritsche, A., et al. (2019). Glucagon-like peptide 1 (GLP-1). *Molecular Metabolism, 30*, 72–130. https://doi.org/10.1016/j.molmet.2019.09.010 (accessed on 22nd July 2025).

25. Murali Krishna, S., Hegde, S. V., Chellathurai, M., Mohandas, N. J. A., Guruswamy, S., Pandit, S., Afra, A., et al. (2024). Correlation between thyroid-stimulating hormone (TSH) and liver function test values in North Karnataka patients admitted to a tertiary care hospital. *Cureus, 16.* https://www.semanticscholar.org/paper/5efe72a04352fa74dec404b768cdc832d8151e2f (accessed on 22nd July 2025).

26. Nøhr, M. K., Hauge, M., Gille, A., Egerod, K. L., Engelstoft, M. S., Husted, A. S., Sichlau, R. M., et al. (2013). GPR41/FFAR3 and GPR43/FFAR2 as cosensors for short-chain fatty acids in enteroendocrine cells vs FFAR3 in enteric neurons and FFAR2 in enteric leukocytes. *Endocrinology, 154*, 3552–3564. https://doi.org/10.1210/en.2013-1142 (accessed on 22nd July 2025).

27. Parkhomenko, L., Strashok, L., & Khomenko, M. (2019). Influence of gastrointestinal hormones on the development of obesity and non-alcoholic fatty liver disease in children. *Problems of Endocrine Pathology*. https://www.semanticscholar.org/paper/eef7d0aa19af500b496abe3d27f2c4c49f08869d (accessed on 22nd July 2025).

28. Pavord, S., Daru, J., Prasannan, N., Robinson, S., Stanworth, S., & Girling, J. (2019). UK guidelines on the management of iron deficiency in pregnancy. *British Journal of Hematology, 188*, 819–830. https://doi.org/10.1111/bjh.16221 (accessed on 22nd July 2025).

29. Raguso, C., & McCullough, A. (2000). Leptin and the gastrointestinal tract. *Current Opinion in Gastroenterology, 16*(2), 160–165. https://www.semanticscholar.org/paper/9b327d590ffc0c3cada4f71a193b964baf4e8e77 (accessed on 22nd July 2025).

30. Schoeler, M., & Caesar, R. (2019). Dietary lipids, gut microbiota and lipid metabolism. *Reviews in Endocrine and Metabolic Disorders, 20*, 461–472. https://doi.org/10.1007/s11154-019-09512-0 (accessed on 22nd July 2025).

31. Sonne, D. (2021). Mechanisms in endocrinology: FXR signaling–a novel target in metabolic diseases. *European Journal of Endocrinology*. https://www.semanticscholar.org/paper/81f83cac6515654be83c091f54165e4a405e48ad (accessed on 22nd July 2025).

32. Stojanov, S., Berlec, A., & Štrukelj, B. (2020). The influence of probiotics on the Firmicutes/Bacteroidetes ratio in the treatment of obesity and inflammatory bowel disease. *Microorganisms, 8*, 1715. https://doi.org/10.3390/microorganisms8111715 (accessed on 22nd July 2025).

33. Tilg, H., Adolph, T. E., & Moschen, A. R. (2020). Multiple parallel hits hypothesis in nonalcoholic fatty liver disease: Revisited after a decade. *Hepatology, 73*, 833–842. https://doi.org/10.1002/hep.31518 (accessed on 22nd July 2025).

34. Tounkara, F., Sara, A., Thanikachalam, K., Noonan, A. M., Mittra, A., Malalur, P., Jin, N., et al. (2025). Predicting immune-related adverse events (irAE) in gastrointestinal malignancies (GI-M): Tumor-specific risk factors (TS-RF), hematological markers (HM), and clinical outcomes. *Journal of Clinical Oncology*. https://www.semanticscholar.org/paper/d8f7723a2c15e181bde17c86fcf38731ef8bb8d7 (accessed on 22nd July 2025).

35. van der Hee, B., & Wells, J. M. (2021). Microbial regulation of host physiology by short-chain fatty acids. *Trends in Microbiology, 29*, 700–712. https://doi.org/10.1016/j.tim.2021.02.001 (accessed on 22nd July 2025).

36. Visseren, F. L. J., Mach, F., Smulders, Y. M., Carballo, D., Koskinas, K. C., Bäck, M., Bénétos, A., et al. (2021). 2021 ESC Guidelines on cardiovascular disease prevention in clinical practice. *European Heart Journal, 42*, 3227–3337. https://doi.org/10.1093/eurheartj/ehab484 (accessed on 22nd July 2025).

37. Wang, L., Wang, N., Zhang, W., Cheng, X., Yan, Z., Shao, G., Wang, X., et al. (2022). Therapeutic peptides: Current applications and future directions. *Signal Transduction and Targeted Therapy, 7*. https://doi.org/10.1038/s41392-022-00904-4 (accessed on 22nd July 2025).

38. Wang, Y., Xu, H., Zhou, X., Chen, W., & Zhou, H. (2024). Dysregulated bile acid homeostasis: Unveiling its role in metabolic diseases. *Medical Review, 4*, 262–283. https://www.semanticscholar.org/paper/ee48be5a38157c8f91b5abda1bed8871eafdae5e (accessed on 22nd July 2025).

39. Yan, M., Man, S., Sun, B., Ma, L., Guo, L., Huang, L., & Gao, W. (2023). Gut-liver-brain axis in diseases: The implications for therapeutic interventions. *Signal Transduction and Targeted Therapy, 8*. https://doi.org/10.1038/s41392-023-01673-4 (accessed on 22nd July 2025).

NEUROENDOCRINOLOGY

13

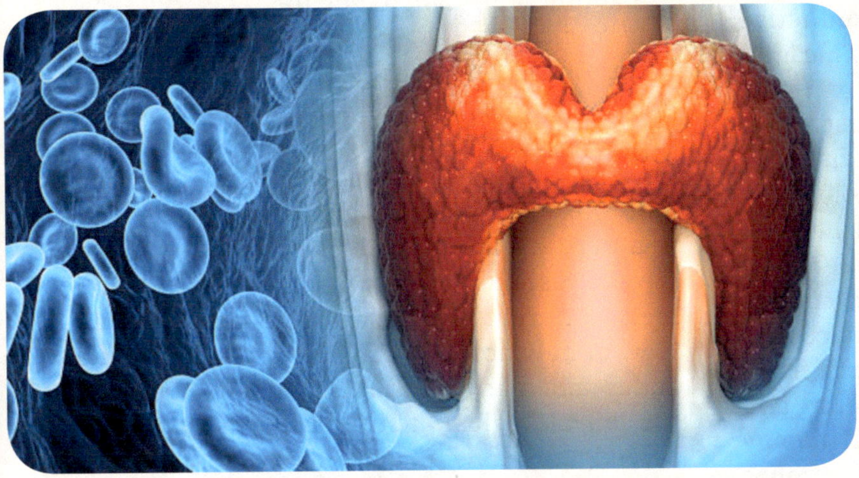

LEARNING OBJECTIVES

After studying this chapter, you will be able to:

1. Understand the interaction between the nervous system and the endocrine system;
2. Describe hormones involved in neuroendocrinology and their functions;
3. Discuss the neuroendocrine regulation of stress;
4. Focus on neuroendocrinology and reproductive health;
5. Deal with neuroendocrinology in metabolism;
6. Explain advances in neuroendocrinology research.

Introduction

Neuroendocrinology is a vital interface between the nervous and endocrine systems, a primary regulator of hundreds of physiological processes. This interdisciplinary field investigates how the brain regulates hormone activity and how the resulting hormones influence brain function and behavior. The hypothalamus is a primary structure for this purpose, integrating the discharge of the pituitary gland's hormones. Through this interaction, neuroendocrinology explores basic functions such as stress response, reproduction, and metabolism. An example of estrous behavior regulation in cattle shows how endocrine functions manage reproductive cycles and how hormones such as estradiol are essential in synchronizing reproduction events and behaviors in the context of broader biological processes (Beerda et al., 2010). Clarification of these intricate interactions is essential to understanding the ways in which diverse physiological systems interact with one another and how their perturbations can lead to a broad spectrum of reproductive and metabolic disorders. Additionally, the field of neuroendocrinology extends its confines to understand the implications of neuroinflammation on reproductive physiology. Research in recent years has established that chronic inflammation, particularly that induced by obesity, exerts considerable effects on neuronal function in reproductive circuits. Neuroinflammation has been found to trigger sex-specific alterations in gonadotropin-releasing hormone (GnRH) neurons, leading to impaired reproductive function in males (Coss et al., 2019). Significantly, the action of inflammatory cytokines on GnRH gene expression provides an illustration of neuroendocrine signaling disruption. By exploring such avenues, neuroendocrinology not only elucidates the physiological underpinnings of reproductive function but also identifies potential targets for therapeutic interventions meant to re-establish hormonal homeostasis in the face of inflammatory injuries. Finally, the contribution of mathematical modeling and systems biology towards neuroendocrinology cannot be overstated. As this discipline continues to grow with the growing complexity of genomic information, the incorporation of physiological responses and computational means represents an effective path toward understanding the complex networks that regulate neuroendocrine functions. Systems biology models, for instance, can describe how hormonal interactions lead to behavioral outcomes by modeling the impact of different hormones on neuronal networks. These types of models are necessary to advance our understanding of the regulation of estrous in dairy cows, as reviewed in the literature (Beerda et al., 2010). Moreover, the ability to work with large datasets ultimately allows for improved predictions and interventions in neuroendocrine function. As the scientific inquiry progresses, these integrative approaches will be centrally involved in uncovering new insight into normal and pathological processes, thereby enhancing our understanding of neuroendocrinology as a whole.

Definition and Scope of Neuroendocrinology

The discipline of neuroendocrinology is characterized by the complex interaction between the nervous and endocrine systems, highlighting how they talk and interact with each other to control different physiological functions. It explores how endocrine glands like the hypothalamus, pituitary gland, and adrenal glands secrete hormones that affect brain functions and behavior. This two-way communication is essential in maintaining homeostasis and reacting to changes in the external environment. For instance, the secretion of cortisol in response to stress not only affects physical measures but also modulates mood and cognition. Thus, neuroendocrinology is a very broad field of study encompassing stress response, reproductive health, and metabolic regulation, so it provides a broad view of how hormonal signaling affects mental states and body health. Beyond its focus on the physiological, neuroendocrinology also investigates how neuroendocrine responses can affect psychological endpoints. Individual variation of chronotype has been found to play a significant role in mental health because of the predisposition of some chronotypes to certain psychiatric illnesses. Evening chronotype, for example, has been found to be a risk factor for depression and alcohol and drug use disorders, whereas morning chronotype is protective against such illnesses. Moreover, understanding of these correlations entails research of the neuroendocrinological mechanisms underlying them, e.g., the way specific hormones and their correlations with psychological processes work. Greater awareness of these correlations highlights the significance of neuroendocrinology in developing targeted therapies for mental illness and underscores the importance of integrating biological and psychological research to achieve optimal well-being (Zou et al., 2022). In addition, the scope of neuroendocrinology reaches into the domain of resilience and adaptation, more specifically in times of stress. Resilience is defined as the ability to sustain well-being by drawing on multicomponent protective and promotive factors across biological, psychological, and environmental contexts. With research advancing in this field, it is important to consider interactions between these systems to better understand the neuroendocrinological foundation of resilience. As one example, population-based studies have shown that biological indicators, such as cortisol and dehydroepiandrosterone, may be linked to psychosocial measures of health in adolescents facing adversity within economically disadvantaged contexts. This integrated model not only enhances our understanding of resilience's operation under stress but also assists in the development of interventions, which could address inequities in health through the integration of neuroendocrinology and social and environmental influences (Ungar et al., 2021) (Figure 13.1).

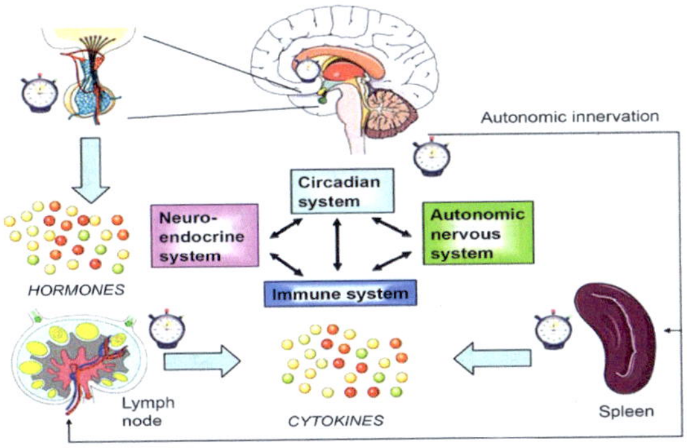

Figure 13.1. Temporal interactions among the neuroendocrine system, the autonomic nervous system, and the immune system as adaptive mechanisms to environmental changes.

Source: https://www.researchgate.net/profile/Vanesa-Jimenez-Ortega/publication/5853415/figure/fig1/AS:506883863973888@1497861938995/Temporal-interactions-among-the-neuroendocrine-system-the-autonomic-nervous-system-and.png.

Historical Background and Key Developments

The field of neuroendocrinology has evolved significantly from its inception during the mid-20th century. Initially, studies on hormones and their interaction with the nervous system were fragmented between disciplines without a unifying framework. Certain influential findings during the 1950s and 1960s, particularly the idea of the hypothalamus' regulatory role over pituitary function, laid the foundation for an integrated understanding of neuroendocrine mechanisms. Experiments by neurobiologists in these decades showed the mechanisms of hypothalamic hormone regulation of anterior pituitary hormone release, demonstrating the intricate interaction between the nervous and endocrine systems. This gave rise to neuroendocrinology as a specialized scientific discipline from this early work, and further work was undertaken to investigate the effects of this interaction on behavior, stress, and overall physiological control. With the coming of age of the field, significant progress in the latter half of the 20th century up to the present has widened the scope of neuroendocrinology. New imaging technologies, such as MRI and PET scans, enabled researchers to visualize brain activity relative to endocrine changes and their impact on diseases like depression and anxiety. Further, with the advent of molecular biology techniques, hormone receptors and pathways have been understood in a better way, and this has resulted in improving the treatment of endocrine disorders. Interestingly, through the addition of neuroendocrinology and developmental biology, how early hormonal influences mold brain development as well as behavior has been realized, significantly impacting our understanding regarding psychological and physiological effects throughout life. This interdisciplinarity underscores the interdependent relationships that neuroendocrinology is now attempting to unravel. The emphasis on diversity and inclusion in health research, as seen in initiatives like the Artificial Intelligence/Machine Learning Consortium to Advance Health Equity and Researcher Diversity (AIM-AHEAD), resonates with the ideals of neuroendocrinology. As the discipline continues to grow, health equity concerns are assuming prominence, particularly in understanding how hormonal impacts can vary across populations based on socio-demographic factors. Studies have linked reproductive health and maternal mortality with socio-economic factors, revealing vast health inequities. In addressing these inequities, neuroendocrinology can assist in developing more just health systems, where investigation and care are attuned to the diversity of populations. Such an equity perspective emphasizes the importance of embracing a holistic definition of neuroendocrinology and encourages the potential for breakthroughs beneficial to the whole population (Kassebaum et al., 2017; Rachele et al., 2023).

Importance of Neuroendocrinology in Modern Science

The transdisciplinary area of neuroendocrinology plays a pivotal role in modern science, bridging the gaps between neuroscience, endocrinology, and psychiatric behavioral medicine. By the investigation of interactions between hormones and the nervous system, researchers are able to uncover the biological substrate for many physiological and psychological processes. The impact of stress and cortisol, the stress hormone, on cognitive processing and emotional regulation is one such field of widespread research. The neuroendocrine reaction to stress has implications for an understanding of such conditions as anxiety, depression, and post-traumatic stress disorder (PTSD). With the progress of science, the gains delivered by neuroendocrinology are also bringing about targeted therapies, optimizing treatment efficiency, and ultimately improved patient outcomes in mental illness. The intricate network of endocrine relationships in the brain underscores the interconnectedness of body functions, maintaining that emotional health is just as important as physical health in holistic scientific research and medical interventions. Aside from mental well-being, neuroendocrinology has evolved as a core field of study about autoimmune diseases, where the immune system erroneously attacks the body's own tissues. Recent studies highlight the intricate interaction of immune mechanisms and neuroendocrine signals, particularly with respect to diseases like multiple sclerosis. As reviewed in the literature, neuroimmunology illuminates the interaction between the immune system and the central nervous system (CNS) and the influence of cytokine and immune cell dysregulation on disease and treatment outcomes. Studies of the neuroimmune axis not only enhance our knowledge of autoimmune pathophysiology but also set the stage for novel therapeutic strategies. Such burgeoning insights reveal the pivotal contribution of integrating neuroendocrinological paradigms into modern clinical research, pushing personalized medicine towards increased innovations that take into consideration the specific demands of each individual and profoundly augment healthcare outcomes. Furthermore, the social implications of neuroendocrinology cannot be overstated, particularly with reference to understanding the biological determinants of men's behavior and mental illness. Studies demonstrate correlations between masculine norms across cultures and elevated suicidal risk among males, and that social expectation and repression of emotion can precipitate intense psychological distress. As indicated in recent qualitative research, returning to these cultural constructs in the context of neuroendocrinological models has the potential to improve male emotional health knowledge and suicide prevention. By promoting holistic interventions that foster emotional sensitivity and interpersonal connections, mental health intervention protocols can be framed better to meet diverse population needs. Lastly, the role of neuroendocrinology in teaching us about the complex interaction between biological, psychological, and social determinants makes it the central focus of the study in the modern science era, paving the way for targeted interventions that augment mental health and social well-being.

13.1. The Nervous System and Endocrine System Interaction

Learning Outcome

1. Discuss the nervous system;
2. Understand the endocrine system;
3. Understand the mechanisms of communication between the two systems.

The complex interaction between the endocrine system and the nervous system is responsible for ensuring homeostasis in the body. Neuroendocrinology, the study of this interaction, emphasizes the way neurons and hormones interact to control the different processes of the body. The interaction is mainly via the hypothalamus, which produces and releases hormones that directly act on the pituitary gland. Through this process, the hypothalamus serves as a crucial intermediary between nervous messages and hormonal responses. Also, there exist feedback mechanisms so that hormonal levels can adjust to varying bodily states, allowing for a speedy change in the presence of stress or metabolic disturbances. This cooperation between the two systems is evidence of the body's complexity in functions, showing an exceptionally developed system of communication for survival and adaptation. One of the interesting features of this dialogue is the role of neurotransmitters within the endocrine environment, that is, reproductive and stress reactions. As a case in point, neurotransmitters such as gamma-aminobutyric acid (GABA) exert not only a primary role in neural communication but also influence endocrine organs. It has been discovered that GABA modulates steroidogenesis in Leydig cells within testicular tissue by means of specific receptor interactions, mediating neuronal action and endocrine response. The finding that these cells express GABA receptors shows how neurotransmitter signaling may impact endocrine function to generate feedback necessary for reproductive health and hormonal homeostasis. Such knowledge can allow for an appreciation of the therapeutic potential for the correction of endocrine disorders based on neural activities and therefore marks the relevance of neuroendocrinology in the clinic. Besides this, ALS pathologies have begun to evidence intricate dysfunctions at the intersection of the endocrine and nervous systems. The study in the Wobbler mouse model that mimics ALS features depicts severe dysregulation in steroid hormones such as corticosterone and testosterone. The elevated corticosterone and decreased testosterone levels evidence how neurodegeneration would disrupt hormonal homeostasis and impact metabolism and neuroprotection. Here, the endocrine response to nervous system change sheds light on adaptive processes that can be initiated in the case of cell degeneration. These findings indicate the importance of examining neuroendocrine dynamics under conditions of neurodegenerative disorder, as they have the potential to lead to new therapeutic strategies targeting both neuronal and hormonal pathways, enhancing patient prognosis in diseases like ALS.

13.1.1. Overview of the Nervous System

The nervous system is a complex and vital component of biological organisms, playing the role of controlling homeostasis regulation and coordination of responses to internal and external stimuli. It is divided into two main divisions: the central nervous system (CNS), comprising the brain and spinal cord, and the peripheral nervous system (PNS), comprising all neural structures other than the CNS. The CNS processes and interprets the senses, while the PNS transmits the signals between the CNS and the body. In this intricate system, the most significant cells are neurons, which serve as the principal units for communication. The cells transmit electric impulses, allowing for rapid responses to stimuli to ensure survival and adaptation. The integrative and coordinative power of the nervous system shows its central role in sustaining life processes and responding to the dynamic world. Neuroendocrinology is the exploration of the relationship between the endocrine system and the nervous system with a focus on how neural impulses regulate endocrine control. In so doing, neuropeptides, a group of protein-like small molecules, regulate the interaction between the two systems and play a central role in regulating physiological processes. For instance, the release of specific neuropeptides can influence the secretion of hormones from other glands and, therefore, govern processes such as growth, metabolism, and stress response. Understanding the intricate interactions and feedback mechanisms involved in these relations is important in understanding how the brain controls body physiology and behavioral responses. This intersection of endocrinology and neurology not only suggests the complexity of body regulation but also points toward the potential implications in the treatment of endocrine disease through neurological pathways and findings brought about by neuroendocrine studies. Research on the neurobiological mechanisms of childbirth is a significant demonstration of how the nervous system regulates endocrine functions, particularly through the action of oxytocin. Studies demonstrate that neurohormonal mechanisms, such as oxytocin release during labor, are at the core of physiological processes but also of the psychological phenomenon of birth. The interplay between sensory inputs and endogenous oxytocin levels illustrates the close connection between nervous system functioning and affective states in maternal behavior and attachment. Moreover, the need for social support during labor further underscores the role of neuroendocrine mechanisms in optimizing maternal well-being. Such an integrative view, encompassing emotional and physiological experiences, illustrates the multifaceted role of the nervous system as a significant force in the direction of not just responses to stimulus but also the highly subjective occurrences concomitant with events of profound life concern, like childbirth, and thereby contributing extensively to the entire study of neuroendocrinology (Alexej, 2019; Fern et al., 2020) (Figure 13.2).

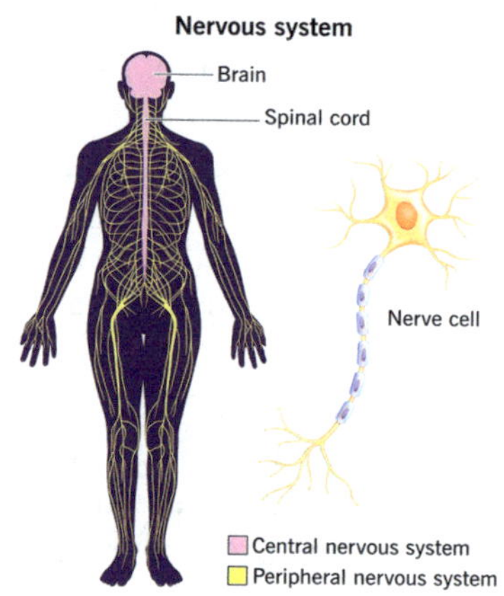

Figure 13.2. Nervous system.

Source: https://my.clevelandclinic.org/-/scassets/images/org/health/articles/21202-nervous-system.

13.1.2. Overview of the Endocrine System

The endocrine system is a sophisticated system of glands and organs that are assigned the task of producing, secreting, and regulating hormones, which play vital functions in the pursuit of achieving homeostasis in the organism. The system involves key components like the pituitary gland, thyroid gland, adrenal glands, and pancreas, each of which performs a specific function in hormone secretion and production. The dynamics of these hormones influence a variety of physiological functions, including growth, metabolism, and reproduction. For instance, the pituitary gland has been referred to as the master gland as it controls most other endocrine glands by secreting stimulating hormones. This system of hierarchy reveals the complexity of the endocrine system, as hormones produced in one location in the body can affect target organs at any other location, highlighting the necessity for physiological processes to be interconnected and the importance of hormonal balance in overall health. Regulation of fertility and sexual behavior is an interesting characteristic of the endocrine system, particularly in dairy cattle. As a byproduct, selection for milk production has led to lower fertility due in part to altered expressions of estrous behavior. Estradiol (E2) and progesterone are key players in the regulation of the estrous cycle, with E2 serving as a primary synchronizer for endocrine and behavioral events. More recent work has begun to define the interplay between hormone signaling and gene expression that underlies these behaviors. Specifically, estrogen induction within single brain regions like the hypothalamus could have a dramatic effect on neural networks involved in the regulation of estrous behavior. This emerging view highlights the interconnection of endocrine mechanisms and reproduction, expanding the broader applications of hormonal regulation in farm animals and potentially in human fertility processes (Beerda et al., 2010). Stress response is also a determining interaction in the endocrine system, controlled by the hypothalamic-pituitary-adrenal (HPA) axis and also mediated primarily by corticotropin-releasing hormone (CRH). It is not only a key regulator of stress responses but also a neuromodulator that influences humoral and behavioral adaptation. Recent work has contradicted the usual perception of CRH signaling, showing that it induces complex cellular processes that trigger physiological responses to stress. Understanding the intricate mechanisms of signaling underlying CRH, including those by cAMP generation and ERK1/2 activation, is significant in an appreciation of how stress impacts neuroendocrine function. Defining the role of CRH within this process is therefore significant for developing specific pharmacologic treatments for disorders with etiology in neuroendocrine dysregulation (Armando et al., 2017).

13.1.3. Mechanisms of Communication Between the Two Systems

The intricate relationship between the nervous and endocrine systems is the foundation of neuroendocrinology. The activity is conveyed by a range of signaling molecules, including hormones and neurotransmitters, that function to mediate responses between and within systems. The hypothalamus plays a key role in this communication by the release of hormones regulating the pituitary gland, thereby influencing a range of endocrine functions in the body. For instance, the release of gonadotropin-releasing hormone (GnRH) from the hypothalamus triggers a cascade that leads to the discharge of luteinizing hormone (LH) and follicle-stimulating hormone (FSH) from the pituitary gland. Such a regulatory process demonstrates the necessary dialogue between endocrine processes and neurobiologic functions, establishing a system that sets the stage for reproductive behavior and health. Understanding these mechanisms is important, especially in the context of the implications that they have for fertility and the physiological response to stressors. The communication networks that commingle the nervous and endocrine systems are also elucidated through hormone action, like that of estradiol, which influences both behavioral and physiological mechanisms. Estradiol has been found to modulate reproductive processes, and it also modulates neuronal networks in regions such as the hypothalamus to determine mammalian estrous behavior. Estradiol, upon binding to its receptors, elicits expression of target genes that reorganize synaptic contacts and neuronal firing. This molecular mechanism delineates how endocrine signals directly reorganize the dynamics of neural circuits, demonstrating the bidirectional nature of interaction between the two systems. These findings are significant as they shed light on the endocrine mechanisms of reproductive cycles and particularly in agricultural-restricted species, where changes in fertility and reproductive behavior can have detrimental economic outcomes, as seen in dairy cattles' estrous behavior regulation (Beerda et al., 2010). Additionally, the merging of several signal pathways even better showcases the intricate nature of communication between the nervous and endocrine systems. For example, recent information on kisspeptin reveals its double role as a neuropeptide and central hormonal messenger in reproductive processes. The peptide is critical for the initiation of the LH surge, estradiol, and neuroprogesterone, organizing the release of kisspeptin within the central nervous system. Such events illustrate the complexity of hormonal control of reproductive behavior across species from birds to mammals. Hormonal messaging, as indicated by the molecular activity of gonadotropin-inhibitory hormone (GnIH), also regulates breeding behaviors by modulating neuroendocrine processes in response to environmental stressors (Bentley et al., 2016). These processes illustrate how neuroendocrinology functions, and the relevance of understanding these processes in order to be able to treat reproductive health conditions as well as infertility (Figure 13.3).

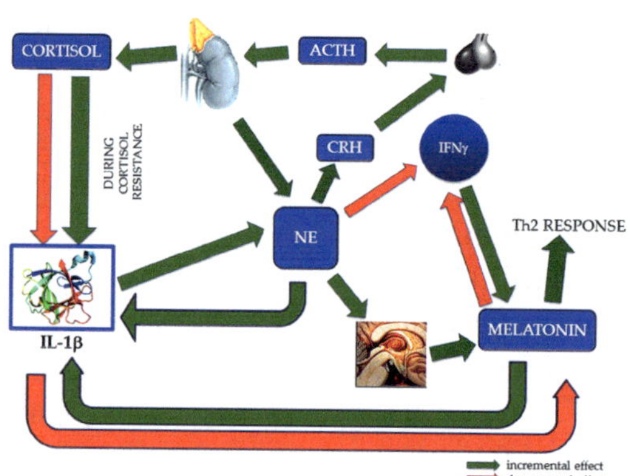

Figure 13.3. Interplay between the central nervous system, the endocrine system, and the immune system.

Source: https://www.researchgate.net/publication/347540420/figure/fig3/AS:11431281172856872@1688671750203/Interplay-between-central-nervous-system-endocrine-system-and-immune-system-Under.png.

Test Your Knowledge

1. What are the key structural and functional differences between the nervous system and the endocrine system?
2. What role does the autonomic nervous system play in modulating hormone release during stress responses?

13.2. Hormones and Their Functions

Learning Outcome

1. Describe types of hormones involved in neuroendocrinology;
2. Explain the role of hormones in regulating physiological processes;
3. Understand the impact of hormones on behavior and mood.

The intricate interplay of hormones in the neuroendocrine axis is at the very core of maintaining homeostasis and body function regulation. Hormones such as gonadotropin-releasing hormone (GnRH) are critical to orchestrating the reproductive axis, which influences the release of other hormones such as luteinizing hormone and follicle-stimulating hormone. However, neuroinflammation can potentially disrupt this fine balance of hormones seriously. Studies have shown that chronic inflammation due to obesity negatively impacts GnRH neurons by reducing their spine density, and this impairs reproductive function only in males (Coss et al., 2019). What is especially interesting about this disruption is the insight it provides into how environmental components can regulate hormonal systems, demonstrating how chronic diseases can stimulate changes in hormone signaling that spread beyond peripheral tissues to impact central reproductive processes. The hypothalamus is the central component of the neuroendocrine system, serving as a center for controlling metabolism and reproduction. Among its various nuclei, the arcuate nucleus stands out as an important mediator of energy homeostasis and feeding. Hormonal signals enter this region, regulating not only metabolism but also the energy reservoirs necessary for reproductive integrity. One is the bidirectional interaction of energy status with the hypothalamic-pituitary-gonadal (HPG) axis, a primary reproductive pathway. The availability of optimal stores of energy is necessary to maintain hormonal homeostasis, highlighting the integration of nutrition, metabolic health, and reproductive competence (Villalobos et al., 2016). The complex interactions of such systems illustrate the manner in which disturbances in metabolic homeostasis may impact broadly on health and biological function. In addition to the direct hormonal actions described in the hypothalamus, the impact of inflammatory cytokines on gene expression is also deserving of important mention. As one illustration, proof has been detected that circulating plasma levels of leukemia inhibitory factor (LIF) during neuroinflammation conditions possess direct capacity to inhibit GnRH gene expression, establishing a mechanistic pathway to reproductive dysfunction (Coss et al., 2019). Moreover, the engagement of specific signaling pathways, such as the MAPK pathway, shows the precise regulation mechanisms governing hormone release and synthesis in response to physiological stressors. These data provide a clearer picture of the neuroendocrine response to inflammation and stress, indicating how disturbances at the molecular level can precipitate large-scale physiological changes. Thus, the study of hormones and their function remains central to the comprehension of the neuroendocrinological landscape, particularly in the context of environmental and metabolic stressors.

13.2.1. Types of Hormones Involved in Neuroendocrinology

The neuroendocrinology study examines the interface of the nervous system and the endocrine system, or how the brain reacts to hormones and vice versa. Of all the various hormones, gonadotropin-releasing hormone (GnRH) is at the core of reproductive regulation through its mechanism of stimulating luteinizing hormone (LH) and follicle-stimulating hormone (FSH) from the pituitary gland. Coordination of GnRH signaling is also critical for reproductive health, as it leads to infertility if this synchrony is disrupted. Classical and non-classical pathways, including the action of estradiol and neuroprogesterone, have been identified as significant areas of research to unravel such mechanisms of control. For instance, LH surge, which is orchestrated through these hormones, demonstrates how neuroendocrine signaling coordinates different physiological systems to produce an orchestrated reproductive outcome (Bentley et al., 2016). Oxytocin (OT) and arginine vasopressin (AVP) are also in the focus of neuroendocrinology, precisely concerning responses to stress and social behavior. OT, long known to be active during delivery and lactation, was discovered to regulate the release of adrenocorticotropic hormone (ACTH) and thereby is implicated in stress regulation. The synergistic effect of OT with corticotropin-releasing factor (CRF) is a testament to the complexity of hormonal interactions of the HPA axis. Experiments demonstrate that OT can promote ACTH release through various mechanisms, primarily intracellular mobilization of calcium. This indicates the major pathways through which OT is involved in triggering physiological responses to stress (Dayanithi et al., 1992). Thus, the intricate regulatory circuits between OT and AVP underscore the major functions of these hormones in regulating neuroendocrine processes. Moreover, the hormonal milieu extends beyond reproductive and stress function to encompass a range of other neuroendocrine processes with respect to metabolism and growth. Hormones like GH and IGF-1 illustrate the contribution of neuroendocrine systems to growth and developmental processes. These hormones act on hypothalamic nuclei that regulate feeding behavior, energy consumption, and thermogenesis. Understanding these interactions holds specific significance for the understanding of metabolic disease, such as diabetes and obesity. As research further uncovers the dynamics of hormone interaction in neuroendocrinology, therapeutic interventions are revealed, potentially improving a variety of health pathologies related to hormonal disruption. In general, these revelations underscore the function of hormones in facilitating conversation between the nervous system and other bodily systems (Bentley et al., 2016) (Figure 13.4).

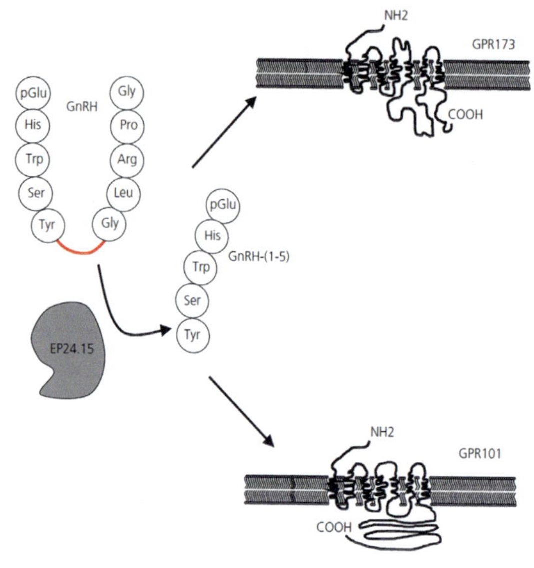

Figure 13.4. Gonadotropin-releasing hormone (GnRH) peptide processing and action.

Source: https://www.researchgate.net/profile/Lauren_Rudolph3/publication/304324298/figure/fig1/AS:391101295939597@1470257223477/Gonadotropin-Releasing-Hormone-GnRH-peptide-processing-and-action-The-decapeptide.png.

13.2.2. Role of Hormones in Regulating Physiological Processes

Hormones play a critical role in regulating a vast array of physiological processes, acting as biochemical messengers to regulate functions across bodily systems. Within the context of neuroendocrinology, the overlap between the nervous and the endocrine systems refers to how hormonal signals stimulate behavior, metabolism, and immune regulation. For instance, the hypothalamus releases releasing hormones that directly stimulate the pituitary gland, which releases hormones regulating vital activities such as growth, stress, and reproduction. The complex interaction illustrates the way that endocrine balance is vital for homeostasis because any disruption may lead to grave health issues. Understanding these regulatory mechanisms is the gateway to appreciating therapeutic strategies for reversing hormonal imbalance and associated disease and, in the end, focusing on the regulating role of hormones in physiological equilibrium. The action of steroid hormones, particularly in relation to reproductive health and neuroendocrine function, transcends traditional boundaries. Recent studies point to how steroid hormones, such as estrogen and testosterone, not only control reproductive tissues but also have significant impacts on the brain. Most notably, these hormones control dopaminergic processes in certain brain regions involved in motivation and reward, with implications for their role in controlling emotional and cognitive process-related behaviors. Studies have shown that alterations in these hormonal levels can potentially alter neural circuitry, and behaviors linked to drug reinforcement and addiction are influenced. As an example, neonatal exposure to estrogen has been reported to enhance dopaminergic neurotransmission later in life and therefore may increase susceptibility to drugs of abuse, pointing to a highly relevant research area in the field of neuroendocrinology (Bonansco et al., 2018). This reveals an intricate interplay between hormones and neural processes, which needs to be better understood in terms of their significance for psychological and behavioral health. Also, the interplay among hormones and various of the body's physiological systems can be viewed in the context of systemic disease, such as COVID-19. Ample evidence suggests that the activity of angiotensin-converting enzyme 2 (ACE2), which is a steroid hormone-regulated receptor, forms the core of the pathophysiology of this disease. Down-regulation of ACE2 by SARS-CoV-2 infection following homeostasis, and correlation with lethal complications like respiratory dysfunction and cardiovascular disorders, have been reported. Understanding how hormones regulate modulation of ACE2 activity in relation to disease severity guides basic therapeutic implications. For instance, manipulation of the levels of steroid hormone can yield a novel therapeutic strategy to improve ACE2 function and minimize severity of disease, indicating the subtlety of hormonal regulation in states of health and disease (Zhang et al., 2020). Such intersection between hormonal regulation and disease mechanism is a vital area of research in neuroendocrinology, in which the promise of novel therapies continues to unfold (Figure 13.5).

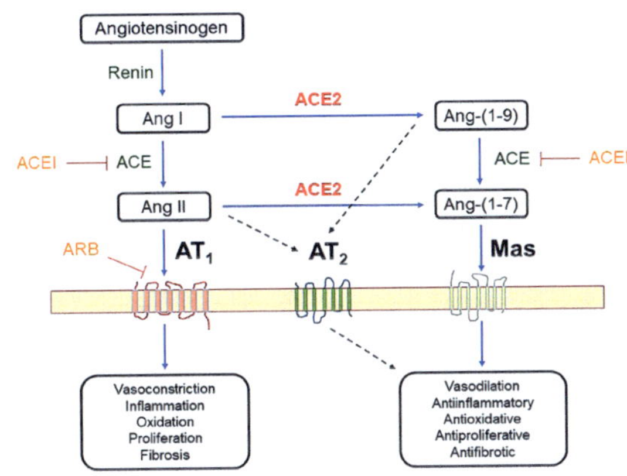

Figure 13.5. Role of angiotensin converting-enzyme-2 (ACE2) in the renin-angiotensin-aldosterone system (RAAS).

Source: https://www.researchgate.net/publication/348139610/figure/fig1/AS:976293038415872@1609777807106/Role-of-angiotensin-converting-enzyme-2-ACE2-in-the-renin-angiotensin-aldosterone.jpg.

13.2.3. Impact of Hormones on Behavior and Mood

The dynamic interaction between hormones and behavior plays an important role in the regulation of mood, showing how hormonal changes can produce extreme shifts in states of emotion. Hormones including cortisol, estrogen, and testosterone have been demonstrated to affect behavior in a direct fashion. For example, elevated levels of cortisol, a hormone generally related to stress, can result in anxiety and depression. This physiologic response is part of the body's greater neuroendocrine system, where stress hormones influence neurotransmitter systems implicated in mood and affective stability. Furthermore, cyclical hormonal changes, as in the menstrual cycle, illustrate how estrogen and progesterone can impact mood, changing emotional responses in women and giving rise to such effects as premenstrual syndrome (PMS). This information highlights the importance of hormonal balance in the maintenance of emotional well-being and suggests therapeutic potential for the treatment of mood disorders. Neuroactive steroids, a group of hormones, have also been noted for their therapeutic potential in modulating behavior and neurotransmission. More specifically, some neuroactive steroids like the 3 alpha-reduced pregnane steroids have been said to act beneficially on the gamma-aminobutyric acid type A (GABA(A)) receptor, enabling inhibitory neurotransmission and producing a state of relaxation and calm. Recent findings, however, indicate another degree of complexity to this interaction in major depression. Dysregulation of these neuroactive steroids is observed to correlate with mood changes; a successful antidepressant therapy has been found to normalize their equilibrium in patients. This finding suggests that neuroactive steroid level changes could be important to the understanding of pathophysiology of mood disorders and that pharmacotherapy could be uniquely efficacious in the correction of hormonal imbalances, and hence create options for more subtle treatment approaches (Akwa et al., 2006). Additionally, the neuroactive steroid interaction with anxiety disorders, such as panic disorder, presents interesting insights into hormonal modulatory effects on mood and behavior. In patients with panic disorder, on the other hand, the opposite changes in neuroactive steroid levels have been observed compared to depressed patients. For example, during panic attacks induced by specific stimuli, substantial decreases in 3 alpha-reduced neuroactive steroids were observed, which may lead to decreased GABAergic tone and heightened anxiety symptoms. This distinction highlights the value of probing hormonal profiles in different states of mind as it can uncover special targets for intervention. As more studies continue to elucidate the mechanisms by which hormones influence mood and behavior, these neuroendocrine profiles may be crucial in optimizing new treatments based on unique hormonal signatures, eventually treating both mood and anxiety disorders more precisely (Mercer et al., 2013) (Figure 13.6).

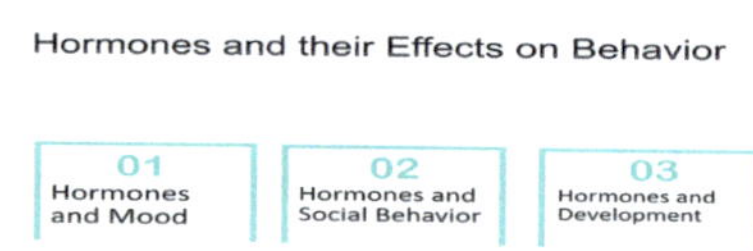

Figure 13.6. Hormones and their effects on behavior.

Source: https://fastercapital.co/i/Neuroendocrinology--Examining-Hormonal-Influences-with-NRD--Hormones-and-their-Effects-on-Behavior.webp.

Test Your Knowledge

1. What are the main classes of hormones involved in neuroendocrinology?
2. How do steroid hormones influence long-term physiological processes such as metabolism and reproduction?

13.3. Neuroendocrine Regulation of Stress

Learning Outcome

1. Understand the basics of hypothalamic-pituitary-adrenal (HPA) axis;
2. Explain the effects of stress hormones on the body;
3. Discuss about long-term consequences of chronic stress.

The neuroendocrine reaction to stress involves intricate interactions between the endocrine and nervous systems, both of which come together to mediate the body's reaction to stressors. The focal point of this mechanism is the HPA axis, which is activated by perceived threats. When activated, the hypothalamus releases corticotropin-releasing hormone (CRH), which causes the release of ACTH from the anterior pituitary gland. This hormone then induces the adrenal cortex to secrete glucocorticoids, in humans, namely cortisol, which prepares the body for a "fight or flight" response by making energy available and halting non-essential activities. Malfunctioning of this axis can result in numerous health issues, such as depression and anxiety, and therefore make one wish to understand neuroendocrine mechanisms of stress regulation in the context of mental illness and overall health. Pharmacologic agents can also have an effect on the HPA axis and stress response regulation. The interaction between medications and neural signaling pathways makes the neuroendocrine response to stress even more complex. For instance, studies showed that the combination of mirtazapine and reboxetine influences cortisol and ACTH release. More specifically, while reboxetine is a noradrenaline reuptake inhibitor that initially stimulates cortisol release, this effect is significantly reduced by co-administration with mirtazapine due to its agonist activity at other neurotransmitter receptors, such as α_2-adrenergic receptors. This counteraction illustrates the efficiency of selective pharmacotherapy in the modulation of endocrine stress responses. These observations highlight the potential of developing therapeutic treatments that target neuroendocrine pathways to enhance coping skills and mitigate stress-induced disease (Baghai et al., 2004). Additionally, reproductive hormone studies identify further complexities involved in the neuroendocrine regulation of stress. The interaction of estradiol and neuroprogesterone with kisspeptin and gonadotropin-releasing hormone (GnRH) illustrates how peripheral hormonal cues can also be manipulated by stress. Research has demonstrated that stress-induced changes in gonadotropin-inhibitory hormone (GnIH) can disrupt normal breeding behaviors by modulating the function of GnRH neurons. These hormonal changes demonstrate that the body's response to stress is not only mediated by nonspecific systems but also has specific implications for reproductive health. These interactions are significant to understand as they embody more general neuroendocrine principles through which stress can both be regulated by and regulate other significant physiological processes, and consequently, the significance of an integrated neuroendocrinology (Bentley et al., 2016).

13.3.1. The Hypothalamic-Pituitary-Adrenal Axis

The HPA axis is a crucial neuroendocrine circuit that mediates the body's response to stress. The network consists of the hypothalamus, which releases corticotropin-releasing hormone (CRH) to activate the pituitary gland's secretion of ACTH. ACTH then influences the adrenal cortex, activating the production of glucocorticoids, primarily cortisol in humans. This chain of hormonal communication is not only required for the body's response to stressors but is critical in maintaining homeostasis. Dysregulation in the HPA axis, however, is associated with many psychiatric illnesses, underscoring the importance of understanding how it works in its optimal state and the consequences of its perturbations in clinical neurobiology and psychology. Research has elucidated that variations in HPA axis function can lead to various pathological states, particularly with disorders of stress such as PTSD and major depressive disorder. Disruptions in the glucocorticoid feedback mechanisms may disrupt the balance of the axis, leading to chronic activation of stress responses. Here, the dynamics of CRH, ACTH, and cortisol secretion can be thought of as basins of attraction of a dynamical system. Investigation of these states shines a light on how the interaction between external stressors and internal homeostasis of hormones can lead to maladaptive behavioral outcomes. Lastly, understanding these mechanisms provides the entry point for therapies that aim to rebalance the HPA axis and address the origins of stress-disordered states (Chou et al., 2016). Moreover, early life stress and HPA axis consequences have been identified as a research priority in neuroendocrinology. Experience during the critical weeks after birth can shape CRH expression and regulation with profound implications for adult stress responses. It has been shown that both the psychological and physiological forms of stress can stimulate transcription factors such as CREB, which enhance CRH gene expression. These molecular changes illustrate how the HPA axis can be altered long-term by early environmental stimuli. As these adaptations can lead to a person becoming more reactive to stress in the future, the establishment of the causal connection between early stress and adult stress disorders is vital to the development of effective preventative strategies (Avishai-Eller et al., 2001). Unraveling these complex associations not only advances the neuroendocrinology but also informs potential clinical interventions for preventing mental health effects of childhood adversity (Figure 13.7).

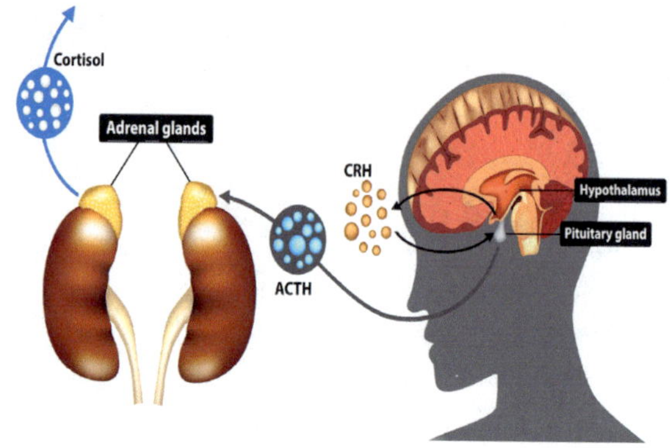

Figure 13.7. Corticotropin-releasing hormone (CRH) stimulating the pituitary gland to secrete adrenocorticotropic hormone (ACTH).

Source: https://www.news-medical.net/image-handler/picture/2019/1/By_Sakurra1.jpg.

13.3.2. Effects of Stress Hormones on the Body

The action of stress hormones on the body is extensive and intricate, acting on numerous disparate physiological processes. Of all the hormones involved, cortisol plays a crucial role in stress responses, acting on metabolism, the immune system, and the cardiovascular system. With stress, the HPA axis comes into play, releasing cortisol from the adrenal glands, enabling various adaptive responses within the body to respond to threatened danger. Chronic exposure to elevated levels of cortisol can have adverse health consequences, such as weight gain, hypertension, and susceptibility to infections. Furthermore, chronic stress is likely to alter neurotransmitter composition and brain activity, potentially causing changes that lead to mood illness or mental deterioration. On this basis, the function of stress hormones is pivotal in neuroendocrinology, particularly as researchers investigate means of reducing their undesirable effects on overall well-being and health. Oxytocin, also commonly known as the love hormone, significantly influences stress and emotional response-related reactions. Its release is brought about by social bonding and stress stimuli, reflecting extensive interaction between social behavior and physiological action. Oxytocin has been identified to be able to modulate the ACTH release and thus cortisol levels. Specifically, oxytocin has been found to enhance ACTH release when combined with other corticotropin-releasing factors such as arginine vasopressin. This underscores the hormone's capacity to promote adaptive stress responses while simultaneously increasing social bonding and reducing anxiety. Additionally, research suggests that maximized oxytocin levels could be a therapeutic target for reversing some of the negative consequences of chronic stress, marking the broader scope of neuroendocrinology in addressing psychological and physiological health issues (Dayanithi et al., 1992). The function of stress hormones in interacting with diverse psychoactive drugs is also significant, particularly their contribution to cortisol levels and overall endocrine function. For instance, the selective noradrenaline reuptake blocker reboxetine has been found to exert significant stimulating effects on cortisol, ACTH, growth hormone, and prolactin secretion. When it is co-administered with mirtazapine, an α_2-blocker, however, the overwhelming stimulation of these hormones is significantly reduced. This reduction demonstrates the mechanisms through which pharmacological manipulation of hormone and neurotransmitter pathways can modulate stress-associated response and cortisol release patterns. These intricate interactions illustrate the necessity to understand neuroendocrinology extensively, inasmuch as therapeutic interventions to alter one aspect of the endocrine system can have a cascading effect along multiple hormonal pathways, ultimately influencing stress resilience and mental health outcomes (Baghai et al., 2004) (Figure 13.8).

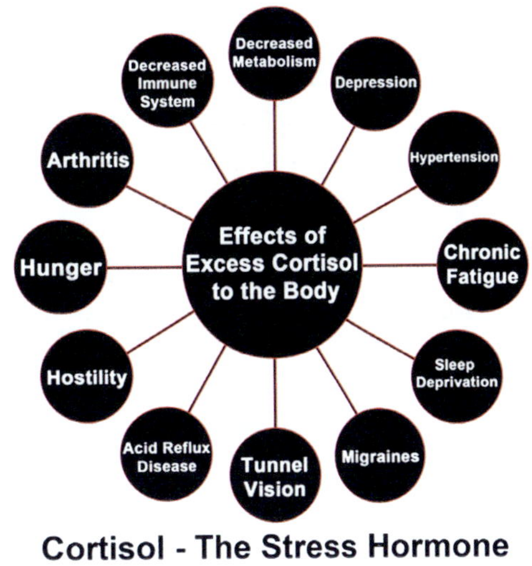

Figure 13.8. Effects of excess cortisol to the body.

Source: https://cdn.shopify.com/s/files/1/0397/5122/1403/files/Cortisol_grande.png?v=1596042286.

13.3.3. Long-Term Consequences of Chronic Stress

Chronic stress profoundly affects the neuroendocrine system and causes a cascade of physiological responses that have a long-lasting effect on mental health and cognitive function. When the body is kept under constant exposure to long-term stress, it constantly releases hormones such as cortisol, which can disrupt normal metabolic functions. With age, elevated cortisol levels contribute to alterations in brain structure and function, particularly in regions such as the hippocampus, which is crucial for learning and memory. It has been found that the neurobiologic responses to chronic stress could differ by biological sex and age and represent a complex interaction influencing vulnerability to stress-related disorder. Understanding such sex differences in neurobiological responses sheds light on the necessity of particular therapeutic measures for minimizing the long-term consequences of chronic stress and prevents the development of stress-related mental illnesses (Shirokova et al., 2025). Chronic stress effects do not remain psychological alone; they manifest in a myriad of physical health conditions as well. Chronic stress has the potential to accelerate cellular aging and immunosenescence, which have been linked to the development of age-related diseases such as neurodegenerative diseases and osteoporosis. For example, there is evidence that chronic stress can lead to alterations in brain structure and neurotransmitter levels, followed by subsequent alterations in behavior and cognitive dysfunction. Animal models have shown that stress is able to induce remarkable histomorphological changes in the hippocampus, eventually affecting neurobehavioral processes.

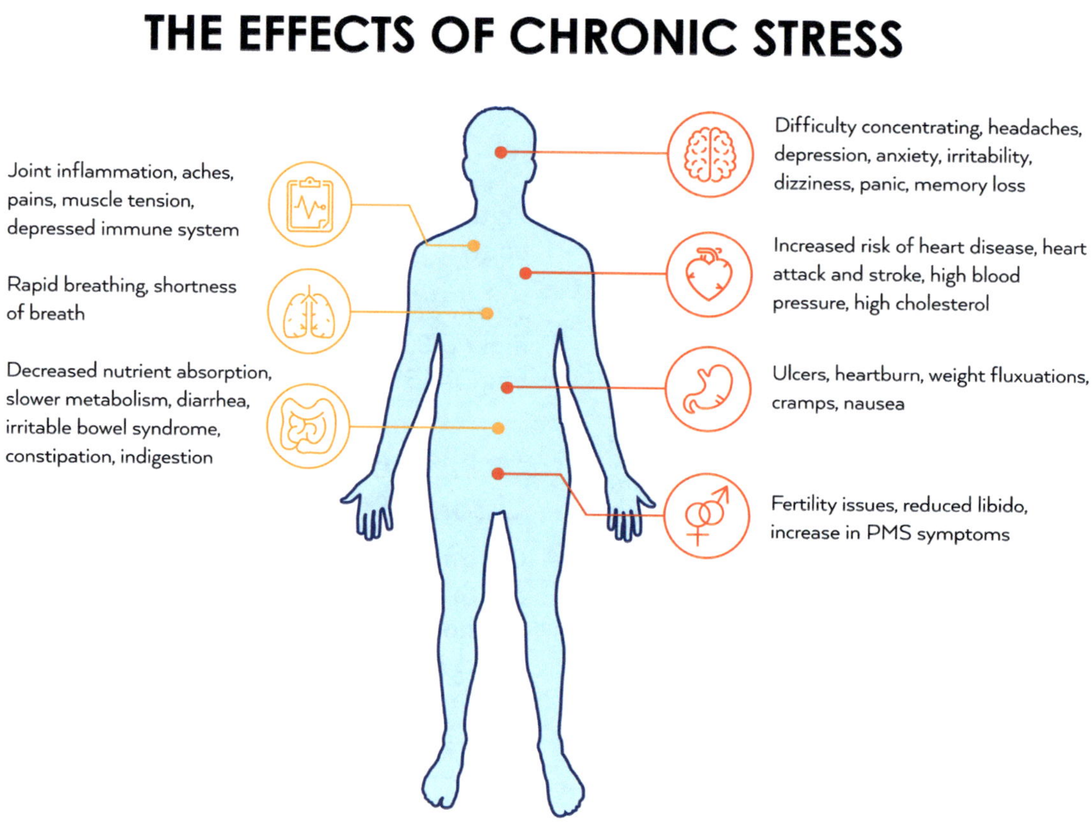

Figure 13.9. The effects of chronic stress.

Source: https://www.researchgate.net/profile/Kelli-Dunlap-2/publication/336208930/figure/fig1/AS:849860148346880@1579633857063/The-effects-of-chronic-stress-according-to-McEwen-2006.png.

The findings point towards the requirement of treating stress not only as a psychological construct but also as a major factor in overall deteriorating health (Adetunji et al., 2024). By addressing the biological origin of stress illnesses, researchers can pave the way for holistic interventions that can forestall such deleterious outcomes. Preventing long-term consequences of chronic stress is a multi-modal process with both behavioral and therapeutic interventions. Recent studies have put into perspective natural adaptogens such as Allium sativum that may offer a protective advantage against stress-induced neurodegenerative changes. Studies indicate that supplementation with these kinds of compounds is able to normalize neurotransmitter levels and enhance biochemical abnormalities induced by chronic stress. Modifying diet, exercise, and social support groups is key to managing stress and its effects. By developing resilience and arming people with healthy coping mechanisms, it is achievable to buffer against chronic stress's long-term destructive effects. With emerging research, the neuroendocrinological aspects of stress will play a central role in designing evidence-based interventions (Adetunji et al., 2024) (Figure 13.9).

Test Your Knowledge

1. What are the key components of the hypothalamic-pituitary-adrenal (HPA) axis, and how do they interact during a stress response?
2. Which hormones are released during acute stress, and what are their immediate physiological effects on the body?
3. How does cortisol help the body adapt to stress, and what mechanisms regulate its secretion?

13.4. Neuroendocrinology and Reproductive Health

Learning Outcome

1. Understand hormonal regulation of reproductive function;
2. Describe neuroendocrine disorders affecting reproduction;
3. Explain the impact of environmental factors on reproductive hormones.

The field of neuroendocrinology is most critical in reproductive health research since it examines the interface between the endocrine and nervous systems. The hormones secreted by the endocrine glands not only regulate various functions of the body but also significantly influence reproductive functions. The hypothalamus releases the gonadotropin-releasing hormone (GnRH), a key regulator of the reproductive axis that stimulates the pituitary gland to release luteinizing hormone (LH) and follicle-stimulating hormone (FSH). These hormones are essential for gametogenesis and control of the menstrual cycle in women, as well as the synthesis of testosterone in men. Dysregulation of the neuroendocrine pathway could result in reproductive diseases, such as PCOS or hypogonadism, and thus the importance of knowledge of these processes for reproductive health. Moreover, the complex interaction between stress and reproductive health is another phenomenon of neuroendocrinology that needs to be tackled. Stress influences the HPA axis, resulting in the secretion of glucocorticoids, such as cortisol. Elevated cortisol levels may disrupt normal reproductive axis function and influence menstrual cycles, ovulation, and fertility. Chronic stress has been shown through research to be linked with infertility and negatively impact pregnancy. Therefore, stress management and neuroendocrine consequences are essential in enhancing reproductive health. As clinicians and researchers continue to explore these connections, there is hope for the creation of targeted interventions that counteract the harmful effects of stress on reproductive function, potentially culminating in better health in those seeking conception. Last, environmental impacts on neuroendocrinology and reproductive health have become more prominent in recent years. Endocrine-disrupting chemicals (EDCs), found in many consumer products, can be harmful to the hormonal messaging and reproductive health. EDCs mimic or compete with hormones to result in adverse reproductive and developmental effects. EDC exposure has been linked to a number of reproductive issues in epidemiological research, including reduced fertility and increased rates of reproductive cancers. Since society is becoming more aware of the possible dangers of these chemicals, measures need to be put in place to minimize exposure, particularly during times of critical development. Merging information from neuroendocrinology and public health policy can be applied in formulating policy to encourage reproductive health in a way that people are protected from the harmful effects of environmental contaminants at all stages of life.

13.4.1. Hormonal Regulation of Reproductive Functions

The intricate interplay of hormones is responsible for regulating the reproductive functions and therefore forms a core theme of neuroendocrinology studies. The focal point of regulating this function is estradiol (E2), which acts as a basic intermediary in coordinating endocrine and behavioral aspects of the reproductive cycle. In dairy cows, for instance, estrous behavior expression is directly related to hormonal fluctuation, particularly under regulation by E2 and progesterone. These hormones not only regulate physiological processes but also affect gene expression engaged in reproductive processes. Understanding mechanistic pathways through which such hormones work is significant, as disrupted hormonal communication can lead to lower fertility, and thus, comprehensive studies taking into account interactions between genes and hormone levels, as seen in recent studies on estrous behavior in animals (Beerda et al., 2010), become imperative. Hormonal responsiveness is also made more complicated by the presence of such factors as metabolic stress and environmental pressures, which disrupt the functioning of hormones. Excessive milk production in dairy cows, while being economically advantageous, leads to decreased fertility due to a metabolic imbalance that affects the pathways of hormonal signals. Excessive E2 concentrations may trigger complex interactions with other hormones, such as gonadotropin-releasing hormone (GnRH) and insulin-like growth factor-1, leading to disturbances in reproductive timing and behavior. The identification of these complexities at the molecular level teaches us the significance of the new agricultural practices on the reproductive well-being of animals and thereby indicates potential intervention that could potentially alleviate fertility issues in high-yielding dairy cows (Beerda et al., 2010). Moreover, the function of the central nervous system in the control of hormones is underscored by research on kisspeptin and its activity in the LH surge required for ovulation. Research using rodent models has identified that E2 and neuroprogesterone stimulate kisspeptin release from key areas of the brain, establishing a feedback system that controls reproductive timing. Moreover, hormonal signaling alterations have been linked with changes in reproductive behavior due to metabolic or stressor impacts, such as the role of gonadotropin-inhibiting hormone in modulating the activity of GnRH neurons in birds. Together, these findings emphasize the need for an integrated neuroendocrinology that considers both peripheral hormonal action and central nervous system messaging, and show the complex array of interactions shaping reproductive processes in a variety of disparate species (Figure 13.10).

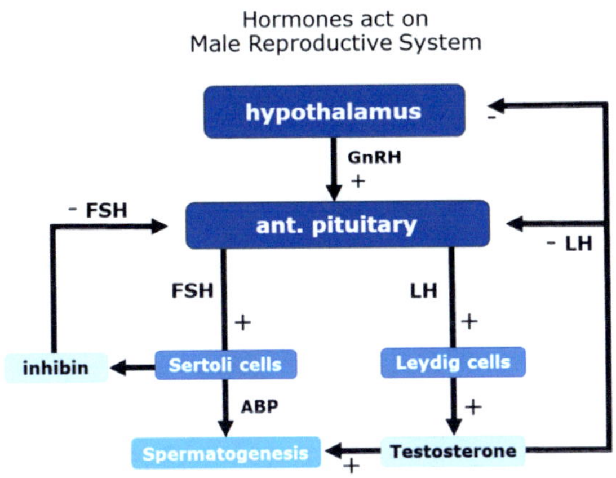

Figure 13.10. Hormonal control of the male reproductive system is mediated by the hypothalamus, anterior pituitary, and testes.

Source: https://iastate.pressbooks.pub/app/uploads/sites/43/2023/02/Slide1-e1701380214733-768x570.png.

13.4.2. Neuroendocrine Disorders Affecting Reproduction

Reproductive neuroendocrine disorders represent a crucial site of overlap between hormonal regulation and neurobiology, profoundly influencing reproductive health and function. The most prevalent of these disorders may be Polycystic Ovary Syndrome (PCOS), which afflicts roughly 10% of women of reproductive age. The condition is characterized by a range of symptoms, including hyperandrogenemia and oligo- or anovulation, and cystic ovaries. The manifestation of these signs is facilitated by neuroendocrine changes, i.e., altered pulsatile release of gonadotropin-releasing hormone (GnRH) from the hypothalamus, which subsequently stimulates luteinizing hormone (LH) release from the pituitary gland. This type of dysregulation creates a cascade effect that influences ovarian function and general reproductive health, thus defining the intricate relationship between neuroendocrine mechanisms and reproductive disease in women with PCOS (Deniselle et al., 2016). The contribution of steroid hormones to neuroendocrine reproductive disorders cannot be overstated. To give an example, estrogens and androgens are both central figures in the hormonal programming that influences reproductive health. Their functions extend beyond sexual differentiation; they modulate neuroendocrine mechanisms that play crucial roles in the regulation of ovarian function. Elevated levels of estrogen, particularly, have been implicated in the etiology of conditions such as PCOS, which is caused by hormonal disturbances. The neuroprotective nature of progesterone in relation to neurodegenerative disorders also highlights the intricacy of these hormones within the neuroendocrine system, as they not only influence reproduction but also impact brain function and health (Deniselle et al., 2016). This multi-dimensional interaction stresses the need for an integrative understanding of how neuroendocrine elements lead to reproductive disorders. Further investigation into the neuroendocrine mechanisms of reproductive disorders reveals significant neuroanatomical and neurochemical changes with PCOS. Experimental studies in animal models revealed alterations in GnRH neuron activity, which bears a relationship to changes in afferent neuronal circuits and points to an underlying neuroendocrine etiology of the disorder. Elevated levels of LH pulsatile release, with hyperactivity of GnRH neural circuits, are a sign of a proliferative state that may exacerbate symptoms of PCOS. In addition, studies have documented high hypothalamic levels of kisspeptin, a potent inducer of GnRH, further clarifying the neuroendocrine pathways involved in the control of reproductive function (Coutinho et al., 2019). With the discovery of each of these hormone and neuron interactions, useful information is being obtained about potential therapeutic approaches for addressing reproductive challenges brought on by neuroendocrine disease (Figure 13.11).

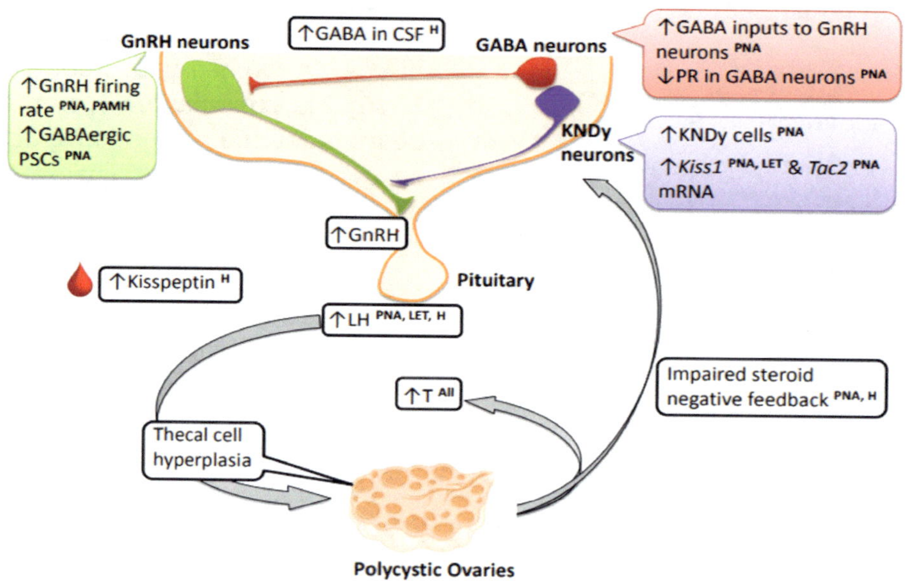

Figure 13.11. Changes in the brain and neuroendocrine reproductive axis in women with PCOS and PCOS-like animal models.

Source: https://www.mdpi.com/medsci/medsci-07-00084/article_deploy/html/images/medsci-07-00084-g001.png.

13.4.3. Impact of Environmental Factors on Reproductive Hormones

Environmental factors play a critical role in the control of reproductive hormones and male and female reproductive health. Probably one of the most basic concerns is exposure to environmental toxins, such as heavy metals and endocrine disruptors, which can have a profound impact on hormonal balance. In women, studies have confirmed that exposure to toxic substances like PM2.5 and other harmful chemicals triggers epigenetic modifications in hormone production and overall reproductive health. Epigenetic modifications like DNA methylation and histone changes have been found to be responsible for causing infertility as well as pregnancy complications, hence the study of environmental factors affecting reproductive health. It is important that these are considered by researchers and clinicians in assessing reproductive health issues and formulating prevention and intervention measures in women's reproductive health (Yu et al., 2024). The impact of endocrine-disrupting chemicals in the environment on reproductive hormones in men is equally astonishing, as disturbed hormone levels significantly compromise reproductive ability. Heavy metals such as lead and mercury are also linked to oxidative stress and hormonal disruption, which subsequently may have adverse effects on spermatogenesis and lead to poor-quality sperm. In addition, fungicide and other pesticide and herbicide exposure have been shown to disrupt the function of necessary reproductive hormones such as testosterone and luteinizing hormone (LH). Endocrine-disrupting chemicals such as these disrupt normal hormone communication and lead to a decrease in male fertility levels. Thus, the impact of such exposures to the environment should be scrutinized with caution and understanding to neutralize adverse reproductive health outcomes (Gautam et al., 2024). To treat the impacts of environmental factors on reproductive hormones, it is important to use a comprehensive strategy that covers lifestyle, eating habits, and exposure identification. Intervention aimed at reducing exposure to harmful chemicals and pollutants can significantly contribute to improved reproductive health outcomes. Public health campaigns must be focused on educating people about the risks associated with certain environmental exposures, such as those associated with agricultural practices and industrial waste. Further research into the pathways through which environmental factors influence reproductive hormones is also required. It will assist in developing optimal therapeutic regimens and interventions for reproductive health maintenance in the context of chronic environmental stress (Gautam et al., 2024; Yu et al., 2024).

Test Your Knowledge

1. Which neuroendocrine hormones are involved in regulating the menstrual cycle and ovulation?
2. How do stress and environmental toxins affect reproductive hormone levels and fertility?

13.5. Neuroendocrinology in Metabolism

Learning Outcome

1. Explain the role of neuroendocrine factors in energy balance;
2. Discuss the hormonal regulation of appetite and satiety;
3. Deal with implications for obesity and metabolic disorders.

The intricate interaction between neuroendocrinology and metabolism is crucial to understanding the body's response to various physiological changes. Neuroendocrinology examines how the endocrine and nervous systems interact to regulate metabolic functions, maintaining homeostasis. The hypothalamus is a significant brain region that facilitates this integration by responding to hormone signals and neurotransmitters to regulate energy balance, hunger, and satiety. Disruption of such neuroendocrine pathways leads to metabolic disease, implying that these interactions are essential to both health and disease. Understanding how the brain regulates hormonal response can lead to better treatments for obesity and diabetes, demonstrating the necessity of a full review of neuroendocrine mechanisms that regulate metabolism. The neuroendocrine regulation of energy intake and expenditure and metabolism merely touches the surface; hormone-controlled glucose and lipid metabolism is a complex interaction. Insulin, glucagon, and leptin are only a few key players within this multidimensional network, affecting how nutrients are metabolized by the body. The release of the hormones is a function modulated by integrating peripheral metabolic signals by the central nervous system (CNS). For instance, insulin secretion by pancreatic beta cells is regulated tightly by the hypothalamus and other regions of the brain's signals. This regulating function is essential because abnormal hormone signaling results in diseases such as insulin resistance and type 2 diabetes. In addition, evidence has emerged of new linkages between lipid metabolism and neuroendocrinology, indicating that neuropeptides regulate cholesterol synthesis and storage, thereby influencing a wide range of metabolic pathways. Advanced research still illuminates the mechanisms by which neuroendocrinology regulates metabolism through mitochondrial function. Mitochondria are pivotal energy-generating structures that are increasingly recognized as destinations for metabolic signaling, affecting many neuroendocrine functions. Importantly, changes in mitochondrial metabolism can affect cholesterol biosynthesis, and current evidence indicates that certain metabolites play pivotal roles in regulating the activity of critical transcription factors of metabolic pathways. For instance, propionate metabolism remodeling in metastasis reflects a profound correlation between energy production and cancer development, as attested in studies of prostate cancer (Li et al., 2025). Such data are supplemented with regards to pathogenesis mechanisms of metabolic disorders and open prospects for therapy aimed at decreasing neuroendocrine impacts on metabolism, demonstrating the merit of an interdisciplinary approach to research in neuroendocrinology in metabolism.

13.5.1. Role of Neuroendocrine Factors in Energy Balance

The role of neuroendocrine components in regulating energy balance is critical to homeostasis within the body. Neuroendocrine signaling involves the coordination between neural and hormonal pathways in the regulation of energy intake, storage, and expenditure. The hypothalamus and various hormones such as leptin, insulin, and ghrelin are some of the key components within this system and transmit nutritional messages to the brain. Leptin, which is a product of adipose tissue, communicates satiety, whereas ghrelin, secreted by the stomach, induces hunger. This complex regulatory mechanism ensures energy balance across varied physiological states. Abnormal regulation of these neuroendocrine mechanisms is the cause of metabolic disease, and thus, they are critical in energy homeostasis. Laying out these determinants is not only essential for the comprehension of obesity but also necessary for the formulation of interventions to restore balance and health. New studies have enlightened our understanding of the functions of Wnt signaling pathways in the neuroendocrine regulation of energy homeostasis. Wnt proteins, already studied within the context of development and cancer, have been identified as critical regulators of hypothalamic function, particularly regarding energy homeostasis. There is evidence that Wnt signaling plays a role in energy balance and glucose homeostasis in the hypothalamus, especially in conditions of diet-induced and genetically induced metabolic stress. Activation of Wnt pathways in specific hypothalamic neurons fine-tunes the function of key neuropeptides, such as pro-opiomelanocortin (POMC) and neuropeptide Y (NPY), which are key to energy intake and expenditure regulation. Information about such pathways can yield clues for treatment intervention in the management of obesity-related metabolic disorders, illustrating the intimate connection between neuroendocrinology and energy regulation within the body (Anagnostou et al., 2016). Moreover, neuroendocrine processes extend from molecular communication to include behavioral adjustments in energy regulation. Hormone-based regulation of behavior is an important determinant of the manner in which organisms respond to fluctuations in available energy. For instance, estradiol has been discovered to affect not just physiological states but also behaviors in terms of influencing the reproductive cycles, such as dairy cow estrous behavior (Beerda et al., 2010). This connection demonstrates how neuroendocrine signals can influence both metabolic processes and the behavioral consequences. As we continue to expand our knowledge of these complex interactions, it is obvious that neuroendocrine control has a major role in training individual health strategies and public health programs attempting to diminish obesity and related disorders. This multi-layered review of the study of the function of neuroendocrinology in energy balance becomes paramount for promoting a comprehensive understanding of how the body maximizes energy resources (Figure 13.12).

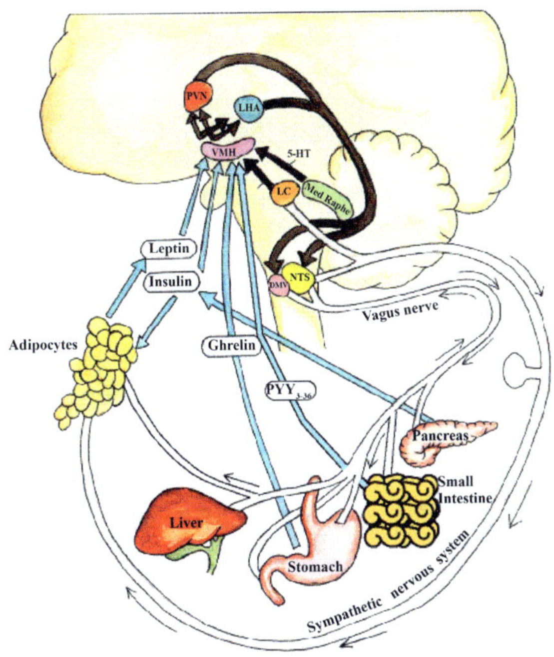

Figure 13.12. Neuroendocrine regulation of energy balance.

Source: https://www.researchgate.net/publication/225087019/figure/fig1/AS:1431281255995037@1719461921271/Neuroendocrine-regulation-of-energy-balance-The-afferent-system-neural-eg-vagal.tif.

13.5.2. Hormonal Regulation of Appetite and Satiety

The complex hormonal control of appetite and satiation is a core concept of neuroendocrinology, with effects on energy homeostasis and general well-being. Peptide YY (PYY), pancreatic polypeptide (PP), leptin, and ghrelin are significant hormones involved in these functions. It is shown through research that the levels of these hormones change with different patterns of diet and physiology. Notably, a study investigating the effect of HP compared with HC meals on postprandial hormone response revealed significant differences. That is, when caloric restriction was instituted, HP meals elicited greater circulating levels of both PP and PYY compared with their HC equivalents, showing that macronutrient composition plays an important function in the modulation of these regulatory hormones. However, subjective hunger and fullness feelings were not different between conditions, demonstrating that subjective perception of hunger and fullness may be independent of endocrine responses (Chockalingam et al., 2013). Leptin and ghrelin are central to appetite regulation with distinct, though complementary, roles in the communication of hunger and satiation. Leptin, secreted predominantly by adipose tissue, signals to the hypothalamus about energy adequacy, hence preventing appetite. It is typically linked with reduced food-seeking behavior, while ghrelin, released in the stomach, is a potent hunger signal that increases before meals and decreases after meals. Surprisingly, it has been shown that the link between these hormones and changes in brain activity is vastly different depending on the fasting status. For instance, higher levels of ghrelin correlated with increased activation of brain areas responsible for food processing during fasting, while the level of leptin negatively correlated with neural activity in areas responsible for satiety after food consumption (Deijen et al., 2012). This dynamic interaction confirms the central role of these hormones in appetite-regulating mechanisms. In addition to hormonal influences, macronutrient distribution and meal timing also contribute significantly to appetite regulation. Research has established that meal timing and protein distribution of a meal can enhance the effectiveness of hormonal satiety signals.

For instance, postprandial fluctuations in PYY and feelings of hunger were greatest for breakfast meals, suggesting that meal timing may be significant to optimize satiety responses. Moreover, liquid meal intake was associated with heightened hormone responses that are potentially linked to more rapid gastric emptying and better delivery of nutrients to the intestine. The results are of important implications for the design of successful weight control regimens and nutritional interventions that are aimed at improving appetite control and more effective eating habits. Understanding the intricate interplay between diet composition and hormone signaling is essential to manage metabolic disease and obesity conditions (Chockalingam et al., 2013) (Figure 13.13).

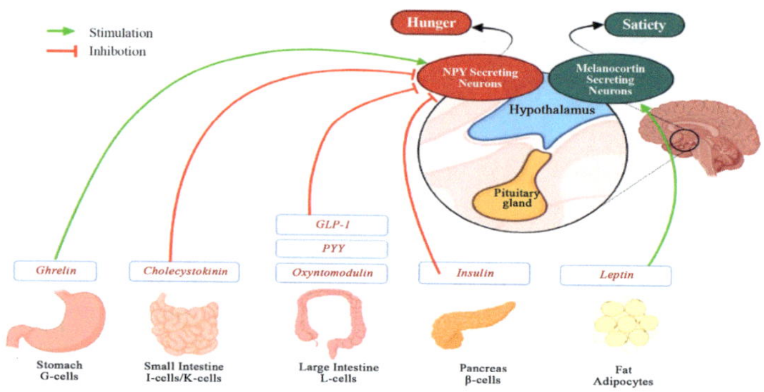

Figure 13.13. Various hormones associated with hunger and satiety.

Source: https://www.researchgate.net/publication/368536149/figure/fig3/AS:11431281123132197@1677641094941/Various-hormones-associated-with-hunger-and-satiety-created-on-Biorendercom.png.

13.5.2. Implications for Obesity and Metabolic Disorders

The intricate interaction of obesity, metabolic disease, and neuroendocrinology is a cause of increasing concern to scholars. Obesity does not happen due to mere overeating of calories or lack of exercise; it is also the outcome of complex endocrine signaling of appetite inhibition and energy homeostasis. Hormones such as leptin and ghrelin play central roles in these mechanisms, whereby leptin signals satiety and ghrelin drives hunger. Disruptions in these hormonal pathways lead to an imbalance, leading to the development of obesity and concomitant metabolic disturbances. Moreover, neuroendocrine alterations brought about by persistent stress have been shown to contribute further to such conditions, increasing the risk for comorbidities such as type 2 diabetes and cardiovascular disease. This highlights the importance of understanding the neuroendocrine mechanisms of obesity to develop effective intervention techniques for combating these conditions (Mercer et al., 2013). The link between neuroendocrinology and metabolic disorders secondary to obesity underlines the vital role of mental health in physical well-being. Research has demonstrated that psychiatric disease, in particular, depression, can add to worsening metabolic derangement by neuroendocrine mechanisms, creating a vicious circle. As an example, depression has been linked with increased adiposity, lipid profile dysregulation, and insulin resistance. Depressive conditions accompanied by inappropriate eating habits or lack of physical activity enhance the risk of obesity and metabolic syndrome by leaps and bounds. Significantly, antidepressant treatment, including Agomelatine, has been found to have a possible therapeutic application for the prevention of such metabolic alterations in animal models, suggesting that treatment of underlying causes of mental health problems can offer a dual advantage to psychological as well as physical health factors (Ionescu et al., 2016). Moreover, demystifying these neuroendocrine interactions would lead to more targeted therapeutic approaches to regulating obesity and related disorders. Knowledge of the biochemical pathways can lead to the development of pharmacologic treatment specifically aimed at hormone dysregulation or metabolic derangements.

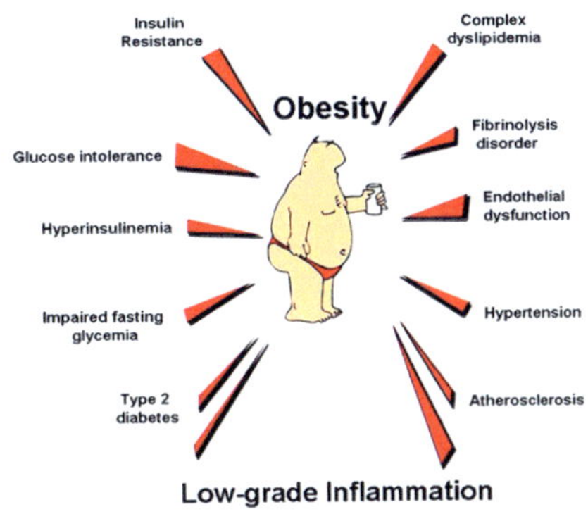

Figure 13.14. Obesity and associated metabolic disorders.

Source: https://www.researchgate.net/profile/Nathalie-Delzenne-2/publication/24427264/figure/fig1/AS:394549311623168@1471079294049/Fig-1-Obesity-and-associated-metabolic-disorders.png.

For instance, measures designed to enhance leptin sensitivity or modulate ghrelin levels may open new avenues for treatment. In addition to pharmacotherapy, dietary and lifestyle changes that try to reduce stress, improve diet quality, and increase physical activity have also been found to trigger favorable neuroendocrine adaptations that can decrease obesity and its metabolic effects. With the integration of neuroendocrinology and research into obesity, clinicians can craft comprehensive interventions that address psychological as well as physiological issues, resulting in enhanced health outcomes among obese individuals and presenting with the associated metabolic complications (Mercer et al., 2013) (Figure 13.14).

Test Your Knowledge

1. Which neuroendocrine signals are involved in regulating appetite and energy expenditure, and where are they produced?
2. What therapeutic strategies target neuroendocrine pathways to treat obesity and other metabolic disorders?

13.6. Advances in Neuroendocrinology Research

Learning Outcome

1. Understand current methodologies in neuroendocrinology studies;
2. Deal with recent findings and breakthroughs in the field of neuroendocrinology;
3. Focus on future directions and potential applications of neuroendocrinology research.

Recent advances in the field of neuroendocrinology research have significantly enhanced our understanding of the complex association between psychological illnesses and neurobiological processes. Of particular focus with respect to eating disorders has been adolescent populations, where the crux of the developmental phase of brain development in relation to the emergence of these conditions has been highlighted. For instance, the neurobiology of anorexia nervosa and bulimia nervosa has been the subject of comprehensive reviews, revealing how brain structure and function changes correlate with cognitive and emotional processes that direct food behavior. The new area of study is trying to shed light on how specific brain circuits contribute to the pathological food intake that characterizes these disorders. These results are crucial in formulating targeted interventions that can improve patient outcomes and prevent the risk of chronicity (DeGuzman et al., 2019). Furthermore, more recent research using newer brain imaging techniques has provided increased illumination on the structural and functional changes of anorexia nervosa. Studies employing larger sample sizes and sophisticated methodologies have begun to clarify the dynamic alterations that occur in the brain after malnutrition and dehydration. Notably, findings indicate that malnutrition-induced structural compromises may be normalized on recovery of weight, suggesting potential avenues of intervention via nutritional rehabilitation. Moreover, studies of learning-associated brain circuits have shown that brain regions involved in reward processing and habit formation can potentially exacerbate food restriction behaviors in the affected (DeGuzman et al., 2019). This information is the basis for possible new therapeutic interventions meant to modify these ingrained habits of behavior, thereby facilitating recovery. Other than the advancement that has occurred in the case of some eating disorders, the research environment in neuroendocrinology today is also heavily concerned with more diffuse issues like interoception—the awareness of internal body states—and its relationship to psychological well-being. It appears that alterations in connectivity between brain regions responsible for processing interoceptive information and social interaction may have a significant impact on an individual's mental well-being. The applicability of this work is particularly significant for the establishment of integrative treatment models that consider not only biological but also psychological and social dimensions of health. By the integration of these apparently differing variables, neuroendocrinology aims to provide an integrative overview of disorders that often intersect, enhancing our capacity to develop effective interventions that are individually tailored to the unique circumstances of those suffering from these complex states (DeGuzman et al., 2019).

13.6.1. Current Methodologies in Neuroendocrinology Studies

Neuroendocrinology is a cross-disciplinary field of investigation focused on the interaction between the nervous system and the endocrine system, and the techniques employed in these studies aptly reflect its complexity. Researchers employ a variety of experimental techniques, ranging from *in vivo* and *in vitro* methods, for the study of the hormonal and neurochemical mechanisms of neuroendocrine regulation. *In vivo* techniques typically utilize animal models, which provide data on both physiological and behavioral responses to neuroendocrine signaling under various stimuli. Concurrently, *in vitro* techniques, like cell culture assays, offer the possibility of manipulated experimentation on individual neural or endocrine cells, and by this, it becomes possible to analyze cellular mechanisms at the molecular level. This methodological pluralism places a premium on firm experimental designs to disentangle the intricate and dynamic interactions observed in neuroendocrinology, subjecting questions from basic science to possible clinical application. In addition, advances in imaging technology and biomarker identification have greatly expanded the methodology toolkit of neuroendocrinology research. Technologies such as functional magnetic resonance imaging (fMRI) and positron emission tomography (PET) allow researchers to study and quantify neuroendocrine function in real time and gain informative knowledge regarding the relationship between brain activity and behavior and neuroendocrine functioning. Further, inclusion of biomarker measurement in blood, saliva, or cerebrospinal fluid offers insight into hormonal fluctuations and their impact on neural substrates.

The use of such cutting-edge methodologies is part of an overall shift towards personalized medicine, with the goal of tailoring interventions to an individual neuroendocrine profile. But it is essential that these methodologies are used uniformly to counterbalance inconsistencies that can result from a non-standardized application of measurement methodologies and analysis protocols. In the goal of achieving a more holistic understanding of neuroendocrinology, interdisciplinary methodologies are essential. Interdisciplinary research among neuroscientists, endocrinologists, and psychologists can yield insights not readily apparent from a single-discipline research effort. For instance, investigating the interplay among stress, hormonal response, and behavior requires a strategy that encompasses physiological, psychological, and environmental elements. Today's research confirms this by employing a range of methodological platforms to address complex questions about the neuroendocrine systems' role in health and disease. As mentioned in recent reviews, e.g., on the interfaces between environmental and mental health, heterogeneity of methods remains essential in approximating the intricate interrelationships in neuroendocrinology as well as filling potential gaps in the literature (Daraojimba et al., 2024; Freymueller et al., 2024). This incorporation not only progresses the field but also emphasizes the imperative for continued innovation in methodological refinement and use.

13.6.2. Recent Findings and Breakthroughs

The field of neuroendocrinology has recently seen great developments that elucidate the intricate relationship between the endocrine and nervous systems. Present findings suggest that neuropeptides, which function as neurotransmitters and hormones, play important roles in the regulation of stress responses as well as emotional behavior. Research has established that specific neuropeptides, such as oxytocin and vasopressin, not only mediate social bonding and attachment but also greatly influence depression and anxiety. The implications of such research have opened up new avenues for therapeutic interventions in the modulation of emotional state through the manipulation of neuropeptides. As scientists are unraveling the neuropeptide signal dynamics, they point to the therapeutic significance of such neuropeptides as drug targets for pharmacotherapy, ultimately paving the way to enhancing clinical tools employed in the management of mood disorders and stress-related diseases. Besides neuropeptide research, there have also been significant advances in the understanding of hormonal regulatory mechanisms in the brain. Recent studies employing cutting-edge imaging techniques have identified new mechanisms through which hormones such as cortisol influence cognition and behavior. As an instance, the intricate interconnection between the HPA axis and cognitive functioning has been well studied and shown to reveal how chronic stress impinges on memory and learning. Key findings indicate that HPA axis activity dysregulation can exacerbate neurodegenerative disorders and cognitive impairments. This new perspective highlights the importance of achieving optimal hormonal balance in maintaining cognitive health, prompting an investigation into methods that promote neuroprotection and resilience against stress-induced neuronal injury. In addition, advances in research on the interaction between circadian rhythms and endocrine function have given profound knowledge to the field of neuroendocrinology. Current evidence indicates that disruption of the circadian rhythm, typically through disruption of sleep patterns or shift work, has a profound effect on the secretion of hormones such as melatonin and cortisol. Circadian disruption can result in a cascade of metabolic disease and psychiatric disorders. Evidence suggests that reversal of circadian rhythm by lifestyle or therapeutic interventions can help reverse some of these negative effects. For instance, ways of enhancing daytime light exposure have been shown to be capable of elevating mood and regulating hormone levels well. Not only has this study enlightened us on the crucial role of biological clocks in the regulation of hormones, but it also points toward the promise of novel treatment modalities based on the application of circadian biology to elevate psychological as well as physical health, bringing neuroendocrinology to a new level (Figure 13.15).

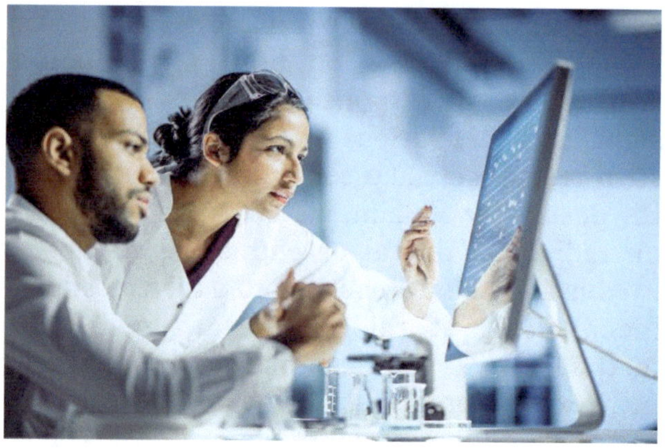

Figure 13.15. The field of neuroendocrinology has recently observed notable breakthroughs that enhance our understanding of the intricate relationship between the nervous and endocrine systems.

Source: https://media.licdn.com/dms/image/sync/v2/D4E27AQGNlmTnccAJ7g/articleshare-shrink_800/articleshare-shrink_800/0/1716931698369?e=2147483647&v=beta&t=3rBchrmSf_nKyvA9J-3v3egG1_UlG_aGWU-B3HwE9P0.

13.6.3. Future Directions and Potential Applications

Following the growth of neuroendocrinology, future research directions are sure to include improved diagnostic strategies and therapeutic interventions for neuroendocrine tumors (NETs). The paucity in imaging strategies and biomarkers has majorly impacted the clinical management of neuroendocrine neoplasia (NEN); hence, it is an urgent imperative to establish improved diagnostic tools. Traditional imaging techniques are often inadequate since they are unable to accurately measure disease progression, which can be slow and silent in nature. According to the vision of experts at an international Delphi consensus meeting, there is a clear requirement for advances in imaging techniques that integrate spatial and functional assessments with circulating biological markers, which may hold the key to defining precise disease status and predicting therapeutic results (Ambrosini et al., 2016). These advances may revolutionize the clinical practice of neuroendocrinology, enhancing patient care through personalized treatment strategies. Similarly, the promising future applications of neuroendocrinology, particularly in the use of circulating biomarkers, including circulating multianalyte mRNA, are a thrilling area of exploration. Early reports suggest the application of multianalyte profiles holds significant clinical utility compared with currently available single-analyte biomarkers that are limited by sensitivity and specificity concerns (Ambrosini et al., 2016). Implementation of these biomarkers in routine clinical practice would enable disease status and treatment response to be monitored in real time, enabling more adaptive management of neuroendocrine tumors. Furthermore, the exploration of circulating RNA as a powerful diagnostic tool aligns with the movement towards personalized medicine. By moving beyond traditional monoanalyte assessment, the field may embrace a more nuanced view of tumor biology and patient response, thereby achieving improved therapeutic outcomes. Beyond diagnostic advances, neuroendocrinology will also stand to benefit from increased interdisciplinary collaboration, particularly in the field of space medicine. The intersection of space science and neuroendocrinology highlights the unique environmental problems that face space travelers and how this can contribute to our understanding on neuroendocrine functions. Products of studies that have been supported by initiatives like the Space Medicine Program highlight the significance of investigating neuroendocrine responses to microgravity, which can yield new knowledge on the regulation of physical and psychological well-being. Future studies that explore these relationships of interaction not only lay the foundation for further advanced therapeutic applications in space but also improve our general understanding of neuroendocrine adaptation under stress. Such information has the potential to promote both terrestrial and extraterrestrial paradigms of health, eventually leading to furtherance of the field in neuroendocrinology as a whole.

Test Your Knowledge

1. What are some of the current techniques used to study neuroendocrine pathways, such as hormone-brain interactions?
2. How is the gut-brain axis influencing emerging research in neuroendocrinology, particularly in metabolic and mood disorders?

SUMMARY

The intersection of neuroendocrinology offers a complicated system of neuroendocrine interactions with the nervous system, emphasizing the relevance of the subject in understanding human physiology and well-being. The coincidence of investigations indicates that neuroendocrinological mechanisms are pivotal in the task of homeostasis maintenance, particularly in stress situations. Brain-orchestrated stress responses not only dictate how a person responds to a perceived threat but also have significant impacts on overall health. Through an unraveling of the dynamic interplay between neural circuits and hormone signals, researchers have enhanced their comprehension of how malfunctions in such systems can lead to pathologies, thereby underscoring the importance of interdisciplinary principles in neuroendocrinology as a unifying paradigm for the health sciences. In addition, neuroendocrinology of the skin is quite important, highlighting the complexity of this organ beyond protective functions. Because the skin interacts with extrinsic stressors—demonstrated by ultraviolet (UV) radiation—it operates as a site where neural and hormonal cues integrate in an effort to modulate systemic function. The activation of local neuroendocrine axes following UV radiation demonstrates the ability of peripheral stimuli to modulate both cutaneous and central nervous system function. Such interaction, besides affording direct immediate physiological compensations, also offers avenues for therapeutic intervention designed to affect disorders underlying immune dysregulation and mood aberrance. This provides compelling reasons for continued research on how the skin and its neuroendocrine interfaces can be harnessed for new therapies, thus expanding the sphere of neuroendocrinology. In conclusion, the evolution of our understanding in the field of neuroendocrinology is central to developing customized interventions for multifaceted health issues. Neuroendocrine systems exhibit significant plasticity, which is the ability to respond to stress and environmental challenges, highlighting their potential for recovery and adaptability, as discussed in the context of allostasis processes. Sex difference detection and the effect of early life experience on neuroendocrine function further highlight the nuanced complexity in the field. Lastly, laying the foundation for interdisciplinary collaborations among researchers, clinicians, and policy-makers will be essential to bridging results with effective health strategies in a bid to improve health outcomes and quality of life. The significance of this new body of knowledge emphasizes the imperative to integrate neuroendocrinology into multidisciplinary models of healthcare so that it can become the cornerstone of modern medical science.

In neuroendocrinology, understanding the intricate interaction between the endocrine system and the nervous system is central to explaining varied physiological processes. Key aspects addressed include how hormones affect the modulation of neurological functions and behavior. For instance, neuropeptides and neurotransmitters such as oxytocin and cortisol possess very potent effects on social behaviors, stress responses, and emotional regulation. The regulation of neuroendocrine signals is vital in providing homeostasis so that the body can deal with internal and external changes. Furthermore, the research on feedback loops in the HPA axis shows how endocrine responses affect neurological effects, further cementing the bidirectional interaction of these two systems. Such a complex process requires more research to better understand how neuroendocrinology helps the mental well-being and overall physical wellness. Moreover, improvements in cellular and tissue technologies have opened up new avenues for the study of neuroendocrine functions, particularly to regenerative medicine. The most recent studies speak of the potential of stem cell therapies for the treatment of neurological disorders that are linked to neuroendocrine malfunction. Such findings emphasize the importance of finding efficient sources of stem cells and new ways to culture them as well as use them in the clinic. Stem cells derived from other tissues, including multipotent mesenchymal cells, possess traits that may be useful for neuroprotective and neuroregenerative processes. By studying the effectiveness of the combination of greater than one stem cell type, researchers try to optimize therapy for disorders such as depression and anxiety that may be induced by aberrant neuroendocrine mechanisms. Such an understanding of therapeutic modalities represents a new frontier in advancing improved interventions in neuroendocrinology. Finally, the consequences of key point analysis (KPA) on distilling in-depth discussions within the field of neuroendocrinology cannot be circumvented. KPA procedures allow for the recovery and quantification of critical pieces of information from vast amounts of literature that could assist scientists in establishing pervasive themes and emergent trends. Using techniques such as aspect sentiment analysis and large language models can enhance the accuracy and applicability of the produced information, offering a structured approach to separating the complexity of neuroendocrine research. The new model guarantees a proper dissemination of significant findings, facilitating inter-consultation and prolonged investigation among the scientific community. As the field of neuroendocrinology advances, incorporating state-of-the-art analytical methods will be critical to continuing innovation and discovering new therapeutic strategies for neuroendocrine interaction-influenced disorders, with the ultimate goal of progressing the aims of modern medical science.

KEY TERMS FROM THIS CHAPTER

- Antidepressant therapy
- Brain activity
- Breeding behaviors
- Central nervous system (CNS)
- Corticotropin-releasing factors
- Dehydroepiandrosterone
- Exposure identification
- GnRH gene expression
- Hormonal communication
- HPA axis consequences
- Maternal mortality
- Metabolic homeostasis
- Methodological pluralism
- Neuroendocrine alterations
- Bidirectional interaction
- Brain-orchestrated stress responses
- Cancer development
- Cognitive function
- Corticotropin-releasing hormone (CRH)
- Developmental biology
- Glucocorticoid feedback mechanisms
- Health inequities
- Hormonal homeostasis
- Immune cell dysregulation
- Metabolic disturbances
- Metabolic stressors
- Neurobiologic responses
- Neuroendocrine dynamics

CRITICAL THINKING QUESTIONS

1. **Which of the following hormones is released by the hypothalamus and plays a central role in the neuroendocrine response to stress?**
   a. Prolactin
   b. Growth hormone
   c. Corticotropin-releasing hormone (CRH)
   d. Luteinizing hormone (LH)
2. **Which neuroendocrine pathway is most directly involved in the regulation of reproductive function?**
   a. HPA axis
   b. HPT axis
   c. RAA system
   d. HPG axis
3. **Which hormone produced by the hypothalamus stimulates the anterior pituitary to secrete thyroid-stimulating hormone (TSH), thus influencing metabolism?**
   a. TRH (Thyrotropin-releasing hormone)
   b. ACTH
   c. Oxytocin
   d. Somatostatin
4. **In neuroendocrinology, what role does the hormone leptin play in the body?**
   a. Promotes glucose uptake in muscles
   b. Regulates appetite and energy balance
   c. Stimulates cortisol release during stress
   d. Enhances calcium absorption in the intestines
5. **Recent advances in neuroendocrinology research have identified which technique as crucial for mapping hormone-sensitive brain circuits?**
   a. EEG
   b. PET imaging
   c. Optogenetics
   d. PCR

Short answer Questions

1. How does the hypothalamus serve as the key interface between the nervous and endocrine systems in neuroendocrinology?
2. What are the primary neurohormones involved in neuroendocrinology, and what roles do they play in physiological regulation?
3. How does the hypothalamic-pituitary-adrenal (HPA) axis regulate the stress response, and what are the consequences of chronic activation?
4. What neuroendocrine mechanisms are involved in the regulation of reproductive health, including the menstrual cycle and sexual behavior?
5. How does the neuroendocrine system influence metabolism, and what roles do hormones like leptin, insulin, and ghrelin play in energy balance?
6. What are some neuroendocrine disorders, and how can dysfunction in the hypothalamus or pituitary gland lead to systemic disease?

Answers to Critical Thinking Questions

1. (c) 2. (d) 3. (a) 4. (b) 5. (c)

REFERENCES

1. Adetunji, O. A., Adegunle, A., Adeoye, B. O., Nwobi, J. C., Fabiyi, O., Akano, O. P., Ogunsanya, S. T., et al. (2024). Chronic stress-induced neurodegenerative changes in Wistar rats: Hippocampal evidence and the mitigating effects of *Allium sativum*. *Babcock University Medical Journal*. https://www.semanticscholar.org/paper/e7d7e6c70743c659ef77b4027a853e211962b163 (accessed on 22nd July 2025).
2. Akwa, Y., Baghai, T. C., Baker, E. R., Barrett-Connor, E., Bicikova, M., Bitran, D., Bloch, M., et al. (2006). Neuroactive steroids in depression and anxiety disorders: Clinical studies. https://core.ac.uk/download/16432473.pdf (accessed on 22nd July 2025).
3. Almajali, T. A. H., Ismail, F. B., Gunnasegaran, P. A. L., Al Shurafa, S. M., & Kazem, H. A. (2024). Exploring the future of solar stills: Recent breakthroughs in performance enhancement. *Separation & Purification Reviews, 54*, 105–127. https://www.semanticscholar.org/paper/67dd9587480f124ab6296be855406571d5a93ef6 (accessed on 22nd July 2025).
4. Ambrosini, V., Baum, R. P., Bodei, L., et al. (2016). Imaging and biomarkers in gastroenteropancreatic neuroendocrine tumor disease management. https://core.ac.uk/download/199417681.pdf (accessed on 22nd July 2025).
5. Anagnostou, G., Bechtold, D. A., Behari, M., Bennett, C., Benzler, J., Benzler, J., Bolborea, M., et al. (2016). Hypothalamic Wnt signaling and its role in energy balance regulation. https://core.ac.uk/download/153514604.pdf (accessed on 22nd July 2025).
6. Aprahamian, F., Cambourg, A., de Nicola, A. F., et al. (2016). Steroid profiling in male wobbler mouse, a model of Amyotrophic Lateral Sclerosis. https://core.ac.uk/download/159290923.pdf (accessed on 22nd July 2025).
7. Armando, N. G., Dos Santos Claro, P. A., Inda, M. C., et al. (2017). Endocrinology and the brain: Corticotropin-releasing hormone signaling. https://core.ac.uk/download/159287854.pdf (accessed on 22nd July 2025).
8. Avishai-Eliner, S., Baram, T. Z., Brunson, K. L., et al. (2001). Neurobiology of the stress response early in life: Evolution of a concept and the role of corticotropin releasing hormone. https://core.ac.uk/download/231897537.pdf (accessed on 22nd July 2025).
9. Baghai, T. C., Laakmann, G., & Schule, C. (2004). Mirtazapine decreases stimulatory effects of reboxetine on cortisol, adrenocorticotropin and prolactin secretion in healthy male subjects. https://core.ac.uk/download/16432476.pdf (accessed on 22nd July 2025).
10. Becu Villalobos, D., Coirini, H., Cornejo, M. P., et al. (2016). Neuroendocrine regulation of metabolism. https://core.ac.uk/download/159290530.pdf (accessed on 22nd July 2025).
11. Beerda, B., Boer, H. M. T., Veerkamp, R. F., et al. (2010). Estrous behavior in dairy cows: Identification of underlying mechanisms and gene functions. https://core.ac.uk/download/pdf/29246031.pdf (accessed on 22nd July 2025).
12. Bennett, S., Robb, K. A., Zortea, T. C., Dickson, A., Richardson, C., & O'Connor, R. C. (2023). Male suicide risk and recovery factors: A systematic review and qualitative meta synthesis of two decades of research. *Psychological Bulletin, 149*, 371–417. https://doi.org/10.1037/bul0000397 (accessed on 22nd July 2025).

13. Bentley, G. E., Calandra, R. S., Micevych, P. E., et al. (2016). Peripheral and central mechanisms involved in hormonal control of male and female reproduction. https://core.ac.uk/download/159295807.pdf (accessed on 22nd July 2025).

14. Bonansco, C., Martínez-Pinto, J., Silva, R. A., Velásquez, V. B., Martorell, A., Martorell, A., Selva, M. V., et al. (2018). Neonatal exposure to oestradiol increases dopaminergic transmission in nucleus accumbens and morphine-induced conditioned place preference in adult female rats. *Journal of Neuroendocrinology, 30*. https://www.semanticscholar.org/paper/d1cde2e297a80583285ad6e57a9286c588e8791d (accessed on 22nd July 2025).

15. Bořkovec, A. B. (2019). *Insect Neurochemistry and Neurophysiology*. CRC Press eBooks. https://doi.org/10.1201/9781351073592 (accessed on 22nd July 2025).

16. Cain, L., Hernández-Cortés, D., Timmins, C., & Weber, P. (2024). Recent findings and methodologies in economics research in environmental justice. *Review of Environmental Economics and Policy, 18*, 116–142. https://www.semanticscholar.org/paper/7b994301f7af4aff8835909bd3536e453f2c619a (accessed on 22nd July 2025).

17. Calandra, R. S., Doepner, R. F. G., Frungieri, M. B., et al. (2003). Evidence for a GABAergic system in rodent and human testis: Local GABA production and GABA receptors. https://core.ac.uk/download/16432477.pdf (accessed on 22nd July 2025).

18. Chockalingam, A., Dellsperger, K. C., Fairchild, T. J., et al. (2013). Liquid meal composition, postprandial satiety hormones, and perceived appetite and satiety in obese women during acute caloric restriction. https://core.ac.uk/download/11244730.pdf (accessed on 22nd July 2025).

19. Chou, T., D'Orsogna, M. R., & Kim, L. U. (2016). Onset, timing, and exposure therapy of stress disorders: Mechanistic insight from a mathematical model of oscillating neuroendocrine dynamics. https://core.ac.uk/download/323078037.pdf (accessed on 22nd July 2025).

20. Coss, D., & Lainez, N. M. (2019). Leukemia inhibitory factor represses GnRH gene expression via cFOS during inflammation in male mice. https://core.ac.uk/download/323083176.pdf (accessed on 22nd July 2025).

21. Coutinho, E. A., & Kauffman, A. S. (2019). The role of the brain in the pathogenesis and physiology of polycystic ovary syndrome (PCOS). https://core.ac.uk/download/323065551.pdf (accessed on 22nd July 2025).

22. Daraojimba, E. C., Nwasike, C. N., Adegbite, A. O., Ezeigweneme, C. A., & Gidiagba, J. O. (2024). Comprehensive review of agile methodologies in project management. *Computer Science & IT Research Journal*. https://www.semanticscholar.org/paper/45dfc420983d9de67043899e9597f74529610de0 (accessed on 22nd July 2025).

23. Dayanithi, G., Föhr, K. J., Gratzl, M., Link, H., et al. (1992). Oxytocin at physiological concentrations evokes adrenocorticotropin (ACTH) release from corticotrophs by increasing intracellular free calcium mobilized mainly from intracellular stores. Oxytocin displays synergistic or additive effects on ACTH-releasing factor or arginine vasopressin-induced ACTH secretion, respectively. https://core.ac.uk/download/12168036.pdf (accessed on 22nd July 2025).

24. DeGuzman, M. C., Frank, G. K. W., & Shott, M. E. (2019). Recent advances in understanding anorexia nervosa. https://core.ac.uk/download/323064386.pdf (accessed on 22nd July 2025).

25. DeGuzman, M. C., Frank, G. K. W., & Shott, M. E. (2019). The neurobiology of eating disorders. https://core.ac.uk/download/288432983.pdf (accessed on 22nd July 2025).

26. Deijen, J. B., Drent, M. L., Jakobsdottir, S., Ruiter, M., et al. (2012). Brain activation by visual food-related stimuli and correlations with metabolic and hormonal parameters: A fMRI study. https://core.ac.uk/download/pdf/15475967.pdf (accessed on 22nd July 2025).

27. Eva, L., Pleș, H., Covache-Busuioc, R. A., Glavan, L. A., Bratu, B. G., Bordeianu, A., Dumitrascu, D. I., et al. (2023). A comprehensive review on neuroimmunology: Insights from multiple sclerosis to future therapeutic developments. *Biomedicines, 11*, 2489–2489. https://doi.org/10.3390/biomedicines11092489 (accessed on 22nd July 2025).

28. Freymueller, J., Schmid, H. L., Senkler, B., Lopez Lumbi, S., Zerbe, S., Hornberg, C., & McCall, T. (2024). Current methodologies of greenspace exposure and mental health research—a scoping review. *Frontiers in Public Health, 12*. https://www.semanticscholar.org/paper/2c36fe80cf2e4d585a11eb088956f7d83e5951ac (accessed on 22nd July 2025).

29. Gautam, R., Priyadarshini, E., Patel, A. K., & Arora, T. (2024). Assessing the impact and mechanisms of environmental pollutants (heavy metals and pesticides) on the male reproductive system: A comprehensive review. *Journal of Environmental Science and Health, Part C, 42*, 126–153. https://www.semanticscholar.org/paper/e97a9e7f54bc4710e151230ed75732fb55e3267a (accessed on 22nd July 2025).

30. Gonzalez Deniselle, M. C., Lara, H. E., Recabarren, S. E., Roselli, C. E., et al. (2016). Developmental and functional effects of steroid hormones on the neuroendocrine axis and spinal cord. https://core.ac.uk/download/159294623.pdf (accessed on 22nd July 2025).

31. Helsper, C., van Gils, C. V., van Erp, N. F., Siepman van den Berg, M. F. R., Rogouti, O., van Asselt, K. V., Maarsingh, O., et al. (2023). Impact of the COVID-19 outbreak—Delayed referral of colorectal and lung cancer in primary care: A national retrospective cohort study. *Cancers, 15*. https://www.semanticscholar.org/paper/f4f6cd37db56a7143204dcd6e0abf3f470c31ede (accessed on 22nd July 2025).

32. Hendricks-Sturrup, R. M., Simmons, M., Anders, S., Aneni, K., Clayton, E. W., Coco, J. R., Collins, B. X., et al. (2023). Developing ethics and equity principles, terms, and engagement tools to advance health equity and researcher diversity in AI and machine learning: Modified Delphi approach. *JMIR AI, 2*. https://www.semanticscholar.org/paper/26cfc0917331dd7e212233c1c96a78b647ee984e (accessed on 22nd July 2025).

33. Ionescu, E., Manea, M. C., Manea, M., Paraschiv, S., et al. (2016). Metabolic alterations in experimental models of depression. https://core.ac.uk/download/144552987.pdf (accessed on 22nd July 2025).

34. Kassebaum, N., Barber, R., Bhutta, Z., Dandona, L., Gething, P., Hay, S. I., Kinfu, Y., et al. (2017). Global, regional, and national levels of maternal mortality, 1990–2015: A systematic analysis for the Global Burden of Disease Study 2015. *Obstetrical & Gynecological Survey*. https://www.semanticscholar.org/paper/1a5d8e3f695a549252b3b8e229440e1eb70f74b0 (accessed on 22nd July 2025).

35. Kyryk, V. (2024). Stem cell therapy for cardiac regeneration: Key points. *Cell and Organ Transplantology*. https://www.semanticscholar.org/paper/6a1b536f3691ad0d162e4187a4a2e2ffd1507b5f (accessed on 22nd July 2025).

36. Li, Z., Liu, S., Kester, O., Jin, W., Chan, U. I., Li, Z., Bullen, N., et al. (2025). Abstract 3802: Isoleucine and valine promote prostate cancer progression via propionyl-CoA-mediated cholesterol metabolism. *Cancer Research*. https://www.semanticscholar.org/paper/a74c64e073d6487b85461d509d703e54ffad9d1a (accessed on 22nd July 2025).

37. Mahindru, V., Sharma, P., & Abrol, V. (2024). Efficiency of biochar with mineral fertilizers on soil properties and crop growth. *International Journal of Advanced Biochemistry Research*. https://www.semanticscholar.org/paper/f723fd1d231cc500d2d22bdc18b68018cddbf1b2 (accessed on 22nd July 2025).

38. McEwen, B. S. (2017). Neurobiological and systemic effects of chronic stress. *Chronic Stress, 1*. https://doi.org/10.1177/2470547017692328 (accessed on 22nd July 2025).

39. Mercer, J. G., & Murphy, M. (2013). Diet-regulated anxiety. https://core.ac.uk/download/19506489.pdf (accessed on 22nd July 2025).

40. Olza Fernández, I., Uvnäs-Moberg, K., Ekström, A., Leahy-Warren, P., Karlsdóttir, S. I., Nieuwenhuijze, M., Villarmea, S., et al. (2020). Birth as a neuro-psycho-social event: An integrative model of maternal experiences and their relation to neurohormonal events during childbirth. *PLoS ONE, 15*, e0230992–e0230992. https://doi.org/10.1371/journal.pone.0230992 (accessed on 22nd July 2025).

41. Pleasant, L. G., & Solberg, J. L. (2025). Space medicine research publications: 1983–1984. https://core.ac.uk/download/pdf/42847043.pdf (accessed on 22nd July 2025).

42. Sefrji, F. O., Abulfaraj, A., Alshehrei, F. M., Al-Andal, A., Alnahari, A. A., Tashkandi, M., Baz, L., et al. (2025). Comprehensive analysis of orthologous genes reveals functional dynamics and energy metabolism in the rhizosphere microbiome of *Moringa oleifera*. *Functional & Integrative Genomics, 25*. https://www.semanticscholar.org/paper/7e84b02013f8c2795eb59be0ef59642827c8f1c5 (accessed on 22nd July 2025).

43. Shirokova, O., Kuzmina, D. M., Zaborskaya, O. G., Shchelchkova, N., Kozliaeva, E., Korotchenko, S. A., Pershin, V. I., et al. (2025). The long-term effects of chronic unpredictable mild stress experienced during adolescence could vary depending on biological sex. *International Journal of Molecular Sciences, 26*. https://www.semanticscholar.org/paper/5f88079764e275fe2c3cbcf38d07d297c6f7eb8d (accessed on 22nd July 2025).

44. Słomiński, A., Żmijewski, M. A., Płonka, P. M., Szaflarski, J. P., & Paus, R. (2018). How UV light touches the brain and endocrine system through skin, and why. *Endocrinology, 159*, 1992–2007. https://doi.org/10.1210/en.2017-03230 (accessed on 22nd July 2025).

45. Tang, A., Zhang, X., Dinh, M., & Cambria, E. (2024). Prompted aspect key point analysis for quantitative review summarization. *ArXiv, abs/2407.14049*. https://www.semanticscholar.org/paper/ed73a37eb5200c4864e622947c4299886cdfe7a1 (accessed on 22nd July 2025).

46. Ungar, M., Theron, L., Murphy, K., & Jefferies, P. (2021). Researching multisystemic resilience: A sample methodology. *Frontiers in Psychology, 11*. https://doi.org/10.3389/fpsyg.2020.607994 (accessed on 22nd July 2025).

47. Yu, X., Xu, J., Song, B., Zhu, R., Liu, J., Liu, Y. F., & Ma, Y. (2024). The role of epigenetics in women's reproductive health: The impact of environmental factors. *Frontiers in Endocrinology, 15*. https://www.semanticscholar.org/paper/9a004e1ad8c9d32515aac0a228232444b17437af (accessed on 22nd July 2025).

48. Zhang, L., Zetter, M. A., Guerra, E. C., Hernández, V., Mahata, S., & Eiden, L. (2020). ACE2 in the second act of COVID-19 syndrome: Peptide dysregulation and possible correction with oestrogen. *Journal of Neuroendocrinology, 33*. https://www.semanticscholar.org/paper/1980e2f815bacb6d90ccc84aaffedaf9ef516cac (accessed on 22nd July 2025).

49. Zou, H., Zhou, H., Yan, R., Yao, Z., & Lu, Q. (2022). Chronotype, circadian rhythm, and psychiatric disorders: Recent evidence and potential mechanisms. *Frontiers in Neuroscience, 16*. https://doi.org/10.3389/fnins.2022.811771 (accessed on 22nd July 2025).

ENDOCRINOLOGY IN CRITICAL ILLNESS AND ICU

14

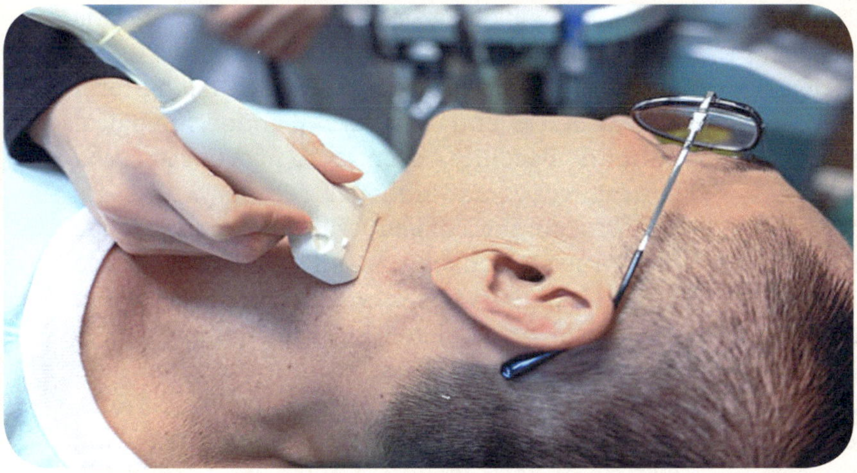

LEARNING OBJECTIVES

After studying this chapter, you will be able to:

1. Explain the role of hormones in critical illness;
2. Describe common endocrine disorders in the ICU;
3. Define hormonal therapies in critical care;
4. Discuss how the hypothalamic-pituitary-adrenal (HPA) axis plays a critical role in the body's response to stress in the intensive care unit (ICU) setting;
5. Deal with endocrine system monitoring in the ICU;
6. Focus on research and advances in endocrinology.

Introduction

The intersection of endocrinology and critical illness is essential to understanding the complex physiological responses that take place in the intensive care unit (ICU). Endocrine disturbance in critical illness can persist to significantly impact patient outcomes, leading to a broad spectrum of hormonal imbalances that govern metabolic processes, glucose regulation, and stress response. The management of such dysfunctions becomes of crucial significance, as they have the potential to complicate recovery trajectories and dictate mortality rates in critically ill patients. For instance, sustaining normoglycemia is one of the challenges in healthcare professionals, and it highlights the significance of evidence-based guidelines for controlling glucose variability effectively. In a compliance study of guidelines of glucose control in a cardiothoracic ICU, compliance remained sub-optimal, highlighting an imminent need to enhance endocrine dysfunction management among critically ill patients (Maharaj et al., 2016). Furthermore, endocrine dysregulation consequences are not restricted to acute glucose control and may encompass more significant hormonal axes that have the potential to be disrupted in severe illnesses. Recent data on diseases such as Long Covid demonstrate that SARS-CoV-2 infection is able to induce deep alterations in hormonal regulation, involving the hypothalamic-pituitary-adrenal (HPA) axis and other essential hormonal systems. Patients can present with varying degrees of adrenal insufficiency with chronic symptoms of dizziness and fatigue. Also, dysregulation of the hypothalamic-pituitary-gonadal (HPG) axis leads to conditions like low testosterone and irregular menstruation, also making it difficult to provide care for the patient in the ICU environment. Knowledge of these endocrine issues is critical for creating more precise therapeutic options that address hormone dysregulation directly among critically ill patients (Abitkar et al., 2025). Approaching endocrinology in critical care holistically not only helps in diagnosing and treating actual conditions but also gives means of improving care for patients in general. The role of healthcare professionals being educated on adhering to protocols for the management of endocrines cannot be overemphasized. Education becomes a priority to enable doctors to respond better to endocrine emergencies that could arise within an ICU. While the extreme variability of glucose and treatment adherence is evident, studies show that ongoing training can lead to improved outcomes. Frequent monitoring of protocol adherence, especially in relation to glucose control, is therefore necessary to ensure optimal care for critically ill patients and reflects a key area for research and improvement in the future (Maharaj et al., 2016).

Importance of Endocrinology in Critical Illness

It is important to recognize the relevance of endocrinology to critical illness to maximize patient management in the intensive care unit (ICU). Endocrine regulation may significantly impact numerous physiological alterations that occur in critical illnesses and determine metabolism, fluid balance, and immune function. Endocrinopathies, including disturbances in cortisol, insulin, and thyroid hormone levels, contribute to worsening the conditions of patients, which results in complications such as hyperglycemia and wound healing defects. This is most obvious in patients who are having severe stress responses, where the hypothalamic-pituitary-adrenal axis gets activated, which results in enhanced production of cortisol. This physiological response, which is adaptive in the short term, can become maladaptive in long-term critical states, and thus, careful endocrinological handling becomes essential to prevent harmful consequences and enhance recovery. As such, the incorporation of endocrinological knowledge into practice can significantly affect the course of critically ill patients. Nutritional support in critical care must be guided by principles of endocrinology since improper nutritional therapy may lead to serious complications. Current studies show that underfeeding during critical illness is linked with less favorable outcomes, and this suggests a multifaceted relationship between nutritional need and hormonal response. For instance, resistance to anabolism has been shown to impede cell repair processes, while hyperglycemia enhances insulin needs, making the management of critical illness patients even more complex. The data from various randomized controlled trials indicate that early high nutrition dosing is not for all and even potentially harmful in the presence of inherent organ dysfunctions (de Man et al., 2024). Physicians thus need to navigate these hormonal nuances to optimize nutrition timing and content for given patient profiles, resulting in enhanced recovery patterns. Furthermore, the recognition of post-intensive care syndrome (PICS) supports the necessity for an endocrinological consideration to approach long-term outcomes in ICU survivors. Since more than one endocrine and metabolic dysregulation contributes to physical, cognitive, and psychological impairments on discharge, a thorough understanding of these relationships is necessary to devise potent rehabilitation protocols. For instance, anabolic resistance and atrophy of muscle have been linked with ICU-acquired weakness, underscoring the importance of early nutritional and hormonal interventions during the recovery process (Voiriot et al., 2022). Similarly, chronic inflammation fueled by hormonal imbalances can be an important feature in avoiding long-term manifestations of PICS. Knowledge of endocrinology's consequences in critical illness ultimately informs elaborate care plans that not only deal with immediate survival, but also enhance quality of life following ICU discharge (Figure 14.1).

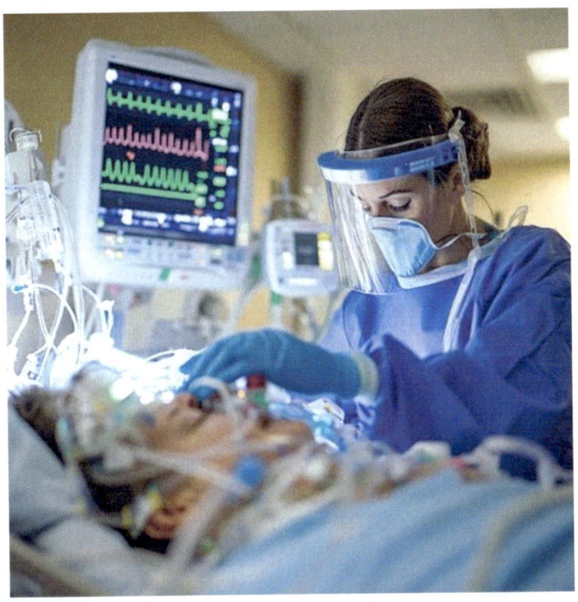

Figure 14.1. Understanding the significance of endocrinology in critical illness is essential for optimizing patient outcomes in the intensive care unit (ICU).

Source: https://images.stockcake.com/public/9/2/c/92c2bb55-92ae-45eb-99ca-e2a83b9ebcef_large/intensive-care-unit-stockcake.jpg.

14.1. The Role of Hormones in Critical Illness

Learning Outcome

1. Discuss stress response and hormone release;
2. Understand the impact of cortisol on metabolism;
3. Focus on thyroid hormone alterations in ICU patients.

The complex interplay of hormones during critical illness is the pivotal mechanism of the body's response to severe physiological stress. Cortisol, catecholamines, and insulin are often deranged in critically ill patients, with an impact on metabolic homeostasis and immune defense. In particular, hypercortisolemia is primarily the result of an abnormal hypothalamic-pituitary-adrenal (HPA) axis that is unable to effectively regulate cortisol release. Research has indicated that plasma ACTH and cortisol concentrations are considerably elevated in ICU patients compared with healthy controls and suggest a defective glucocorticoid feedback mechanism. The hypercortisolemia may plausibly be involved in inappropriate consequences, particularly in glucose homeostasis and immunosuppression. Awareness of these endocrine changes can inform therapy, highlighting the importance of modulating hormonal imbalance to improve patient outcomes in ICU (Allolio et al., 1993). The contribution of the gut microbiota to the modulation of hormones in critical illness cannot be excluded either. Gut microbiome abnormalities in ICU patients, a frequent feature, lead to the shift to ultra-low-diversity microbial communities. These changes are typically complemented by the use of broad-spectrum antibiotics and by stress-related hormonal mechanisms, leading to decreased microbial diversity. Interestingly, certain gut microbes possess a bimodal capacity for pathogenic and commensal life, which impacts the host's endocrine processes. In situations of stress, e.g., opioid exposure, this microbiota may have the capacity to shift towards pathogenicity, which in turn may influence hormone balances as well as immune function. The complexity of such a connection points to the significance of including microbiome management in the treatment protocols for endocrine therapy among critically ill patients, which might prevent the adverse effects of hormonal dysregulation (Alverdy et al., 2014). Finally, the interaction between stress hormones and inflammatory disorders among critically ill patients suggests a two-way interaction, adding intricacy to the management of patients. Increased pro-inflammatory cytokine levels in the context of critical illness may lead to increased secretion of glucocorticoids, which is considered a protective mechanism to restrict the inflammatory process. However, this increased glucocorticoid response in turn can be immunosuppressive and affect metabolism and hence be a cause of the development of sequelae such as hyperglycemia and increased susceptibility to infection. Such continuous monitoring and regulation of hormonal responses can be crucial in the management of critically ill patients, as hormone therapy has the potential to provide specific support to enable homeostasis. By elucidating the intricate functions of hormones during critical illness, medical professionals can provide more effective treatment protocols that target both metabolic and hormonal regulation, thereby improving patient prognosis in ICU settings (Allolio et al., 1993).

14.1.1. Stress Response and Hormone Release

The stress response of the body, particularly in the context of critical illness, is an intricate interplay of neuroendocrine pathways that promote survival. The HPA axis primarily governs stress response and facilitates the secretion of corticosteroids, namely cortisol. Cortisol secretion plays an important role in modulating inflammation and maintaining metabolic homeostasis in the context of the ICU. Hypersecretion of cortisol can enhance gluconeogenesis and influence immune response, both of which are vital in physiological stresses such as surgical operations or septicemia. While such responses are essential for survival, inappropriately elevated cortisol has negative effects, such as immunosuppression and hyperglycemia, and adds to the complications of patient care in the critical care environment. Systemic inflammation also has a profound impact on the release of stress hormones, as evidenced in studies involving the measurement of cytokine levels during surgery. Inflammatory reactions that induce high cytokines can further activate the HPA axis, generating a cascade of endocrine changes that may include increased secretion of adrenocorticotropic hormone (ACTH). These genetic differences have been shown in research to influence this hormonal response, such as SNPs of the toll-like receptors (TLRs), for instance. In cardiac surgery patients with TLR4 SNPs, it has been reported that levels of ACTH decrease during inflammation, revealing a nuanced understanding of the extent to which genetic factors can modulate the endocrine stress response in critical illness (Boehm et al., 2011). Such recognition is particularly important because it highlights the need for individualized strategies in personalized medicine for critical care. In addition, the physiological substrates for stress reactions extend beyond hormone release to encompass broader metabolic and immunologic effects. In critically ill individuals, HPA axis dysfunction may cause a relative inability to respond to stressors, expressed as adrenal insufficiency. This state may exacerbate the patient's underlying pathology and result in complications such as septic shock and acute respiratory distress syndrome (ARDS). The endocrine alterations are not isolated occurrences; they have cross-talking effects on various organ systems, impacting recovery patterns as a whole. Understanding these processes is crucial to successfully treating critically ill patients, as therapeutic maneuvers to modulate the endocrine response may improve outcomes (Brém et al., 2020). Encouraging an in-depth knowledge of the endocrine response to stress will enhance the ability to manage the complexities of ICU patient care (Figure 14.2).

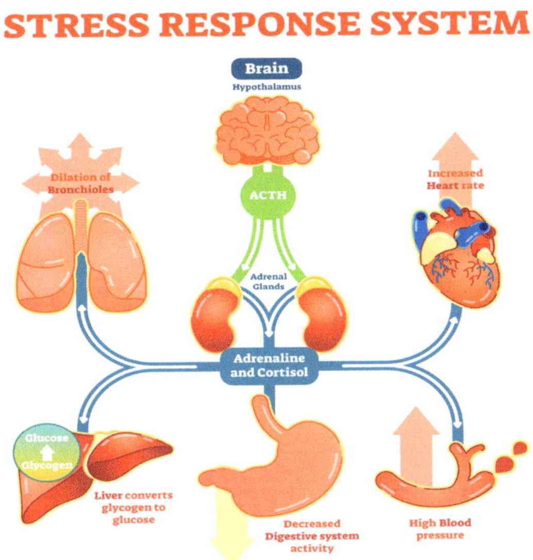

Figure 14.2. Stress response system.

Source: Bhttps://hcahealthcaretoday.com/wp-content/uploads/2019/04/GettyImages-923451074.jpg.

14.1.2. Impact of Cortisol on Metabolism

Cortisol, the major glucocorticoid secreted from the adrenal glands, is a major regulator of metabolism, particularly during critical illness. Elevated cortisol levels are common among patients in ICUs, where the pathophysiologic stress of illness demands greater energy availability. Cortisol influences many metabolic processes, facilitating gluconeogenesis in the liver and stimulating lipolysis. Above all, its powerful effect on glucose production is critical to preserving energy during severe stress. However, long-term exposure to cortisol can lead to deleterious metabolic consequences, including insulin resistance, making it challenging to control blood glucose levels in the critically ill. As dysregulation of the HPA axis is prevalent among this population, familiarity with cortisol's metabolism-altering factors is important so that proper treatment strategies can be developed in critical care units (Allolio et al., 1993). It has been revealed by studies that critically ill patients with elevated cortisol levels demonstrate a remarkable alteration in insulin sensitivity. This sensitivity is significantly blunted in the presence of glucocorticoids, enhancing the risk of hyperglycemia related to stress, a ubiquitous clinical issue in ICUs. Such alterations in metabolic control can complicate glucose control and outcomes with recovery. An observational study of critically ill patients on glucocorticoids demonstrated a median reduction in insulin sensitivity by 31% compared to controls, attesting to the significant influence that cortisol has upon the regulation of metabolism within critical illness. The increased release of cortisol, especially as a reaction to surgical stress or critical infection, aggravates this phenomenon, generating a vicious cycle of metabolic derangements that can postpone patient recovery and prolong ICU stay (Pretty et al., 1997). Cortisol's interaction with other hormones and metabolic pathways further underscores its role in the complexity of critical care. Particularly, the interaction of cortisol with catecholamines enhances the stress response of the body, raising the metabolic rate and leading to increased energy expenditure. Not only does it influence glucose metabolism, but it also influences protein catabolism and fat utilization, resulting in a state of catabolism exhibited by critically ill patients. Understanding these metabolic dynamics is crucial for healthcare providers as they navigate the intricate balance of modulating cortisol levels and managing the resulting metabolic disturbances. Recognizing the multifaceted nature of cortisol, clinicians can better individualize interventions aimed at stabilizing metabolism and enhancing patient outcomes within the ICU (Allolio et al., 1993; Pretty et al., 1997) (Figure 14.3).

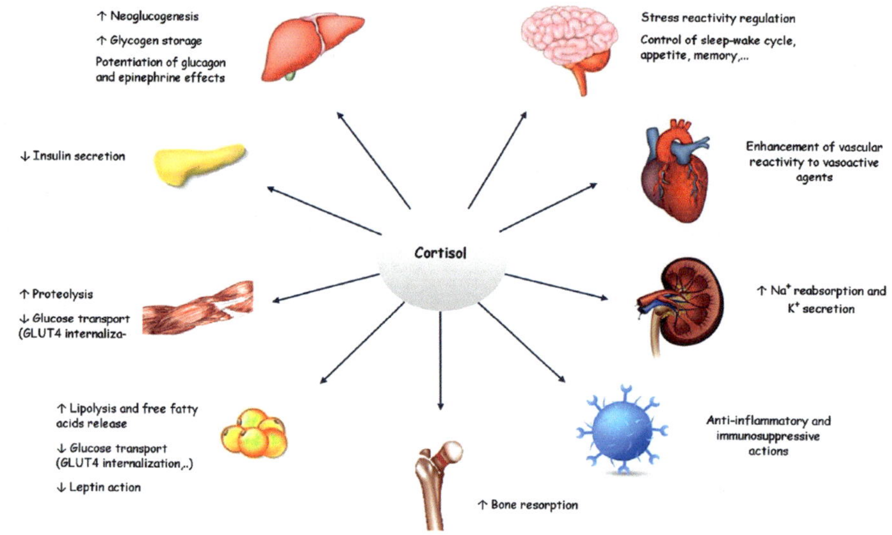

Figure 14.3. Physiological effects of cortisol.

Source: https://www.researchgate.net/publication/330836812/figure/fig1/AS:11431281136552216@1680537446241/Physiological-effects-of-cortisol.tif.

14.1.3. Thyroid Hormone Alterations in ICU Patients

Dysfunctions of thyroid hormones are a significant cause of concern among critically ill patients, particularly those admitted to ICUs. Thyroid illness is commonly associated with low levels of thyroxine (T4) and elevated thyroid-stimulating hormone (TSH) and is termed non-thyroidal illness syndrome (NTIS). This impact is particularly obvious in ICU patients who are subjected to numerous stressors, including inflammation, which can suppress the hypothalamic-pituitary-thyroid (HPT) axis. These alterations may lead to an inaccurate interpretation of thyroid function tests, thereby complicating the treatment. Knowledge of the mechanisms underpinning these hormonal changes is crucial to enable clinicians to implement the most optimized therapy for ICU patients, alongside addressing the overall implications on their recovery and eventual long-term health outcomes. There is supporting evidence for an intimate connection between changes in thyroid profiles and increased morbidity and mortality in hospital patients. A retrospective study conducted on older patients revealed that those with low T4 and high TSH levels had unfavorable clinical outcomes, highlighting the prognostic significance of thyroid function in acute settings. Elevated morbidity was defined in terms of such parameters as prolonged hospitalization and the need for ICU admission, which helped to highlight the clinical relevance of monitoring thyroid hormone levels. ICU patients also have an aberrant response to hormones that could otherwise stimulate recovery and metabolic homeostasis; therefore, detection of such alterations helps tailor appropriate treatment regimens (Brenta et al., 2012). Lack of proper intervention during these hormone disturbances might cause prolonged critical illness and make recovery patterns complicated. Besides, alterations of glucocorticoid feedback in critical illness also increase the complexity of thyroid hormone alterations. ICU patients typically present with higher plasma ACTH and cortisol levels, which can cross-talk with thyroid hormone metabolism. It has been noted in studies that the raised cortisol levels do not suppress ACTH as would be expected, providing evidence of an adaptive rather than a simple failure of the HPT axis in critical illness. Such intricate endocrine interactions serve to demonstrate how variability in thyroid hormone is enmeshed within the complex hormonal milieu in critically ill patients. They need to be understood in order to come up with particular strategies to control thyroid function and achieve better patient outcomes in the ICU setting (Allolio et al., 1993). An investigation of these correlations can unlock the intricacies of endocrinology in the critical care setting (Figure 14.4).

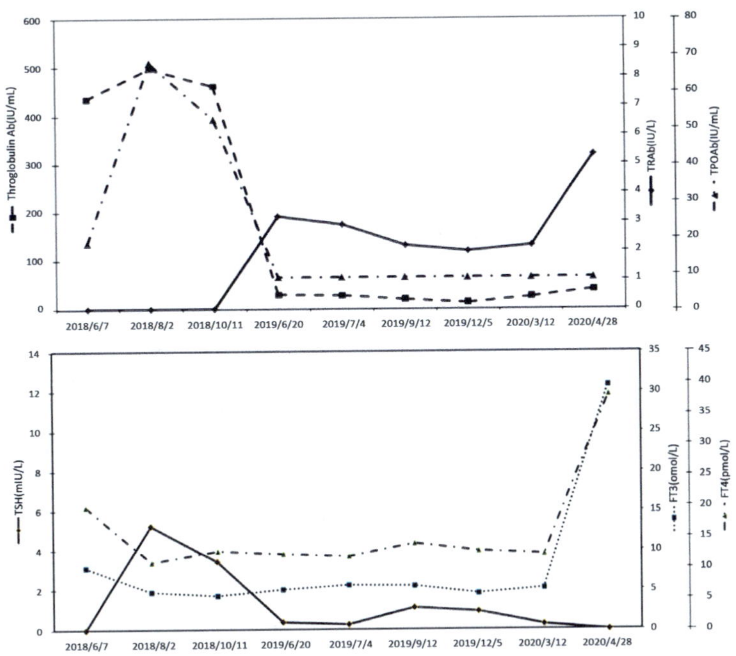

Figure 14.4. Alterations in the patient's serum thyroid hormone levels (left) and thyroid autoantibody titers (right) during a 20-month observation period.

Source: https://www.researchgate.net/publication/369971183/figure/fig1/AS:11431281161845669@1685073961604/Alterations-in-the-patients-serum-thyroid-hormone-levels-left-and-thyroid-autoantibody.jpg.

Test Your Knowledge

1. How does critical illness trigger the neuroendocrine stress response and what hormones are primarily involved during ICU admission?
2. What effects does elevated cortisol have on glucose metabolism and immune function in ICU patients?
3. What are the common patterns of thyroid hormone alterations observed in critically ill patients?

14.2. Common Endocrine Disorders in the ICU

Learning Outcome

1. Manage diabetes mellitus in critically ill patients;
2. Understand adrenal insufficiency in critically ill patients;
3. Focus on thyroid dysfunction in the intensive care setting.

Critically ill patients in the ICU frequently present with a range of endocrine disorders, which can complicate treatment and outcome. These conditions include adrenal insufficiency, thyroid disease, and derangements of glucose metabolism. Adrenal insufficiency, most commonly resulting from acute stress, sepsis, or chronic corticosteroid treatment, can produce severe hemodynamic instability. This stresses the need for early detection and management, as uncontrolled adrenal crisis is associated with increased morbidity and mortality. The response to stress also results in a condition generally referred to as sick euthyroid syndrome, which is characterized by an altered thyroid hormone value not always indicative of standard criteria for diagnosis. These alterations may prolong recovery and complicate critical care management, thus making this fact significant to the focus of extensive endocrine testing in the ICU setting. Thyroid hormone alterations are particularly significant in the ICU because alterations can influence metabolic processes, cardiovascular stability, and overall outcomes. Research has shown that alterations in triiodothyronine (T3) and thyroxine (T4) levels can be easily identified in critically ill patients, even in those with no prior history of thyroid-related disease. This relationship between patient survival and the interaction is intriguing, as found in studies where certain thyroid dysfunction has been found to predict mortality in ICUs. Alterations in Free T4 and T4, for instance, were discovered to possess strong predictive capability with regards to survival rates in ICU patients, and this evaluation of thyroid function potentially becomes critical during illness. Thus, understanding these endocrine responses is crucial in optimizing treatment and patient outcomes in critically ill patients. In addition, hyperglycemia is a prevalent problem in ICU patients that often complicates the recovery from critical illness. The stress response elicited by critical illness has the potential to lead to insulin resistance and increased glucose production, favoring hyperglycemic states. Subsequent hyperglycemia has been implicated in adverse outcomes, including longer ICU admission and increased mortality. Therefore, control of blood glucose becomes a core aspect of critical care that needs to be carefully monitored and treated. Several studies indicate that more stringent glycemic control can significantly enhance survival, and that there is an intricate interplay between endocrine function and patient well-being in the ICU. As evidenced by studies illustrating a direct correlation between worse functional status at discharge and higher post-hospital mortality, the control of endocrine disorders such as hyperglycemia plays a pivotal role in maximizing post-ICU recovery (Amrein et al., 2016; Bartolović et al., 2024).

14.2.1. Diabetes Mellitus and Its Management

Diabetes mellitus in the critically ill patient is very difficult to manage, particularly with regard to the interaction between hyperglycemia, insulin resistance, and the intrinsic stress of critical illness. Hyperglycemia, typically due to stress responses, has the potential for severe adverse outcomes, including increased rates of morbidity and mortality. The impact of baseline dysglycemia needs to be recognized, as individuals with elevated glycated hemoglobin (HbA1c) concentrations have a sharply increased risk of in-hospital mortality. Specifically, research has shown that those patients with

HbA1c levels above the 9.3% level experience a mortality risk that is substantially heightened in relation to patients who present with lower levels. Glycemic control plays a crucial role in acute care settings, as it can prevent secondary complications associated with high blood glucose levels, thereby emphasizing the importance of careful monitoring and management within the ICU setting (Fabbrin et al., 2014). Intraoperative blood glucose monitoring and control are important not only during the early critical period, since dysglycemia might continue to affect postoperative outcomes. There is evidence that operative diabetic patients are at risk for intraoperative dysglycemia and that could be exacerbated by the operative duration. In an investigation of elderly surgical patients, diabetic patients had a far higher likelihood of having blood glucose levels outside the range that was set during surgery.

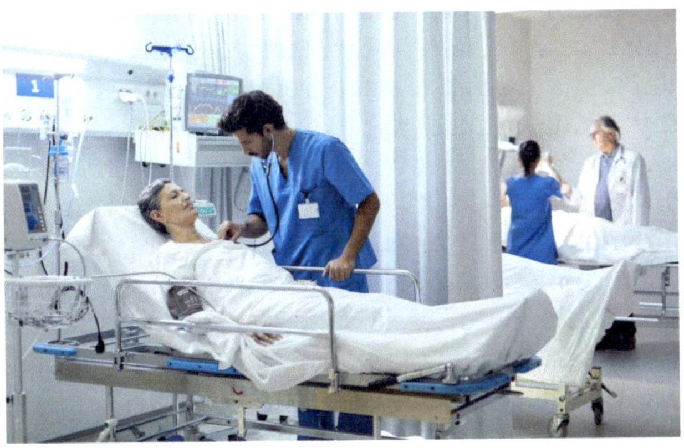

Figure 14.5. The management of diabetes mellitus in critically ill patients presents significant challenges.

Source: https://i0.wp.com/glytec.com/wp-content/uploads/2021/09/xcc5.jpg?fit=1058%2C675&ssl=1.

These dysglycemic events not only complicate the immediate postoperative course of recovery but are also associated with longer ICU and hospital length of stay, underlining the need for meticulous glycemic control guidelines according to the individual patient risk factor profiles (Knaak et al., 2019). Effective control of diabetes mellitus in critically ill patients involves both pharmacological and non-pharmacological interventions that ensure blood glucose stability.

Insulin infusion is the mainstay of glucose management in the ICU, where continuous infusion regimens have been shown to be more effective at maintaining target glucose levels. In addition, education and awareness among healthcare workers for risk factors of dysglycemia, such as existing diabetes and anticipated surgical duration, are key to preventing unwarranted outcomes. This proactive approach, in addition to correcting the immediate problems posed by disrupted metabolic conditions in critically ill patients, also emphasizes the importance of an active, team-oriented approach to the treatment of diabetes when a patient is critically ill, thus enhancing patient outcomes as well as healthcare efficiency (Fabbrin et al., 2014; Knaak et al., 2019) (Figure 14.5).

14.2.2. Adrenal Insufficiency in Critically Ill Patients

Adrenal insufficiency is a critical problem in the management of patients in the ICU, particularly those who are critically ill. Physiological stressors of severe illness have the potential to badly damage the HPA axis and subsequently cause relative adrenal insufficiency. It is characterized by an insufficient secretion of cortisol in the context of stress, with negative impacts on hemodynamic stability, immunity, and metabolism. In patients who are critically ill, the ability to respond well to stress is most critical; therefore, the early identification of adrenal insufficiency can be paramount in the prevention of complications, particularly in cases with septic shock or profound underlying pathologies that need to be closely watched and managed. The use of etomidate for RSI in critically ill patients has been a cause for specific concern regarding the impact on adrenal function. Being an extremely potent anesthetic, etomidate can inhibit 11β-hydroxylase, a key enzyme in cortisol synthesis, and hence plummet cortisol levels precipitously even after a single dose. Steroidogenesis suppression is risky and can be especially hazardous in patients with underlying adrenal insufficiency or in those who were not adequately screened for adrenal function prior to intubation. Thus, etomidate administration can contribute to an exaggerated state of stress-induced adrenal insufficiency, increasing morbidity and mortality in patient populations already at risk. Clinicians must weigh the risks against the benefits when choosing induction agents in critically ill settings, particularly when adrenal support is under threat (Soleimanpour, 2023).

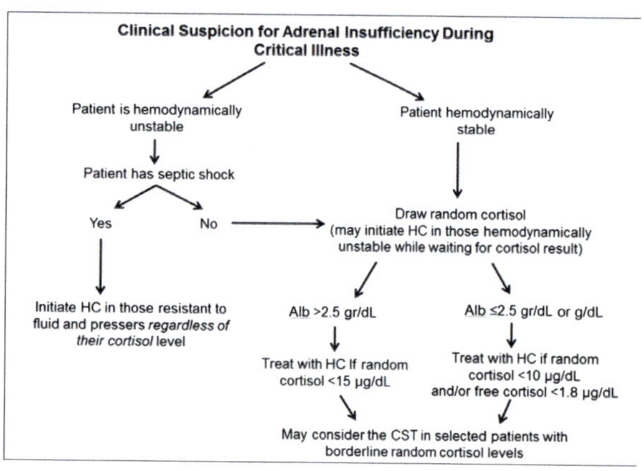

Figure 14.6. Clinical suspicion for adrenal insufficiency during critical illness.

Source: https://ars.els-cdn.com/content/image/1-s2.0-S1530891X20358109-gr2.jpg.

Adrenal insufficiency in critically ill patients is managed by a multidimensional approach involving early detection and management. Being vigilant about manifestations such as hypotension, altered mental status, and profound fatigue is useful in making an early diagnosis of adrenal crisis. Equally important is the initiation of therapeutic measures such as corticosteroid replacement therapy in managing adrenal insufficiency effectively. The dosage and timing of glucocorticoid therapy must be individually adjusted with care, particularly in the acute illness setting where HPA axis dysregulation may be quite pronounced. In addition, appreciation of the multifactorial importance of adrenal insufficiency in the critically ill, especially in obstetric and non-obstetric emergencies, underscores the necessity of a team approach to optimize outcomes and minimize the risk of endocrine dysfunction-associated adverse events (Khanum et al., 2024) (Figure 14.6).

14.2.3. Thyroid Dysfunction in the Intensive Care Setting

Thyroid dysfunction is a frequent and complex presentation in critically ill patients in ICUs. The interaction between acute illness and thyroid hormone levels can lead to significant alterations in thyroid function, either in the guise of hyperthyroidism or hypothyroidism. This syndrome, better referred to as non-thyroidal illness syndrome (NTIS), is well known to manifest with decreased serum levels of T3 and T4, with the level of TSH typically normal or suppressed. These changes can compromise metabolic homeostasis and amplify the challenge of treating critically ill patients. Identification and monitoring of thyroid function are therefore significant in the comprehensive management of ICU patients. Assessment of thyroid dysfunction not only aids in explaining the pathophysiological mechanisms of such changes but is also crucial in optimizing therapeutic strategies for patient care during recovery. Of special interest in thyroid disease is the interaction with other endocrine axes, the HPA axis. The HPA axis is activated in the acute stress state of the critically ill, leading to increased secretion of cortisol and increased levels of ACTH, which directly influence thyroid hormone availability and metabolism. Elevated levels of ACTH can inhibit peripheral conversion of T4 into T3 and thereby play a role in the formation of NTIS. Moreover, disrupted feedback mechanisms within the HPA axis can render it challenging to evaluate and treat thyroid pathology in such individuals. For example, heightened levels of cortisol can inhibit signs of thyroid deficiency, and as such, clinicians are tasked with consideration of the entirety of the patients endocrine profile when diagnosing and treating thyroid complications in the ICU (Allolio et al., 1993). Thyroid dysfunction in the ICU also often demands a particular strategy that acknowledges the particular dynamics present with critically ill patients. Thyroid hormone replacement therapy can be undertaken in certain cases; nonetheless, appropriate caution is required while considering the patient's overall clinical profile, including potential interactions with other hormonal therapies and effects on outcomes of recovery. The requirement to consider underlying pathologies, including traumatic brain injury (TBI), becomes more pertinent as TBI is strongly associated with secondary hypopituitarism, which can affect thyroid hormone production and regulation (Attard et al., 2015). Finally, creating a nuanced understanding of thyroid disease in critical illness is most critical to maximize patient outcomes, justifying ongoing study to define optimal treatment paradigms and ascertain probable pitfalls of error in the interpretation of thyroid hormone values in the ICU setting.

Test Your Knowledge

1. What are the challenges of managing diabetes mellitus in critically ill patients?
2. How is adrenal insufficiency diagnosed in ICU patients, and what are the implications for treatment during critical illness?
3. What types of thyroid dysfunction commonly occur in the ICU, and how do they differ from primary thyroid disease?

14.3. Hormonal Therapies in Critical Care

Learning Outcome

1. Discuss the use of glucocorticoids in sepsis;
2. Explain insulin therapy for glycemic control;
3. Understand thyroid hormone replacement strategies.

Hormonal therapies play an important role in the practice of critical care, particularly for managing patients presenting with endocrine dysregulation secondary to critical illness. The response to stress in critically ill patients causes changes in the secretion of hormones, specifically adrenal hormones such as cortisol. The subsequent dysregulation can result in acute adrenal insufficiency, which is associated with adverse clinical outcomes. Glucocorticoid treatment has been shown to improve the course of relative adrenal insufficiency in these patients by inducing hemodynamic stability and potentially decreasing the mortality rates. Further, patient-specific dosing of glucocorticoids can be evaluated to enhance therapeutic performance, particularly in patients with prolonged ICU stays, where, over time, the hormonal counterregulation could be affected, as has been theorized based on studies demonstrating a decline in prognostic function of acute illness parameters in such patients (Vijayaraghavan et al., 2025). Another important area of hormonal manipulation in the ICU is thyroid hormone regulation, especially in relation to critical illness. Critical illness is known to cause a state called non-thyroidal illness syndrome (NTIS), where the metabolism of thyroxine (T4) to its active metabolite, triiodothyronine (T3), is reduced. This hormonal alteration has also been described by low levels of T3 and raised reverse T3, which actually may reflect the degree of illness but not the major thyroid dysfunction. Therapeutic use of thyroid hormones in carefully chosen patients can affect metabolic control and potentially have beneficial influences on recovery and mortality. However, this intervention needs to be researched more so that the appropriate protocols can be set up, so as not to compromise potential complications with hormone replacement in critically ill patients (Clarke et al., 2024). In addition, care needs to be taken regarding the psychological effects of critical illness and the ensuing hormonal changes. Patients who are discharged from an ICU typically experience deep psychological distress, a problem that is compounded by hormonal disturbances that take place while they are hospitalized. The provision of psychological therapy has been identified as an essential component in post-ICU rehabilitation, where comprehension of the experience of critical illness can lead to emotional recovery. Psychological interventions can support patients to make sense of their ICU experience and reintegrate into daily life, thus integrating endocrinological and psychological healing processes. The coordination of hormonal therapies and psychotherapy requires that a multidisciplinary approach be implemented within the ICU, both for physical recovery and general well-being of the patient to support inclusive rehabilitation protocols (Clarke et al., 2024).

14.3.1. Use of Glucocorticoids in Sepsis

In sepsis, glucocorticoid use is of critical therapeutic value, largely due to their anti-inflammatory action. Sepsis's pathophysiology is associated with a systemic inflammatory response that may lead to diffuse organ dysfunction. Glucocorticoids control such a response by suppressing the production of pro-inflammatory cytokines as well as reducing the effect of inflammation on target tissues. Evidence indicates that septic shock patients usually have adrenal insufficiency or critical illness-related corticosteroid insufficiency (CIRCI), impairing the ability to develop an effective response to stress and hence the need for glucocorticoid treatment for maximal management. Its use in these circumstances not only alleviates adrenal insufficiency but may also improve hemodynamic stability and patient clinical outcomes, as reflected by many critical care studies, and the clinical benefit of glucocorticoid therapy for septic patients. Glucocorticoids are found to improve septic patient outcomes, particularly in patients who are vasopressor dependent. One study reported that patients with adrenal insufficiency treated with hydrocortisone experienced a significant reduction in the requirement of norepinephrine as compared to untreated patients with glucocorticoids, indicating the importance of addressing adrenal function in critical illness. Such a therapeutic approach suggests that there must be vigilant monitoring of cortisol in septic patients with severe sepsis, so that timely glucocorticoid therapy is administered. However, the onset of glucocorticoid treatment must be weighed cautiously with attention to the adverse effects associated with long-term corticosteroid exposure, such as immunosuppression and impaired wound healing. Maintaining a careful balance between taking advantage of the therapeutic effects of glucocorticoids without enhancing probable harm is a consideration to make in sepsis treatment in the ICU. Furthermore, the complexities of glucocorticoid treatment in sepsis are highlighted by new insights into the dysregulation of the HPA axis in critical illness. Experiments have shown that sepsis can cause abnormalities of cortisol metabolism and produce a state of relative glucocorticoid resistance, with target tissues being refractory to elevated cortisol levels. This pathophysiologic environment supports the need for glucocorticoid replacement therapy in patients who exhibit CIRCI, since their bodies may be incapable of initiating an adequate endogenous response. Additionally, knowledge of how sepsis-related stress and glucocorticoid therapy interact is critical as clinicians sift through the difficulties of caring for critically ill patients. Lastly, glucocorticoid use in sepsis remains a topic of ongoing interest in the field of endocrinology, with more study needed to optimize treatment options within the ICU population, specifically regarding the potential morbidity of undertreated adrenal insufficiency in this high-risk population (Acton et al., 2005; Annane et al., 2017) (Figure 14.7).

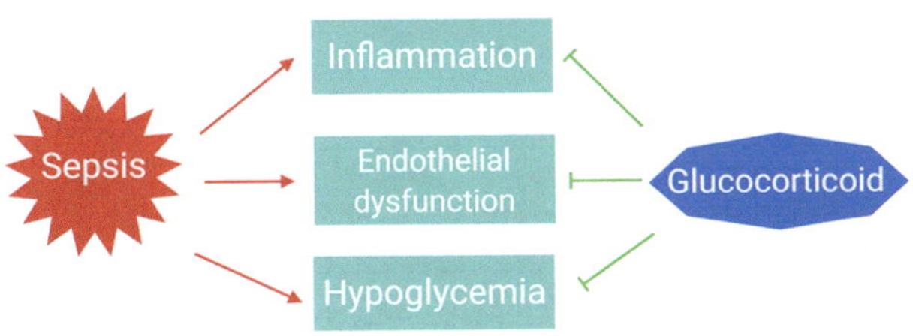

Figure 14.7. The essential roles of glucocorticoids to tolerate sepsis.

Source: https://www.researchgate.net/publication/343105262/figure/fig2/AS:11431281250511607@1717868960557/The-essential-roles-of-glucocorticoids-to-tolerate-sepsis-In-sepsis-patients-the-immune.tif.

14.3.2. Insulin Therapy for Glycemic Control

In intensive care, the control of blood glucose with insulin therapy is essential to maximize outcomes in patients. Hyperglycemia and worsening morbidity go hand in hand, and therefore glycemic control becomes inevitable, particularly in critically ill patients with stress hyperglycemia. Insulin therapy not only normalizes blood glucose but also may be utilized to neutralize the adverse effects of high sugar, such as inflammation and immunosuppression. This type of therapy is particularly marked in environments like the ICU, where patients could have underlying diseases requiring precise metabolic management. Effective insulin therapy allows clinicians to stabilize the glycemic status step by step, thus making the recovery process smoother and reducing the negative effects of uncontrolled hyperglycemia. There is growing evidence pointing to the need for technology to maximize insulin therapy for glycemic control. The recent introduction of continuous glucose monitoring (CGM) systems into clinical practice provides real-time data on glucose fluctuations, enabling tailored insulin administration that can significantly enhance therapeutic outcomes. For instance, a trial among liver transplant recipients revealed that real-time CGM plus standard care notably improved glycemic control. Patients receiving active CGM spent a longer period within the target glucose level compared to those receiving therapy alone, highlighting the role of technology as an adjunct to drug treatment. This adaptability serves to reflect not merely enhanced proficiency within the sphere of endocrinology but also aligns with the general objective of personalized medicine for ICUs, where individualization of the patient is critical for therapy success (Hagerf et al., 2025). Besides, the function of insulin therapy becomes increasingly recognized in the context of diseases like COVID-19, in which patients are exposed to specific metabolic stress. The glycemic response to critical diseases, like those caused by COVID-19, has significant results on insulin requirements and overall patient management in the ICU. Research indicates that insulin therapy may be crucial in achieving optimal glycemic control during such severe infection, which otherwise complicates the course of hospitalization and increases the risk of mortality. As highlighted in the latest review, achieving optimal blood glucose levels in critically ill patients is not only beneficial for recovery but also associated with improved survival, underscoring the critical role of endocrinology in the broader context of critical illness management (Soltani et al., 2024). Careful scrutiny of insulin therapy for glycemic control, therefore, remains a foundation of effective ICU practice (Figure 14.8).

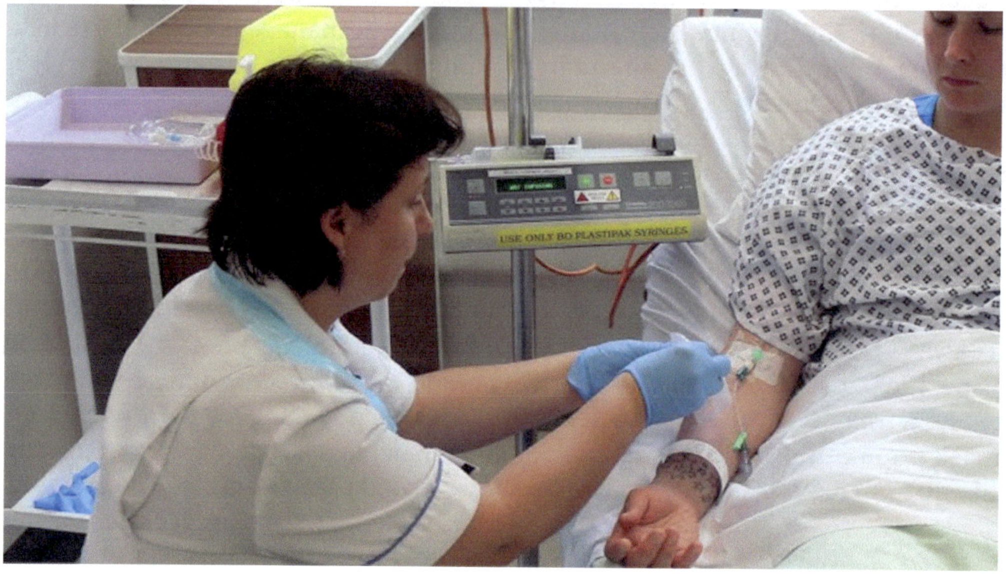

Figure 14.8. Regulating blood glucose levels through insulin therapy is vital for improving patient outcomes.

Source: https://i.ytimg.com/vi/8VH9UINEI24/hq720.jpg?sqp=-oaymwE7CK4FEIIDSFryq4qpAy0IARUAAAAAGAElAADIQj0AgKJD8AEB-AH-CYAC0AWKAgwIABABGGUgXyhXMA8=&rs=AOn4CLBdQYN1ycYdPlrit6TxKT8PJisR2g.

14.3.3. Thyroid Hormone Replacement Strategies

In endocrinology, particularly in ICU and critical illness scenarios, thyroid hormone replacement therapy administration is a decisive factor influencing the outcomes of patients. Thyroid hormones play an essential role in regulating metabolism, cardiovascular function, and overall homeostasis, particularly in patients experiencing an acute stress response. In critically ill individuals, altered thyroid hormone levels can worsen derangements in metabolism and lead to such complications as hypothermia and blunted contractility of the heart. Therefore, the early identification of thyroid dysfunction and appropriate replacement hormone therapy can also have a profound influence on the recovery process. The decision-making process for initiating and the dose of thyroid hormone replacement is established upon careful evaluation of the patient's clinical condition, including their endocrine response to acute illness. In addition, the timing and dose of thyroid hormone replacement are key to successful treatment outcomes in the ICU environment. Synthroid, or levothyroxine, is usually the drug of choice because of its pharmacokinetic profile, which is compatible with the requirements of critically ill patients. It is important to monitor serum thyroid-stimulating hormone (TSH) and free thyroxine (FT4) levels around the clock to adjust the replacement regimen to individual physiological responses. Each patient's unique metabolic and hormonal constitution necessitates an individualized response, considering the intricate interaction of thyroid hormones with the remaining endocrine axes. Intravenous administration may be one of the methods employed, particularly in those unable to be administered orally, in a bid to achieve therapeutic levels quickly.

These individualized therapies aim to reverse metabolic stressors and promote the healing of patients in the ICU setting. In particular, multidisciplinary team management is of utmost importance in developing thyroid hormone replacement therapy in critically ill patients. Endocrinologists, intensivists, and pharmacists need to work together closely to continuously monitor and adjust thyroid hormones, so that each profession is working towards an integrated treatment plan. Most particularly in those with pre-existing hypopituitarism or other endocrine illnesses, the subtleties of thyroid hormone management are more significant since these diseases may enhance metabolic derangement (Andereggen et al., 2024). As has been contended, hypopituitarism can produce additive morbidity with metabolic dysfunction, and thus thyroid hormone replacement needs to be included in more global management regimens for these high-risk populations. Effective communication and mutual care among specialists function to optimize thyroid function, thereby optimizing overall patient outcomes in critical care settings.

Test Your Knowledge

1. What is the role of glucocorticoid therapy in the management of sepsis and septic shock in critically ill patients?
2. How is insulin therapy optimized in the ICU to achieve glycemic control without increasing the risk of hypoglycemia?
3. When is thyroid hormone replacement indicated in critically ill patients with thyroid dysfunction?

14.4. The Hypothalamic-Pituitary-Adrenal (HPA) Axis

Learning Outcome

1. Understand the function of the HPA axis in stress response;
2. Discuss dysregulation of the HPA axis in critical illness;
3. Focus on the clinical implications of HPA axis dysfunction.

The HPA axis is also accountable for the body's stress response, integrating neuroendocrine inputs to modulate a variety of physiological mechanisms. In severe illness, the HPA axis acts to provide homeostasis through the release of glucocorticoids in the form of cortisol. Cortisol mediates the body's stress response through augmenting glucose metabolism, decreasing inflammation, and modulating immune response. Understanding the HPA axis is crucial in the ICU setting because failure of the axis can increase the severity of illness and determine recovery outcome. For instance, acute illness or critical illness can lead to dysregulation of the HPA axis and hence underproduction of cortisol, which plays a significant role in physiologic adaptation to stressors of critical health occurrences. The changes in the HPA axis during critical illness have the potential to impact a patient's prognosis. Dysregulation of cortisol levels has the potential to cause complications such as adrenal insufficiency, which typically makes it challenging to treat critically ill patients. This highlights the state of reduced adrenal function, which can impair the body's ability to handle stress optimally, leading to heightened vulnerability to septic shock and death. It is evidenced that patients with diseases such as COVID-19 can have distinctive adrenal function alterations depending on the severity of the virus and its systemic effect on the endocrine system. The COVID-19 reviews have shown that adrenal gland weakness not only makes the underlying glucocorticoid illness harder but also raises the demand for continuous monitoring of the HPA axis in critically ill patients, especially in the setting of systemic illnesses like COVID-19 (Cozzolino et al., 2023).

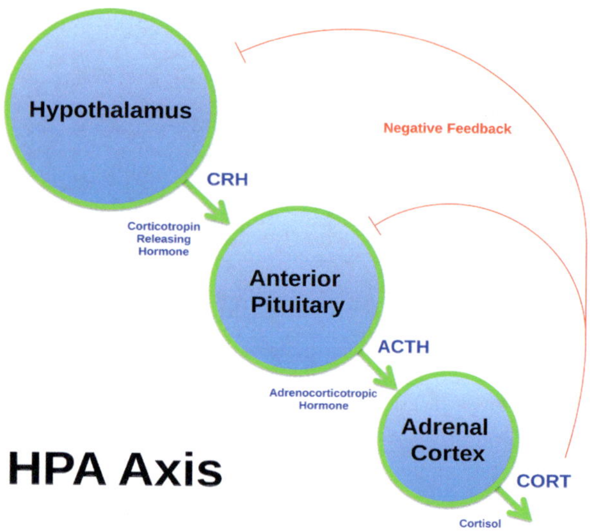

Figure 14.9. Schematic of the HPA axis [CRH: Corticotropin-releasing hormone; and ACTH: adrenocorticotropic hormone].

Source: https://upload.wikimedia.org/wikipedia/commons/thumb/e/ee/HPA_Axis_Diagram_%28Brian_M_Sweis_2012%29.svg/800px-HPA_Axis_Diagram_%28Brian_M_Sweis_2012%29.svg.png.

The critically ill patients typically require corticosteroid therapy to counteract the impact of HPA axis abnormalities. The interventions are aimed at the restoration of homeostasis and the minimization of morbidity from deficient hormonal responses. Corticosteroids can be of therapeutic benefit in severe states of inflammation in disease, e.g., in severe COVID-19. The use of such medications has to be tightly controlled to avoid side effects like immunosuppression and secondary infection. Latest studies highlight the necessity of an in-depth understanding of the endocrine disturbances in critical illness because these not only influence the immediate outcome of patients but also that of recovery in the long run. How COVID-19 affects the HPA axis is a good example of the necessity for particular therapy that will reverse these endocrine alterations, thereby improving the overall management and outcome of critically ill patients (Esmaeilzadeh et al., 2022) (Figure 14.9).

14.4.1. Function of the HPA Axis in Stress Response

The HPA axis is the central component of the body's stress response, particularly in the setting of critical illness scenarios in the ICU. The process of activation of this axis begins with the release of corticotropin-releasing hormone (CRH) by the hypothalamus, which stimulates the anterior pituitary gland to release ACTH. ACTH stimulates the adrenal cortex to release cortisol, a key glucocorticoid that is in charge of controlling the stress response. Cortisol maintains homeostasis during times of stress through control of metabolism, immune processes, and cardiovascular function. Pathologic regulation of the HPA axis can lead to conditions such as critical illness-related corticosteroid insufficiency (CIRCI), which makes patient management and outcome in the ICU complicated. Complications of the HPA axis function reveal significant implications for patients with critical illness. Studies have revealed that systemic inflammation induces Toll-like receptor (TLR) signaling pathways, thus initiating the endocrine stress response. Elevated cytokine levels during the process are able to modulate ACTH and cortisol response, thereby influencing the patient's overall recovery.

Patients, for instance, with some genetic polymorphisms of TLR, e.g., TLR4 SNP, have been reported to exhibit varying levels of ACTH and cortisol, as well as cytokine variability, in the perioperative state (Boehm et al., 2011). These findings underscore the necessity of clarifying the interaction between genetic factors and the HPA axis to optimize therapeutic management in critical care settings, addressing stress-induced dysregulation in particular.

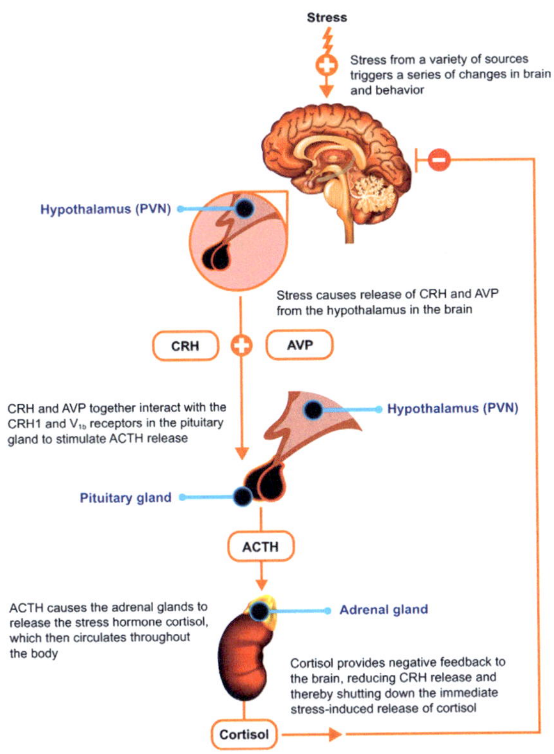

Figure 14.10. Key elements of the HPA axis stress response.

Source: https://www.researchgate.net/publication/370132959/figure/fig2/AS:11431281256966210@1719584590036/Key-elements-of-the-HPA-axis-stress-response.jpg.

Exploring the function of the HPA axis in critical illness not only informs us about endocrine responses but also points to the potential development of targeted interventions. Because HPA axis dysregulation can be an etiology of CIRCI and tissue glucocorticoid resistance, clinicians should be vigilant for diagnosis and treatment of this complex status (Annane et al., 2017). The complex interaction between the immune system and the HPA axis further complicates the expression of stress responses, making an interdisciplinary approach to patient care in the ICU necessary. By using a sophisticated knowledge of these mechanisms, clinicians can enhance the outcomes of critically ill patients and customize interventions that restore balance within the endocrine milieu essential to patient recovery (Figure 14.10).

14.4.2. Dysregulation of the HPA Axis in Critical Illness

Dysregulation of the HPA axis is the cause of critical illness pathology and has significant prognostic and therapeutic implications in treating patients in the ICU. In the healthy subject, the HPA axis is tasked with the regulation of homeostasis through the modulation of cortisol release that is fundamental to stress responses. In critical illness, there is a relative failure of normal regulation, resulting in relative adrenal insufficiency (RAI). This condition is a component of a state of corticosteroid insufficiency-related critical illness (CIRCI), which complicates inflammatory reactions and hinders recovery. Dysregulation in the HPA axis has been associated with poorer outcomes in critically ill patients, illustrating the importance of early identification and management in improving survival in this population, as stressors of illness inappropriately stimulate the HPA axis (Abitkar et al., 2025). Dysregulation of the HPA axis in critical illness has been noted to dramatically alter cortisol levels, adversely impacting many physiological systems. Research indicates that decreased cortisol production in accordance with signs of dizziness and fatigue can be a marker of adrenal insufficiency (Abitkar et al., 2025). An imbalance of the hormones may enhance the clinical presentation by playing a role in the development of complications like hypotension and impaired metabolism. In addition, variability in cortisol and ACTH levels observed among systemic inflammatory response syndrome (SIRS) patients emphasizes HPA axis variability and the complexity of response during critical illness. Identification of optimal cortisol response patterns is important because such dysregulation necessitates therapeutic management, i.e., corticosteroid therapy, to restore balance and facilitate patient recovery in the ICU context (Stewart et al., 2018). In addition to cortisol dysregulation, persistent consequences of HPA axis derangement in critical illness can be a major limiting factor for recovery. Studies in survivors of severe illness, such as COVID-19, show persistent endocrine disturbances, specifically low testosterone and altered adrenal function, to be the cause of chronic fatigue and other disabling features (Abitkar et al., 2025). Additionally, the convergence of the HPA axis with other endocrine axes, such as the hypothalamic-pituitary-gonadal (HPG) axis, further complicates the course of recovery in critically ill patients. Thus, an understanding of the intricacy in the dysregulated endocrine response is crucial for devising all-encompassing therapeutic maneuvers. Assessment of endocrine dysfunction in an integrated manner within critical care will enable clinicians to optimize patient outcomes and address the multifaceted problems presented by dysregulated hormonal reactions (Stewart et al., 2018).

14.4.3. Clinical Implications of HPA Axis Dysfunction

Dysfunction of the HPA axis has significant clinical consequences, particularly in critical illness when endocrine homeostasis is crucial for maintaining homeostasis. In critically ill patients, a condition known as critical illness-related corticosteroid insufficiency (CIRCI) exists and is best characterized by inadequate cortisol synthesis, leading to relative adrenal insufficiency. This condition is particularly perilous in the sense that it can exacerbate the patient's underlying condition, diminished ability to cope with stressors such as infections or traumatic injuries. Detection and prompt treatment of CIRCI are critical because studies have indicated that intervention prior to a point where the patient would otherwise have died can significantly increase survival rates in critically ill patients, emphasizing the importance of strict monitoring of adrenal function in the ICU setting (Abitkar et al., 2025). Moreover, HPA axis dysfunction clinical presentations extend beyond adrenal insufficiency as expressed in the course of a variety of endocrine abnormalities complicating ICU patient care. By way of illustration, evidence indicates that long COVID patients may experience interference in their endocrine systems, including alterations in the HPA axis as evidenced by decreased cortisol levels and concomitant symptoms such as fatigue and hypotension (Abitkar et al., 2025). These endocrine dysfunctions have been correlated with prolonged recovery times and decreased quality of life, creating obstacles for clinicians treating both the physiological as well as psychologic effects of these dysfunctions. Therefore, the recognition of these endocrine alterations is imperative to the establishment of successful therapeutic interventions involving both hormonal and supportive care in critically ill individuals. In addition to adrenal dysfunction, the relationship between metabolic dysregulation and HPA axis abnormalities presents a further hurdle to critical care practice. Insulin resistance and hyperglycemia are also commonly occurring in patients and complicate blood sugar control and predict poorer outcomes (Stewart et al., 2018). The prognostic value of these changes in predicting outcome is critical; for example, elevated cortisol and ACTH levels in certain critically ill patients have been correlated with non-survival. This highlights the significance of not only tracking hormonal levels but also instituting specific treatment protocols to correct metabolic derangements. By addressing the clinical consequences of HPA axis disruption effectively, healthcare clinicians can enhance patient outcomes, underscoring the necessity of a well-rounded approach with endocrinology as a central part of the healthcare paradigm in the ICU (Figure 14.11).

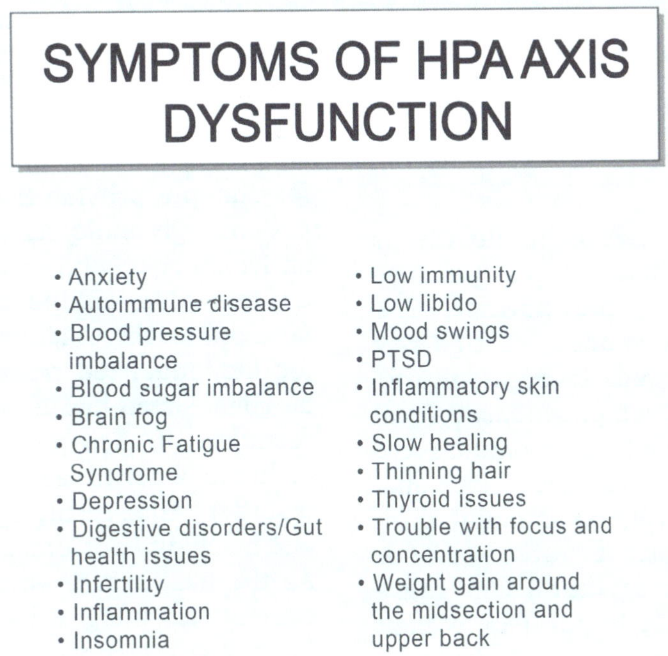

Figure 14.11. Symptoms of HPA-axis dysfunction.

Source: https://i0.wp.com/drchristinemaren.com/wp-content/uploads/2021/07/Symptoms-of-HPA-axis-dysfunction.png?resize=549%2C549&ssl=1.

Test Your Knowledge

1. What is the physiological role of the HPA axis in regulating the body's response to acute stress?
2. How does critical illness affect the normal functioning of the HPA axis, and what mechanisms contribute to its dysregulation?

14.5. Endocrine System Monitoring in the ICU

Learning Outcome

1. Explain the importance of hormonal level assessments;
2. Describe techniques for monitoring endocrine function;
3. Deal with challenges in interpreting hormonal data.

Endocrine system monitoring in the ICU is critical since critical illness places immense physiological stress on the patient. The intricate balance of hormones, particularly during critical illness, needs to be monitored closely in order to avoid complications. Critical illnesses such as sepsis, trauma, and severe surgery have the capability to disrupt hormonal balance, leading to disturbances in metabolism that can aggravate patient outcomes. For instance, HPA axis dysregulation can cause adrenal insufficiency that jeopardizes patient recovery. Endocrine surveillance is crucial for instituting interventions as needed, such as glucocorticoid administration, with the aim of stabilizing the hormonal equilibrium in the patient and improving clinical outcomes in the ICU, thereby emphasizing the pivotal role of endocrinology within the ICU setting. Moreover, the interprofessional team model of ICU healthcare teams enhances the efficiency of monitoring the endocrine system. Pharmacists, intensivists, nurses, and other medical care providers each utilize their unique expertise to contribute complete patient evaluations. The team model assures the dynamic monitoring of hormonal imbalances that inform treatment, with final effects on medication management and nutritional support plans among critically ill patients. For example, routine thyroid hormone testing may have an effect on metabolic control, while glucose monitoring has critical roles in diabetes control and prevention of hyperglycemia-related complications. The emphasis on interprofessional practice within the ICU promotes effective communication and timely intervention steps toward treating endocrine disorders and ensuring maximal patient outcomes, emphasizing enhanced patient care provided with maximal interprofessional practice (Kleinpell et al., 2021). Further, technological advances in monitoring have significantly enhanced the ability to assess endocrine function in real-time. CGM devices, for example, provide critical data regarding the patient's glycemic status and allow for more anticipatory insulin treatment. New diagnostic devices also enable clinicians to monitor hormone levels with increased accuracy, allowing for individualized treatment interventions to be constructed based on the unique hormonal response of each patient. These advances in technology permit early diagnosis of endocrine disorders, thus resulting in improved mortality and morbidity outcomes in critically ill patients. As the health care environment continues to evolve with integrative technology as well as improved interprofessional relationships, the need for careful monitoring of the endocrine system in the ICU continues to be central to the effective management of critically ill patients (Christopher et al., 2022).

14.5.1. Importance of Hormonal Level Assessments

In critical care settings, endocrine hormonal measurements are important in the diagnosis of underlying endocrine dysfunction that is frequently seen with critical disease. In critically ill patients, stress response causes profound changes in hormone levels, such as glucocorticoids, catecholamines, and insulin. The changes in hormones can produce a dramatic effect on metabolic pathways, immune responses, and final patient outcome. For instance, elevated cortisol due to physiological stress can condition glucose metabolism and has been associated with deleterious outcomes, such as the requirement for prolonged ventilation and increased mortality. Habitual monitoring of hormones thus not only reflects the physiological status of the patients but also maximizes therapeutic care and follows up on patterns of recovery. Tending to hormonal derangements with appropriate, timely evaluation will do much to improve the quality of care in the ICU. Also, measurements of hormonal levels play a crucial role in the management of specific endocrine disease states frequently induced by critical illness, such as adrenal insufficiency and thyroid disease. Conditions such as adrenal crisis may occur because of an insufficient level of glucocorticoids during stress, leading to hemodynamic instability. Regular monitoring of hormone levels, most notably cortisol, enables clinicians to identify these deficiencies early, with early interventions that can prevent complications. In the same way, thyroid hormone disorder is not uncommon among critically ill patients, with alterations impacting metabolism and affecting the patient's outcome of recovery. Thyroid hormone monitoring helps guide individualized treatment protocols for these deficiencies, thereby enhancing the patients chances of a successful recovery. Hence, the clinician's capacity to detect and rectify such hormonal imbalances is critical to optimizing outcomes in critically ill patients. In addition, hormonal assessment can serve as an effective prognostic marker in the ICU, enabling risk stratification and therapy decision-making. For example, high levels of inflammatory mediators and hormonal indicators such as high-sensitivity C-reactive protein and interleukin-6 have been linked with unfavorable outcomes in critically ill patients. By assessing such indicators and extrapolating the same with respect to hormone levels, the clinicians can make a more accurate prognosis of the patients recovery prospects and schedule treatment accordingly. Such a multi-parameter strategy facilitates the application of preventive measures to counter complications and maximize the recovery strategy. With the evidence that endocrine levels are a significant contributing factor in morbidity and mortality within critical illness, endocrine examination must be prioritized among the routine screening of ICU patients by medical professionals (Maharaj et al., 2016; Wong et al., 2022). It not only facilitates personalized medicine but also signifies the juncture of endocrinology and critical care medicine (Figure 14.12).

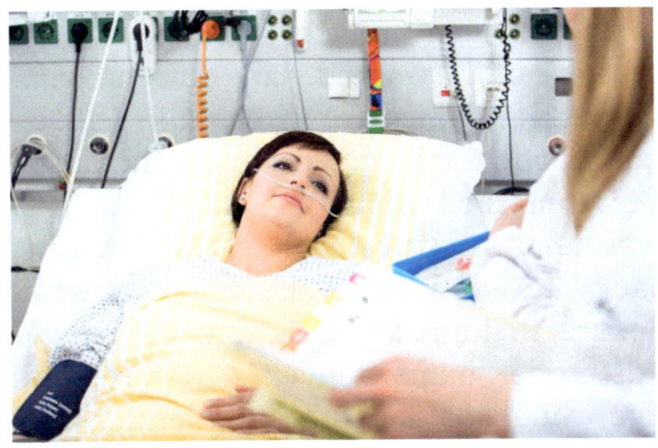

Figure 14.12. Hormonal level assessments are pivotal for understanding the underlying endocrine dysfunctions that frequently accompany severe illnesses.

Source: https://medlineplus.gov/images/CriticalCare_share.jpg.

14.5.2. Techniques for Monitoring Endocrine Function

Endocrine function monitoring in the critically ill is necessary to address hormonal imbalance resulting from acute illness, drug therapy, or stress of hospitalization. Various tests are employed to evaluate the status of endocrine glands like blood test for hormone concentration, which identifies alterations in the HPA axis, thyroid hormones, and insulin. Immunoassays and mass spectrometry are essential to accurate measurement of hormones, and they are markers for diseases such as adrenal insufficiency and thyroid disease. In the same way, dynamic testing protocols, measuring the hormonal reaction of the body to stressors, are also important in quantifying the capability of the endocrine system to function during acute states. Therefore, the integration of routine endocrine assessment into critical care management is essential to optimize patient outcomes and tailor hormone replacement therapy when necessary. In addition to routine blood sampling, imaging modalities add valuable information on the structural composition of endocrine glands. Ultrasound, CT, and MRI can precisely define pathologic alterations of the thyroid gland, adrenal glands, and pancreas, which are involved in endocrine disturbances. For instance, ultrasound is a non-invasive method commonly used for thyroid assessment in critically ill patients with the capacity to allow quick assessments without exposure to ionizing radiation. CT and MRI, on the other hand, deliver a high-resolution image which has the ability to identify masses or lesions that compromise endocrine function. The combination of biochemical analysis and imaging modalities enables reliable diagnosis of pathologies underlying, enabling timely intervention in critical care, where the hormonal status of patients is necessary for effective recovery. Another promising approach for endocrine monitoring is through the use of CGM systems, necessary in diabetic patient and steroid-treated patients, who can impact glucose metabolism. CGM devices provide immediate glucose readings, and it is possible to initiate immediate adjustments in insulin therapy and diet management. It is particularly helpful in the ICU setting, where blood glucose concentration can fluctuate due to stress and illness, potentially resulting in fulminant complications. Wearable technology has more recently become a part of endocrine monitoring and provides data on various hormonal parameters using sophisticated sensors. With the evolving critical care setting brought about by advances in technology, the application of these monitoring techniques will serve to better tailor treatments and improve overall endocrine disorder care in critically ill patients, eventually resulting in better outcomes.

14.5.3. Challenges in Interpreting Hormonal Data

Hormonal measurement interpretation in critically ill patients is fraught with numerous difficulties that complicate endocrine function determination and metabolic status. Stress reaction, trauma, and basic pathophysiology can alter hormone levels and their relationships with clinical outcomes. For instance, cortisol levels are commonly elevated during critical illness and can create a misleading impression of adrenal function in such patients. Moreover, inherent feedback mechanisms of endocrine control can be disturbed and produce abnormal patterns that are misleading for caregivers. Demanding clarity in this kind of relationship is the reason hormonal information must be evaluated within the overall clinical presentation of patients. Particularly, awareness of these distinctions is crucial to the practice of evidence-based recommendations, such as those reported by Maharaj et al. (2016), to emphasize the value of compliance and regular reassessment of hormonal values to optimize ICU management. Additionally, the lack of a commonly agreed-upon set of reference ranges for hormonal tests in critically ill patients is an important barrier to rational interpretation of hormonal findings. Therefore, normal ranges typically derived from healthy controls may not be applicable to the diseased patients with acute illnesses, leading to delayed and inappropriate diagnoses. As an example, variations in thyroid hormone levels that are relatively easily encountered in the non-thyroidal illness syndrome would make the assessment process cumbersome. Additionally, variations in laboratory procedures, sample handling, and processing would create variations in hormone measures, further obscuring the clinical picture. These flaws also increase the heterogeneity of clinical practice, as these differences can potentially cause differential decision-making in treatment. The findings emphasized by Ali et al. (2022) highlight the absolute need for robust clinical guidelines and education for clinicians to overcome the effects of these hormones on patients. Finally, the interaction of multiple hormones with each other in the context of critical illness can create a complex matrix that is difficult to unravel. For instance, alterations in insulin and glucose metabolism can lead to severe complications in critical illness patients, particularly concerning glucose control protocols.

Data suggest hormonal reactions can be significantly dissimilar in day and night shifts, affecting compliance with protocols drawn up, as was described by Maharaj et al. (2016). In addition, the interaction of various endocrine axes—such as the HPA axis and the thyroid axis—requires an integrated approach for sound interpretation. Clinicians must recognize the significance of interactions and develop a comprehensive understanding of the nuances of hormonal responses in critical illness. Therefore, an interdisciplinary insight is required for improved patient management in the ICU and successful hormonal assessment in the face of ongoing challenges (Figure 14.13).

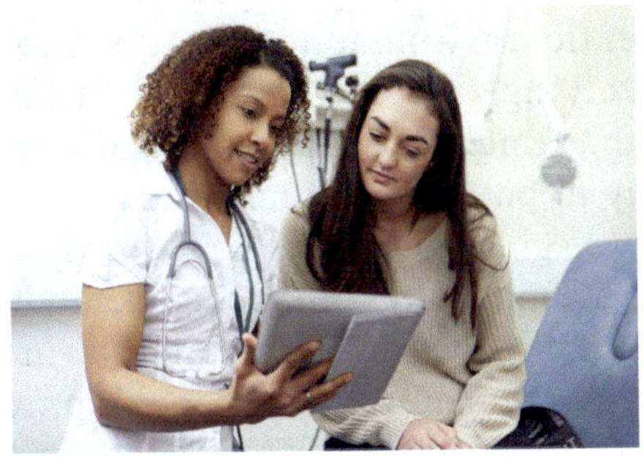

Figure 14.13. The interpretation of hormonal data in critically ill patients presents numerous challenges that complicate the assessment of endocrine function and metabolic status.

Source: https://www.marionguckclinic.com/wp-content/uploads/2023/01/shutterstock_284569505.jpg.

Test Your Knowledge

1. Why is monitoring endocrine function important in critically ill patients admitted to the ICU?
2. What are the common laboratory techniques and biomarkers used to assess hormonal levels in the ICU setting?
3. What challenges do clinicians face when interpreting hormonal data in critically ill patients?

14.6. Research and Advances in Endocrinology

Learning Outcome

1. Focus in recent studies on endocrine function in critical care;
2. Discuss about emerging therapies and their potential impact;
3. Deal with future directions for research in endocrinology.

Endocrinological studies have made significant advances in the area of hormonal response in critical illness, with emphasis on the seismic effect of endocrine impairment on the patient's outcome in ICU. The research has explained how acute stressors induce hormonal changes, particularly in the HPA axis, to lead to abnormal levels of cortisol that complicate recovery. These endocrine fluctuations not only influence metabolism but also manage immune functions, further contributing to the tenuous balance required for recuperation. Recent studies have centered on the endocrine dysregulation observed in conditions such as sepsis and trauma, where the cycle of hormone release can result in amplified inflammation and organ dysfunction. Understanding these mechanisms improves clinical practice through more specialized therapeutic regimens that address both the endocrine and the metabolic problems that critically ill patients suffer. The therapeutic environment of endocrinology is also evolving, most significantly related to the management of adrenal insufficiency in critically ill patients. Research has proven that the use of glucocorticoids in a timely fashion aids in dramatically enhancing hemodynamic stability and lowering mortality from septic shock. Furthermore, the development of biomarkers for identifying patients at risk of adrenal insufficiency is an exciting leap for personalized medicine. The biomarkers could play a role in more balanced interventions that not only improve endocrine function but also overall patient treatment in the ICU. Apart from glucocorticoids, innovative therapies for other endocrine pathways, such as thyroid and insulin signaling, are currently under investigation, placing endocrinology at the vanguard of life-saving innovation within critical care. All of this progress necessitates that critical care clinicians stay current with these advancements to optimize patient care. Moreover, understanding immune-related adverse events (irAEs) associated with cancer immunotherapy has generated additional avenues of research within endocrinology. The incidence of endocrinopathies such as adrenalitis and thyroid disease has been increasing in patients treated with checkpoint inhibitors and CAR T-cell therapy, which is particularly challenging in the management of critically ill patients. Literature indicates that these side effects necessitate a greater awareness, particularly within the ICU context, where early treatment and diagnosis can significantly influence clinical course. Physicians also have to identify such complications at an early stage since they may also manifest as other life-threatening disorders, such as sepsis. With more and more boundaries between endocrinology and oncology changing due to the development of better care strategies, interprofessional team practice is required to treat patients with both endocrine dysfunctions and serious illness (Brém et al., 2020; Klucznik et al., 2019).

14.6.1. Recent Studies on Endocrine Function in Critical Care

The cross-talk between critical illness and endocrine function has become an area of increasing priority in recent investigations. The action of stress on the HPA axis is especially critical to understand the hormonal changes observed in critically ill subjects. Hypercortisolemia is frequently encountered, representing a stress-related physiological response. However, long-term hypercortisolemia has also been found to bring about complications such as immunosuppression and metabolic derangements, which include glucose metabolism disturbances. Recent findings suggest that these endocrine changes can exacerbate the severity of disease in critically ill patients by affecting immune function and recovery patterns. Therefore, understanding these hormonal dynamics can inform the development of effective management strategies that can mitigate the potentially detrimental consequences of critical illness in the ICU. They have also addressed the interaction between endocrine dysfunctions and some diseases, such as diabetes mellitus (DM) and COVID-19. There appears to be a two-way interaction between these diseases, particularly at advanced stages. Patients with DM are at higher risk for serious disease upon SARS-CoV-2 infection. Conversely, COVID-19 can induce metabolic dysregulation and lead to new-onset DM or worsening of existing ones. Notably, the virus binding to ACE2 receptors on both endothelial and pancreatic cells suggests an initial impact on glucose homeostasis. These findings underscore the need for the integration of endocrinology with critical care practice, in that it may refine treatment protocols and improve patient outcomes within the context of complex pathophysiologic associations (Kazakou et al., 2022). Besides, recent guidelines from multidisciplinary expert groups recognize the need to address immune-related adverse events (irAEs) in critically ill patients receiving immune checkpoint inhibitor (ICPi) therapy. Though ICPis hold revolutionary potential in oncology, they are associated with a range of endocrinopathies that require careful monitoring and management. Endocrine insufficiency and thyroid abnormalities are particularly challenging because these can mask or complicate the clinical course of critically ill patients. The current guidelines advocate for individualized treatment approaches, modulating management according to the grade of the adverse events without withholding essential therapies. Open communication among healthcare teams is important in a bid to optimize results and minimize complications. With the development of the field, continued research into the subtleties of endocrine regulation in critical illness will be pivotal in developing global care strategies (Bryan et al., 2021).

14.6.2. Emerging Therapies and Their Potential Impact

The practice of endocrinology in critical illness is being transformed with the advent of newer treatments. New approaches to glucose management have shown promising outcomes in ICUs. Model-based glycemic control uses advanced algorithms to individualize treatment, customizing it based on the patient's individual needs. They are very effective, achieving target levels of glucose within hours with very few hypoglycemic events, thereby enhancing patient safety. Of specific interest, studies to date have demonstrated an association between stringent glycemic control and improved clinical outcomes, warranting the promise of such sophisticated methodologies as part of routine ICU practice. With the rejection of conventional ad-hoc approaches in favor of a more formalized, model-based approach, the risk of uncertainty regarding patient outcome can be significantly reduced, presenting a tailored route for hyperglycemia management in severe illness (Chase et al., 1998). In addition to this, research into adipokines as drug targets is another fruitful area of intervention in the care of critically ill patients. Adipose tissue is increasingly being recognized as an active endocrine organ that secretes bioactive substances that influence metabolic and inflammatory processes. In particular, the anti-inflammatory adipokine adiponectin has been of interest due to its link with metabolic and immune responses in critical illness. The studies have indicated that HMW adiponectin levels increase with clinical recovery from sepsis, and it has been suggested to exert a protective role against inflammatory reaction and insulin resistance (Alison et al., 2014). These new discoveries about the role of adipokines can provide access to therapies tailored to modulate these pathways, a novel approach to the treatment of critically ill patients, alongside fulfilling their complex metabolic needs. Finally, the incorporation of new biomarkers and treatments into clinical practice has enormous potential to optimize patient care in the ICU. The evaluation of new adipokines, such as zinc-alpha2-glycoprotein (ZAG), is particularly important, given emerging evidence of its interaction with adiponectin during the recovery process of sepsis. The elevated level of ZAG during patient recovery suggests that it may play a role in the pathophysiology of sepsis and metabolic derangement (Alison et al., 2014). Through the identification and application of these biomarkers, physicians can develop personalized therapies that promote not only metabolic stability but also overall patient outcomes in the critical care environment. Ultimately, the integration of such advanced therapeutic modalities and biomarker-guided strategies into endocrinologic practice has the promise to revitalize the quality of care for critically ill patients, enabling a greater understanding of the intricate interrelationship between endocrine function and critical illness (Figure 14.14).

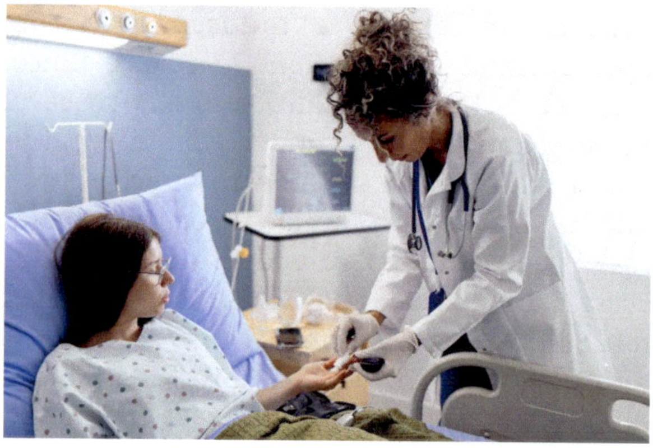

Figure 14.14. Model-based methods for glycemic control use advanced algorithms to personalize treatment, addressing individual patient needs.

Source: https://e8oujf7rsur.exactdn.com/wp-content/uploads/2024/12/Doctor-Patient.jpg?strip=all&lossy=1&ssl=1.

14.6.3. Future Directions for Research in Endocrinology

The field of endocrinology has much room for further development, particularly in ICU and critical illness settings. The future will bring more intense scrutiny of how the endocrine systems react to stressors such as sepsis and multi-organ failure. These are conditions that can disrupt hormonal control, yielding complication that affects the outcome of patients. A promising direction of investigation is the role of glucocorticoids and their impact on inflammation in critical illness. Understanding how these hormones influence both metabolic and immune functions may uncover new therapeutic pathways tailored to each patient. Furthermore, research into biomarkers of endocrine disturbance may provide the key to earlier diagnosis and treatment, potentially enhancing the management of fatal diseases classically presenting with complex hormonal derangement, as reviewed in recent literature. Immune-related adverse events (irAEs) as a result of advanced cancer therapy also deserve meticulous attention in endocrinology studies in the ICU environment. As cancer treatment becomes more advanced, so does the endocrine health concern in critically ill patients. Investigations are increasingly beginning to identify what types of irAEs manifest as endocrine dysfunctions that are contributing to the body of knowledge about post-treatment dysfunction. For instance, conditions such as adrenal insufficiency and thyroid dysfunction have the potential to complicate recovery, which makes early diagnosis and management a necessity. Research examining the pathophysiology of such irAEs can potentially inform the development of protocols to prevent endocrine complications in patients undergoing novel cancer therapy. The relationship between immunotherapy and endocrinology is significant, particularly as checkpoint inhibitors and CAR T-cell therapy are increasingly employed in clinical practice, necessitating a unifying approach to the management of such patients within the ICU (Brém et al., 2020). Moreover, patient satisfaction is a critical field of research, especially in the context of effective endocrine interventions in critical care. The perception of health care quality is a significant determinant of patient outcomes, and endocrinology clinicians must be attuned to satisfaction determinants. Investigations can assess the impact of effective management of endocrine disorders on overall ICU patient experience, such as compliance and recovery rates. Care barriers like poor communication of treatment regimens or a lack of empathy from clinicians can significantly reduce patient confidence and satisfaction. By addressing these service failures, endocrinologists can not only improve the clinical management of such serious conditions but also enhance the overall patient experience, ultimately leading to improved healthcare provision and greater congruence with patient expectations (Mohiuddin et al., 2020) (Figure 14.15).

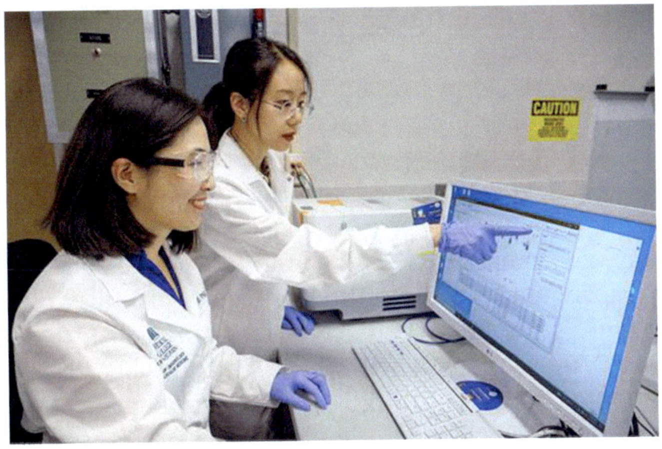

Figure 14.15. Future research endeavors are likely to encompass a deeper exploration of the endocrine system's response to stressors such as sepsis and multi-organ failure.

Source: https://www.mcw.edu/-/media/MCW/Departments/Medicine/Endocrinology/Research-and-Labs/Endocrinology-Research.jpg?h=400&w=600&hash=D035DABB3FE596C79AF6B73DD14CA225.

Test Your Knowledge

1. What recent studies have enhanced our understanding of endocrine function and hormonal regulation in critically ill patients?
2. How are emerging therapies shaping the management of endocrine disorders in critical care?

SUMMARY

The intricate interaction between endocrinology and critical illness determines the necessity of a thorough understanding of the regulation of hormones in the ICU. Endocrine dysregulation of more than one hormonal axis is often the result of critical illness, which has the potential to make significant impacts on patient outcomes. Studies have shown that dysregulation in levels of hormones in certain areas, namely stress response, metabolism, and growth, are contributors towards extended ICU stay and mortality. Management of these endocrine dysregulations with targeted interventions, e.g., hormone replacement therapy or glycemic control, may improve recovery and quality of life of patients following ICU discharge, as measured by scores with instruments like the EQ-5D-5L and WHODAS 2.0, which directly measure health-related quality of life and disability among these patients (Buse et al., 2025). The consequences of glycemic control in critical illness extend beyond mere survival; they also encompass overall recovery and functional status. A systematic review indicated that glucose variability, typified by multiple measures of glycemic variability, is strongly related to short-term mortality. Increased glycemic variability is likely to be adverse in critically ill patients and should be measured and treated with vigilance within the ICU environment. Such attention to endocrinological factors underscores the importance of integrated metabolic management in optimizing patient care and, potentially, preventing adverse outcomes due to endocrine uncertainty (Brett et al., 2024). Ultimately, the integration of endocrinological knowledge with critical care guidelines can lead to improved prognostic capacity and therapeutic strategy. With advancements in endocrinology, further research is needed to develop standardized protocols for assessing and managing hormonal imbalances in critically ill patients. The potential for improving such techniques with ongoing research and securing the place of endocrinology in critical care makes it imperative for an interprofessional approach by healthcare practitioners. By embracing this comprehensive model, enhancement can be realized to enhance recovery paths, address long-term health problems, and eventually redefine the ICU care environment (Brett et al., 2024; Buse et al., 2025).

In critically ill patients, the gut microbiota dynamics are heavily impacted, resulting in greater susceptibility to infection and complications. In a study involving fecal samples collected from ICU patients, the development of ultra-low-diversity bacterial communities with prevalent densities of merely a single to four bacterial taxa, e.g., Enterococcus and Staphylococcus, was identified. These changes in microbial populations are of concern since they have been linked with the presence of pathogenic fungi like *Candida albicans* and *C. glabrata* in a considerable number of instances. These revolutionary changes imply that antibiotic treatment and host physiologic stress during critical illness can trigger the overgrowth of multidrug-resistant pathogens that need novel therapeutic interventions to restore normal intestinal flora and possibly prevent sepsis and other infections (Alverdy et al., 2014). Metabolic dysregulation is another critical dimension of endocrinology in critical illness, as beautifully illustrated by the role of leptin, an adipocyte-produced cytokine. One investigation of critically ill patients highlighted the correlation between elevated leptin levels and systemic inflammation, insulin resistance, and hyperglycemia —common metabolic disturbances in these patients. To everyone's surprise, neither serum leptin nor its receptor was found to differ significantly in the patients—yes, including those with and without sepsis—yet interestingly, there were positive correlations between leptin levels and disease conditions like obesity and diabetes. This identifies the importance of leptin not just as a marker of metabolic well-being but also as an indicator of the advanced interaction between inflammation and metabolic physiology in critical illness and its impact on patient outcomes (Koch et al., 2010). The understanding of the intricate interaction between the microbiome and the metabolic hormone, such as leptin, is crucial to improve clinical outcomes in the critically ill patient. The ability of ultra-low-diversity microbial communities to alternate between commensal and pathogenic modes in response to the environment highlights the need for targeted interventions in the ICU. Similarly, the role of leptin as a predictor of outcome highlights the need for monitoring metabolic status as part of ICU treatment. Collectively, these findings of the mutual relationship between the gut microbiota and endocrine responses in severe disease emphasize the need for an integrated strategy to ensure endocrinology and its implications on patient management and outcome in the ICU.

KEY TERMS FROM THIS CHAPTER

- Calcium-related symptoms
- Chronic hormonal hyperstimulation
- Endocrine tumors
- Genetic markers
- Genetic predispositions
- Germline mutations
- Hormone-secreting glands
- Individualized screening regimens
- Medullary thyroid carcinoma
- MEN-1 syndrome
- Neuroendocrine neoplasms
- Neuroendocrine tumors
- Non-functioning tumors
- Pathophysiological mechanisms
- Patient-clinician relationship
- Pheochromocytoma
- RET mutation
- RET proto-oncogene mutations
- Symptomatic agents
- Thyroid tumors
- Cardiovascular syndromes
- Chronic ramifications
- Evidence-based guidelines
- Genetic mutations
- Genetic susceptibility
- Hormonal disorders
- Hypercalcemia
- Intensity-modulated radiation therapy
- MEN syndromes
- Multiple endocrine neoplasia (MEN)
- Neuroendocrine system
- Non-endocrine symptoms
- Pancreatic neuroendocrine tumors (pNETs)
- Patient management
- Peptide receptor radionuclide therapy (PRRT)
- Prophylactic thyroidectomies
- RET proto-oncogene
- Surgical procedures
- Thyroid carcinomas
- Tumor architecture

CRITICAL THINKING QUESTIONS

1. **Which of the following hormones is primarily responsible for mediating the stress response via the hypothalamic-pituitary-adrenal (HPA) axis in critically ill patients?**
   a. Insulin
   b. Cortisol
   c. Thyroxine (T4)
   d. Growth hormone
2. **In critically ill patients, which endocrine disorder is most commonly observed and may require hormonal therapy in the ICU?**
   a. Primary hypothyroidism
   b. Hyperparathyroidism
   c. Critical illness (CIRCI)
   d. Acromegaly
3. **What is the role of the hypothalamic-pituitary-adrenal (HPA) axis in the intensive care unit setting?**
   a. To regulate calcium metabolism
   b. To maintain glucose homeostasis during stress
   c. To initiate the systemic inflammatory response and provide cortisol for stress adaptation
   d. To increase secretion of thyroid hormones
4. **Which hormone therapy is commonly used in septic shock patients with relative adrenal insufficiency?**
   a. Levothyroxine
   b. Hydrocortisone
   c. Insulin
   d. Somatostatin
5. **Monitoring which of the following endocrine parameters is crucial in critically ill patients to guide therapy and prognosis?**
   a. Serum calcium and phosphate
   b. Serum aldosterone only
   c. Serum parathyroid hormone (PTH)
   d. Serum cortisol and blood glucose levels

Short answer Questions

1. What roles do hormones such as cortisol, catecholamines, and insulin play in the physiological response to critical illness?
2. What are the most common endocrine disorders encountered in ICU patients, and how do they affect patient management and outcomes?
3. How are hormonal therapies, including glucocorticoids, insulin, and thyroid hormone replacement, utilized in critical care settings to improve patient prognosis?
4. How does the hypothalamic-pituitary-adrenal (HPA) axis regulate the stress response in critically ill patients, and what are the consequences of its dysregulation in the ICU?
5. What are the key challenges and best practices in monitoring endocrine function and hormone levels in ICU patients?

Answers to Critical Thinking Questions

1. (b) 2. (c) 3. (c) 4. (b) 5. (d)

REFERENCES

1. Abitkar, A. S., Bala, P., Kutbudeen, A., Puthooran, S., et al. (2025). From infection to imbalance: The endocrine puzzle of long COVID. https://core.ac.uk/download/656543382.pdf (accessed on 22nd July 2025).
2. Acton, A., Annane, D., Baranova, I., Beishuizen, A., Borkowski, T., et al. (2005). The hepatoadrenal syndrome: A common yet unrecognized clinical condition. https://core.ac.uk/download/12205621.pdf (accessed on 22nd July 2025).
3. Ali, A. M., & Kunugi, H. (2021). Screening for sarcopenia (physical frailty) in the COVID-19 era. *International Journal of Endocrinology, 2021*, 1–16. https://doi.org/10.1155/2021/5563960 (accessed on 22nd July 2025).
4. Ali, G. C., Argente Oliver, J., Dattani, M., Francombe, C., et al. (2022). Challenges and improvement needs in the care of patients with central diabetes insipidus. https://core.ac.uk/download/519719255.pdf (accessed on 22nd July 2025).
5. Allolio, B., Reincke, M., Winkelmann, W., Würth, G., et al. (1993). The hypothalamic-pituitary-adrenal axis in critical illness. https://core.ac.uk/download/12167813.pdf (accessed on 22nd July 2025).
6. Alverdy, J. C., Garfield, K., Gilbert, J. A., Kade, M., et al. (2014). Membership and behavior of ultra-low-diversity pathogen communities present in the gut of humans during prolonged critical illness. https://core.ac.uk/download/323064638.pdf (accessed on 22nd July 2025).
7. Amrein, K., Christopher, K. B., Horkan, C. M., Mogensen, K. M., et al. (2016). Functional status in ICU survivors and out of hospital outcomes: A cohort study. https://open.bu.edu/bitstream/2144/30064/3/nihms753357.pdf (accessed on 22nd July 2025).
8. Andereggen, L., Christ, E. R., & Ebrahimi, F. (2024). Morbidities and mortality among hospitalized patients with hypopituitarism: Prevalence, causes and management. https://core.ac.uk/download/610613672.pdf (accessed on 22nd July 2025).
9. Annane, D., Arlt, W., Balk, R. A., Beishuizen, A., et al. (2017). Critical Illness-Related Corticosteroid Insufficiency (CIRCI): A narrative review from a multispecialty task force of the Society of Critical Care Medicine (SCCM) and the European Society of Intensive Care Medicine (ESICM). https://core.ac.uk/download/211704962.pdf (accessed on 22nd July 2025).
10. Attard, C., & Vella, S. (2015). Hypopituitarism following traumatic brain injury. https://core.ac.uk/download/46603761.pdf (accessed on 22nd July 2025).
11. Bartolović, D., Jovičić, S., & Terzić, B. (2024). Uloga hormona tiroidne žlezde u proceni preživljavanja bolesnika u odeljenjima intenzivne nege. https://core.ac.uk/download/613179589.pdf (accessed on 22nd July 2025).
12. Boehm, O., Bornstein, S. R., Grotemeyer, D., Hamann, A., et al. (2011). Genetic variation of TLR4 influences immunoendocrine stress response: An observational study in cardiac surgical patients. https://core.ac.uk/download/14521219.pdf (accessed on 22nd July 2025).
13. Brém, E., Koyfman, A., & Long, B. J. (2020). Oncologic emergencies: Immune-based cancer therapies and complications. https://core.ac.uk/download/305124082.pdf (accessed on 22nd July 2025).

14. Brenta, G., Brites, F. D., Faingold, C., Fossati, P., et al. (2012). High TSH and low T4 as prognostic markers in older patients. https://core.ac.uk/download/158838184.pdf (accessed on 22nd July 2025).

15. Chase, J. G., Hann, C. E., Shaw, G. M., Wong, J., et al. (1998). Overview of glycemic control in critical care – Relating performance and clinical results. https://core.ac.uk/download/pdf/35459323.pdf (accessed on 22nd July 2025).

16. Clarke, R., Weare, V., Chow, H., Bowering-Sheehan, L., & Hitchcock, C. (2024). "It saved me": A thematic analysis of experiences of psychological therapy following critical illness and intensive care. *Journal of the Intensive Care Society, 25*, 288–295. https://www.semanticscholar.org/paper/9bf38fa9e6be0c044238d4c77640198778190e74 (accessed on 22nd July 2025).

17. Cozzolino, A., Hasenmajer, V., Newell-Price, J., & Isidori, A. M. (2023). COVID-19 pandemic and adrenals: Deep insights and implications in patients with glucocorticoid disorders. *Endocrine, 82*, 1–14. https://doi.org/10.1007/s12020-023-03411-w (accessed on 22nd July 2025).

18. de Man, A. D., Gunst, J., & Reintam Blaser, A. (2024). Nutrition in the intensive care unit: From the acute phase to beyond. *Intensive Care Medicine, 50*, 1035–1048. https://www.semanticscholar.org/paper/1cb11e88d1fcc20a85a1e585c9b13fa5e6fe72bf (accessed on 22nd July 2025).

19. Esmaeilzadeh, A., Elahi, R., Siahmansouri, A., Jahani Maleki, A., & Moradi, A. (2022). Endocrine and metabolic complications of COVID-19: Lessons learned and future prospects. *Journal of Molecular Endocrinology, 69*, R125–R150. https://doi.org/10.1530/jme-22-0036 (accessed on 22nd July 2025).

20. Fabbrin, A. R., Gerchman, F., Gross, J. L., Canani, L. H., Santos, M. F., Viana, M. V., Moraes, R. B., et al. (2014). Contrasting effects of preexisting hyperglycemia and higher body size on hospital mortality in critically ill patients: A prospective cohort study. https://core.ac.uk/download/pdf/81732111.pdf (accessed on 22nd July 2025).

21. Hagerf (Voglová), B., Protuš, M., Németová, L., Mráz, M., Girman, P., Haluzík, M., Franeková, J., et al. (2025). 2016-LB: Implementing rtCGM in early postoperative intensive care of liver transplant recipients treated with insulin comprehensively improves glycemic control. *Diabetes*. https://www.semanticscholar.org/paper/f16e6f7f95236b54076be6f61194f1bb7f5a55b2 (accessed on 22nd July 2025).

22. Hall, A. M., Bing, C., Ding, C., Welters, I. D., & Leuwer, M. (2014). Circulating anti-inflammatory adipokines High Molecular Weight Adiponectin and Zinc-α2-glycoprotein (ZAG) are inhibited in early sepsis, but increase with clinical recovery: A pilot study. https://core.ac.uk/download/pdf/81169848.pdf (accessed on 22nd July 2025).

23. Hryciw, B. N., Ghossein, J., Rochwerg, B., Meggison, H., Fernando, S., Kyeremanteng, K., Tran, A., et al. (2024). Glycemic variability as a prognostic factor for mortality in patients with critical illness: A systematic review and meta-analysis. *Critical Care Explorations, 6*. https://www.semanticscholar.org/paper/1b7353c5c762bbafd1dc85241686d86af3ce4566 (accessed on 22nd July 2025).

24. Kazakou, P., Lambadiari, V., Ikonomidis, I., Kountouri, A., Panagopoulos, G. N., Athanasopoulos, S., Korompoki, E., et al. (2022). Diabetes and COVID-19; a bidirectional interplay. *Frontiers in Endocrinology, 13*. https://doi.org/10.3389/fendo.2022.780663 (accessed on 22nd July 2025).

25. Khanum, E., Ara, G., & Islam, M. A. (2024). Management of critically ill obstetric patients admitted in intensive care unit of Enam Medical College Hospital, Savar, Dhaka. *Journal of Enam Medical College*. https://www.semanticscholar.org/paper/6427d90a935931847597e4de979950b7fee635ad (accessed on 22nd July 2025).

26. Kleinpell, R., Grabenkort, W. R., Boyle, W. A., Vines, D., & Olsen, K. M. (2021). The Society of Critical Care Medicine at 50 Years: Interprofessional practice in critical care: Looking back and forging ahead. *Critical Care Medicine, 49*, 2017–2032. https://doi.org/10.1097/ccm.0000000000005276 (accessed on 22nd July 2025).

27. Klucznik, C. (2019). *Baystate Medical Center Nursing Report–2019*. https://core.ac.uk/download/327145544.pdf (accessed on 22nd July 2025).

28. Knaak, C., Kuenz, S., Kurpanik, M., Lachmann, B., et al. (2019). Risk factors of intraoperative dysglycemia in elderly surgical patients. https://core.ac.uk/download/225124691.pdf (accessed on 22nd July 2025).

29. Koch, A., Sanson, E., Tacke, F., Trautwein, C., et al. (2010). Relevance of serum leptin and leptin-receptor concentrations in critically ill patients. https://core.ac.uk/download/pdf/8454782.pdf (accessed on 22nd July 2025).

30. Maharaj, D. (2016). Evaluation of adherence to the glucose control protocol in a cardiothoracic ICU. https://core.ac.uk/download/188772806.pdf (accessed on 22nd July 2025).

31. Mohiuddin, A. K. (2020). Patient satisfaction with healthcare services: Bangladesh perspective. https://core.ac.uk/download/480549859.pdf (accessed on 22nd July 2025).

32. Murray, C. J. L., Ikuta, K. S., Sharara, F., Swetschinski, L. R., Robles Aguilar, G., Gray, A. P., Han, C., et al. (2022). Global burden of bacterial antimicrobial resistance in 2019: A systematic analysis. *The Lancet, 399*, 629–655. https://doi.org/10.1016/s0140-6736(21)02724-0 (accessed on 22nd July 2025).

33. Pretty, C. G., Chase, J. G., Lin, J., Shaw, G., et al. (1997). Impact of glucocorticoids on insulin resistance in the critically ill. https://core.ac.uk/download/pdf/35466847.pdf (accessed on 22nd July 2025).

34. Ramakrishnan, R. K., Kashour, T., Hamid, Q., Halwani, R., & Tleyjeh, I. M. (2021). Unraveling the mystery surrounding post-acute sequelae of COVID-19. *Frontiers in Immunology, 12*. https://doi.org/10.3389/fimmu.2021.686029 (accessed on 22nd July 2025).

35. Ribet Buse, E., Grunow, J. J., Spies, C. D., Weiss, B., & Paul, N. (2025). Health-related quality of life correlates with patient-reported and proxy-reported disability in critical illness survivors: A secondary analysis of the ERIC trial. *Critical Care, 29*. https://www.semanticscholar.org/paper/fbfa7ea72b38c23ddab210b5d574700536405a37 (accessed on 22nd July 2025).

36. Schneider, B. J., Naidoo, J., Santomasso, B., Lacchetti, C., Adkins, S., Anadkat, M. J., Atkins, M. B., et al. (2021). Management of immune-related adverse events in patients treated with immune checkpoint inhibitor therapy: ASCO guideline update. *Journal of Clinical Oncology, 39*, 4073–4126. https://doi.org/10.1200/jco.21.01440 (accessed on 22nd July 2025).

37. Soleimanpour, H. (2023). The magical role of vitamin C on adrenal insufficiency subsequent to etomidate administration: Ongoing challenges in the management of trauma patients. *International Journal of Drug Research in Clinics*. https://www.semanticscholar.org/paper/46075399d11d3ecbd47b3e6e657c0712dabdd23b (accessed on 22nd July 2025).

38. Soltani, N., Häbel, H., Balintescu, A., Lind, M., Grip, J., Thobaben, R., Nelson, D., et al. (2024). Insulin requirement trajectories during COVID-19 versus non-COVID-19 critical illness—A retrospective cohort study. *Acta Anesthesiologic Scandinavica, 69*. https://www.semanticscholar.org/paper/293919d48265e3a160c6a32ec75d72473d9eb284 (accessed on 22nd July 2025).
39. Stewart, A. (2018). Endocrine response to illness in sick horses. https://core.ac.uk/download/211564876.pdf (accessed on 22nd July 2025).
40. Tirupakuzhi Vijayaraghavan, B. T., Rashan, A., Ramakrishnan, N., Haniffa, R., Beane, A., Adhikari, N. K., Lone, N. I., et al. (2025). Persistent critical illness among intensive care patients in India: A registry-embedded cohort study. *Critical Care Medicine*. https://www.semanticscholar.org/paper/d4d02ded4fe10091892eee13b0f81a99639f93bd (accessed on 22nd July 2025).
41. Voiriot, G., Oualha, M., Pierre, A., Salmon-Gandonnière, C., Gaudet, A., Jouan, Y., Kallel, H., et al. (2022). Chronic critical illness and post-intensive care syndrome: From pathophysiology to clinical challenges. *Annals of Intensive Care, 12*. https://www.semanticscholar.org/paper/dd8fba8de3a46c1485b64ac7ca9a3a9dbee72457 (accessed on 22nd July 2025).
42. Wong, C. M. H. (2022). Musculoskeletal outcomes among older adults following hospitalization for COVID-19: A pilot study. https://core.ac.uk/download/519836771.pdf (accessed on 22nd July 2025).

ENDOCRINE TUMORS AND MULTIPLE EN DOCRINE NEOPLASIA (MEN)

15

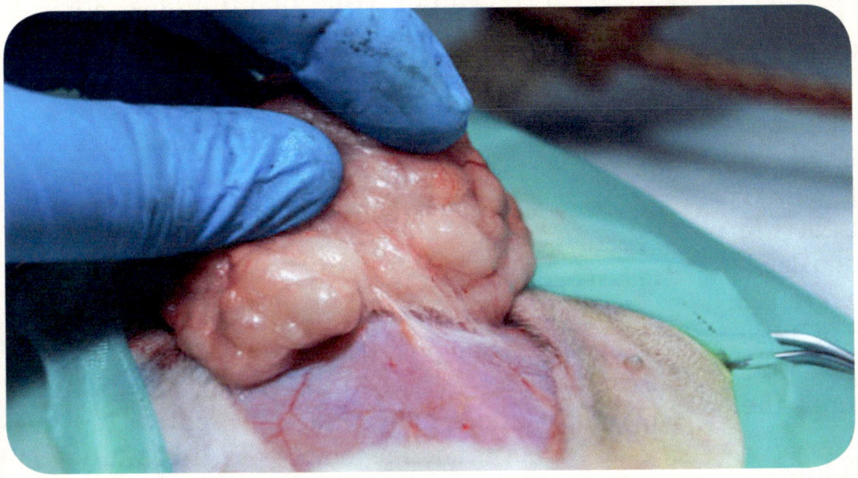

Introduction

The study of endocrine tumors and their relation to multiple endocrine neoplasia (MEN) is significant in de-mystifying the simplicity of these conditions. Endocrine tumors share the unique characteristic of occurring in hormone-secreting glands such as the thyroid, adrenal glands, and pancreas. Amongst these tumors, those that belong to the class of MEN syndromes are hereditary diseases that consist of a set of endocrine cancers. MEN syndromes result in a wide range of tumors, which have profound effects on the quality and length of life. The tumors should be diagnosed and treated early since they can be present simultaneously or sequentially and complicate diagnosis and treatment. It is this chapter's intention to discover the intricate landscape of endocrine tumors paying close attention to MEN syndromes and their varied forms, namely MEN1 and MEN2, in light of the advancements in genetic screening and therapeutic management that would improve the outcomes of patients (COLAO et al., 2011). Understanding MEN syndromes

LEARNING OBJECTIVES

After studying this chapter, you will be able to:

1. Explain the types of endocrine tumors;
2. Understand the pathophysiology of endocrine tumors;
3. Describe multiple endocrine neoplasia (men) syndromes;
4. Discuss how to diagnose endocrine tumors;
5. Define treatment options for endocrine tumors;
6. Deal with the prognosis for patients diagnosed with endocrine tumors.

is important since they have a genetic origin and are susceptible to developing more than one tumor. MEN1, for example, is characterized by tumors in the pancreas, parathyroid glands, and pituitary gland, indicating a state of proliferation in the neuroendocrine system (Camera et al., 2014). On the other hand, MEN2 typically presents with primary hyperparathyroidism, pheochromocytomas, and medullary thyroid carcinoma, which indicates the varied presentations of these syndromes. Interestingly, the occurrence of such tumors usually requires surgical procedures, with progress in biotherapy having developed as effective adjuncts to surgery. The role of somatostatin analogues as a therapeutic application, for example, in the management of symptoms and tumor development of pancreatic neuroendocrine tumors in MEN patients has been emphasized, thereby reinforcing the use of an integrative treatment strategy. Through elucidation of these clinical and genetic particulars, the chapter aims to enhance understanding about the possibilities for treating patients with endocrine tumors of MEN. Moreover, the importance of early diagnosis through genetic screening in hereditary syndromes cannot be emphasized enough. Indications highlight that preclinical genetic screening holds the potential of reducing the severity and improving prognostic outcomes for patients with hereditary neuroendocrine tumors (Colao et al., 2011). For instance, genetically diagnosed individuals prior to clinical tumor onset are likely to exhibit less advanced disease stages as well as better overall survival. They highlight the need for individuals at risk of developing MEN syndromes to be identified through genetic testing in order to make timely interventions that could even reduce the load of the disease. Therefore, this chapter aims to discuss the implications of genetic screening and how it revolutionizes clinical management toward better patient care and even reduced mortality in families with these complicated diseases.

Definition of Endocrine Tumors

Endocrine tumors are neoplasms derived from the endocrine system cells, which are responsible for producing and regulating hormones. They consist of the thyroid gland, pituitary gland, adrenal glands, and the pancreas. The tumors may either be functional or non-functional. Functional tumors produce hormones actively, leading to hormone-dependent syndromes and associated clinical presentations such as hyperglycemia with insulinomas or hypercalcemia with parathyroid adenomas. Non-functional tumors are not secretory but can cause symptoms either from mass effects or invasion. The distinction between these two groups is of vital importance in management and diagnosis, since functional tumors might have to be treated with specific therapy for the associated hormonal disturbances, while non-functional tumors might be treated with surgery or oncology to decrease the impact on surrounding structures. In the broad context of endocrine tumors, MEN syndromes represent a special type of endocrine tumors with hereditary predispositions towards multiple endocrine cancers. Types 1 and 2 MEN, for instance, are linked with some gene mutations that put the patient at higher risk of having a variety of tumors, including pituitary adenomas, medullary thyroid carcinoma, and pheochromocytomas. The genomics of such syndromes illustrate how single-gene mutation can disrupt normal endocrine function and make tumorigenesis possible. Specifically, the RET gene in MEN2 is of interest since mutations lead to the development of medullary thyroid carcinoma and other tumors, underscoring the link between genes and tumor development in endocrine mechanisms. For this purpose, these genetic processes are significant in risk estimation, screening strategies, and personalized treatment plans for patients with inherited endocrine tumor syndromes (Bondi et al., 2010). Clinical importance of endocrine tumors extends beyond categorization because timely diagnosis and treatment can significantly alter the outcome for patients. In MEN syndromes, patients may have variable clinical manifestations due to the varying expressivity of the underlying genetic mutations. Clarification of the phenotypic effects of mutations can lead to heightened surveillance regimens whereby early intervention can be initiated prior to otherwise asymptomatic tumors becoming apparent. In addition, the integration of multidisciplinary approaches to the treatment of such tumors will optimize care quality. These could involve resection, medical therapy, and genetic consultation aimed at tailoring treatment to patient-specific risk and tumor behavior. Knowledge of the metabolic effect and long-term implications of these disorders thus becomes increasingly important (Dreijerink et al., 2012) (Figure 15.1).

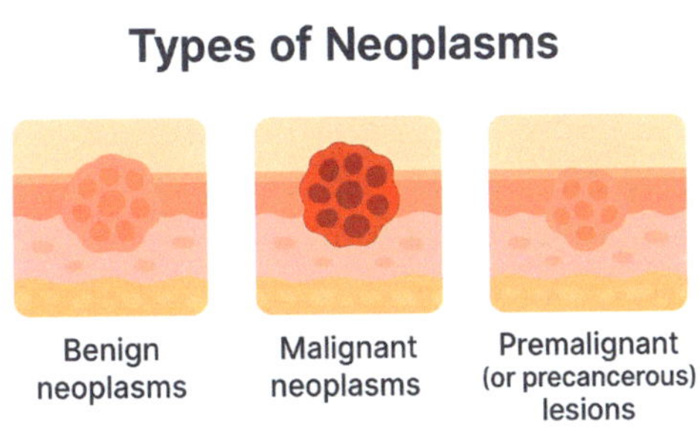

Figure 15.1. Types of neoplasms.

Source: https://oncodaily.com/pub/uploads/2025/05/Types_of_Neoplasms_OncoDaily.jpg.

Overview of Multiple Endocrine Neoplasia

MEN is a syndrome of familial disorders characterized by the simultaneous occurrence of neoplasms of more than one endocrine gland. The best recognized forms of MEN are MEN1, MEN2A, and MEN2B, each of which is associated with specific gene mutations. MEN1, or Wermer's syndrome, is most commonly related to hyperplasia or tumors of the parathyroid glands, pancreatic islet cell tumors, and anterior pituitary tumors. Conversely, MEN2A and MEN2B include medullary thyroid carcinoma, pheochromocytomas, and other tumors, with MEN2B appearing more aggressively and often being associated with mucosal neuromas. Proper classification of these subtypes is crucial since it determines genetic counseling and surveillance strategies in the affected patient and families. The genetic nature of MEN syndromes is now well understood, enhancing diagnosis and management. In particular, genetic screening has demonstrated its value in identifying individuals at risk before clinical disease develops. Studies have illustrated that precocious genetic testing can yield desirable outcomes; that is, patients detected with the aid of genetic screening had fewer advanced tumors than those diagnosed on clinical grounds alone. In cohort research, surgical rates for MEN-related neoplasms were considerably higher in individuals who had undergone diagnosis following identification of genetic origin, proving the efficacy of anticipatory management in hereditary syndromes (Colao et al., 2011). This highlights the importance of genetic counseling for families with histories of such illnesses, facilitating early detection and treatment. Beyond genetic predispositions, the clinical presentation of MEN syndromes requires an interprofessional management strategy. These typically involve endocrine surgeons, medical oncologists, geneticists, and endocrinologists in collaboration. An example is the treatment of pheochromocytomas arising in MEN2, which includes careful planning of the timing of surgical therapy and pre-operative management to minimize hypertensive crises. Genetic studies have also characterized specific germline mutations for bilateral and malignant pheochromocytomas with increased risk, suggesting the requirement for individualized screening regimens in afflicted families (Cranston et al., 2017). With regard to the complexities of these disorders, an integrated treatment approach that considers genetic backgrounds and patient profiles is critical in an attempt to improve prognosis and quality of life for MEN syndrome patients (Figure 15.2).

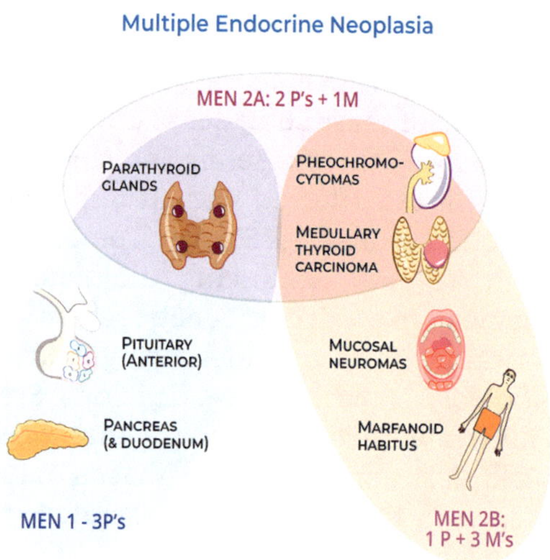

Figure 15.2. Multiple endocrine neoplasia (MEN).

Source: https://d1j63owfs0b5j3.cloudfront.net/term/images/multiple-endocrine-neoplasia-5831.png.

Importance of Studying Endocrine Tumors and MEN

The importance of studying endocrine tumors and MEN cannot be overstated, as it also significantly helps to enhance our understanding of complex pathological mechanisms and aid in the treatment of the patients. Endocrine tumors, even though they are uncommon, are a heterogenous group of neoplasms which may result in life-threatening complications if not diagnosed and treated appropriately. MEN, which encompasses a variety of genetic syndromes producing multiple endocrine tumors, highlights the need for high-level expertise and facilities in the laboratory and bedside. In N/A (2018), they point out that due to the rarity of the diseases, it is difficult to create evidence-based guidelines, thus there is a necessity to carry out studies that can serve as basis for clinical management and improve patient outcomes. Thus, meticulous investigation in these states not only contributes individually to patient management but also optimizes the wider field of endocrine science. In endocrine tumors and MEN, specifically, advances in diagnostic technologies and classification systems are pivotal in delineating treatment regimens. The current WHO classification of Neuroendocrine tumors (NETs) is a prime example in demonstrating how systematic classification guides therapeutic regimen and prognosis. This classification identifies various tumor types based on histopathological features, thus informing the selection of the optimal treatment regimens, as defined by Cuccurullo et al. (2021). By understanding variations between functional and non-functional tumors, healthcare providers can create interventions that address the unique biological behaviors of the tumors. Consequently, such information signifies the value of ongoing research on endocrine tumors, which not only enhances diagnosis accuracy but also ensures the application of precise and effective therapy modality.

Furthermore, research into endocrine tumors and MEN furnishes insight into the genetic and molecular mechanisms underlying these diseases necessary to engineer targeted treatment regimens. The majority of endocrine tumors, particularly those of the MEN syndromes, have been associated with some genetic mutations that are relevant to understanding their pathogenesis. As foregrounded in N/A (2018), the emphasis on observational studies on affected patient populations is crucial in the discovery of such genetic markers and their influence on the behavior of such tumors. Such information paves the way for new treatment methods, such as gene therapy and targeted therapy, which can potentially enhance outcomes for patients. Furthermore, it makes it possible for clinicians to have the means of conducting efficient risk assessment of members of the family for MEN syndromes, paving the way for preventive treatment and increased monitoring for timely detection. This holistic approach illustrates the ongoing need for studies and training in endocrine tumors, reaffirming the importance of this field to the development of medical science and patient treatment.

15.1. Types of Endocrine Tumors

Learning Outcome

1. Define pituitary tumors;
2. Describe thyroid tumors;
3. Classify adrenal tumors.

Endocrine tumors are varied in their cause and presentation and are generally classified by gland of origin. The main categories are pituitary, adrenal, and thyroid tumors, each with distinctive biologic activity and clinical presentation. Pituitary tumors are typically functioning, producing hormone that can be responsible for syndromes such as Cushing's disease or acromegaly, depending on whether they produce ACTH or growth hormone. Thyroid tumors can be benign such as follicular adenomas or malignant such as papillary and medullary thyroid carcinoma. Interestingly, the benign and malignancy status of the tumors makes them unique, necessitating specific diagnostic and treatment modalities that are appropriate to their functional status and histological typing. It should be noted to know these differences, especially for syndromes inherited through family such as MEN, wherein genetic background increases the risk of developing specific endocrine tumors (Diaz et al., 2012). Of all endocrine tumors, pheochromocytomas are noteworthy because of their distinctive pathophysiological mechanisms and their clinical significance. These tumors are from the adrenal medulla and are due to hypersecretion of catecholamines, resulting in spells of hypertension, palpitations, and anxiety. Pheochromocytomas can be sporadic or in familial syndromes, notably in association with MEN 2, in which they occur with medullary thyroid carcinoma and hyperparathyroidism. Genetic testing can identify underlying RET proto-oncogene mutations that allow early diagnosis and treatment. Furthermore, understanding the family nature of pheochromocytomas has prognostic value for surveillance and prevention in at-risk individuals. This is a reason for genetic screening in the recognition of families with predisposition to these tumors, allowing early interventions that can significantly influence patient management (Crossey et al., 1996). Neuroendocrine tumors (NETs) represent another crucial group of endocrine neoplasms that are arising from neuroendocrine cells throughout the body, but predominantly in the gastrointestinal tract and pancreas. These tumors exhibit a variability of behavior ranging from functional tumors that secrete hormones like insulin or gastrin to insidiously presenting non-functioning ones. They are heterogenous and thus hard to diagnose, which causes them to present late when the symptoms become more pronounced. In MEN, especially in MEN 1 where pancreatic NETs are one of the triad's essential parts, knowledge of this tumor types of clinical relevance is important. Treatment of the majority of NETs is typically in the form of a multidisciplinary treatment strategy, which involves surgical removal, medical therapy, and vigilant follow-up for tumor reappearance or metastasis. This combined model of care is especially significant in view of the potential for high morbidity with advanced-stage NETs, necessitating urgent research and development in their treatment (Diaz et al., 2012).

15.1.1. Pituitary Tumors

Pituitary adenomas are the most prevalent pituitary tumors and create a significant issue in endocrinology since they possess the potential to produce hormonal dysregulation and invasive growth. They may be functional or non-functioning tumors, and the functioning tumor can secrete hormones, which disrupt the normal endocrine balance of the body. Examples of functioning types include prolactinomas leading to hyperprolactinemia and acromegaly due to overproduction of growth hormone. Their impact extends beyond bodily manifestations, often disturbing the psychological condition of patients via hormonal imbalance and treatment stress. Considering such complicacies, timely identification and accurate diagnosis are crucial for effective management, rendering the role of comprehensive endocrine evaluation in patients with presumed pituitary pathologies significant. The association of pituitary adenomas with genetic syndromes, particularly MEN, complicates their clinical presentation even further. MEN1 patients, caused by MEN1 gene mutations, are predisposed to developing aggressive pituitary adenomas earlier in life that remain refractory to conventional medical therapies. In contrast, AIP gene mutations are seen with familial isolated pituitary adenomas, suggesting an inherited susceptibility that requires genetic testing in susceptible populations. The inclusion of genetic risk factors in the assessment of patients remains relevant, as understanding these inherited patterns guides surveillance and intervention. In addition, such genetic information refers us to the value of individualized treatment that takes into consideration the specific characteristics of the tumor and the individual's own personal map, especially in cases of early-onset or aggressive presentation. New advances in diagnostic modalities, including serum markers such as Chromogranin A (CgA), have enhanced our understanding of neuroendocrine tumors, including pituitary adenomas. Although CgA has been reported to be implicated in the diagnosis and follow-up of neuroendocrine tumors, its specificity is not total, and hence careful interpretation in clinical practice. Elevated CgA levels have also been observed in other neuroendocrine tumors, and thus its potential use; however, correlation with tumor size and type renders it a candidate for judicious use in the diagnostic workup. Importantly, while plasma CgA levels are informative, they cannot substitute detailed imaging and hormonal evaluations necessary in the diagnosis of pituitary adenomas. Therefore, the combination of serum markers with conventional diagnostic techniques is a promising area for enhancing clinical results for such multifaceted endocrine tumors (Figure 15.3).

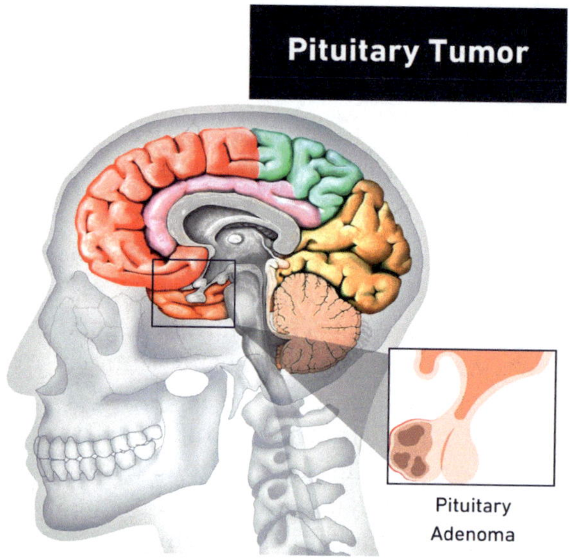

Figure 15.3. Diagram showing pituitary tumor.

Source: https://www.princetonbrainandspine.com/wp-content/uploads/2024/07/pituitary-tumor.jpg.

15.1.2. Thyroid Tumors

Thyroid tumors are a significant category of endocrine tumors with their heterogeneity of histological structure and clinical presentation. Thyroid tumors can be benign or malignant, with the latter classified into papillary, follicular, medullary, and anaplastic thyroid carcinomas. The prognosis and treatment also differ immensely based on the tumor type; for instance, papillary thyroid carcinoma has a favorable prognosis, while anaplastic thyroid carcinoma is associated with a poor prognosis. Risk factors involved in the development of these tumors include genetic predispositions, such as mutations of the RET proto-oncogene, which is somewhat specific for patients presenting with MEN type 2. The combination of genetic predisposition and environmental exposure complicates the image of thyroid oncogenesis, and therefore, a complete understanding of these dynamics is required to allow efficient treatment and intervention. Thyroid tumors' association with several endocrine neoplasia syndromes is also indicative of the complexity of endocrine tumors. Patients with MEN2 often develop medullary thyroid carcinoma, and this should be monitored and treated early. Studies show that early genetic screening can profoundly alter the outcome of hereditary neuroendocrine tumor syndromes by providing an opportunity to discover tumors before they become clinically evident. For example, one study revealed a significant difference in patient outcomes between those diagnosed previously and those diagnosed later, highlighting the need for proactive genetic examination and counseling. Proactive management is able to improve surgical outcomes and reduce mortality rates due to disease, indicating the possible benefits of genetic tests for hereditary thyroid and other endocrine tumors, as with MEN syndromes (Colao et al., 2011). In addition, the treatment modalities for thyroid tumors are influenced to a great extent by the biological behavior of the tumor and its association with genetic syndromes. For hereditary disorders like MEN2, treatment is mostly prophylactic thyroidectomies to make the patient devoid of the risk of medullary thyroid carcinoma. Genetic counseling and individual mutation-based treatment planning are imperative to maximize results. For patients who are diagnosed with obvious subtypes of thyroid tumors, the treatment will involve surgery, radioactive iodine treatment, and targeted therapies, depending on histology and stage of the tumor. The evolving image of treatment, particularly for aggressive forms of thyroid tumors, requires ongoing investigations and clinical trials to delineate improved management protocols, thereby enhancing the survival rate and quality of life in the patients (Iuliis et al., 2016) (Figure 15.4).

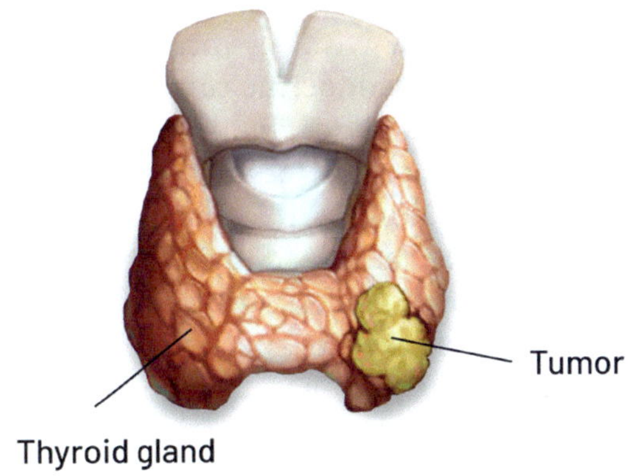

Figure 15.4. Tumor in thyroid gland.

Source: https://www.saintjohnscancer.org/endocrine/wp-content/uploads/sites/3/2023/01/Thyroid-cancer-diagram.png.

15.1.3. Adrenal Tumors

Classification of adrenal tumors is important in understanding their etiology and treatment in the realm of endocrine disease. They may be classified into broad groups of functional and non-functional tumors, of which the functional tumors have a tendency to produce profound cortisol disturbances. For instance, adrenal adenomas may secrete excess cortisol and produce Cushing's syndrome, while pheochromocytomas secrete catecholamines that result in episodic hypertension and other cardiovascular syndromes. The intricate interaction of these tumors with the endocrine system highlights the need for an integrated strategy towards diagnosis and management, especially in those patients who present with MEN syndrome symptoms. In MEN syndromes, the predisposition to several endocrine tumors highlights the importance of early diagnosis and early intervention to minimize morbidity and mortality associated with adrenal neoplasms, as they may be part of a multifold endocrine dysfunction that requires multimodal treatment approaches. Genetic susceptibility is of particular significance in the pathogenesis of adrenal tumor formation in the context of hereditary syndromes, such as MEN1 and MEN2, which are also associated with an increased risk of developing various endocrine tumors. In MEN1, patients are at risk of developing tumors of the endocrine glands of the pituitary, parathyroid, and pancreas, along with adrenal tumors. Genetic screening could lead to earlier diagnosis and treatment of individuals, thereby improving clinical outcomes. In patients with hereditary NET syndromes, patients diagnosed at the preclinical stage prior to tumor development clinically did better and had improved survival compared to those diagnosed after symptom development. Specifically, surgical intervention frequency was clearly higher in the preclinical genetic test-receiving group, which bears witness to the profound impact of early diagnosis on the alleviation of the severity of adrenal tumors and complications, as can be seen from the data of group A and group B (Colao et al., 2011). Pheochromocytomas, adrenal tumors originating in chromaffin cells, offer a pertinent example of the complex interplay between tumor biology and genetics. Pheochromocytomas are most commonly located in the adrenal medulla and are characterized by the overproduction of catecholamines, resulting in hyperadrenergic manifestations. Recent research indicates that specific genetic pathways, such as the Rb/p16 tumor-suppressive pathway, may be most critical to tumor progression in these tumors. Disabling genes such as p16 can disrupt normal cell cycle control, leading to uncontrolled growth and cell division. This genetic mutation not only reiterates the significance of genetic factors in pheochromocytoma etiology but also reasserts the necessity of genetic testing in high-risk groups, particularly in the case of MEN syndromes, where multiple endocrine tumors can coexist and need to be under close observation along with targeted therapy for optimal management (Brewer et al., 2006) (Figure 15.5).

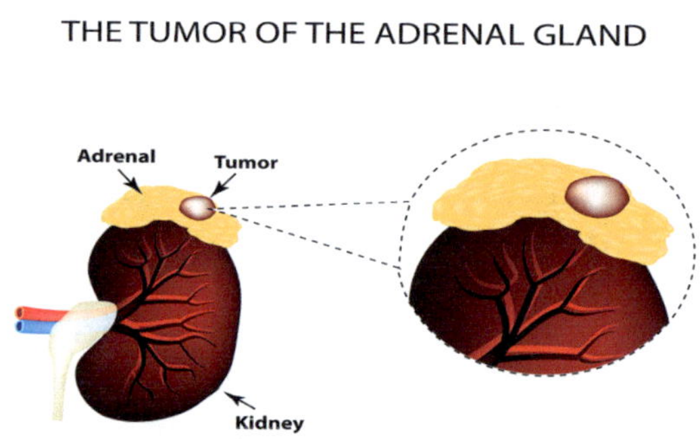

Figure 15.5. The tumor of adrenal gland.

Source: https://medanta.s3.ap-south-1.amazonaws.com/blogs/July2024/q1lzRwK8B6ukAceDAnkzkEeWPBv6K8-metaQ3JhY2tpbmcgdGhlIEhhY2sgb2YgQWRyZW5hbCBHbGFuZCBUdW1vcnMgQmVpbmcgQ2FuY2Vyb3VzIG9yIE5vdC5qcGc=-.jpg.

Test Your Knowledge

1. What are the common types of pituitary tumors, and how do they affect hormone production?
2. What symptoms might suggest an adrenal tumor?

15.2. Pathophysiology of Endocrine Tumors

Learning Outcome

1. Understand the mechanisms of tumor formation;
2. Discuss about hormonal dysregulation in understanding the pathophysiology of endocrine tumors;
3. Describe genetic mutations associated with endocrine tumors.

The pathophysiology of endocrine tumors is a multifaceted interaction between cellular, molecular, and genetic processes. These tumors most commonly arise from hormone-secreting glandular cells. Gene mutations, such as those occurring in tumor suppressor genes like MEN1, play a pivotal role in tumor development and progression. Loss of function in these genes will result in abnormal cell growth, characterized by the formation of functional or nonfunctional tumors with variable endocrine effects. In conditions such as MEN type 1, individuals may present with multiple endocrine tumors, particularly in the parathyroid, pituitary, and pancreatic tissues. The distinction between sporadic and hereditary presentations of these neoplasms is important since it impinges on prognosis as well as therapy, underlining the importance of understanding basic pathophysiological mechanisms in the treatment of endocrine tumors. Insulinomas, the most common of pancreatic neuroendocrine tumors (PNETs), are a classic illustration of the intricacy of the pathophysiology of endocrine tumors. These tumors occur most frequently due to hypersecretion of insulin, leading to episodes of hypoglycemia that can significantly impact the quality of a patient's life. The pathophysiology of insulinomas usually involves their hereditary aspects, as in the case of being associated with MEN-1 syndrome. In this familial setting, insulinomas have a tendency to present earlier and in the multicentric form rather than as solitary sporadic tumors, which are usually benign. Biochemically, the diagnosis of insulinomas relies on specialized tests that measure insulin levels during fasting; knowledge of these levels aids in identifying the effect of the tumors on metabolic processes. Surgical resection is usually the most effective type of treatment, but new treatments like endoscopic ultrasound-guided therapy are becoming increasingly significant for dealing with small, solitary tumors, a hallmark of the evolving nature of treatment modalities in endocrine oncology. The heterogeneity of pancreatic neuroendocrine tumors, particularly in MEN-1 patients, presents severely challenging clinical management. Aggressive metastasizing non-functioning PNETs are typically not diagnosed until they are advanced and thus pose challenges to prognosis and planning for treatment. The malignant potential has been noted to be correlated with the size of the tumor, and large threshold values have been inferred for surveillance strategies. Advanced imaging technologies, such as contrast-enhanced multi-detector CT scans, have enhanced diagnostic precision by allowing assessment of tumor vascularity and grading according to proliferation indices like Ki-67. In MEN-1 patients, the multifocal nature of these tumors necessitates diligent follow-up since the existence of lesions with different enhancement features can complicate treatment planning. It is essential to realize these pathophysiological nuances to tailor individual patient management strategies and maximize outcomes in endocrine tumor scenarios, particularly within the MEN spectrum (Camera et al., 2023; Rychlewska-Duda et al., 2025).

15.2.1. Mechanisms of Tumor Formation

Tumor growth is a complex biological process that involves a cascade of epigenetic and genetic alterations. In endocrine tissues, such modifications may lead to the oversecretion of hormones and uncontrolled cell growth, as in the case of MEN. Mutations of tumor suppressor genes and oncogenes are the shared underlying mechanisms by which normal cells are transformed into cancer cells. One of the primary avenues of research has identified the roles of G-proteins—i.e., their mutant forms—in activating cancerous processes. Point mutations in the alpha chain of Gs, the adenylyl cyclase–activating G-protein, have been implicated in GH-secreting pituitary tumors, for instance, demonstrating how a single genetic mutation can have systemic effects on cellular responses and overall hormone regulation (Chrousos et al., 1933). Chronic hormonal hyperstimulation and signal pathway dysregulation are also critical factors in the process of tumor development. In adrenocortical neoplasms, the signal pathways towards abnormally proliferating cells can be caused by chronic elevation of a number of hormonal precursors, i.e., proopiomelanocortin-derived peptides. Pathologies like ACTH-dependent Cushing's syndrome indicate a direct correlation between the imbalance of hormones and the occurrence of neoplasms. Furthermore, recent findings suggest the role of somatic mutations in the spontaneous transformation of adrenal cells. Through examination of the clonal organization of tumors, researchers have found that the majority of adrenocortical adenomas are of a monoclonal nature, therefore indicating that such tumors develop from one mutated cell (Abdelhamid et al., 1994). This one-cell origin model further explains the pathogenesis underlying adrenocortical tumors and suggests potential therapeutic targets. The tumorigenesis model in endocrine tissues highlights the complexity of genetic instability, growth factor signaling, and hormonal control. The genetic identity of the tumor could incorporate a variety of mutations beyond those identified in G-proteins, making the processes of tumor formation complex. For example, the contribution of X chromosome inactivation patterns gives a critical clue to distinguishing polyclonal from monoclonal tumors, and our understanding of tumor evolution. Clonal analysis findings reveal that while some endocrine tumors result from a single genetic abnormality, conditions such as adrenal hyperplasia may be more heterogeneous in their composition, with diverse genetic predispositions and reactions to hormonal stimulation. In combination, these mechanisms are ongoing in shedding light on clinical management and therapeutic approaches against endocrine tumors and the treatment of MEN syndrome patients (Figure 15.6).

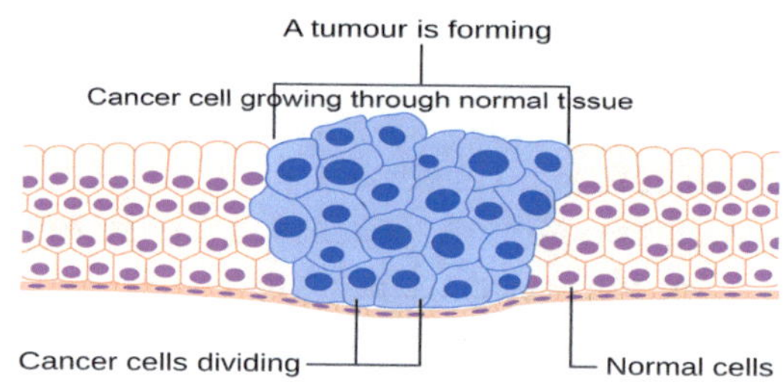

Figure 15.6. A depiction of tumor formation.

Source: https://www.researchgate.net/profile/Nicholas_Kerna/publication/335858313/figure/fig1/AS:804067492237317@1568716037940/A-depiction-of-tumor-formation-Note-Figure-in-the-public-domain.ppm.

15.2.2. Hormonal Dysregulation

Dysregulation of hormones is an integral part of the pathogenesis of endocrine tumors, particularly of MEN. The condition is represented by excessive growth of neuroendocrine cells, potentially leading to ectopic secretion of hormones. In MEN type 1, for example, the most frequently encountered tumors are those of the parathyroid glands, pancreas, and pituitary gland, whose combined effect is a dysregulated hormonal state. Hyperparathyroidism, with its associated hypercalcemia and accompanying symptoms of kidney stones and muscular weakness, can be caused by elevated parathyroid hormone levels as in clinical presentations in MEN1 patients. The associated pancreatic neuroendocrine tumors can also secrete insulin or other hormones to complicate the clinical picture. This harmony of tumor behavior and endocrine disturbance underscores the importance of early detection and meticulous management in maximizing patient outcomes, highlighting the intricate complexities of hormonal dysregulation in MEN. The findings related to hormonal dysregulation in MEN syndromes are similarly relevant to the diagnosis and treatment of patients with metastatic neuroendocrine tumors (NETs). A retrospective analysis of MEN patients treated with peptide receptor radionuclide therapy (PRRT) provides information regarding the repercussions of hormonal imbalance and tumor formation. The majority of patients with MEN have a variety of hormonal disorders, including hyperparathyroidism and pituitary adenomas, alongside the formation of multifocal gastroenteropancreatic tumors. This hormonal deregulation has a significant impact on the effectiveness of treatments such as PRRT, which targets tumor cells based on their neuroendocrine activity. As revealed in current studies, PRRT has also proven to be fairly effective in diminishing tumor burden and clinical symptomatology in patients who are battling with hormonal dysregulation, thereby highlighting the interaction of treatment with hormone levels and therapeutic measures, especially in a group of patients with MEN. The study of the role of hormonal dysregulation highlights the need for integrated management strategies in the treatment of MEN syndromes. Hormonal disturbances not only affect the clinical presentation and course of endocrine tumors but also regulate patients' reactions to therapy. For instance, elevated levels of tumor-released hormones can lead to disabling symptoms that require a multimodal approach to treatment, such as endocrinological evaluation and oncological treatment. In addition, monitoring procedures such as serial measurement of serum calcium and PTH levels are essential in the early detection and management, particularly in patients with a history of recurrent nephrolithiasis, as this may be suggestive of parathyroid adenoma involvement typical of MEN1. Finally, identification and management of hormonal dysregulation as the basis for MEN care offers a model for improved patient prognosis and quality of life, affirming the interconnectedness of endocrine function and tumor behavior in this particular patient population.

15.2.3. Genetic Mutations Associated with Endocrine Tumors

Genetic mutations are the cause of endocrine tumor pathogenesis, particularly in the instance of MEN syndromes. MEN syndromes represent hereditary illnesses characterized by the association of tumors in multiple endocrine glands. Each MEN syndrome has associated specific genetic alterations; for instance, mutations in the *MEN1* gene are commonly encountered in MEN type 1, which leads to hyperparathyroidism, pancreatic endocrine tumors, and pituitary adenomas. The pathogenic process often involves the disruption of tumor suppressor genes, which otherwise regulate cell growth and proliferation. Mutation in these genes allows uncontrolled cell growth and proliferation, ultimately leading to tumorigenesis. As is demonstrated through several clinical cases, genetic testing can reveal such mutations, but in a seeming paradox, patients can present with nonfunctional neuroendocrine tumors without a positive genetic result, suggesting the complexity of the genetic correlations in these conditions (Deng et al., 2023). Outside of the known MEN syndromes, additional genetic mutations continue to be identified as significant contributors to endocrine tumorigenesis. Of these, mutation of the CDKN1B gene has been linked with MEN type 4 and has shown parathyroid and anterior pituitary tumor associations, and also a possible association with other tumors, including adrenal and renal neoplasms. This highlights the intricate set of genetic factors inducing susceptibility to endocrine tumors and stresses the need for extensive genetic profiling in subjects who present with more than one tumor phenotype. Furthermore, in published cases of MEN 4, despite the absence of mutations in known genes such as RET, researchers have found variants of unknown significance (VUS) that can implicate as yet to be defined risk pathways.

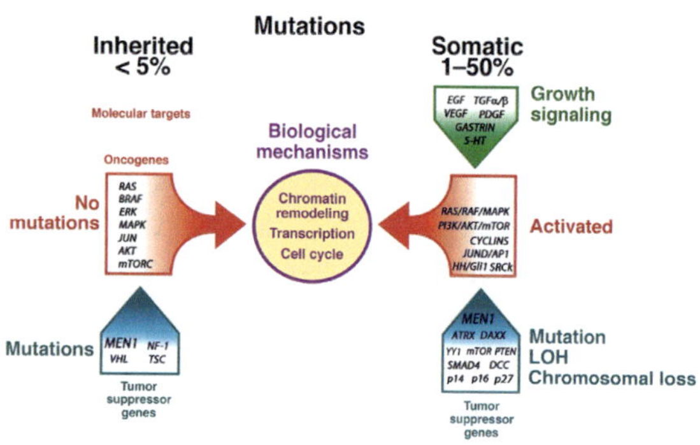

Figure 15.7. Inherited mutations have only been identified in tumor-suppressor genes (TSGs) and occur in fewer than 5% of all gastroenteropancreatic neuroendocrine neoplasms (GEP-NENs).

Source: https://www.researchgate.net/profile/Mark-Kidd/publication/271726350/figure/fig1/AS:267477649195093@1440783049714/Inherited-mutations-have-only-been-identified-in-tumor-suppressor-genes-TSGs-and-occur.png.

This again highlights that genetic mutation profiles hold the potential to affect clinical management and prognostic outcomes in patients presenting with multiple endocrine tumors (Soe et al., 2020).

Clinical uses of genetic mutation in endocrine tumors extend beyond identification alone; they affect therapeutic modalities and follow-up strategies as well.

Patients frequently require immediate intervention for symptom control in the case of hyperfunctioning tumors or addressing malignant transformation. Genetic mutations are used in therapeutic modality selection, particularly for patients who possess mutations responsive to targeted therapy.

For instance, in certain pheochromocytomas, somatic NF1 gene mutations have been reported to correlate with the tumors biochemical phenotype. This correlation highlights the importance of identifying genetic underpinnings to optimize patient outcomes through personalized medicine approaches.

In addition, genetic counseling comes into play, particularly in people with a family history of endocrine tumors, since the identification of hereditary inclinations can result in earlier diagnosis and intervention strategies (Deng et al., 2023) (Figure 15.7).

Test Your Knowledge

1. What are the common mechanisms that lead to the formation of endocrine tumors?
2. How does hormonal dysregulation occur in functioning endocrine tumors?

15.3. Multiple Endocrine Neoplasia (MEN) Syndromes

Learning Outcome

1. Describe MEN type 1 (Wermer's syndrome);
2. Understand MEN type 2A (Sipple syndrome);
3. Explain multiple endocrine neoplasia (MEN) Type 2B.

MEN syndromes are inherited diseases characterized by tumor development in greater than one endocrine gland. MEN syndromes are primarily of two categories: MEN1 and MEN2. MEN1, or Wermers syndrome, typically results in tumors of the pancreas, parathyroids, and pituitary gland, while MEN2 has two forms: MEN2A, with medullary thyroid carcinoma, pheochromocytoma, and primary hyperparathyroidism, and MEN2B, with identical features along with mucosal neuromas and a typical marfanoid habitus. The genetic nature of the syndromes is strong, including MEN1 mutations for MEN1 and RET proto-oncogene for MEN2. Identification of the genetic predisposition associated with MEN syndromes is thus essential for early diagnosis and treatment, which can preclude the development of virulent disease phenotypes. Clinical presentations of MEN syndromes are more than simple genetic identification; they significantly affect patient treatment and therapy outcome. Risk of tumor development necessitates life-long follow-up and anticipatory intervention strategies. As a case in point, individuals with MEN2 are shielded by prophylactic thyroidectomies against the formation of medullary thyroid carcinoma, a critical step considering the often-aggressive nature of the malignancy. Patient care complexity is also increased by heterogeneity among tumor types and initial symptoms, which require modified treatment approaches. Recent research emphasizes that an early genetic diagnosis can enable better clinical outcomes because the proof of significantly smaller tumor stage and improved survival rate in the gene-diagnosed patients before any onset of clinical symptoms evidently attests (Colao et al., 2011). In addition to that, the association between MEN syndromes and the development of neuroendocrine tumors (NETs) has also been of interest to the medical society. NETs may arise sporadically or as part of inherited syndromes, illustrating the requirement for genetic screening in at-risk subjects. Surgical rates and tumor stage were considerably improved in patients with hereditary syndromes of NET in a study group that had already been identified through previous genetic screenings (Colao et al., 2011). These findings underscore the importance of vigilance in patient surveillance with a family history of MEN syndromes because early treatment has the potential to reduce morbidity and mortality significantly. Moreover, the intricate interplay between genetic predisposition and tumor development suggests a general need for continued exploration of therapies targeted to specific sites and prophylactic interventions aimed at optimizing long-term outcomes in patients with MEN syndromes.

15.3.1. MEN Type 1 (Wermer's Syndrome)

MEN type 1, or Wermers syndrome, is a hereditary syndrome characterized by the occurrence of tumors in multiple endocrine glands concomitantly. The syndrome is most frequently associated with three large glands: the pituitary, parathyroid, and pancreas. The presenting symptom in the majority of patients is hyperparathyroidism, and this can manifest as calcium-related symptoms due to an elevation of parathyroid hormone (PTH). Also, functioning pancreatic neuroendocrine tumors, such as insulinomas or gastrinomas, are common, and they lead to serious metabolic disturbances. The presence of these tumors not only complicates patient management but also demands an extensive understanding of their biochemical and histological profiles for proper diagnosis and therapy. Imaging studies play a significant role in the diagnosis of MEN Type 1, particularly when neuroendocrine-main pancreatic tumors are under consideration. As demonstrated by recent publications, improvements in CT imaging can also characterize the nature of these lesions, suggesting differences in their histological types and vascularity. Specifically, pattern analysis of enhancement can assist clinicians in distinguishing benign from malignant lesions and accordingly guide treatment decisions. Another investigation found that different patterns of lesion enhancement were statistically related to malignancy; for instance, lesions with early enhancement were most frequently benign, but lesions that continued to enhance in delayed stages were likely to be malignant (Novaria et al., 2012). These findings point towards the importance of integrating imaging outcomes with clinical evaluation to optimize patient management in MEN Type 1. Surgery, and specifically parathyroidectomy, is considered optimal treatment for managing associated hyperparathyroidism in MEN Type 1. Surgery is advised, especially in symptomatic individuals, though currently it is realized that carefully chosen asymptomatic individuals may also be operated on for prevention of cumulative morbidity. Besides, the management of pancreatic neuroendocrine tumors will also vary, as some may require surgical resection while others may be treated with observation and nothing else, depending on how big they are and how functional (Bandeira et al., 2016). MEN Type 1 is complex and thus demands an inter-disciplinary management by all means where all facets of the patients' health are addressed while watching for new tumor development during their lifespan. This model of holistic care is essential for promoting prognosis and quality of life in persons with this disorder (Figure 15.8).

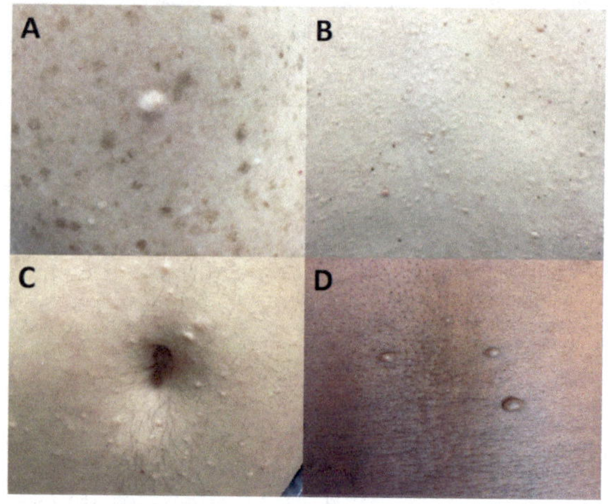

Figure 15.8. Multiple endocrine neoplasia type 1-associated collagenomas, which are benign connective tissue nevi with a dominant collagen component. They are hypopigmented or skin-colored and usually found on the neck, shoulder, and trunk. (A) 46-year-old woman with multiple collagenomas in addition to pigmented nevi on the arm. (B) 46-year-old man with innumerable collagenomas on the back. (C) 33-year-old man with multiple peri-umbilical collagenomas. And (D) 46-year-old man with truncal collagenomas.

Source: https://www.researchgate.net/publication/364445553/figure/fig2/AS:11431281258692365@1720125257649/Multiple-endocrine-neoplasia-type-1-associated-collagenomas-which-are-benign-connective.tif.

15.3.2. MEN Type 2A (Sipple Syndrome)

In learning about MEN type 2A, or Sipple syndrome, it is crucial to note its genetic origin and manifestations. MEN 2A is defined by the triad of medullary thyroid carcinoma (MTC), pheochromocytomas, and primary hyperparathyroidism. The development of these tumors comes from the disruption of the RET proto-oncogene, an important gene involved in cell signaling and proliferation. As Sipple syndrome is inherited, a family history of MEN 2A increases the risk of development of the disease, and hence genetic testing for high-risk subjects is essential. Early screening of the genetic mutation of MEN 2A allows surgeons to take aggressive surgical interventions, which will lead to better outcomes and survival of patients. Pheochromocytomas are a feature of MEN 2A and are neuroendocrine tumors typically developing in the adrenal glands and causing hypersecretion of catecholamines with resultant hypertensive crises and other cardiovascular illnesses. The impact of these tumors also extends beyond immediate physiological effects as they may complicate the management of other manifestations of MEN 2A, particularly medullary thyroid carcinoma. Diagnosis typically requires combined biochemical testing, imaging studies, and prolonged clinical assessment to identify the tumor's presence and size. Treatment of pheochromocytomas is imperative, as adrenalectomy for tumor removal is undertaken in patients, avoiding severe hypertension and related complications. Both clinical presentation and genetic susceptibility emphasize the difficulty of managing MEN 2A patients. The benefit of a multidisciplinary treatment regimen for MEN 2A cannot be overstated. Treatment options most commonly involve endocrinologists, surgeons, and genetic counselors who collaboratively practice integrated care. Systematic screening regimens in patients with diagnosed RET mutations are mandatory in the identification of MTC and pheochromocytomas prior to the onset of symptoms. Screening for primary hyperparathyroidism is also critical, as untreated individuals may develop complications like osteoporosis and kidney stones. As research in MEN 2A continues to advance, having knowledge of the disease's biology, including the RET gene and tumor suppressor pathways, is imperative. Further research is important to plan specialized therapy and enhance the overall care of patients afflicted by this rare but serious genetic disorder (Brewer et al., 2006; Sherad et al., 2024) (Figure 15.9).

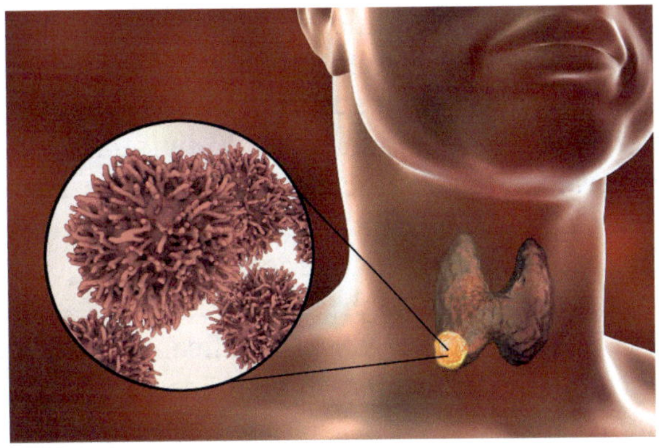

Figure 15.9. MEN 2A is characterized by the of medullary thyroid carcinoma (MTC).

Source: https://www.rarediseaseadvisor.com/wp-content/uploads/sites/25/2021/07/Medullary-Thyroid-Cancer-Differential-Diagnosis-909255562.jpg.

15.3.3. MEN Type 2B

The MEN category also includes MEN Type 2B, a rare hereditary disorder which is predominantly caused by mutations of the RET proto-oncogene. The clinical presentation of MEN Type 2B patients predominantly involves medullary thyroid carcinoma, pheochromocytoma, and mucosal neuromas, all of which collectively describe the multiform impact of the disorder on the endocrine system. Patients usually come with early-medullary thyroid carcinoma, most commonly diagnosed in young adulthood or childhood, necessitating aggressive screening and prophylactic thyroid surgery. Detection of RET mutations is the cornerstone of early diagnosis and management and serves to emphasize the necessity of genetic counseling in affected kindreds for the prevention of cancer. Pheochromocytomas in MEN Type 2B are particularly challenging, both with inherited and sporadic presentations of the disease. Genetic testing shows that a significant proportion of patients harbor germline mutations with frequencies of 6.8% for RET mutations; these findings are particularly relevant to patients with bilateral or malignant pheochromocytomas.

Screening for germline mutations in patients with pheochromocytomas can guide treatment and the need for surgery. More recently, researchers have found that individuals with bilateral pheochromocytomas are more likely to have mutations in the germline level, thus close monitoring and genetic testing is required among those at a higher risk (Cranston et al., 2017). These measures will significantly enhance surveillance and assist in risk assessment for families involved. MEN Type 2B is also associated with an increased incidence of the development of other tumors, like gastrointestinal stromal tumors (GISTs). Recent research also reveals that certain genetic mutations are associated with recurrence rates, which influence the surgical planning and postoperative care. These associations allow the medical teams to implement a tailored surveillance and intervention policy. For instance, those with obvious residual tumors following surgery require more vigilant monitoring since they are at increased risk of recurrence (Bergsneider et al., 2019). Therefore, the intricacies involved in the management of MEN Type 2B require a multidisciplinary team to involve genetic counseling, periodic surveillance, and early treatment, which maximizes the results for patients managing the difficulties presented by this endocrine disorder (Figure 15.10).

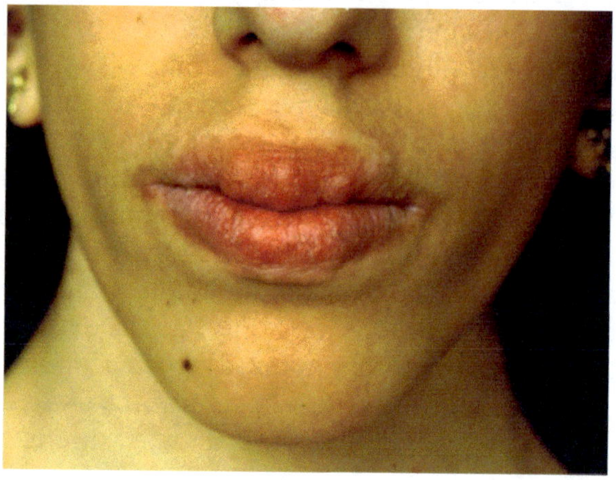

Figure 15.10. Characteristic phenotype of MEN 2B including thickened lips with bumps.

Source: https://www.researchgate.net/profile/Sergio-Bernasconi/publication/221722590/figure/fig1/AS:216370064171008@1428598051194/Characteristic-phenotype-of-MEN-2B-including-thickened-lips-with-bumps.png.

Test Your Knowledge

1. What are the primary endocrine tumors associated with MEN type 1 (Wermer's syndrome)?
2. Which gene is mutated in MEN type 2 syndromes, and what type of mutation is it?
3. How does MEN type 2B differ clinically from MEN 2A?

15.4. Diagnosis of Endocrine Tumors

Learning Outcome

1. Describe imaging techniques in the diagnosis and management of endocrine tumors;
2. Understand biochemical tests for hormone levels;
3. Discuss about histopathological examination.

Diagnosis of endocrine tumors involves a multidisciplinary approach that combines clinical evaluation, imaging investigations, and biochemical testing. The assessment begins usually with a thorough history and physical examination of the patient to identify hormonal imbalance signs and symptoms, for example, hypercalcemia with parathyroid tumors and unexpected weight loss in thyroid cancer. In line with this, various imaging modalities such as ultrasound, computed tomography (CT), and magnetic resonance imaging (MRI) play significant roles in localizing the tumors and identifying their nature. This is a very significant step because it will distinguish benign and malignant lesions in endocrine tissues, which may have a very strong bearing on treatment strategy. The combination of these tests is essential in making an early and accurate diagnosis, which is essential in maximizing patient outcomes, particularly in the case of endocrine neoplasias, wherein early intervention is of prime importance. Biochemical testing is also essential in the diagnostic hierarchy of endocrine tumors, enabling the quantification of specific hormone levels associated with specific types of tumors. For instance, the patients presenting with manifestations of MEN may have inappropriately elevated calcitonin levels in medullary thyroid carcinoma or increased catecholamines in pheochromocytomas. The hormone assays not only guide the clinicians to the diagnosis of the endocrine tumor but also distinguish among the different neoplastic conditions. Furthermore, the advent of genetic testing has transformed the diagnostic landscape, particularly in establishing inherited syndromes such as MEN1 and MEN2. These conditions are worthy of understanding as their knowledge cycles back into surveillance tactics and into family genetic counseling, with a valuable framework for the management of endocrine tumors in familial contexts (Romanet et al., 2024). In the MEN 2B condition, a syndrome of some endocrine tumors, diagnosis typically relies on genetic mutations such as the RET mutation. Early identification of such mutations is also important in the prevention of the dangers of medullary thyroid carcinoma and pheochromocytoma, since patients typically deserve early surgery for optimum outcomes. The multiple interaction of non-endocrine symptoms, including mucosal neuromas and typical phenotypic features, further complicates diagnosis. Due to the often-subtle presentation of these non-endocrine symptoms, the risk of delayed diagnosis exists, and thus, emphatic clinical examination is emphasized in suspected cases (Aynaou et al., 2024). With increasing science, the reliance on use of a mixture of genetic evaluation and judicious clinical assessment remains pivotal in rendering correct diagnoses for patients with endocrine tumors and related syndromes.

15.4.1. Imaging Techniques (CT, MRI, Ultrasound)

The use of imaging techniques is crucial in the diagnosis and management of endocrine tumors, particularly among patients with MEN. Among all imaging modalities, ultrasonography (US) computed tomography (CT), and magnetic resonance imaging (MRI) are recognized for their effectiveness in the detection of pancreatic tumors among MEN patients. CT, particularly multidetector-row CT, is highly preferred as a first-line imaging modality due to its ability to obtain in-depth visualization of the pancreatic organ, differentiation between solid and cystic lesions. Meanwhile, MRI complements CT images through enhanced contrast resolution, required in the characterization of complicated masses. Given that a considerable percentage of pancreatic tumors can be multifocal in origin, these imaging modalities, taken together, allow for proper staging and assessment of tumors as well as the surrounding soft tissue structures, thereby impacting treatment planning and management accordingly (Baccari et al., 2016). In MEN patients, particularly those with pancreatic endocrine tumors, multifocal disease is also exacerbated by the limitations of traditional imaging modalities. While MRI and endoscopic ultrasound (EUS) play an important role in tumor detection, they have been found to underestimate the extent of disease. For instance, EUS will typically detect more tumors than MRI; however, both techniques can miss lesions detected at pathology. Underestimation has critical implications on surgical planning as well as on postoperative outcome because it may lead to inadequate tumor resection. Therefore, extensive preoperative assessment by multiple modalities must be utilized to better approximate the degree of disease and tailor surgical interventions for patients (Adkisson et al., 2012). Lastly, the imaging modality combination enhances diagnostic performance in treating endocrine tumors of MEN. For example, accurate interpretation of imaging analyses is important to establish the level of surgical resection that should be achieved. Where multifocality is observed, for example, in pancreas cases, complete excision of involved tissue can be crucial in avoiding recurrence at the expense of maintaining endocrine function. As the outcomes of recent studies confirm, complete pancreatectomy could be the option for surgeons where the disease is highly multifocal, hence validating comprehensive imaging prior to intervention. Therefore, the choice of imaging techniques not only facilitates the detection of endocrine tumors but also plays a crucial role in surgical planning, thereby demonstrating their vital contribution to the overall treatment of patients with MEN (Adkisson et al., 2012; Baccari et al., 2016) (Figure 15.11).

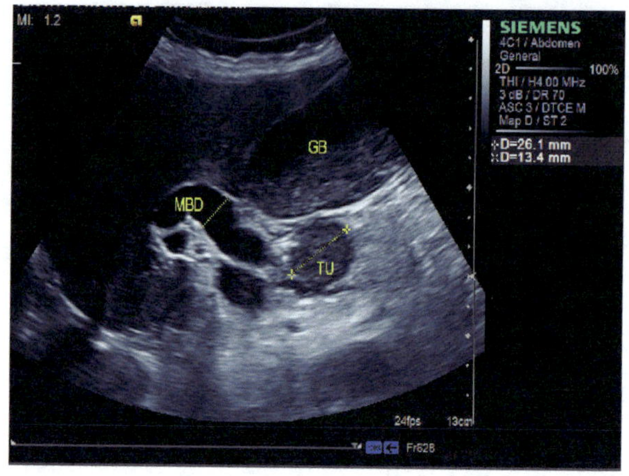

Figure 15.11. Neuroendocrine tumor in the pancreatic head. Standard US: hypoechoic mass (TU); dilated main biliary duct (MBD); GB: gallbladder.

Source: https://www.researchgate.net/profile/Roxana-Sirli/publication/317145962/figure/fig7/AS:498200152293376@1495791580447/Neuroendocrine-tumor-in-the-pancreatic-head-standard-US-hypoechoic-mass-TU-Dilated.png.

15.4.2. Biochemical Tests for Hormone Levels

Biochemical hormone assays play a significant role in the diagnosis and management of endocrine tumors and MEN syndromes. The assays allow clinicians to quantitate the blood level of some hormones, which can indicate the presence of tumor-associated abnormalities. A higher level of catecholamines and metabolites, metanephrine and normetanephrine, for example, can be quantitated by some assays in the case of pheochromocytoma. Such biochemical markers not only assist in establishing the diagnosis but also facilitate follow-up of patients post-treatment. These investigations are invaluable tools in the clinician's arsenal, providing a more nuanced understanding of endocrine disease and facilitating therapeutic care by rendering treatment strategies more tailored to hormone profiles, thereby optimizing patient management. Other than catecholamines, glucagonomas are also difficult to detect biochemically due to their nature and the variability of symptoms that they can cause. Glucagonomas, or tumors of pancreatic alpha cells, result in measurable elevations of glucagon detectable in blood tests. Rarely, the syndrome of glucagonoma with necrolytic migratory erythema, hyperglycemia, and weight loss makes diagnosis difficult. In the diagnosis of glucagonoma-suspected patients, biochemical testing not only quantifies levels of hormones but also provides information regarding the metabolic changes that are seen in these patients. Biochemical evidence of elevated glucagon levels is crucial in making the correct diagnosis and distinguishing glucagonoma syndrome from other causes of hyperglycemia, and this emphasizes the importance of precise biochemical testing in treating such difficult cases (Bano et al., 2017).

Development of biochemical diagnostic techniques has also significantly enhanced the early detection of endocrine tumors and subsequently, treatment plans and patient prognosis. As a result of the evolution of extremely sensitive immunoassays and mass spectrometry, doctors are able to identify hormonal profiles with greater specificity and sensitivity. This is particularly significant in MEN syndrome conditions when multiple endocrine organs are involved. For example, in MEN 1, biochemical measurement of the tumor burden and surgical decision-making can be highly useful in measuring the levels of parathyroid hormone, insulin, and gastrin. Continuing advances in these testing modalities not only improve diagnostic performance but also aid in individualized treatment planning, which ultimately leads to improved patient management of endocrine tumor patients and their syndromes (Bratu et al., 2019).

15.4.3. Histopathological Examination

Histopathological examination forms the cornerstone of the diagnosis and management of endocrine tumors, including those of MEN syndromes. Histopathological examination involves microscopic study of tissue samples to identify cellular characteristics that are characteristic of a specific type of tumor and its connotation of behavior. In MEN, as patients harbor more than one tumor in various endocrine glands, accurate histopathological examination gains importance. For instance, the classification of neuroendocrine tumors as different types, such as pancreatic neuroendocrine tumor (pNET), requires astute evaluation to guide therapeutic management. Merging of histopathological findings with clinical details provides the opportunity to obtain a complete understanding of tumor biology capable of profoundly influencing treatment strategy and patient outcomes. The histopathologic diagnosis of endocrine tumors often involves using immunohistochemical analysis to contribute to the diagnostic data. These tests utilize particular antibodies for the detection of markers characteristic of various types of tumors and render diagnoses more specific. In MEN syndromes, in which there are overlapping tumor types, i.e., medullary thyroid carcinoma and pancreatic neuroendocrine tumors, immunohistochemistry plays a significant role in establishing tumor origins. The complexities of such syndromes call for a collaborative effort from pathologists, endocrinologists, and oncologists toward fostering a multidisciplinary culture that guides appropriate management measures. With accurate histological analysis, not only can tumoral differentiation be achieved, but so too can the understanding of genetic mutations, even those covering the RET proto-oncogene, thus maximizing prognostic prediction and treatment modes (IULIIS et al., 2016). Aside from diagnostic analysis, histopathological study aids in assessing tumor aggressiveness and metastasis, which is highly significant in the management of endocrine tumors. For example, the detection of lymphovascular invasion or high mitotic activity could indicate aggressive tumor characteristics necessitating stricter treatment protocols. With complex presentations, as with synchronous tumors of MEN patients, careful histopathological evaluation becomes a component of understanding relationships between different sites of tumors and their implications on therapy. A systematic approach to managing the difficulty posed by such diverse tumor milieus is required, including rigorous histological work-up and advanced imaging. This multimodal strategy ensures that patients receive site-specific therapies tailored to their individual tumor profile, thereby necessitating specialized care networks for treating rare but aggressive conditions (Caplin et al., 2017) (Figure 15.12).

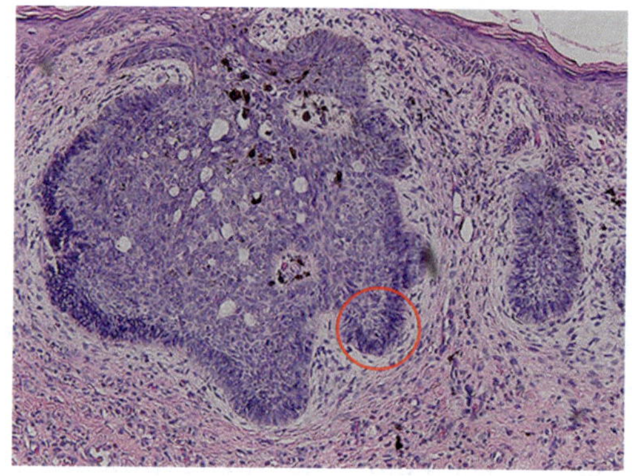

Figure 15.12. Histopathological examination showing that the tumor cells form a palisading structure (red circle).

Source: https://www.researchgate.net/publication/372076626/figure/fig3/AS:11431281256484779@1719536216621/Histopathological-examination-showing-that-the-tumor-cells-formed-a-palisading-structure.jpg.

Test Your Knowledge

1. Which imaging modalities are most commonly used for detecting pituitary, thyroid, and adrenal tumors, and why?
2. What biochemical tests are useful for diagnosing functioning pituitary tumors?
3. How are thyroid nodules evaluated using both imaging and laboratory tests?

15.5. Treatment Options for Endocrine Tumors

Learning Outcome

1. Focus on surgical interventions in the management of endocrine;
2. Understand medical management (hormonal therapy, chemotherapy);
3. Focus on radiation therapy in managing various types of tumors.

The treatment paradigm for endocrine tumors, with particular focus on neuroendocrine tumors (NETs), utilizes an array of treatment modalities based on the tumor's profile, including histology, stage, and the patient's status. Surgical removal is the cornerstone treatment for localized malignancies, which is most likely to yield long-term remission. However, when tumors are metastatic or nonsurgical, systemic therapies take center stage. Somatostatin analogues such as octreotide and lanreotide have been shown to be of benefit in the control of symptoms in carcinoid syndrome and in inhibiting tumor growth in certain groups of patients. It has been proven by clinical trials like PROMID and CLARINET that octreotide LAR and lanreotide are beneficial in treating well-differentiated metastatic NETs, highlighting both their use in symptom control and treatment of the disease (Baldelli et al., 2018). For more advanced pNETs, targeted treatment provides additional options. Everolimus has also become a significant therapeutic alternative for advanced pNETs, exhibiting improved rates of progression-free survival in treated patients. Similarly, sunitinib is administered in patients with progressing gastrointestinal stromal tumors demonstrating intolerance to imatinib, as represented by randomized trials confirming its benefit for overall and progression-free survival in advanced pNET. The treatment of more virulent or treatment-resistant NETs presents a challenge, and research into other therapeutic agents, such as pasireotide, has been helpful in patients who remain symptomatic despite standard treatment, testifying to growing interest in new therapies for this specialty area (Baldelli et al., 2018). Additionally, the treatment of pancreatic neuroendocrine neoplasms requires a multidisciplinary, team-based approach because of the complexity of these neoplasms and the variety of treatment modalities required. The complexity of these tumors frequently demands specialized biochemical investigations and sophisticated radiological studies to allow for adequately informed treatment decisions. Given multiple surgical and medical treatment modalities, optimization of outcomes requires the provision of comprehensive care within an integrated network of care. It is essential to have an understanding of the unique biology and behavior of these tumors since they develop slowly. Thus, implementing an ensemble that combines these resources can significantly enhance the treatment process for endocrine tumor patients.

15.5.1. Surgical Interventions

Surgery is the cornerstone of treating endocrine tumors, particularly for MEN. The primary aim of surgery is the excision of tumor tissue entirely, a step that not only eliminates symptoms but also significantly reduces the risk of metastasis and subsequent complications. In MEN patients, where multiple endocrine glands may be affected, a multimodal strategy has to be employed in planning surgery. Tumor sizes, locations, and types dictate expertise-specific methodologies, with the goal of enhancing the survival and quality of life of patients through tumor resection. As MEN syndromes have a hereditary component, genetic counseling is also included in the preoperative assessment, which allows for intelligent decision-making regarding the indications and timing of surgery (N/A, 2018). The intricacy of surgery in MEN further necessitates the use of advanced imaging and diagnostic modalities. Such modalities not only allow for tumor detection but also for localization within the endocrine system. The integration of techniques such as endoscopic surgery and minimally invasive surgery has revolutionized the landscape of surgery for endocrine tumors by decreasing patient recovery and postoperative complications. Moreover, prospective outcome data collection of patients also better defines how efficient various surgical techniques are. This is particularly true for rare disorders like MEN, where inadequate data might hinder the generation of evidence-based guidelines. Multidisciplinary management by healthcare professionals ensures the patient has tailored management plans according to individual tumor characteristics and the patient's own wishes (Brandi et al., 2017). After surgery, surveillance remains essential for MEN patients because the risk of tumor recurrence or development of new tumors remains. It is common to have follow-ups that incorporate biochemical markers and imaging investigations to monitor for evidence of regrowth or new tumors. Clinical guidelines for individualized follow-up strategy are more relevant in the context of the inheritable nature of MEN and its effects on families. Coordination among endocrinologists, oncologists, and surgeons also enhances long-term patient management, leading to improved outcomes in morbidity and mortality. As surgical techniques and postoperative care are constantly getting better due to developments in medical science, an increased awareness of such treatments will further translate into better overall management of endocrine tumors in MEN patients with the long-term aim of a higher quality of life and improved survival rates (N/A, 2018) (Figure 15.13).

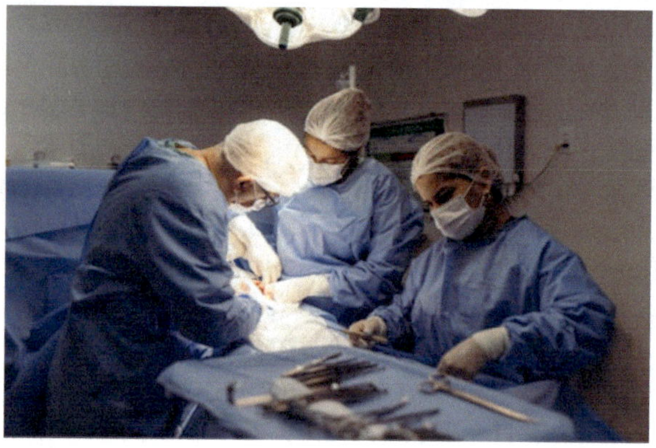

Figure 15.13. Surgical interventions play a pivotal role in the management of endocrine tumors, particularly within the context of multiple endocrine neoplasia (MEN).

Source: https://images.unsplash.com/photo-1703809047974-4de2c5276087?crop=entropy&cs=tinysrgb&fit=max&fm=jpg&ixid=M3w3MDgyMDR8MHwxfHNlYXJjaHwxfHxlbmRvY3JpbmUlMjBzdXJnZXJ5JTJDJTIwYW5lc3RoZXNpYSUyQyUyMHN1cmdpY2FsJTIwdGVjaG5pcXVlc3xlbnwwfDB8fHwxNzUwMDAzOTY2fDA&ixlib=rb-4.1.0&q=80&w=500&?utm_source=numberanalytics&utm_medium=referral.

15.5.2. Medical Management (Hormonal Therapy, Chemotherapy)

Both hormonal therapy and chemotherapy play critical roles in the medical management of endocrine tumors, particularly for the normalization of the hormonal imbalances and tumor growth that typify the cancers. Therapy generally begins with control of the excess hormonal secretion, which tends to occur in a variety of manifestations and syndromes. For instance, in patients with neuroendocrine tumors (NETs), it is crucial to manage hormone-related symptoms effectively, thereby improving the quality of life for these patients. Hormonal treatments such as somatostatin analogues and other targeted therapies are commonly employed so that hypersecretion of the hormones can be avoided in patients. These treatments are also applicable in the control of the course of the disease, particularly when surgery alone is inadequate or when tumors occur at a metastatic level. The treatment program thus needs to be multidisciplinary in nature, involving both the surgical and medical treatments for maximum gain (Eijck et al., 2004). Chemotherapy is also a critical component of the management of endocrine tumors when surgery by itself is not sufficient to control the disease burden. While surgical resection is the preferred treatment for localized endocrine tumors, it is only when there is metastatic disease that chemotherapy is employed. Multiple regimens of chemotherapy have been employed, based on the type of tumor, stage, and factors that are specific to the patient. Specifically, MEN1 patients present unique challenges due to the multiplicity and malignancy of their neuroendocrine tumors. As demonstrated in recent publications, MEN1 patients and pancreatic neuroendocrine tumors (pNETs) are best treated with surgery and chemotherapy, especially at advanced disease where tumor invasiveness is an absolute risk (Camera et al., 2014). Therefore, not only does chemotherapy have an important role in reducing the tumor, but it also maximizes the outcome of subsequent surgical procedures. The association of hormonal therapy and chemotherapy highlights the importance of multi-professional collaboration between specialists in addressing endocrine tumors, particularly in relation to the MEN syndromes. Because of the complexity of these diseases, treatment is often a multidisciplinary effort between endocrinologists, oncologists, and surgeons to give comprehensive care. For example, in treating patients with disseminated pNETs, the employment of symptomatic agents, hormonal therapy like lanreotide, and chemotherapy can best manage endocrine syndromes and tumor growth. Optimal patient outcomes are achieved through individualized treatment plans that consider patient preferences, therapeutic response, and potential side effects (Camera et al., 2014; Eijck et al., 2004). The individualized treatment permits effective disease control without excessively impairing the patient's global quality of life, highlighting the importance of subtle medical management in treating endocrine tumors (Figure 15.14).

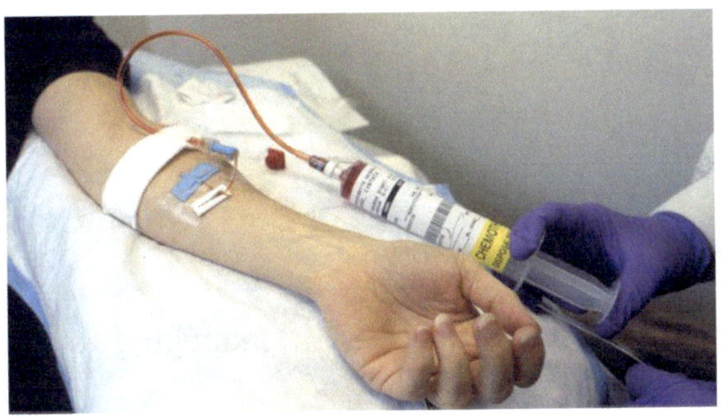

Figure 15.14. Chemotherapy plays crucial roles, particularly in addressing the hormonal imbalances and tumor growth associated with these malignancies.

Source: https://i0.wp.com/ronnyallan.net/wp-content/uploads/2015/04/chemo.jpg?fit=624%2C351&ssl=1.

15.5.3. Radiation Therapy

Radiation therapy has now become a leading treatment option in the treatment of various forms of tumors, particularly when concerning endocrine disorders such as MEN. Advances in radiation techniques, including stereotactic radiosurgery and intensity-modulated radiation therapy, have allowed the use of treatment with exact lesion targeting with minimal damage to adjacent normal tissues. In endocrine tumors, where the tumors are also frequently observed with abnormal growth patterns and endocrine secretion, accuracy in radiation therapy is crucial. Current evidence suggests that the application of radiation not only serves to control tumor growth but may even affect the indigenous genetic constitution of the tumor, which decides its resistance and risk of recurrence. With treatment modalities in view among clinicians, understanding the role of radiation therapy within the multifaceted paradigm of MEN is essential to optimum patient outcomes. Radiation therapy has been linked to profound mutational perturbations of tumor architecture, with relevant implications for long-term management strategies. Evidence suggests that radiation treatment has the potential to contribute significantly to the mutational burden and diversification of the subclonal architecture of the tumor, but not necessarily to the eradication of the original founding tumor clone. This is consistent with observations in other brain tumors, in which incomplete eradication of the tumor clone often results in treatment-resistant relapses. As stated in the case of ependymomas, the interactions between radiation treatment and tumor genomic evolution require careful planning for treatment, especially for individuals with MEN who are predisposed to developing more than one endocrine cancer. This correlation necessitates ongoing genomic monitoring and potentially adaptive treatment plans to optimize long-term outcomes. Moreover, newer developments in combining radiation therapy with other modalities have begun to alter treatment approaches to endocrine tumors of MEN. For instance, a combination of somatostatin analogues (SSAs) and PRRT together with radiation has been identified as a promising method for enhancing treatment outcomes. The combination of these treatments may potentially lead to increased response rates and longer progression-free survival rates. With promising phase III trials already establishing that these combinations are effective, the exploration of polytherapeutic regimes becomes increasingly relevant in the clinical management of neuroendocrine tumors. Ultimately, the ongoing discovery and understanding of how radiation interacts with other medications will be crucial to creating integrated treatment models for patients battling endocrine tumors and the complexity of MEN syndromes (Figure 15.15).

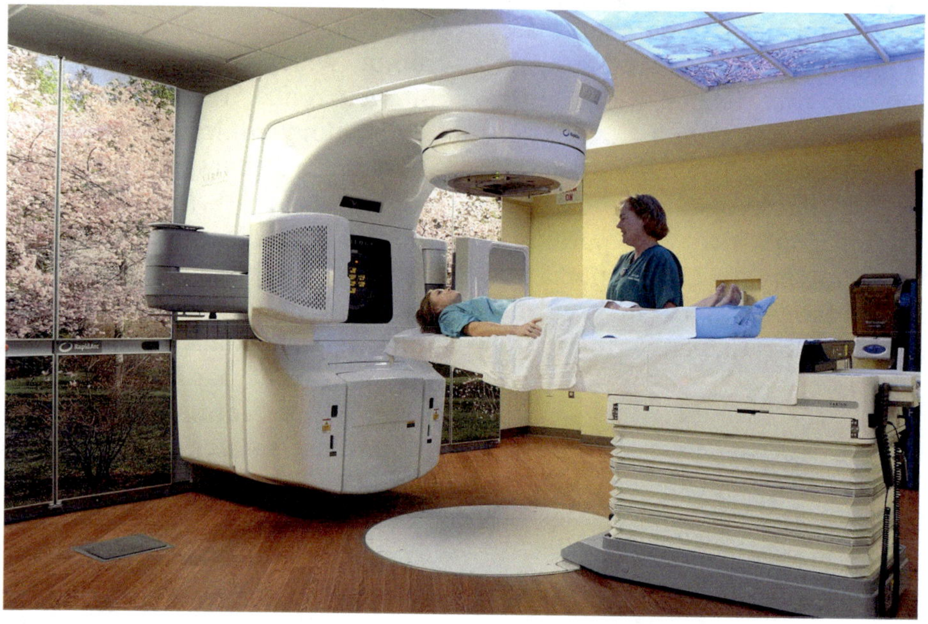

Figure 15.15. Radiation therapy has emerged as a pivotal treatment modality in managing various types of tumors.

Source: https://www.datocms-assets.com/30187/1620664918-cancerswetreathero.jpg?auto=format&w=1600.

Test Your Knowledge

1. What is the primary treatment for most localized endocrine tumors, and why?
2. Which medications are commonly used to manage hormone-secreting pituitary tumors?
3. When is radiation therapy indicated in endocrine tumors?

15.6. Prognosis and Outcomes

Learning Outcome

1. Describe factors influencing prognosis in patients with endocrine tumors;
2. Deal with long-term management of patients with endocrine tumors;
3. Focus on quality of life (QoL) considerations in the treatment and management of endocrine tumors and multiple endocrine neoplasia (MEN).

Prognosis in the endocrine tumor patient, particularly within the context of the MEN syndrome, depends mainly on the histological characteristics, location, and extent of the tumors. Neuroendocrine tumors (NETs), for instance, exhibit a very variable behavior directed to a great extent by these variables, basically dictating prognosis as well as therapy. Cancers such as well-differentiated pancreatic neuroendocrine neoplasms (pNETs) have been shown to be linked with improved prognoses if detected early and treated accordingly. Therapeutic management, for instance, with targeted therapies such as everolimus in advanced pNETs, has been shown to have positive effects on progression-free survival (PFS), hence the need for early treatment in ensuring patient outcomes in such complex situations (Baldelli et al., 2018). Ideal management of neuroendocrine tumors requires a tailored treatment plan, particularly in the context of heterogeneity of tumor behavior in the MEN. Clinical studies like PROMID and CLARINET highlight the advantage of somatostatin analogs, i.e., octreotide and lanreotide, to inhibit the growth of tumors and relieve carcinoid syndrome symptoms (Baldelli et al., 2018). The results of these investigations demonstrate that tailored therapeutic regimens will significantly enhance PFS and, in some cases, overall survival. However, pre-existing MEN conditions most commonly complicate the prognosis, with intense evaluation of each patient's unique clinical presentation necessary to optimize treatment modalities and improve long-term outcomes. Furthermore, the incorporation of multidisciplinary teams into specialized networks is necessary to approach the complexity of endocrine tumors in MEN. The complexity of these tumors, along with the diverse diagnostic and therapeutic needs, necessitates that experts handle patients to provide them with comprehensive care. In accordance with recent studies, the use of sophisticated biochemical tests and advanced radiological imaging enhances diagnostic precision, which is crucial in delineating the most suitable treatment pathways. Utilizing a network approach not only facilitates best practice dissemination but also facilitates patient support and education, ultimately achieving more favorable prognostic outcomes in patients afflicted by MEN and associated endocrine tumors.

15.6.1. Factors Influencing Prognosis

Prognosis in patients with endocrine tumors, particularly neuroendocrine tumor (NET) patients, is based on numerous factors, including tumor histology, site of origin, and stage at diagnosis. Endocrine tumors are characterized by their variable biological behavior, making it difficult to treat and predict prognosis. Well-differentiated NETs, for instance, typically confer a better prognosis than their poorly differentiated counterparts, which have a propensity to grow aggressively and be chemoresistant. Moreover, the tumor cells' proliferative index, as a measure of cell proliferation rate, is a major prognostic factor, seen in the successful management approaches used in trials such as PROMID, which studied somatostatin analogs for tumor growth control in metastatic NETs (Baldelli et al., 2018). Prognostic factors such as these must thus be carefully evaluated to ensure effective modulation of treatment protocols and improvement in patient outcomes. Another significant prognostic factor in endocrine tumors is the presence of underlying genetic syndromes, i.e., MEN syndromes. MEN1 syndrome, which typically presents as parathyroid, enteropancreatic, and pituitary tumors, alters the patient's clinical course due to its hereditary nature and associated tumor aggressiveness. The likelihood of several tumors developing concurrently delays diagnosis and treatment because such tumors tend to have a more aggressive course compared to sporadic tumors. Statistical observations indicate that the illness typically manifests early in life for most patients and is progressing at the time of diagnosis (Rossier et al., 2015). Thus, early detection through genetic testing and enhanced vigilance in family environments becomes essential towards effective control and even the prevention of adverse effects associated with MEN syndrome (Rossier et al., 2015). Lastly, comorbidities and the general condition of the patient are the key determinants that can heavily influence the prognosis of endocrine tumors. The patients with comorbid conditions might have a more complex treatment process with adverse results. Conditions such as cardiovascular disease, obesity, or diabetes would adversely affect a patient's ability to tolerate certain treatments, thus yielding lower therapeutic efficiency. Moreover, psychological factors, including patient motivation and compliance with treatment, also have a deep impact on the overall prognosis. Interventions aimed at supportive care for these psychosocial issues are all part of an overall holistic management approach. By emphasizing the multifaceted nature of the prognosis of endocrine tumors, healthcare workers are better able to individualize interventions that take both medical and psychological interventions into account for optimal overall patient outcomes and quality of life.

15.6.2. Long-Term Management of Patients

Management of long-term endocrine tumor patients, particularly MEN-associated ones, calls for a multi-disciplinary approach balancing effective tumor control with minimizing harm due to therapy. In the MEN1 condition, where patients are apt to harbor numerous subcentimeter pNETs, the use of somatostatin analogs such as octreotide can be of pivotal value. Literature has documented instances where treatment with octreotide resulted in a remarkable decline in levels of pancreatic polypeptide (PP), but long-term results remain uncertain. Importantly, care must be exercised while following up because the treatment may be discontinued with patient tolerance and resulting increase in hormone levels, thus necessitating individualized treatment strategies based on efficacy and quality of life (Kemm et al., 2019). The treatment of children with pituitary adenomas, particularly those associated with genetic syndromes like MEN1, is a particular challenge that should be addressed. Pediatric presentations usually have significant complications either because of delayed or inappropriate diagnosis, and thus should be managed with a multi-modal approach using genetic screening and counseling. Refractory forms of the tumor, like in some of the early-onset patients, may need active interventions like surgical debulking or radiotherapy. The concomitant long-term morbidities that result from these treatments, including syndromes like panhypopituitarism, highlight the requirement of long-term care that not only addresses tumor management but also endocrine deficiency management and overall patient well-being (Gan et al., 2015). Ultimately, the long-term care for endocrine tumor patients and MEN patients must be carried out on a cooperative basis by multidisciplinary groups to ensure continuous care involving surveillance, symptomatic management, and psychosocial support. Clinicians should closely monitor for potential recurrence or emergence of new tumors, along with the patient's desire and quality of life. Patient-clinician relationship maintained throughout ensures a setting where the patient is able to freely express concerns regarding the condition and treatment, allowing for more adaptive coping with complex management therapy. By prioritizing a holistic approach in the context of professional guidelines, health professionals can improve patient outcomes and quality of life for patients who live with the chronic ramifications of endocrine tumors and MEN syndromes. Therefore, continued interaction with patients is critical in effectively treating the intricacies of long-term care (Figure 15.16).

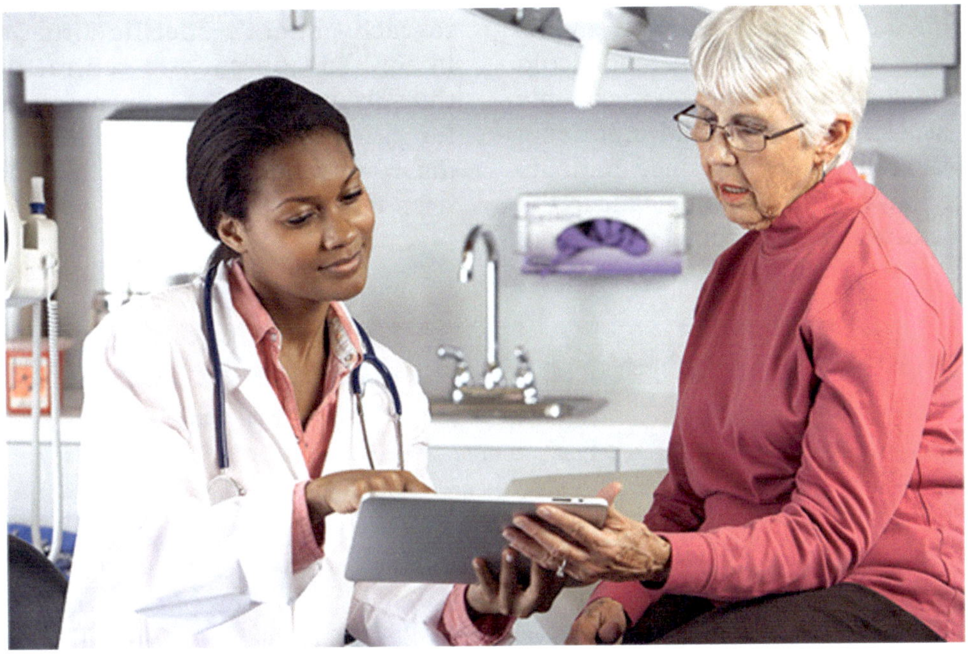

Figure 15.16. The long-term management of patients with endocrine tumors.

Source: https://expertperspectives.com/wp-content/uploads/2024/02/Topic3_web.jpg.

15.6.3. Quality of Life Considerations

Quality of life (QoL) problems are of utmost priority in the treatment and management of endocrine tumors and MEN. Both diseases pose a severe threat to physical health, but also influence the psychological and emotional well-being of the patients. Patients with endocrine tumors experience fatigue, pain, and hormonal imbalance, which can diminish their quality of life. The treatment regimens should therefore not only prioritize the physical excision of tumors but also supportive care strategies addressing psychiatric disease, nutritional disturbances, and lifestyle modifications. This broad-spectrum approach would immensely enhance patient satisfaction and adherence to treatment, ultimately enhancing health outcomes and quality of life in this high-risk patient cohort. Further, the psychological burden of a diagnosis of endocrine tumors or MEN is the worry of ongoing surveillance for potential recurrence and the fear of metastatic disease. Fear may also be experienced by patients with complex treatment regimens, including surgeries, hormone replacement therapy, and medications. These can be dealt with well by proper communication and patient education to ease distress and create an optimistic outlook. Moreover, caregivers and family members should be consulted for their input on QoL, as they play a vital role in psychological resilience. Consequently, integrating mental health care support, stress reduction strategies, and open communication within the treatment system may help develop a positive environment to foster psychological and physical recovery. Research has found that the optimal management of hormone-related disorders associated with endocrine tumors can have significant positive effects on quality of life. For instance, the regulation of excess hormones not only brings relief from physical symptoms but also increases psychological health. For instance, treatments that are capable of regulating glucocorticoid excess in adrenocortical carcinoma are capable of reversing associated fatigue and emotional distress and overall QoL. Also, since patients with MEN may have more than one cancer, the treatment protocols may become multiform, multifactorial, and coordinated. Guidelines encourage multidisciplinary team collaboration, involving oncologists, endocrinologists, dietitians, and mental health professionals to formulate individualized care plans tailored to each patient's specific situation. Such an integrated approach is central to improving the survival rate and improving quality of life for patients with such complicated endocrine disorders, and this results in a superior long-term outlook.

Test Your Knowledge

1. What are the key factors that influence prognosis in patients with endocrine tumors?
2. Why is long-term follow-up essential for patients with endocrine tumors, even after treatment?
3. What are common quality of life (QoL) issues for patients living with endocrine tumors?

SUMMARY

The study of endocrine tumors and the complexity of MEN has yielded critical details regarding patient management and treatment efficacy. The prognosis of patients with MEN varies according to the specific subtype and implies the need for customized therapeutic intervention. Notably, PRRT has produced optimistic results in MEN patients with metastatic or unresectable neuroendocrine tumors (NETs). As is illustrated in the research, 177Lu-DOTATATE reported favorable results, with a cumulative response rate of 43% and median progression-free survival of 32.6 months, establishing the status of 177Lu-DOTATATE as a successful treatment modality in advanced NETs in this group of patients (Aggarwal et al., 2025). In total, these advances in the understanding and management of MEN are a silver lining, and the call for ongoing research in the field is imperative. Gender impact on the presentation and outcome of MEN, particularly MEN-1, should be mentioned in endocrine tumor literature. Recent studies have not found any gender-related differences in clinical presentation or survival among MEN-1 patients. Male and female patients were shown to have similar mean age at diagnosis and similar progression-free and overall survival within a series seen at the "Federico II" University of Naples. This lack of disparity means that screening protocols and subsequent treatment need to be standardized, and without gender discrimination, to provide equal treatment. The identical results across genders ensure that clinical practices need to focus on individual risk factors and tumor characteristics and not demographic groups (Modica et al., 2024). The findings, hence, encourage an inclusive approach in the treatment of MEN patients to ensure maximum efficacy of treatment protocols. Summarily, the relationship between endocrine tumors and MEN is a complicated spectrum that needs more research and clinical evaluation. The positive outcomes associated with advanced therapeutic regimens, such as PRRT, provide an important foundation for managing patients with aggressive forms of NETs, potentially improving their quality of life and survival. The gender-neutral findings into clinical presentation underpin more precise planning for patient treatments, with an emphasis on bespoke therapies that consider patient-specific environments. Future studies need to build on these findings by examining larger cohorts and multicentric studies to cross-validate treatment protocols, ultimately advancing the broader care environment for individuals suffering from endocrine tumors and MEN (Aggarwal et al., 2025; Modica et al., 2024).

The study of endocrine tumors and MEN encompasses a broad array of neoplasms characterized by their relationship with specific hormonal secretions and genetic predispositions. MEN encompasses a series of diseases, such as MEN1 and MEN2, that are both hereditary syndromes and the development of multiple endocrine tumors. MEN1 primarily leads to parathyroid gland, pancreatic, and pituitary gland tumors, while MEN2 includes medullary thyroid carcinoma, pheochromocytoma, and primary hyperparathyroidism. Apart from affecting the endocrine system, these disorders also have a significant role in influencing the quality of life in patients as they typically necessitate complex monitoring and management regimens. The intersection of clinical symptoms and genetic mutations in patients who present with MEN highlights the need for a knowledge of the physiological and psychological impact that these tumors exert on individuals. Psychological implications of MEN, particularly anxiety and quality of life, are crucial aspects to examine. Studies have shown that MEN1 patients have increased anxiety surrounding their genetic status and implications for family transmission, as evidenced by significant correlations between anxiety and quality of life measures. Patients may worry about passing the predisposition to their offspring and, therefore, develop emotional distress requiring attention beyond clinical control. Genetic counseling becomes a valuable asset, one that can, nonetheless, also increase the level of anxiety for some individuals. Although genetic counseling offers priceless guidance and information, it is necessary to be capable of managing the emotional climate that is created through genetic counseling, so the benefits of such counseling do not then unintentionally engender additional stress for the patient (Akihiro et al., 2024). Furthermore, a key aspect of managing MEN patients is identifying the environmental factors that affect the growth of endocrine tumors. New evidence suggests that exposure to certain environmental toxins with hormonal activity may be linked to the increasing number of reproductive and endocrine diseases. This underscores the multifactorial nature of neoplasia in which both genetic and environmental determinants converge to affect health outcomes. This interaction necessitates an interdisciplinary research strategy involving epidemiological studies and clinical experience. Clarification of the etiology and risk factors for endocrine tumors is conducive to the development of enhanced prevention strategies and targeted interventions, ultimately leading to improved patient care for diseases like MEN. An emphasis on minimizing environmental risks, along with a robust infrastructure of endocrine surveillance for hormonal well-being, is central to the battle against these endocrine neoplasms (Giwercman et al., 1996).

KEY TERMS FROM THIS CHAPTER

- Calcium-related symptoms
- Chronic hormonal hyperstimulation
- Endocrine tumors
- Genetic markers
- Genetic predispositions
- Germline mutations
- Hormone-secreting glands
- Individualized screening regimens
- Medullary thyroid carcinoma
- MEN-1 syndrome
- Neuroendocrine neoplasms
- Neuroendocrine tumors
- Non-functioning tumors
- Pathophysiological mechanisms
- Patient-clinician relationship
- Pheochromocytoma
- RET mutation
- Cardiovascular syndromes
- Chronic ramifications
- Evidence-based guidelines
- Genetic mutations
- Genetic susceptibility
- Hormonal disorders
- Hypercalcemia
- Intensity-modulated radiation therapy
- MEN syndromes
- Multiple endocrine neoplasia (MEN)
- Neuroendocrine system
- Non-endocrine symptoms
- Pancreatic neuroendocrine tumors (pNETs)
- Patient management
- Peptide receptor radionuclide therapy (PRRT)
- Prophylactic thyroidectomies
- RET proto-oncogene

CRITICAL THINKING QUESTIONS

1. **Which of the following is a common type of endocrine tumor found in Multiple Endocrine Neoplasia type 1 (MEN1)?**
   a. Medullary thyroid carcinoma
   b. Pheochromocytoma
   c. Parathyroid adenoma
   d. Papillary thyroid carcinoma
2. **What is the pathophysiological mechanism behind most endocrine tumors in MEN syndromes?**
   a. Autoimmune destruction of endocrine glands
   b. Germline mutations in tumor suppressor genes
   c. Viral infections causing neoplastic transformation
   d. Nutritional deficiencies leading to hyperplasia
3. **Which of the following is typically associated with MEN2A syndrome?**
   a. Insulinoma
   b. Prolactinoma
   c. Growth hormone-secreting adenoma
   d. Medullary thyroid carcinoma
4. **What is the most appropriate initial test for diagnosing a suspected pheochromocytoma?**
   a. Serum calcium level
   b. Serum cortisol level
   c. Plasma free metanephrines
   d. TSH (thyroid-stimulating hormone)
5. **What is the mainstay of treatment for most localized endocrine tumors?**
   a. Surgical resection
   b. Chemotherapy
   c. Radiation therapy
   d. Hormonal replacement therapy

Short Answer Questions

1. What are the main types of endocrine tumors, and which glands do they typically affect?
2. What is the underlying pathophysiology of hormone-secreting endocrine tumors?
3. What are the key features of multiple endocrine neoplasia (MEN) type 1 and type 2 syndromes?
4. How are hormone levels used to diagnose functioning endocrine tumors?
5. What imaging modalities are typically used to localize endocrine tumors?
6. What role does genetic testing play in the diagnosis of MEN syndromes?
7. What are the main treatment strategies for endocrine tumors?
8. How does long-term management differ between sporadic endocrine tumors and those caused by MEN syndromes?

Answers to Critical Thinking Questions

1. (c) 2. (b) 3. (d) 4. (c) 5. (a)

REFERENCES

1. Abdelhamid, S., Allolio, B., Beuschlein, F., Chrousos, G. P., et al. (1994). Clonal composition of human adrenocortical neoplasms. https://core.ac.uk/download/12167841.pdf (accessed on 22nd July 2025).
2. Adkisson, C. D., Asbun, H. J., Bowers, S. P., Raimondo, M., et al. (2012). What extent of pancreatic resection do patients with MEN-1 require? https://core.ac.uk/download/619642430.pdf (accessed on 22nd July 2025).
3. Aggarwal, P., Satapathy, S., Kaur, G., Sood, A., Bhadada, S., Walia, R., Gupta, R., et al. (2025). Safety and efficacy of peptide receptor radionuclide therapy in multiple endocrine neoplasia syndrome: A single-center experience. *Clinical Nuclear Medicine, 50*, 605–611. https://www.semanticscholar.org/paper/79fe63e2c1928c8bcec3e1399af79f292e9b045e (accessed on 22nd July 2025).
4. Amthauer, H., Jann, H., Kayser, A., Roderburg, C., et al. (2019). Somatostatin analogues in the treatment of neuroendocrine tumors: Past, present and future. https://core.ac.uk/download/288114008.pdf (accessed on 22nd July 2025).
5. Aynaou, H., & Salhi, H. (2024). Exploring multiple endocrine neoplasia type 2B: Key findings from a case report. *International Journal for Multidisciplinary Research*. https://www.semanticscholar.org/paper/d8ee3020b65c54cd893696ac677d79e69f45d2a2 (accessed on 22nd July 2025).
6. Baccari, P., Cappabianca, S., D'Andrea, A., Falcone, L., et al. (2016). Pancreatic tumors imaging: An update. https://core.ac.uk/download/98333045.pdf (accessed on 22nd July 2025).
7. Baldelli, R., Campana, D., Di Giacinto, P., Isidori, A., et al. (2018). Chromogranin A: From laboratory to clinical aspects of patients with neuroendocrine tumors. https://core.ac.uk/download/188822602.pdf (accessed on 22nd July 2025).
8. Bandeira, F., Bhadada, S. K., Bilezikian, J. P., Bollerslev, J., et al. (2016). Primary hyperparathyroidism: Review and recommendations on evaluation, diagnosis, and management. A Canadian and international consensus. https://core.ac.uk/download/46664932.pdf (accessed on 22nd July 2025).
9. Bano, G., Beharry, N., Du Parc, J., Khalid, J. M., et al. (2017). Glucagon secreting tumors and glucagonoma syndrome. https://core.ac.uk/download/82918934.pdf (accessed on 22nd July 2025).
10. Bergsneider, M., Dabbagh, A., Heaney, A. P., Linetsky, D., et al. (2019). Residual tumor confers a 10-fold increased risk of regrowth in clinically nonfunctioning pituitary tumors. https://core.ac.uk/download/323079920.pdf (accessed on 22nd July 2025).
11. Bondi, F., Boscaro, M., Bottici, V., Brandi, M. L., Cappai, A., Cappelli, C., Castagna, M. G., et al. (2010). Multiple endocrine neoplasia type 2 syndromes (MEN 2): Results from the ItaMEN network analysis on the prevalence of different genotypes and phenotypes. https://core.ac.uk/download/53617916.pdf (accessed on 22nd July 2025).
12. Bouillon, R., Coopmans, W., de Herder, W. W., Krenning, E. P., et al. (1997). Chromogranin A as serum marker for neuroendocrine neoplasia: Comparison with neuron-specific enolase and the alpha-subunit of glycoprotein hormones. https://core.ac.uk/download/19185434.pdf (accessed on 22nd July 2025).

13. Bouillon, R., Marcocci, C., Carmeliet, G., Bikle, D. D., White, J. H., Dawson-Hughes, B., Lips, P., et al. (2018). Skeletal and extra skeletal actions of vitamin D: Current evidence and outstanding questions. *Endocrine Reviews, 40*, 1109–1151. https://doi.org/10.1210/er.2018-00126 (accessed on 22nd July 2025).

14. Brandi, M. L., Giusti, F., Marini, F., Tonelli, F., et al. (2017). Management impact: Effects on quality of life and prognosis in MEN1. https://core.ac.uk/download/301573649.pdf (accessed on 22nd July 2025).

15. Bratu, O. G., Diaconu, C. C., Gaman, M. A., Manea, M., et al. (2019). Pheochromocytoma–Clinical manifestations, diagnosis and current perioperative management. https://core.ac.uk/download/232440325.pdf (accessed on 22nd July 2025).

16. Brewer, A. (2006). Genetic characteristics of pheochromocytomas: An analysis of p16 tumor suppressor gene inactivation. https://core.ac.uk/download/76295549.pdf (accessed on 22nd July 2025).

17. Camera, L., Boccadifuoco, F., Modica, R., Messerini, L., Faggiano, A., Romeo, V., Gaudieri, V., et al. (2023). Gastrinomas and non-functioning pancreatic endocrine tumors in multiple endocrine neoplasia syndrome type-1 (MEN-1). *Endocrine*. https://www.semanticscholar.org/paper/6a9502dc2ddcc02450915a6ea18d5782dfa2d944 (accessed on 22nd July 2025).

18. Camera, L., Carratù, A., Colao, A., de Luca di Roseto, F., et al. (2014). Combined biological therapy with lanreotide autogel and cabergoline in the treatment of MEN-1-related insulinomas. https://core.ac.uk/download/pdf/154848802.pdf (accessed on 22nd July 2025).

19. Cano González, D. A., Flores Martínez, Á., & Venegas Moreno, E. (2019). AIP and MEN1 mutations and AIP immunohistochemistry in pituitary adenomas in a tertiary referral center. https://core.ac.uk/download/299806478.pdf (accessed on 22nd July 2025).

20. Caplin, M., Falconi, M., Fusai, G. K., Lykoudis, P., et al. (2017). Treatment challenges in and outside a specialist network setting: Pancreatic neuroendocrine tumors. https://core.ac.uk/download/168403284.pdf (accessed on 22nd July 2025).

21. Chrousos, G. P., Karl, M., Reincke, M., Travis, W. D., et al. (1933). No evidence for oncogenic mutations in guanine nucleotide-binding proteins of human adrenocortical neoplasms. https://core.ac.uk/download/12167815.pdf (accessed on 22nd July 2025).

22. Colao, A., Di Somma, C., Milone, F., Faggiano, A., et al. (2011). Clinical and prognostic implications of the genetic diagnosis of hereditary NET syndromes in asymptomatic patients. https://core.ac.uk/download/55058929.pdf (accessed on 22nd July 2025).

23. Cranston, T., Grossman, A. B., Isidori, A., Jafar-Mohammadi, B., et al. (2017). Routine genetic screening with a multi-gene panel in patients with pheochromocytomas. https://core.ac.uk/download/153364956.pdf (accessed on 22nd July 2025).

24. Crossey, P. A., Engelhardt, D., Frilling, A., Höppner, W., et al. (1996). Isolated familial pheochromocytoma as a variant of von Hippel-Lindau disease. https://core.ac.uk/download/12175991.pdf (accessed on 22nd July 2025).

25. Cuccurullo, V., Iacomino, A., & Marino, A. (2021). Neuroendocrine tumors: From anatomopathological to clinical presentation. https://core.ac.uk/download/534976287.pdf (accessed on 22nd July 2025).

26. Dahiya, S., Dunn, G. P., Fulton, R. S., Li, H., et al. (2018). Resistance-promoting effects of ependymoma treatment revealed through genomic analysis of multiple recurrences in a single patient. https://core.ac.uk/download/231816709.pdf (accessed on 22nd July 2025).

27. De Iuliis, F., Lanza, R., Lunardi, G., Menghi, A., et al. (2016). Synchronous primary papillary breast cancer, medullary thyroid carcinoma and neuroendocrine tumor in postmenopausal woman. https://core.ac.uk/download/188828824.pdf (accessed on 22nd July 2025).

28. Deng, J., Liao, X., & Cao, H. (2023). Neuroendocrine tumors in a patient with multiple endocrine neoplasia type 1 syndrome: A case report and review of the literature. *Medicine, 102*. https://www.semanticscholar.org/paper/97dd82391a027d166e0bacd89258d4ff876762e7 (accessed on 22nd July 2025).

29. Diaz, R. E., & Wohllk, N. (2012). Multiple endocrine neoplasia: The Chilean experience. https://core.ac.uk/download/pdf/8711910.pdf (accessed on 22nd July 2025).

30. Dreijerink, K. M., Höppener, J. W. M., Links, T. P., Lips, C. J., et al. (2012). Recent results of basic and clinical research in MEN1: Opportunities to improve early detection and treatment. https://core.ac.uk/download/518762163.pdf (accessed on 22nd July 2025).

31. Faßnacht, M., Assié, G., Baudin, E., Eisenhofer, G., de la Fouchardière, C., Haak, H. R., de Krijger, R. R., et al. (2020). Adrenocortical carcinomas and malignant phaeochromocytomas: ESMO–EURACAN clinical practice guidelines for diagnosis, treatment and follow-up. *Annals of Oncology, 31*, 1476–1490. https://doi.org/10.1016/j.annonc.2020.08.2099 (accessed on 22nd July 2025).

32. Gan, H. W., Bulwer, C., Jeelani, O., Levine, M., Korbonits, M., & Spoudeas, H. (2015). Treatment-resistant pediatric giant prolactinoma and multiple endocrine neoplasia type 1. *International Journal of Pediatric Endocrinology, 2015*. https://www.semanticscholar.org/paper/897328fbd8cbeba3e71e6a99aeb29e2c1bf46590 (accessed on 22nd July 2025).

33. Giwercman, A., Ansell, P. E., Avellan, L., Jégou, B., Baird, D. D., Baumrucker, G. O., Berkowitz, G. D., et al. (1996). Male reproductive health and environmental xenoestrogens. https://core.ac.uk/download/337395.pdf (accessed on 22nd July 2025).

34. Kemm, M., Manly, C., Hoang, T., Mai, V., & Shakir, M. (2019). Octreotide use in a patient with MEN-1 syndrome and multifocal pancreatic neuroendocrine tumors: A case report and review of the literature. *Case Reports in Gastrointestinal Medicine, 2019*. https://www.semanticscholar.org/paper/9bf75557a16fd69e29f3ab41cd197fa52c76c16b (accessed on 22nd July 2025).

35. Modica, R., Liccardi, A., Minotta, R., Benevento, E., Cannavale, G., Di Iasi, G., & Colao, A. (2024). Neuroendocrine tumors and survival rates in multiple endocrine neoplasia type 1 patients: Impact of gender difference. *Neuroendocrinology, 115*, 364–370. https://www.semanticscholar.org/paper/1200cdefff6dc805191fedfecf61800c5d3307f2 (accessed on 22nd July 2025).

36. Novaria, L. (2012). Characterization of the neuroendocrine pancreatic tumor's nature by MDCT enhancement pattern: A radio-pathological correlation. https://core.ac.uk/download/14704148.pdf (accessed on 22nd July 2025).

37. Romanet, P., Charnay, T., Sahakian, N., Cuny, T., Castinetti, F., & Barlier, A. (2024). Challenges in molecular diagnosis of multiple endocrine neoplasia. *Frontiers in Endocrinology, 15*. https://www.semanticscholar.org/paper/2cc531e3599ae90d32c2894deab1988ef7249c85 (accessed on 22nd July 2025).

38. Rossier, S. (2015). Clinical and genetic characteristics of multiple endocrine neoplasia type 1 (MEN 1) syndrome in a small cohort of Swiss patients. https://core.ac.uk/download/84058640.pdf (accessed on 22nd July 2025).

39. Rychlewska-Duda, J., Lisiecka, J., Janik, M., Ufnalska, B., Konarska, A., Fabijański, A., Machowiak, A., et al. (2025). Insulinomas: Comprehensive review of epidemiology, pathophysiology, clinical manifestations, diagnostic approaches, and treatment options. *Quality in Sport*. https://www.semanticscholar.org/paper/64ae9c3faebfed938fe4398653fbd25356933417 (accessed on 22nd July 2025).

40. Sakurai, A., Suda, K., Ito, M., Masanori, T., et al. (2024). Psychological impact and genetic counseling in patients with multiple endocrine neoplasia type 1 (MEN1): Addressing quality of life concerns. https://core.ac.uk/download/622036003.pdf (accessed on 22nd July 2025).

41. Sherad, M., Rohuma, M., Mira, R., & Mira, R. (2024). Sipple syndrome: From diagnosis to management–A case report. https://core.ac.uk/download/596400885.pdf (accessed on 22nd July 2025).

42. Soe, M., Cheng, C., & Liu, C. (2020). SAT-LB310 A mysterious multiple endocrine neoplasia (MEN) like syndrome. *Journal of the Endocrine Society, 4*. https://www.semanticscholar.org/paper/e8a32053053f8e31de5b0956394f5871ecfc06d9 (accessed on 22nd July 2025).

43. Sun, M., Chang, X., Huang, X., Chen, L., Peng, M., & Zhong, X. (2025). Case report: A novel likely pathogenetic variant of the MEN1 gene in multiple endocrine neoplasia type 1. *Frontiers in Endocrinology, 16*. https://www.semanticscholar.org/paper/8c2face7b26c13365b93e07ed19a02cf05b742d2 (accessed on 22nd July 2025).

44. van Eijck, C. H. J., de Herder, W. W., Krenning, E. P., Lamberts, S. W. J., et al. (2004). Considerations concerning a tailored, individualized therapeutic management of patients with (neuro) endocrine tumours of the gastrointestinal tract. https://core.ac.uk/download/18512572.pdf (accessed on 22nd July 2025).

INDEX

C

D

E

F

G

I

J

K

L

M

N

O

P

R

S

T

U

V

W